POCKET
NOTEBOOK

Pocket ANESTHESIA

T0200301

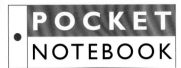

POCKET NOTEBOOK

Pocket ANESTHESIA

Fourth Edition

Edited by

RICHARD D. URMAN, MD, MBA, FASA, FAACD
Associate Chair for Dana-Farber Cancer Institute
Medical Director, Sedation for Interventional Medicine
Director (Anesthesia), Center for Perioperative Research
Fellowship Director, Perioperative Medicine
Associate Professor of Anesthesia, Harvard Medical School
Department of Anesthesiology, Perioperative and Pain Medicine
Brigham and Women's Hospital
Boston, Massachusetts

JESSE M. EHRENFELD, MD, MPH, FASA, FAMIA
Senior Associate Dean and Director
Advancing a Healthier Wisconsin Endowment
Professor, Anesthesiology
Medical College of Wisconsin
Milwaukee, Wisconsin

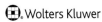
Wolters Kluwer

Philadelphia · Baltimore · New York · London
Buenos Aires · Hong Kong · Sydney · Tokyo

Acquisitions Editor: Keith Donnellan
Development Editor: Ashley Fischer
Editorial Coordinator: Blair Jackson
Marketing Manager: Phyllis Hitner
Production Project Manager: David Saltzberg
Design Coordinator: Holly McLaughlin
Manufacturing Coordinator: Beth Welsh
Prepress Vendor: Aptara, Inc.

4th edition
Copyright © 2021 Wolters Kluwer.

9 8 7 6 5 4

Printed in China

978-1-9751-3679-6
Library of Congress Cataloging-in-Publication Data
available upon request

Library of Congress Control Number: 2020904447

CCS1123

CONTRIBUTORS

Brian F. S. Allen, MD
Assistant Professor
Department of Anesthesiology
Vanderbilt University Medical Center
Nashville, Tennessee

Megan Graybill Anders, MD
Assistant Professor, Associate Chair for Safety and Quality
Department of Anesthesiology
University of Maryland School of Medicine
Baltimore, Maryland

Joshua H. Atkins, MD, PhD
Associate Professor of Anesthesiology and Critical Care
Director of Anesthesia for Head and Neck Surgery
Co-Director of Penn-China Anesthesia Program
Perelman School of Medicine at the University of Pennsylvania
Philadelphia, Pennsylvania

Jeanette R. Bauchat, MD, MS
Division Chief, Obstetric Anesthesiology
Associate Professor
Department of Anesthesiology
Vanderbilt University Medical Center

Melissa L. Bellomy, MD
Clinical Fellow in Critical Care and Cardiothoracic Anesthesiology
Department of Anesthesiology
Vanderbilt University Medical Center
Nashville, Tennessee

Frederic T. Billings, IV, MD, MSc
Associate Professor
Department of Anesthesiology
Vanderbilt University Medical Center
Nashville, Tennessee

Jason Bouhenguel, MD
Fellow
Critical Care/Cardiothoracic Anesthesia
Stanford Health Care
United States, California

Eric R. Briggs, MD
Assistant Professor of Clinical Anesthesiology
Vanderbilt University Medical Center
Nashville, Tennessee

Manuel Cavazos, MD
Anesthesiology Resident
Department of Anesthesiology
Vanderbilt University Medical Center
Nashville, Tennessee

Francis X. Dillon, MD
Attending Anesthesiologist
Department of Anesthesiology
Indiana University Health Ball Memorial Hospital
Muncie, Indiana

Kurt F. Dittrich, MD
Assistant Professor
Department of Anesthesiology
Vanderbilt University School of Medicine
Nashville, Tennessee

David A. Edwards, MD, PhD
Assistant Professor
Department of Anesthesiology
Vanderbilt University Medical Center
Nashville, Tennessee

Jesse M. Ehrenfeld, MD, MPH, FASA, FAMIA
Senior Associate Dean and Director
Advancing a Healthier Wisconsin Endowment
Professor, Anesthesiology
Medical College of Wisconsin
Milwaukee, Wisconsin

Julie K. Freed, MD, PhD
Department of Anesthesiology
Medical College of Wisconsin
Milwaukee, Wisconsin

Robert E. Freundlich, MD, MS, MSCI
Assistant Professor of Anesthesiology and Biomedical Informatics
Anesthesiology Critical Care Medicine
Medical Director
Vanderbilt Anesthesiology & Perioperative Informatics
Vanderbilt University Medical Center
Nashville, Tennessee

Chad R. Greene, DO
Department of Anesthesiology
Vanderbilt University Medical Center
Nashville, Tennessee

Robert Hsiung, MD
Staff Anesthesiologist
Department of Anesthesiology
Virginia Mason Medical Center
Seattle, Washington

Elisabeth M. Hughes, MD
Associate Professor
Department of Anesthesiology
Vanderbilt University School of Medicine
Associate Professor
Pediatric Anesthesiology
Monroe Carell Jr. Children's Hospital at Vanderbilt
Nashville, Tennessee

Christina Jelly, MD
Assistant Professor
Anesthesiology Critical Care Medicine, Cardiothoracic Anesthesiology,
    Multispecialty Adult Anesthesiology
Vanderbilt University Medical Center
Nashville, Tennessee

Daniel W. Johnson, MD
Assistant Professor and Division Chief, Critical Care
Department of Anesthesiology
University of Nebraska Medical Center
Omaha, Nebraska

Jimin Kim, MD
Fellow
Department of Anesthesiology, Perioperative and Pain Medicine
Brigham and Women's Hospital
Harvard Medical School
Boston, Massachusetts

Adam B. King, MD
Department of Anesthesiology
Vanderbilt University Medical Center
Nashville, Tennessee

Meredith A. Kingeter, MD
Assistant Professor
Cardiothoracic Anesthesiology
Vanderbilt University Medical Center
Nashville, Tennessee

I. Matthew Kynes, MD
Assistant Professor
Department of Anesthesiology
Vanderbilt University School of Medicine
Nashville, Tennessee

Ryan J. Lefevre, MD
Assistant Professor
Cardiothoracic Anesthesiology
Vanderbilt University Medical Center
Nashville, Tennessee

Michael C. Lubrano, MD, MPH
Resident Physician
Anesthesia and Perioperative Care
University of California, San Francisco Medical Center
San Francisco, California
Cleveland, Ohio

Matthew D. McEvoy, MD
Associate Professor of Anesthesiology
Vanderbilt University Medical Center
Nashville, Tennessee

David A. Nakata, MD, MBA
Associate Professor of Clinical Anesthesia
Indiana University Medical Center
Indianapolis, Indiana

Alexander Nguyen, MD
Virginia Mason Medical Center
Seattle, Washington

Jonathan A. Niconchuk, MD
Anesthesiology Resident
Department of Anesthesiology
Vanderbilt University School of Medicine
Nashville, Tennessee

Joseph R. Pawlowski, MD
Department of Anesthesiology
University of Nebraska Medical Center
Omaha, Nebraska

Amanda J. Rhee, MD
Assistant Professor
Department of Anesthesiology
Mount Sinai Hospital
New York, New York

Amy C. Robertson, MD
Assistant Professor of Anesthesiology
Vice Chair for Clinical Affairs, Department of Anesthesiology
Vanderbilt University School of Medicine
Nashville, Tennessee

Thomas M. Romanelli, MD, FAAP
Assistant Professor of Clinical Anesthesiology
Vanderbilt University Medical Center
Nashville, Tennessee

Ramsey Saba, MD
Anesthesiology Resident
Department of Anesthesiology
Brigham and Women's Hospital
Boston, Massachusetts

Michael W. Sanford, MD
Assistant Professor of Anesthesiology
Indiana University School of Medicine
Indianapolis, Indiana

Linda Shore-Lesserson, MD, FAHA, FASE
Director
Cardiovascular Anesthesiology
North Shore University Hospital
Manhasset, New York

Kara K. Siegrist, MD
Cardiothoracic Anesthesiology Fellow
Vanderbilt University Medical Center
Nashville, Tennessee

Michael N. Singleton, MD
Department of Anesthesiology
Hospital for Special Surgery
New York, New York

Alyssa K. Streff, MD
Department of Anesthesiology
Vanderbilt University Medical Center
Nashville, Tennessee

Muoi A. Trinh, MD
Assistant Professor of Anesthesiology
Mount Sinai Medical Center
New York, New York

Richard D. Urman, MD, MBA, FASA, FAACD
Associate Chair for Dana-Farber Cancer Institute
Medical Director, Sedation for Interventional Medicine
Director (Anesthesia), Center for Perioperative Research
Fellowship Director, Perioperative Medicine
Associate Professor of Anesthesia, Harvard Medical School
Department of Anesthesiology, Perioperative and Pain Medicine
Brigham and Women's Hospital
Boston, Massachusetts

Jenna Walters, MD
Assistant Professor
Department of Anesthesiology
Vanderbilt University Medical Center
Nashville, Tennessee

Jonathan P. Wanderer, MD, MPhil
Associate Professor
Department of Anesthesiology
Vanderbilt University Medical Center
Nashville, Tennessee

PREFACE

Written by residents, fellows, and attending staff, this newest edition of *Pocket Anesthesia* provides a practical, concise, up-to-date source of information for management of the most common perioperative conditions facing today's anesthesia provider. Our goal in writing this popular pocket guide was to give you a useful, evidence-based reference which providers can refer to, in order to quickly find the most relevant information they need.

For this fourth edition, we updated much of the information to reflect current knowledge and significantly expanded regional anesthesia and chronic pain management chapters. We also expanded coverage of enhanced recovery after surgery, ultrasonography, and echocardiography. We are grateful for the support of all our contributors from many different institutions across the country. With its basic and advanced content, this book is intended for a wide audience, from students and resident trainees to experienced practitioners.

We are especially indebted to a number of individuals whose unending support and encouragement made this work possible. We would like to thank the Wolters Kluwer staff, including Ashley Fischer, Keith Donnellan, and Blair Jackson.

Finally, a very special thanks to our parents and families, including Mr. Judd Taback, Drs. Katharine Nicodemus, David Ehrenfeld, and Zina Matlyuk-Urman for their continued encouragement, love, and support. We hope that you find the fourth edition of *Pocket Anesthesia* a valuable resource in your clinical practice.

RICHARD D. URMAN, MD, MBA
BOSTON, MASSACHUSETTS

JESSE M. EHRENFELD, MD, MPH
MILWAUKEE, WISCONSIN

CONTENTS

APPENDIX

INDEX

PREOPERATIVE PATIENT EVALUATION

J. MATTHEW KYNES • JESSE M. EHRENFELD

INTRODUCTION

	ASA Physical Status Classification	Example
I	No organic/physiologic/psychiatric problems	Healthy pt, nonsmoker
II	Controlled medical conditions with mild systemic effects, no limitations in functional ability	Controlled HTN/smoker/obesity/controlled diabetes
III	Medical conditions with severe systemic effects, limitations in functional ability	Controlled CHF/stable angina/morbid obesity/COPD/chronic renal insufficiency
IV	Poorly controlled medical conditions associated with significant impairment in functional ability that is potential threat to life	Unstable angina/symptomatic COPD or CHF
V	Critical condition, little chance of survival without surgical procedure	Ruptured AAA, massive trauma, or multisystem organ failure
VI	Brain dead, undergoing organ donation	
E	Emergency	Delay in treatment would cause significant ↑ in threat to life or limb

Preoperative Interview	
Current Issue	Indication for Surgery
Past medical history	Presence & severity of medical comorbidities
ROS	Focus on general functional capacity
CV	Angina, SOB, exercise tolerance, activity level and limiting factors, dyspnea on exertion
Pulmonary	Hx of asthma, smoking, inhaler use, baseline O_2 use, obstructive sleep apnea
Neurologic	TIA, stroke, pain, depression, anxiety, neurologic dz, neuropathies
GI	GERD symptoms, NPO status
Renal/GU/OB	Possibility of pregnancy, UTIs
Heme	Easy bruising, easy bleeding, hx of anemia, clotting d/o
Musculoskeletal	Cervical range of motion, bone or muscle d/o
Endocrine	Diabetes, thyroid dz
Surgical history	Previous surgeries, including complications/outcomes
Anesthetic history	Examine old records for hx of difficult airway management, PONV, any family hx suggestive of malignant hyperthermia
Social history	Tobacco/alcohol/illicit drug use
Allergies	Drug allergies (anaphylaxis, airway swelling, hives, pulmonary reactions) vs. side effects/intolerance, latex allergy
Medications	Especially cardiovascular meds, insulin, anticoagulation meds

PREOPERATIVE PHYSICAL EXAMINATION

- Vital signs: Resting heart rate, BP, SpO_2 height, weight, body mass index
- CV & pulm: Heart & lung sounds, JVD, pulm/periph edema, carotid bruits
- Airway examination:
  - Mallampati score (see Fig. 1-1)
  - Thyromental distance: Have pt extend neck & measure space between mental prominence and thyroid cartilage; <6 cm may indicate difficult intubation
  - Cervical spine flexion/extension: Examine pt for ↓ range of motion that might limit head movement into sniffing position during intubation
  - Miscellaneous: Oral opening, size of mandible (micrognathia) & tongue (macroglossia), dentition (loose, missing, prostheses)

Mallampati Scoring System

Pt in an upright position, mouth open as wide as possible, not sticking tongue out

Grade View	Visible Structures	Intubation
1	Tonsillar pillars, soft palate, entire uvula	Unlikely difficult
2	Pillars & soft palate, only part of uvula	Unlikely difficult
3	Soft palate & base of uvula	Possibly difficult
4	Hard palate only	Difficult/impossible

Figure 1-1 Mallampati classification of the oropharyngeal structures.

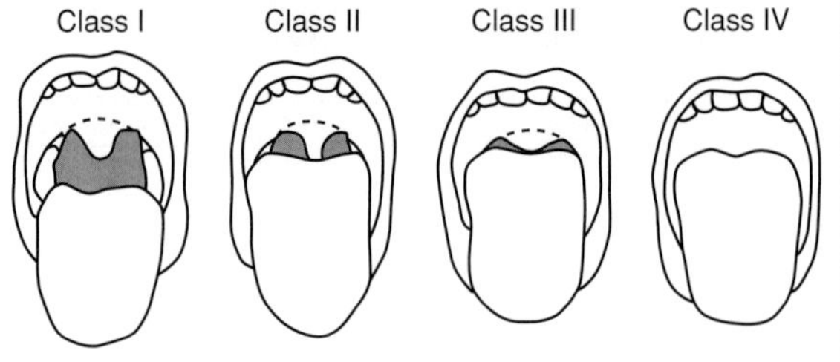

Class I   Class II   Class III   Class IV

(From Samsoon GLT, Young JRB. Difficult tracheal intubation, a retrospective study. *Anaesthesia* 1987; 42:487–490, with permission.)

Consensus (Minimum) Fasting Guidelines

Solid food, milk, infant formula	6 h
Breast milk	4 h
Clear liquids (water, soda, juices, black coffee)	2 h
Emergency cases	Rapid sequence intubation

PREOPERATIVE LABORATORY TESTING

- No test is absolutely required for anesthesia, especially for healthy pts
  - Consider **pregnancy testing** if possibility of pregnancy (childbearing age, no previous BSO or hysterectomy)
  - Consider **creatinine** if contrast will be used
  - Order **HCT/Hgb, type & screen** if significant blood loss anticipated

Suggested Metrics for Preoperative Testing

ASA	Low-Risk Surgery[1]	Elevated-Risk Surgery[2]
I & II	None	Creatinine/glucose, Hgb/Hct/platelets (especially in older pts), consider type & screen
III & IV	None required, testing based on comorbidities and procedure	Creatinine/glucose, Hgb/Hct/platelets, type & screen

Additional Suggested Laboratory Testing Based on Specific Comorbidities

Diabetes/renal dz/endocrine d/o	Electrolytes, creatinine, glucose[3]
Cardiovascular dz	Electrolytes, creatinine, glucose[4]
Severe obesity	Electrolytes, creatinine, glucose[5]
Significant liver dz unexplained bleeding	CBC, platelets, PT/PTT, LFTs
Hematologic d/o/malignancy	CBC, platelets, PT/PTT

[1]See table below on page 3: Validated Cardiac Risk Prediction Tools for low-/elevated-risk calculation.
[2]See table below on page 3: Validated Cardiac Risk Prediction Tools for low-/elevated-risk calculation.
[3]Often cheaper to order a lab "bundle" with electrolytes, rather than separate creatinine/glucose.
[4]Often cheaper to order a lab "bundle" with electrolytes, rather than separate creatinine/glucose.
[5]Often cheaper to order a lab "bundle" with electrolytes, rather than separate creatinine/glucose.

Other Testing	Notes
Chest x-ray	Rarely useful unless pt has *abnormal breath sounds*, suspected CHF, substernal goiter, or low SpO_2 Usually obtained as baseline prior to *cardiothoracic surgery*
Pulmonary function testing	Not useful for risk stratification unless pt is being considered for *lung resection*
Echocardiogram	Recommended for *murmurs* other than clearly functional ones, or pt with *CHF/unexplained dyspnea*
Carotid Doppler	Obtained for *symptomatic bruits* (TIAs) Often obtained prior to high-risk surgery (CABG, AAA)
Flexion–extension c-spine films	Consider in *longstanding RA, Down* syndrome if not previously screened (controversial if asymptomatic)
Noninvasive cardiac testing	See Figure 1-2. Perioperative cardiac assessment algorithm for CAD

ELECTROCARDIOGRAM (ECG) TESTING

- Need diagnosis other than "preoperative eval"; age-based ordering not reimbursed
- ECG indicated for:
  - **Symptoms or findings:** Such as chest pain, syncope, palpitations, dyspnea, irregular pulse, murmur, peripheral edema, rales, suspected or recent MI/unstable angina
  - **Risk stratification/modification:**
    - Pts with known CAD, significant arrhythmia, PVD, CVD, or other significant heart dz except in low-risk surgery
- ECG NOT indicated in asymptomatic pt undergoing low-risk surgery

CARDIAC RISK STRATIFICATION

Preop Management Recommendations for Cardiac Conditions (Non-CAD)	
Condition	**Recommendation**
Heart failure	Assess LV function for worsening dyspnea or change in clinical status
Arrhythmias	Investigate cause of preop arrhythmia, esp for high-grade AV block, 3rd-degree AV block, Mobitz II, or supraventricular arrhythmias
Moderate or greater valvular dz	Preop echo if there has been none within 1 y, or a significant change in symptoms/exam since last eval

Source: Fleisher LA, et al. ACC/AHA 2014 guideline on perioperative cardiovascular evaluation. *Circulation* 2014. doi:10.1016/j.jacc.2014.07.944.

Validated Cardiac Risk Prediction Tools	
(1) Revised Cardiac Risk Index (RCRI) (*Circulation* 1999;100(10):1043-9)	
Summary	Risk of MI, pulmonary edema, complete heart block, or ventricular fibrillation based on pt and surgical factors
Criteria	(1) High-risk surgery (open intraperitoneal, intrathoracic, suprainguinal vascular); (2) Hx of MI/positive stress test; (3) Hx of CHF; (4) Hx of TIA or stroke; (5) DM managed with insulin; (6) preop creatinine >2 mg/dL
Calculation Method	0–1 point = low (<1%) risk; 2–6 points = elevated risk
(2) ACS NSQIP MICA (*Circulation* 2011;124(4):381–7)	
Summary	Risk of cardiac arrest or MI based on pt and site-specific surgical factors
Criteria	Age, creatinine >1.5 mg/dL, functional status, surgery type (21 options)
Calculation Method	Web-based or spreadsheet (http://www.surgicalriskcalculator.com/miorcardiacarrest)
(3) ACS NSQIP Surgical Risk Calculator (*J Am Coll Surg* 2011;217(5):833–42)	
Summary	Risk of major adverse cardiac event, death, and 8 other outcomes based on specific operation and pt factors
Criteria	Name of operation, ASA physical status, wound class, ascites, systemic sepsis, ventilator dependent, disseminated cancer, steroid use, HTN, previous cardiac event, sex, dyspnea, smoker, COPD, dialysis, acute kidney injury, BMI, emergency case
Calculation Method	Web-based (http://www.riskcalculator.facs.org)

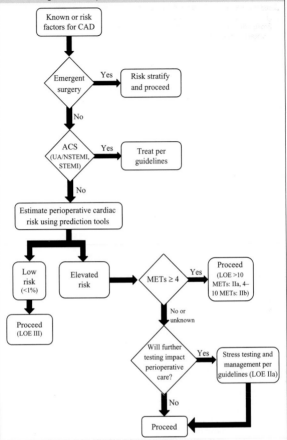

Figure 1-2 Perioperative cardiac assessment algorithm for CAD.

Cardiac eval algorithm for noncardiac surgery based on combined surgical/clinical risk and functional status for pts with known or risk factors for CAD. See tables in this section for Cardiac Risk Prediction Tools, Metabolic Equivalents, and Preop Management Recommendations for Cardiac Conditions (Non-CAD). UA, unstable angina; MET, metabolic equivalent; LOE, level of evidence.

(Adapted from Fleisher LA, et al. ACC/AHA 2014 guideline on perioperative cardiovascular evaluation. *Circulation* 2014. doi:10.1016/j.jacc.2014.07.944.)

Metabolic Equivalents (METs)		
Poor (<4 METs)	Moderate (4–7 METs)	Excellent (>7 METs)
Eating, bathing, dressing	Climbing a flight of stairs	Washing floors
Slow walking (2 mph)	Fast walking (4 mph)	Playing tennis (singles)
Vacuuming	Weeding, bicycling	Jogging, squash

Source: Fletcher GF, et al. Exercise standards. *Circulation* 1995;91:580–615.

INFECTIVE ENDOCARDITIS (IE) ANTIBIOTIC PROPHYLAXIS

- Based on risk of developing IE & severity of outcome if IE were to occur
- Highest-risk pts (those requiring prophylaxis) include those with:
  - Prosthetic cardiac valve or previous IE
  - Congenital heart dz
  - Repaired CHD with residual defect at site
  - Previous cardiac transplantation with subsequent cardiac valvulopathy

Note: Guidelines no longer include pts with common valve lesions (bicuspid aortic valve, acquired aortic/mitral valve dz, mitral valve prolapse, hypertrophic cardiomyopathy)

Recommended Antibiotic Regimen (30–60 min Prior to Surgery)		
	First-Line Antibiotic	**Alternative Antibiotic (PCN-Allergic Pts)**
Oral	Amoxicillin 2 g Cephalexin 2 g	Clindamycin 600 mg Azithromycin 500 mg Clarithromycin 500 mg
IV/IM	Ampicillin 2 g IV/IM Cefazolin 2 g IV/IM Ceftriaxone 1 g IV/IM	Clindamycin 600 mg IV/IM

Source: Adapted from Wilson W, et al. Prevention of infective endocarditis. *Circulation* 2007;116(15):1736–1754.

PERIOPERATIVE β-BLOCKER THERAPY

- Perioperative β-blockers may ↓ cardiac events and mortality, but may ↑ risk of stroke, hypotension and bradycardia, and uncertain effect on surgical mortality *(Circulation 2014;130:2246–64)*
  - Pts already on β-blocker therapy should continue time of initiation of β-blocker and specific dose still controversial but should not start on day of surgery
  - Consider initiation of β-blocker therapy in pts with 3 or more RCRI risk factors *(2014 ACC/AHA guideline)*

STATINS

- Continue in the perioperative period, *including day of surgery* *(2014 ACC/AHA Perioperative Guidelines)*

STENTS & ANTIPLATELET AGENTS

- *Angioplasty:* Continue aspirin at least 14 d *(2014 ACC/AHA Perioperative Guidelines)*
- *Bare metal stent:* Clopidogrel & aspirin (dual antiplatelet) therapy should be continued for ≥4 wk
- *Drug-eluting stent:* Need ≥6 mo of dual antiplatelet therapy for 2nd-generation DES
- Aspirin (≥81 mg qd) should be continued perioperatively if clopidogrel is discontinued *(J Am Coll Card. Cardiovasc Interv 2010;3(2):131-112)*
- Pts with stents who discontinue antiplatelet agents before surgery have higher risk of major cardiac events and MI (7.3% & 4%) compared to those who continue them (0.3% & 0%); risk of significant bleeding is the same *(Thromb Haemost 2015;113(2):272–282)*

CONDITIONS WHICH MAY REQUIRE DELAY OF SURGERY FOR OPTIMIZATION

- Recent MI, unstable cardiac rhythm, uncontrolled or malignant hypertension
- Coagulopathy
- Hypoxia or respiratory insufficiency
- Untreated hyperthyroidism

MEDICATIONS REQUIRING SPECIAL CONSIDERATIONS IN THE PERIOPERATIVE PERIOD

- **Anticoagulants:** Aspirin, clopidogrel, coumadin, argatroban—*especially if coronary stents are present or regional is being considered* (see **Stents and Antiplatelet Agents** above). Factor Xa inhibitors (rivaroxaban, apixaban, edoxaban) may be held 2–3 d prior to surgery. Prasugrel is a platelet inhibitor which should be stopped 7 d prior to surgery.
- **Diabetic medications:** Insulin, metformin (see Diabetes, 27-2)
- **Antihypertensives:** Ace inhibitors, angiotensin receptor blockers, β-blockers

MEGAN GRAYBILL ANDERS

INTRODUCTION

Potent inhalational agents: **Mechanism of action** still undetermined. Experimental evidence for $GABA_A$ receptor/K^+ channel potentiation by volatile agents; NMDA inhibition with N_2O. Anesthetic binding might significantly modify membrane structure.

INHALED ANESTHETIC UPTAKE

- Agent levels in the brain depend on agent levels (partial pressure) in the alveolus
- Goal is to achieve rise in Fa (alveolar anesthetic concentration)/Fi (inspired anesthetic concentration)
- ↑ Fa/Fi →↑ speed of induction (Fig. 2A-1)

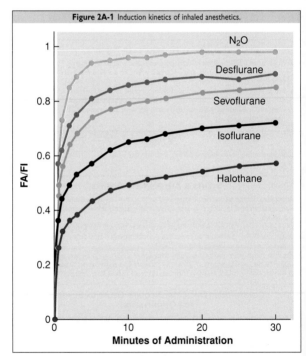

Figure 2A-1 Induction kinetics of inhaled anesthetics.

(From Ebert TJ, Naze SA. Inhaled Anesthetics. In: Barash PG, Callan MK, Cullen BF, Stock MC, Stoelting RK, Ortega R, Sharar SR, Holt N, eds. *Clinical Anesthesia*. 8th ed. Philadelphia, PA: Wolters Kluwer; 2018:463.)

MAJOR FACTORS AFFECTING UPTAKE

Solubility

- Partition coefficients express relative solubility of anesthetic gas at equilibrium
- Lower partition coefficients imply ↓ solubility, faster equilibration of partial pressure (alveolus ↔ blood ↔ brain), *rapid* induction (e.g., desflurane)

- Higher partition coefficients imply ↑ solubility, slower equilibration as more molecules are dissolved in blood, *prolonged* induction (e.g., halothane)
- Tissue: Blood partition coefficient = time for equilibrium of tissue with arterial blood

Cardiac Output

- Increased cardiac output results in faster uptake but ↓ alveolar concentration (Fa) and, therefore, slower induction (more blood passing through lungs – anesthetic is carried away faster)
- Effect is less pronounced for insoluble agents

Note: Slower induction with R → L cardiac shunt due to no uptake of agent in shunted blood → dilution of arterial concentration despite faster ↑ in alveolar concentration (Fa); least soluble agents are affected most

Alveolar–Venous Concentration Gradient

- Depends on uptake by desired (brain) and undesired (fat, muscle) tissues
- Tissue uptake is determined by partition coefficients and regional blood flow
- Less tissue uptake means blood returns to alveolus with higher partial pressure; thus alveolar concentration (Fa) can ↑ faster

---

OTHER FACTORS INFLUENCING UPTAKE

Concentration effect: Increasing the inspired concentration of a gas results in a disproportionate ↑ in the alveolar concentration (Fa); most clinically significant with N_2O, as can be used at ↑↑ inspired concentrations than volatile anesthetics.

Second gas effect: Large-volume uptake of the first gas (classically N_2O) causes ↓ total gas volume in alveolus, thereby ↑ alveolar concentration/accelerating uptake of second gas (volatile agent).

					Vapor Pressure		
Agent	Blood/ Gas	Brain/ Blood	Muscle/ Blood	Fat/ Blood	(mmHg, 20°C)	MAC (%) 30–60 y	MAC (%) >65 y
Nitrous oxide	0.46	1.1	1.2	2.3	—	104	
Halothane	2.5	1.9	3.4	51	243	0.75	0.64
Isoflurane	1.5	1.6	2.9	45	238	1.2	1.0
Desflurane	0.42	1.3	2.0	27	669	6.6	5.2
Sevoflurane	0.65	1.7	3.1	48	157	1.8	1.45

Pharmacologic Properties of Common Inhaled Anesthetic Agents

Source: Adapted from Barash PG, Cullen BF, Stoelting RK. *Clinical Anesthesia*. 6th ed. Philadelphia, PA: Lippincott Williams & Wilkins; 2009:415.

Factors That Speed Rate of Induction (↑ Fa/Fi)

- Use of agents with ↓ solubility (low partition coefficients)
- Low cardiac output with minimal R → L shunt and preserved cerebral blood flow
- Increased alveolar minute ventilation, ↑ inspired concentration of agent, ↑ fresh gas flow rate (replaces anesthetic taken up in bloodstream)
- Pediatric pts → faster induction due to ↑ alveolar ventilation, ↓ FRC, ↑ % of blood flow to brain

---

ELIMINATION/RECOVERY

- Reduction of anesthetic in brain tissue is via exhalation >> biotransformation > transcutaneous loss
- Biotransformation via P-450 enzymes more important for halothane (20%) than sevoflurane (5%), isoflurane (0.2%), or desflurane (<0.1%)
- Recovery expedited by high fresh gas flows, elimination of rebreathing, low absorption by the circuit, decreased solubility, high cerebral blood flow, and ↑ minute ventilation
- Context-sensitive elimination time: Longer duration of anesthetic is associated with longer time to recovery; over longer time more anesthetic is deposited in undesired tissues and must be "washed out"; effect more pronounced with ↑ solubility of agent (Fig. 2A-2)

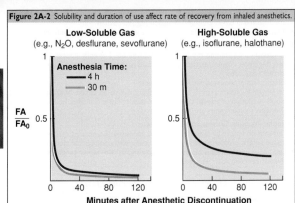

Figure 2A-2 Solubility and duration of use affect rate of recovery from inhaled anesthetics.

(Adapted from Epstein RM, Rackow H, Salanitre E, et al. Influence of the concentration effect on the uptake of anesthetic mixtures: the second gas effect. *Anesthesiology.* 1964;25:364. In: Barash PG, Callan MK, Cullen BF, Stock MC, Stoelting RK, Ortega R, Sharar SR, Holt N, eds. *Clinical Anesthesia.* 8th ed. Philadelphia, PA: Wolters Kluwer; 2018:465.)

DIFFUSION HYPOXIA

- High concentrations of relatively insoluble gases (N_2O) diffuse out of the blood and enter the alveolus, displacing and reducing alveolar concentration of O_2 and CO_2
- Dilution of alveolar O_2 can lead to hypoxia, dilution of CO_2 can ↓ ventilatory drive and worsen hypoxia
- Administer high-flow 100% O_2 for 5–10 min after discontinuation of N_2O

MINIMUM ALVEOLAR CONCENTRATION (MAC)

- Unitless value comparing potency of inhaled anesthetic agents
- Reference point (1 MAC) = alveolar concentration at which 50% of pts will not move in response to a standardized surgical stimulus; analogous to ED_{50}
- MAC values are roughly additive (i.e., 0.5 MAC of N_2O plus 0.5 MAC of sevoflurane ≈ 1.0 MAC)
- MAC is greatest at 1 y of age and reduced by 6% per decade of life
- At MAC 1.3, 95% of pts will not move in response to surgical stimulus
- MAC-BAR (1.5–2.0 MAC): Concentration which Blocks Adrenergic Response to nociceptive stimuli
- MAC-Aware (estimated 0.4–0.5 MAC): Concentration at which 50% of pts will not be forming long-term memory
- MAC-Awake (0.15–0.5 MAC): Concentration at which 50% of pts open eyes on command

Factors That ↓ MAC (↑ Potency)	
Acidosis	Intravenous anesthetics
Acute alcohol use	Hypotension (severe)
Advanced age	Hypothermia
Anemia	Hypoxia
Benzodiazepines	Opiates
Increased altitude	Pregnancy

Factors That ↑ MAC (↓ Potency)
Chronic alcohol abuse
Very young age (closer to 1 y of age)
Increased temperature (>42°C)
Decreased altitude
Drugs: MAOIs, TCAs, cocaine, acute amphetamine use

CLINICAL CONSIDERATIONS OF INHALED ANESTHETICS

- Volatile agents may trigger malignant hyperthermia (MH) (see Appendix C)
- Agents in current use are nonflammable at clinical concentrations
- All potentiate neuromuscular blockade, degree varies with combinations of drugs/agents; effect of volatiles > N_2O
- Volatile agents associated with prolongation of QT interval
- Carbon monoxide formed in reaction of volatile agents with desiccated CO_2 absorbent (desflurane > isoflurane >> halothane, sevoflurane); CO production ↑ with Baralyme, dry granules (classic example is Monday AM after O_2 flows left on), ↑ temperature, ↑ concentration of absorbent
- Exothermic degradation reaction of sevoflurane in the presence of desiccated Baralyme linked to rare absorbent canister fires
- Inhaled anesthetics (especially desflurane, N_2O) are greenhouse gases

SYSTEMIC EFFECTS OF INHALED AGENTS

- **Cardiovascular:**
  - All volatile agents are dose-dependent CV depressants, though mechanism of ↓ BP differs (see Table—Differential Physiologic Effects of Inhaled Anesthetics)
  - Heart rate effects vary with MAC and inspired concentration rate of change
- **Pulmonary:**
  - All agents cause ↑ RR with ↓ TV, overall volatile agents cause ↓ in minute ventilation and ↑ resting $PaCO_2$
  - All blunt ventilatory response to hypoxemia (even at 0.1 MAC), volatile agents ↓ response to hypercarbia
  - Volatile agents are potent bronchodilators
  - Minimal inhibition of hypoxic pulmonary vasoconstriction (HPV)
- **Neurologic:**
  - All agents ↑ cerebral blood flow causing ↑ ICP (especially halothane) and impair autoregulation of vascular tone (least with sevoflurane at <1 MAC)
  - Volatile agents ↓ cerebral metabolic rate, N_2O may ↑
  - Desflurane and isoflurane at <1 MAC can suppress status epilepticus while ↑ sevoflurane concentrations are associated with epileptiform EEG Δ
  - All agents ↓ SSEP/MEP signals
- **Hepatic:** Halothane causes both hepatic artery vasoconstriction and ↓ portal vein flow (potential for hypoxic hepatic injury, ↑ LFTs), others preserve vascular supply better with ↑ in hepatic artery flow compensating for ↓ portal vein flow
- **Renal:** All cause ↓ renal blood flow, ↓ GFR, ↓ urine output; untreated hypotension can cause acute kidney injury

Differential Physiologic Effects of Inhaled Anesthetics					
	Nonvolatile N_2O	Volatile			
		Halothane	Isoflurane	Sevoflurane	Desflurane
HR	↔ or ↑	↔ or ↓	↑	↔	↑
SVR	↔ or ↑	↔	↓	↓	↓
CO	↔ or ↑	↓↓	↔	↔	↔
Contractility	↔ or ↓	↓↓	↓	↓	↓
HBF	↓	↓↓	↓	↓	↓

HR, heart rate; SVR, systemic vascular resistance; CO, cardiac output; HBF, hepatic blood flow; ↑ and ↓, slight or mild change; ↓↓, significant decrease; ↔, no change.

INHALATIONAL ANESTHETICS, SPECIFIC COMMENTS

Nitrous Oxide (N_2O)
- Key features: MAC of 104% precludes use as solo agent for surgical anesthesia; used at 30–70% concentration as adjuvant to IV or potent inhaled anesthetics. Low solubility = rapid onset/offset of action. Nonpungent, has analgesic properties.
- Disadvantages: Rapidly diffuses into and expands air-containing cavities → avoid in air embolism, pneumothorax (75% N_2O doubles size in 10 min), bowel obstruction, pneumocephalus, middle ear and retinal procedures; monitor ETT cuffs and PAC balloons for expansion. Important greenhouse gas with >100 y atmospheric lifetime

- Prolonged exposure → inhibits B_{12}-dependent enzymes responsible for myelin and nucleic acid synthesis; megaloblastic bone marrow Δ possible with >12–24 h use; neurotoxicity with repeated exposures (abuse)
- Increased homocysteine levels theorized to ↑ postop MI, but ENIGMA-II trial found no ↑ in death or CV events (Lancet 2014;384(9952):1446–54).
- Teratogenic in animal models, no evidence in humans at clinical doses
- Not flammable, although does support combustion
- ↑ PONV
- CV effects: Sympathomimetic, though direct myocardial depressant effect may prevail in hypovolemia, cardiac dx; ↑ PVR especially in pts with pre-existing pulmonary HTN

Isoflurane
- Key features: Inexpensive; slower onset/offset of action, pungent. Versatile use
- Disadvantages: Coronary vasodilator, potential for coronary "steal" effect (flow diverted away from vessels with fixed lesions) of uncertain clinical significance

Desflurane
- Key features: Most rapid onset/offset of action among volatiles; very pungent
- Disadvantages: High vapor pressure requires an electrically heated vaporizer (eliminates variation in delivery owing to Δ in ambient temperature). Pungency may be irritant in pts prone to bronchospasm. Rapid ↑ or high concentration may cause transient but significant sympathetic stimulation. Potent greenhouse gas

Sevoflurane
- Key features: Least pungent (best choice for inhalational induction); fast onset/offset of action; causes ↓ tachycardia than desflurane or isoflurane; does not sensitize myocardium to catecholamines
- Disadvantages: Controversial potential for nephrotoxicity due to metabolic production of fluoride ion and degradation to Compound A (nephrotoxic in animals). Compound A production ↑ with low flows, high concentrations of sevoflurane, desiccated barium lime absorbent; minimizing exposure recommended although studies have not shown nephrotoxicity in humans (if using flow rate of 1–2 L limit exposure to <2 MAC h; use >2 L for longer cases)

Halothane
- Key features: Low pungency (ideal for gas induction), inexpensive, ↑ cerebral blood flow > other volatiles, especially potent bronchodilator
- Disadvantages: Use ↓↓ due to rare but fulminant postop autoimmune hepatitis, CV depression, and myocardial sensitization to catecholamines (↑ ventricular dysrhythmias)

Heliox (Helium–Oxygen Combination)
- Nonanesthetic gas mixture, commonly 70–79% helium + 21–30% O_2
- Lower density of gases (up to 2/3 ↓ than air + O_2) promotes laminar flow, reduces turbulence in upper airway obstruction, asthma, COPD
- Helps ↓ pressures needed to ventilate pts with small-diameter ETTs; ↓ work of spontaneous breathing

MEGAN GRAYBILL ANDERS

INTRODUCTION

Pharmacology of Common Noninhaled Anesthetics							
	Induction/Bolus Dose[a]	Onset	Duration of Action (min)	VD (L/kg)	Protein Binding (%)	$t_{1/2}$ Elimination (h)	Infusion Dose
Propofol	1–2.5 mg/kg	15–45 s	5–10	2–10	98	2–24	GA: 100–200 mcg/kg/min; Sedation: 25–75 mcg/kg/min
Etomidate	0.2–0.3 mg/kg	15–45 s	3–10	4–4.5	75	3–5	GA: 10 mcg/kg/min[c]
Thiopental	3–5 mg/kg	15–30 s	5–10	1.6–8	72–86	12	GA: 30–70 mcg/kg/min
Methohexital	1–2 mg/kg	15–30 s	5–10	1.9–2.2	73	4	GA: 50–150 mcg/kg/min
Ketamine	1–2 mg/kg IV; 4–6 mg/kg IM; 6–10 mg/kg PO	30–60 s IV; 3–4 min IM; 20–40 min PO	5–10 IV; 12–25 IM	2–3	69	2–4	GA: 30–90 mcg/kg/min; Adjunct: 0.1 mg/kg/h
Dexmedetomidine	1 mcg/kg[b]	—	—	1.6	94	2–3	Sedation: 0.2–1.4 mcg/kg/h

[a]Reduce dose up to 50% for elderly, chronically or critically ill, hypovolemic, or heavily premedicated pts.
[b]Loading dose over 10 min for sedation infusion.
[c]With N_2O and opiate; limit duration due to adrenal suppression.

Clinical Considerations of Common Noninhaled Anesthetics

	Propofol	Etomidate	Thiopental	Ketamine	Dexmede-tomidine	Midaz-olam
Myoclonus	+	+++				
Antiepileptic	+++	↓	+++	+		+++
Burst suppression	+++	+	+++			
Nausea/vomiting	↓	++				↓
Painful injection	++	+++	+			
Analgesia			↓	+++	+ or ++	

+, mild association; ++, moderate association; +++, strong association; ↓, reduction.

Physiologic Changes with Common Noninhaled Anesthetics

	Propofol	Etomidate	Thiopental	Ketamine	Dexmedeto-midine	Midazolam
HR	↔ or ↓	↔	↑	↑↑	↑ (bolus); ↓ (infusion)	↔ or ↓
MAP	↓↓↓	↔ or ↓	↓↓	↑↑	↑ (bolus); ↓ (infusion)	↔ or ↓
Myocardial contractility	↓	↔	↓↓	↓	↔	↔
CBF	↓↓↓	↓↓	↓↓	↑	↓	↓
CMRO₂	↓↓↓	↓↓	↓↓	↑	↓	↓
ICP	↓↓↓	↓↓	↓↓	↔ or ↑	↔	↔
MV	↓↓↓	↔	↓↓	↓	↔ or ↓	↔ or ↓
Ventilatory drive	↓↓↓	↓	↓↓↓	↔	↔ or ↓	↓

↔, no change; ↑, increase; ↓, decrease; HR, heart rate; MAP, mean arterial pressure; CBF, cerebral blood flow; CMRO₂, cerebral metabolic rate of oxygen; ICP, intracranial pressure; MV, minute ventilation.

GENERAL PRINCIPLES

- Lipophilic drugs produce rapid induction of general anesthesia
- Most IV anesthetics exert effect through activation or augmentation of postsynaptic GABA_A receptors (↑ chloride influx → hyperpolarization → ↓ neuronal excitability)
- An ideal anesthetic drug provides amnesia, analgesia, immobility, and hypnosis; "balanced anesthesia" uses combinations of drugs to achieve these aims
- Infusions may be used for maintenance of GA; this total intravenous anesthesia (TIVA) is a useful, though costly, option in selected scenarios (e.g., MH susceptibility, severe PONV)
- Low-dose infusions/small incremental boluses used for procedural sedation, regional anesthesia adjunct
- Most IV anesthetics are capable of causing transient apnea with induction doses; respiratory depressant effects ↑ by co-administration of narcotics
- Direct myocardial depressant properties "unmasked" by hypovolemia, critical illness, or catecholamine depletion; use caution and adjust dosing accordingly
- Agents with varying extent and route of metabolism show similar duration of action after bolus (induction) dosing because termination of effect is due to redistribution to skeletal muscle or fat
- Drugs bound to plasma proteins are unavailable for uptake by target organs; dosing for highly protein-bound drugs may need adjustment in dz states with ↓ protein production (CHF, malignancy, renal or hepatic failure)

PROPOFOL (DIPRIVAN)

- Widely used for anesthetic induction, though associated with CV depression
- Reduce/titrate dose for elderly, critically ill, hypovolemic (↓ central distribution volume, ↓ clearance → ↑ myocardial depression)
- Infusion common for MAC and TIVA; rapid clearance makes context-sensitive half-life <40 min for infusions up to 8 h

- Hepatic and extra-hepatic clearance to inactive metabolites; minimal kinetic changes in renal/liver dz
- Insoluble alkylphenol formulated in lipid emulsion containing egg yolk lecithin (per AAAAI, can use for egg- and soy-allergic pts without special precautions)
- Lipid emulsion supports bacterial growth linked to sepsis; observe aseptic technique and use within 12 h of opening
- Prolonged infusion linked to rare but lethal syndrome of arrhythmias, lipemia, metabolic acidosis, rhabdomyolysis

ETOMIDATE (AMIDATE)

- Favored for induction in hemodynamically unstable pts due to minimal direct myocardial depression, though may still cause hypotension in hypovolemic pts
- Adrenal suppression (blocks hydroxylases in cortisol pathway) limits use as infusion; importance of transient effect after single dose is highly controversial, may affect outcome in sepsis (Intensive Care Med 2011;37(6):901–910)

SODIUM THIOPENTAL (PENTOTHAL)

- Barbiturate with favorable neurologic profile, used for neuroprotection during ↓ cerebral perfusion
- Generally ↑ CV stability than propofol, though effect varies markedly based on cardiac function, volume status, autonomic tone
- Alkaline solution precipitates with acids (e.g., neuromuscular blockers); severe tissue injury with extravasation (rx with local anesthetic infiltration) or intra-arterial injection (rx with papaverine, regional sympathetic block)
- Unavailable in USA after controversy over use for capital punishment (ASA Statement on Sodium Thiopental's Removal from the Market. January 21, 2011)

METHOHEXITAL (BREVITAL)

- Barbiturate with cardiorespiratory and injection considerations similar to thiopental
- More rapid hepatic clearance than thiopental → ↓ elimination $t_{1/2}$
- Uniquely activates epileptic foci facilitating electroconvulsive therapy and identification of seizure foci during ablative surgery

KETAMINE (KETALAR)

- Phencyclidine derivative with unique action through NMDA receptor
- Produces analgesia, unique dissociative hypnosis (limb movement, eye opening common), potent bronchodilation
- Perioperative adjuvant dosing associated with ↓ postoperative opiate use (Cochrane Database Syst Rev 2018;12:CD012033)
- Relative preservation of respiratory and CV function (sympathomimetic)
- Adverse effects include ↑ cardiac work, ↑ oral secretions, direct myocardial depressant effect seen with catecholamine depletion (sepsis, trauma)
- Dose-dependent psychomimetic effects (e.g., hallucinations), ↓ with co-administration of benzodiazepines
- Oral and IM routes useful for noncooperative pts

DEXMEDETOMIDINE

- Selective $\alpha 2$ adrenergic agonist with sedative, amnestic, analgesic effects
- Approved for procedural and short-term (generally <24 h) ICU sedation and fiberoptic intubation; slower onset/offset than propofol
- Desirable for sedation with very minimal respiratory depression, maintenance of arousability
- Perioperative opioid use ↓ when used as adjunct
- Adverse qualities include dose-dependent hypotension and bradycardia, ↑ cost

BENZODIAZEPINES (SEE TABLE—PHARMACOLOGY OF COMMONLY ENCOUNTERED BENZODIAZEPINES)

- Effective premedication (usually midazolam); produce anxiolysis and amnesia
- Associated with ↓ respiratory depression than barbiturates; unique ability to be antagonized by flumazenil

- Potent anticonvulsants useful for status epilepticus, alcohol withdrawal, local anesthetic toxicity
- Duration of effect depends on hepatic clearance rate (midazolam >> lorazepam > diazepam)
- Midazolam used for infusion; caution due to association with ↑ delirium, renal excretion of active metabolite
- Diazepam, lorazepam cause pain on injection due to propylene glycol solvent
- Large (GA induction) doses of midazolam may cause ↓ preload and afterload, prolonged sedation

Pharmacology of Commonly Encountered Benzodiazepines							
	Protein Binding (%)	Volume (L/kg)	Elimination $t_{1/2}$ (h)	Route	Adult Dosing[a]	Onset (min)	Peak (min)
Midazolam (Versed)	97	1–3	1.8–6.4 (mean = 3); active metabolites	PO[b] IV (premed) IV (induction)	0.25 mg/kg (max 20 mg) 1–2 mg 0.2–0.4 mg/kg	15–30 1–3 0.5–1.5	20–50 3–5 3–5
Lorazepam (Ativan)	89–93	1.3	11–22	PO IV IM	1–4 mg 1–4 mg 1–4 mg	30–60 1–5 15–30	60–360 15–20 90–120
Diazepam (Valium)	98	0.8–1	20–50 +; active metabolites	PO IV IM	2–10 mg 2–10 mg 2–10 mg	20–40 1–5 10–20	60–120 15–30 30–90

[a]Incremental dosing with titration to effect recommended for all IV benzodiazepines.
[b]Oral midazolam premedication use more common in pediatrics (0.5 mg/kg dose), IV formulation can be added to juice for PO use.

MEGAN GRAYBILL ANDERS

OPIOIDS (SEE ALSO CHAPTER 13, ACUTE PAIN MANAGEMENT)

General Comments
- Suppress pain through action on mu, kappa, delta opioid receptors
- Directly inhibit ascending nociceptive transmission and activate descending pain control circuits
- Dose-dependent analgesia and sedation; amnesia at large doses (unreliable)
- Differences in lipid solubility affect pharmacokinetic variability
- Very wide variation in dose requirements to achieve analgesia
- Pts will report improved comfort but are still aware of pain (contrast to nerve block)
- May cause pruritus (especially neuraxial dosing), rx with mixed agonist/antagonist
- Abuse, addiction, diversion potential though concerns should not supersede proper management of pain.

Physiologic Effects of Opiates		
Cardiovascular		
Heart rate	Generally CNS-mediated ↓ with high doses; meperidine causes ↑ due to atropine-like structure	May impair compensatory sympathetic response (↑ orthostatic hypotension)
Contractility	↓ with meperidine, otherwise no change	
Blood pressure	May ↓ due to ↓ sympathetic outflow; vasodilation with histamine-releasing agents (morphine, meperidine)	
Respiratory		
Respiratory rate	↓↓; may still breathe on command	May cause chest wall rigidity, vocal cord closure with high bolus doses (impairs ability to ventilate). Central antitussive effect. Respiratory depression may peak after analgesic effect.
Resting pCO_2	↑↑; supplemental O_2 may mask hypoventilation	
Response to hypercarbia	↓↓; may outlast analgesic effects and ↓ of respiratory rate	
Response to hypoxia	↓	
Airway reflexes	↓	
Neurologic		
$CMRO_2$	Modest ↓	CBF and ICP may ↑ with hypercarbia; support ventilation adequately. No effect on sensory evoked potentials.
CBF	↓ when administered with N_2O	
ICP	↓	
Seizures	↑ with accumulation of meperidine metabolite in renal insufficiency; possible ↑ focal neuroexcitation after ↑ doses potent opioid	
Gastrointestinal		
Motility	↓ gastric emptying and peristalsis, ↑ ileus	No tolerance to constipating effect
Nausea/vomiting	↑; complex mechanism includes stimulation of chemoreceptor trigger zone, ↑ vestibular sensitivity	
Common bile duct pressure	↑ with fentanyl, morphine, meperidine	
Urologic		
Urinary retention	↑	Especially with intrathecal use

Fentanyl (Sublimaze IV, Fentora Buccal, Actiq Lozenge, Duragesic Transdermal)

Dose:	
Premed/regional adjunct: 25–100 mcg/dose GA adjunct: Intraoperative dose range 2–20 mcg/kg (1–3 mcg/kg as intubation adjunct); infusion of 2–10 mcg/kg/h High dose (20–50 mcg/kg) is used rarely, e.g., open heart surgery (up to 150 mcg/kg as sole GA agent) Intrathecal*: 10–25 mcg (1 mcg/kg peds) Epidural*: 2–10 mcg/mL local anesthetic PACU*: 25–100 mcg/dose	Sedation/analgesia*: 0.5–1 mcg/kg (load); 0.5–2 mcg/kg/h (maint)

*Off-label uses

Clearance: Liver by CYP-450 3A4; 10% unchanged in urine, metabolite norfentanyl detectable up to 48 h

Comments: High lipid solubility causes rapid redistribution to inactive sites (fat, skeletal muscle); therefore, quick onset and quick redistribution below therapeutic index. Duration of action ↑ with large and repeated doses. Peak respiratory depression occurs at 5–15 min (lags behind analgesic effect). Less emetic effect than morphine

Remifentanil (Ultiva)

Induction: 1 mcg/kg over 30–60 s GA adjunct: Loading dose: 1 mcg/kg; bolus 0.5–1 mcg/kg; maint: 0.05–2 mcg/kg/min	Sedation: 0.5–1 mcg/kg load over 30–60 s; 0.025–0.2 mcg/kg/min maint (titrate carefully, respiratory depression ↑ with propofol) *May bolus 0.5–1 mcg/kg when changing infusion rates*

Clearance: Unique, rapid metabolism of ester linkage by nonspecific blood and tissue esterases (NOT plasma cholinesterase)

Comments: Bolus produces profound transient analgesia and suppression of autonomic response to noxious stimulus. Rapid recovery observed after infusion regardless of duration (short context-sensitive half-time). May cause bradycardia, chest wall rigidity, hypotension; some data suggest acute opioid tolerance with ↑ postoperative opioid requirements. Do not administer concomitantly with blood as esterases may metabolize. Must dose other analgesics very soon after stopping infusion. Initial dose based on ideal body weight in obese pts.

Sufentanil (Sufenta)

Dose:	
GA adjunct (minor proc): 1–2 mcg/kg load (induction/intubation), then 10–50 mcg/kg prn GA adjunct (moderate proc): 2–8 mcg/kg load, then 10–50 mcg prn or infusion 0.3–1.5 mcg/kg/h	GA (major proc): 8–30 mcg/kg load, then 10–50 mcg prn or infusion 0.5–2.5 mcg/kg/h Sedation*: Load: 0.1–0.5 mcg/kg; infusion 0.2–0.5 mcg/kg/h Epidural: 10–15 mcg/10 mL of 0.125% bupivacaine

*Off-label

Clearance: Liver CYP3A4 metabolism, renal/biliary excretion

Comments: Produces hypnosis at doses ≥8 mcg/kg (cardiovascular, neurosurgery). Calculate dose on ideal body weight. Provides analgesic effect after discontinuation of infusion. When used as GA adjunct, total dosage recommendation of ≤1 mcg/kg/h of anesthesia; up to 75% given at induction.

Alfentanil (Alfenta)

Dose:
Incremental GA adjunct: 20–50 mcg/kg at induction, then 5–15 mcg/kg q5–20min (up to 75 mcg/kg total). Infusion GA adjunct: Spontaneous/assisted ventilation: 8–20 mcg/kg load, then 0.5–1 mcg/kg/min; total dose 8–40 mcg/kg. Controlled ventilation: 50–75 mcg/kg load, then 0.5–3 mcg/kg/min (avg 1–1.5 mcg/kg/min). Reduce infusion rates 30–50% for initial h after induction. GA: 130–245 mcg/kg induction over 3 min (with muscle relaxant), then 0.5–1.5 mcg/kg/min MAC: Load 3–8 mcg/kg, then 3–8 mcg/kg IV q5–20min or 0.25–1 mcg/kg/min; total dose 3–40 mcg/kg.

Clearance: Liver CYP3A4 (widely variable)

Comments: Rapid peak effect useful for blunting response to single, brief stimulus (similar to remifentanil). Produces hypnosis as single agent at high dose. Erythromycin, protease inhibitors, others inhibit clearance. Initial dose based on ideal body weight in obese pts.

Morphine (Astramorph, Duramorph, MS Contin, Others)

Dose:	Infusion: 0.8–10 mg/h (Peds: Sickle cell/cancer pain
Sedation/analgesia: 2–10 mg IV	0.025–2 mg/kg/h; postop: 0.01–0.04 mg/kg/h)
(Peds: 0.02–0.1 mg/kg IV)	Intrathecal: 0.1–0.5 mg (Peds: 0.01 mg/kg)
Analgesic dosing: 2–20 mg q2–4h	Epidural: 2–6 mg q8–24h (bolus); 0.08–0.16 mg/h
IV, IM, SC	(infusion); max 10 mg/24 h; (Peds: 0.03–0.05 mg/kg, max:
	0.1 mg/kg or 5 mg/24 h)

Clearance: Primarily renal; metabolites: Morphine-3-glucuronide (55–75%, inactive) and morphine-6-glucuronide, active

Comments: Crosses blood–brain barrier slowly, peak effect may be delayed 10–40 min, complicating titration. Adjust dosing in renal failure. Greatest histamine release of commonly administered opiates. Sustained-release PO preparations available

Hydromorphone (Dilaudid)
Dose: Analgesic dosing: 0.4–2 mg IV (Peds: 0.005–0.02 mg/kg)
Clearance: Liver metabolism, urine/bile excretion; metabolites: Liver glucuronidation 3-glucuronide (major) and 6-hydroxy (minor)
Comments: Useful alternative to morphine; less histamine release, safer in renal impairment, shorter time to peak effect

Meperidine (Demerol)
Indication: Moderate–severe pain. Also used for postoperative shivering
Dose: Sedation/analgesic dosing: 50–150 mg
IV/IM q3–4h (Peds: 0.5–2 mg/kg IV, IM)
Infusion: 0.3–1.5 mg/kg/h; postoperative shivering: 12.5–25 mg IV
Clearance: Liver metabolism, urinary excretion
Comments: Direct myocardial depressant, may ↑ HR due to structural similarity to atropine. Metabolite: Normeperidine linked to CNS excitation, seizure caution in elderly, renal impairment, chronic dosing. Administration with MAOI may result in delirium or hyperthermia (serotonin syndrome). Antishivering action may be result of kappa receptor agonism. Shorter duration of action than morphine (see Fig. 2C-1)

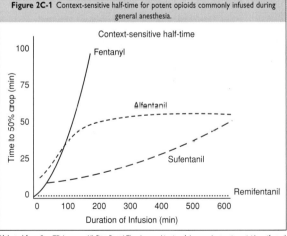

Figure 2C-1 Context-sensitive half-time for potent opioids commonly infused during general anesthesia.

(Adapted from Egan TD, Lemmens HJ, Fiset P, et al. The pharmacokinetics of the new short-acting opioid remifentanil (GI87084B) in healthy adult male volunteers. *Anesthesiology.* 1993;79(5):881–892.)

Pharmacologic Properties of Intravenous Analgesics

Drug	Onset (min)	Duration of Action[a]	Part. Coeff.	Vd (L/kg)	Protein Binding (%)	Potency (Relative to Morphine)
Fentanyl	1–3	30–60 min	820	4	84	100
Remifentanil	0.5–1.5	4–6 min	17.9	0.3–0.4	70	80–100[b]
Sufentanil	1.5–3	20 min	1,750	2.5	93	500–4,000
Alfentanil	1.2–5	15 min	130	0.86	90	10–25
Morphine	5–20	2–3 h	1.4	3–4	20–40	1
Hydromorphone	15	2–3 h	1.3	3.7	8–19	5–7
Meperidine	15	2–3 h	21	3–4.5	70	0.1

[a]After single (bolus) dose; see the chart for infusion context-sensitive half-times.
[b]Slightly less potent than fentanyl in most references, others describe higher potency.

Typical PCA Parameters for Adult Pts[a]

	Morphine	Hydromorphone	Fentanyl
Concentration	1 mg/mL	0.2 mg/mL	10 mcg/mL
Clinician bolus	2 mg (1.2–3 mg)	0.4 mg (0.2–0.6 mg)	20 mcg (20–40 mcg)
Clinician bolus/h	1–2	1–2	1–2
PCA dose	1 mg (0.6–1.5 mg)	0.2 mg (0.1–0.3 mg)	10 mcg (10–20 mcg)
Lockout	8–10 min	8–10 min	8–10 min
Limit	6 demand doses + basal rate (if applicable)		
Basal[b]	0.5–1 mg/h	0.1–0.2 mg/h	10–30 mcg/h

[a]Suggested dose for adult pts with normal renal function. Use reduced doses for elderly, renally insufficient, or opioid sensitive (e.g., OSA) pts. Upper limit of range provided not appropriate for opioid naive pts.
[b]Not recommended for starting PCA. Consider adding as 1/3 of average hourly usage if PCA use > 3×/h and unable to sleep, after demand dose/h limit titration.

Typical PCA Parameters for Pediatric Pts <50 kg

	Morphine	Hydromorphone	Fentanyl
Concentration	1 mg/mL	0.2 mg/mL	10 mcg/mL
Clinician bolus	40–80 mcg/kg	8–15 mcg/kg	0.5–1 mcg/kg
Clinician bolus/h	2	2	2
PCA dose	10–20 mcg/kg	2–4 mcg/kg	0.25–0.5 mcg/kg
Lockout	10 min	8–15 min	10 min
Limit	100 mcg/kg/h	20 mcg/kg/h	3 mcg/kg/h
Basal (optional)	5–20 mcg/kg/h	1–5 mcg/kg/h	0.15–0.5 mcg/kg/h

Methadone (Dolophine)

Indications: Chronic pain, opioid withdrawal
Dose: Adults, opiate-naive: Start 2.5–10 mg PO or 2.5–5 mg IV/IM/SC q8–12h; titrate up q3–5d. Dose conversion: 5 mg IV = 10 mg PO.
Mechanism: Opiate agonist and NMDA receptor antagonist
Clearance: Hepatic, renal excretion (use 50–75% of dose in renal impairment)
Comments: Major adverse effect is respiratory depression (peaks later/longer than analgesic effect). Very long/variable half-life (13–100 h) although many pts require dosing q6–8h to maintain analgesia. Use caution when converting long-standing opiate users to methadone, as paradoxically ↓ dose conversion ratios are required (incomplete cross-tolerance) (see Table—Conversion of Oral Morphine Equivalent to Oral Methadone, Opiate-Tolerant Pt). Requires careful titration; deaths reported even in opioid tolerant pts. QT prolongation possible, more common in >200 mg/d; consider ECG when initiating/titrating. Use for detoxification may require participation of licensed opiate agonist therapy program.

Conversion of Oral Morphine Equivalent to Oral Methadone, Opiate-Tolerant Pt

Daily Oral Morphine Equivalent (mg)	Conversion Ratio Morphine:Methadone
<30	2:1
31–99	4:1
100–299	8:1
300–499	12:1
500–999	15:1
1,000	20:1

Use caution. Considerable individual variation and long half-life of methadone can result in dangerous dose escalation if sufficient time (~5 d) is not allowed between dose changes. These tables should NOT be used in reverse (converting from methadone to morphine).
Source: From Fisch M, Cleeland C. Managing cancer pain. In: Skeel RT, ed. Handbook of Cancer Chemotherapy. 6th ed. Philadelphia, PA: Lippincott Williams & Wilkins; 2003:66.

Conversion of IV Morphine to IV Methadone

Daily IV Morphine Dose (mg)	Estimated Daily IV Methadone Dose (As % of Daily Morphine Dose)
10–30	40–66
30–50	27–66
50–100	22–50
100–200	15–34
200–500	10–20

Source: Methadone injection [package insert]. Lake Forest, IL: Bioniche Pharma USA LLC; 2009.
For Equianalgesic Opioid Dosage Table, see Chapter 13-4.

Common PO Opioid Analgesics

Generic	Brand name
Hydrocodone + acetaminophen*	Norco Lortab Vicodin
Hydrocodone + ibuprofen	Vicoprofen
Codeine + acetaminophen	Tylenol with codeine # 3, 4
Codeine + acetaminophen, butalbital, caffeine	Fioricet with codeine
Oxycodone	Roxicodone OxyIR
Oxycodone (controlled release)	OxyContin
Oxycodone + acetaminophen	Percocet Roxicet
Morphine	Roxanol
Morphine (sustained release)	MS Contin Avinza Kadian Oramorph SR
Oxymorphone (extended release)	Opana ER
Tramadol	Ultram

*FDA requested manufacturers limit acetaminophen in combination tablets to 325 mg/tablet (2011), may impact available formulations.

Oxycodone

Indications: Moderate–severe pain

Dose: Opioid naïve adults: 5–15 mg (immediate release) PO q4–6h; 10 mg (controlled release) q8–12h, titrate by 25–50% q1–2d

Mechanism: Metabolized to oxymorphone via CYP2D6, poor metabolizers may not achieve adequate effect

Comments: Extended treatment for severe pain to involve scheduled doses of sustained-release, prn availability of immediate-release dose for "breakthrough" pain (similar to other drugs available in immediate/sustained forms). Do not crush or administer sustained-release tablets through feeding tube. Rapid metabolizers (to active form) may have ↑ toxicity. High-abuse potential, available in "abuse-deterrent" preparations

Codeine

Indications: Mild–moderate pain, cough suppression

Dose: Adult: 15–60 mg PO q4–6h (max 120 mg/d); Peds: 1–1.5 mg/kg/d divided q4–6h (max 30 mg/d ages 2–6, 60 mg/d ages 6–12)

Mechanism: Metabolized to morphine by cytochrome P450 CYP2D6

Comments: Significant genetic/ethnic variability in metabolism—may cause insufficient analgesia in poor metabolizers (5–10% of pts) or life-threatening toxicity in ultra-metabolizers (1–2% of pts). Avoid in breastfeeding women, and in children after tonsillectomy/adenoidectomy.

Mixed Opiate Agonists–Antagonists				
Drug	Dose Equianalgesic to Morphine 10 mg IV	Onset	Duration (h)	Typical Dosing/ Comments
Buprenorphine (Buprenex, IM/IV, Suprenex SL)	0.3–0.4 mg q6–8h IM/IV (May repeat initial dose in 30–60 min ×1. >0.3 mg/dose should only be given IM)	5–15 min	6–8	**2–12 y/o:** 2–6 mcg/kg IM/IV q4–6h, max 6 mcg/kg/dose **>13 y/o:** 0.3 mg IV/IM q6–8h, max 300 mcg/dose Epidural: 0.3 mg
Buprenorphine/ naloxone (Suboxone)	See Chapter 2H-52			
Butorphanol (Stadol)	2 mg IM/IV q3–4h	5–30 min	3–4	1 mg IV or 2 mg IM. Max 4 mg/dose IM Nasal spray: 1 mg in 1 nostril q3–4h **As anesthesia adjunct,** 2 mg IV before induction then 0.5–1 mg IV prn
Nalbuphine (Nubain)	10 mg IV/IM/SC q3–6h	3–15 min	3–6	Max 20 mg/dose, 160 mg/d. For opioid-induced pruritus: 2.5–5 mg q6h or 60 mcg/kg/h
Morphine/ naltrexone (Embeda)		7.5 h (peak levels)	29 (half-life)	20 mg/0.8 mg PO q24h, titrate q1–2d. Do not administer more than bid.

Indications: Mild to moderate pain, esp headaches

Mechanism: Bind to mu receptors with limited response (partial agonist) or no effect (competitive antagonist) and often kappa/delta receptor agonism as well

Comments: Agonist–antagonist can ↓ efficacy of subsequently administered opiates. Advantage is that these have limited respiratory depression and ↓ potential for physical dependence. Unlike pure opiate agonists, agonist–antagonists have a ceiling effect in their dose–response relationship (not recommended when pain may ↑). Antagonist effects of these drugs may precipitate withdrawal in opiate-dependent pts. Butorphanol (not nalbuphine) ↑ systolic blood pressure, pulmonary artery blood pressure, and cardiac output. Milder effects on GI and biliary systems then with morphine. Butorphanol commonly used in obstetrics; nalbuphine (low-dose bolus or infusion) effective in relieving neuraxial opioid-related pruritus without affecting pain control

NMDA RECEPTOR ANTAGONIST & OPIATE AGONISTS

Ketamine (Ketalar)

See also Chapter 2B and Chapter 13

Indications: Used for (1) pre-incision, intraoperative ("pre-emptive") analgesia; (2) postoperative opioid adjunct; (3) adjunct in regional and neuraxial anesthesia

Dose[1]: (1) Bolus of 0.15–0.5 (up to 1) mg/kg and/or infusion at 0.1–0.6 mg/kg/h; (2) 3 mcg/kg/min × 48 h; or 120 mcg/kg/h × 24 h, then 60 mcg/kg/h × 48 h or longer;

[1]Studied doses listed, no strong consensus on optimal dose and timing for analgesic adjunct indications.

(3) *Epidural:* 30 mg or 0.25–0.5 mg/kg via epidural before incision; *Caudal:* 0.5 mg/kg; *Intra-articular:* 10 mg; *Brachial plexus block:* 30 mg.

Comments: Potent analgesic with unique mechanism of action. Incremental bolus may be used for short, painful procedures (e.g., burn dressing changes). Evidence for ↓ in postoperative opioid requirements when low doses used as adjunct. Emerging uses under investigation include sub-anesthetic doses for rescue analgesia in PACU, infusion to improve analgesia in highly opioid-tolerant pts, and oral dosing for complex regional pain syndrome as well depression and neuropathic, ischemic, phantom limb, and cancer pain.

Tramadol (Ultram)

Dose: Start at 25 mg qAM, increasing 25 mg qd to 25 mg qid, then 50 mg/d × 3 d to 50 mg qid. Max 400 mg/d or 300 mg/d if age >75. May skip dose titration if immediate onset desired.

Mechanism: Dual: (1) Opiate agonist (2) spinal inhibition of pain (similar to tricyclics) via inhibition of serotonin/norepinephrine reuptake. Active metabolite M1 has 200× ↑ affinity for mu opioid receptor

Clearance: Hepatic metabolism, renal excretion

Comments: Less resp and GI motor effects. May cause seizures, caution in renal dz, alcohol use, stroke, head injury. Potential for life-threatening serotonin syndrome with serotonergic drugs, P450 inhibitors. CYP2D6 poor metabolizers have 20% ↑ tramadol, 40% ↓ M1 levels; genotyping available. Not completely antagonized by naloxone.

OPIATE ANTAGONISTS (SEE CHAPTER 2H)

TRANSDERMAL/TOPICAL MEDICATIONS

Fentanyl Transdermal (Duragesic)

Indications: Sustained-release opiate therapy, treatment of chronic pain

Dose: See Table—Opiate to Fentanyl Patch Conversion

Mechanism: Opiate agonist

Clearance: See Fentanyl above

Comments: Available from 12.5–100 mcg/h patches. Time to peak efficacy 12 h. Change every 72 h. See Fentanyl, 2C-15, for side effects. Conversion from total daily dose of morphine to fentanyl complicated with multiple possible formulas (see Table—Opiate to Fentanyl Patch Conversion). Contraindicated for postoperative pain relief in opiate naïve pts as high risk for respiratory depression. Concurrent use of P450 3A4 inhibitors including some antimicrobials causes ↑ fentanyl levels

Opiate to Fentanyl Patch Conversion*				
Current Analgesic	**Daily Dosage (mg/d)**			
Oral morphine	60–134	135–224	225–314	315–404
IM/IV morphine	10–22	23–37	38–52	53–67
Oral oxycodone	30–67	67.5–112	112.5–157	157.5–202
Oral hydromorphone	8–17	17.1–28	28.1–39	39.1–51
IV hydromorphone	1.5–3.4	3.5–5.6	5.7–7.9	8–10
Oral methadone	20–44	45–74	75–104	105–134
	↓	↓	↓	↓
Recommended fentanyl patch*	25 mcg/h	50 mcg/h	75 mcg/h	100 mcg/h

Oral 24-h Morphine (mg/d)	Fentanyl Patch (mcg/h)
405	See above
405–494	125
495–584	150
585–674	175
675–764	200
765–854	225
855–944	250
945–1,034	275
1,035–1,124	300

*Do not use tables to convert to fentanyl patch to other therapies because conversions listed here are conservative.
Source: Duragesic [package insert]. Mountain View, CA: Janssen Pharmaceutica Products, LP; 2003.

Lidocaine Patch, 5% (Lidoderm)
Indications: Neuropathic pain, local inflammatory conditions
Dose: 1–3 patches q24h with 12 h on and 12 h off typical usage although >3 patches and 24-h usage have been studied and found to be safe and well tolerated
Mechanism: Sodium channel blockade
Comments: Produces analgesia but not anesthesia. Minimal systemic absorption. Main side effect is local skin irritation (e.g., burning, dermatitis, pruritus, rash)

NONSTEROIDAL ANTI-INFLAMMATORY DRUGS (NSAIDS)

General comments: Produce analgesic, anti-inflammatory, antipyretic effects. Generally have a ceiling effect (unlike opiates) beyond which further analgesia does not occur, but side effects worsen. Mechanism via inhibition of cyclooxygenase (COX) → decreased formation of inflammatory mediators (i.e., prostaglandins). See Figure 2C-2. COX-1 inhibition associated with majority of side effects: GI mucosal ulceration, ↓ renal perfusion, and ↓ platelet aggregation. Inhibition of prostaglandin synthesis suspected mechanism for NSAID-induced bronchospasm. NSAIDs, particularly selective COX-2 inhibitors, may ↑ risk of MI and CVA, which can be fatal. Perioperative use in orthopedic surgery requires caution and communication with surgeons; NSAIDs inhibit bone healing in vitro, although clinical significance is controversial and under investigation.

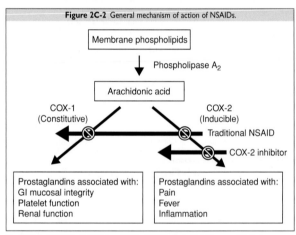

Figure 2C-2 General mechanism of action of NSAIDs.

(From Ballantyne JC, Salahadin AS, Fishman SM. *The MGH Handbook of Pain Management.* 2nd ed. Philadelphia, PA: Lippincott Williams & Wilkins; 2002.)

NONSELECTIVE COX INHIBITORS

Acetaminophen (Tylenol, Paracetamol, Ofirmev)
Indications: Mild–moderate pain, fever
Dose: *Adults:* **PO/PR:** 325–650 mg q4–6h, or 1,000 mg q6–8h (max 4 g/d, some recommend max 3 g/d). **IV:** *Adults >50 kg:* 650 mg q4h or 1,000 mg q6h over 15 min, max 4 g/d; *adults <50 kg* 12.5 mg/kg q4h or 15 mg/kg q6h max 750 mg/dose or 3.75 mg/d. *Peds:* See Table—Dosing of Commonly Used Propionic Acid NSAIDs
Onset: 5 min (IV) 10 min (PO)
Mechanism: Unclear, possibly inhibition of COX-2
Clearance: Liver
Comments: Lacks significant anti-inflammatory effect (not a true NSAID). Favorable side effect profile: does not produce GI irritation, affect platelet aggregation. Major toxicity in overdose (single dose or cumulative use): Hepatic necrosis due to depletion of antioxidant glutathione, formation of *N*-acetyl-*p*-benzoquinone. Acetylcysteine may substitute for glutathione and prevent hepatotoxicity if administered within 8 h

Selected Adjunct Medications in Treatment of Chronic Pain

Drug	Starting Dose (Adult)	Dose Range (mg/d)	Mechanism	Evidence for Efficacy	Selected Adverse Effects
Membrane Stabilizers					
Gabapentin (Neurontin)	100–300 mg qhs-tid	900–3,600, divide tid	Binds voltage-gated Ca channel	Neuropathic pain, fibromyalgia, spinal stenosis	Dizziness, sedation, weight gain, nausea
Pregabalin (Lyrica)	50 mg bid	50–450, divide bid-tid	Binds voltage-gated Ca channel	Neuropathic pain, fibromyalgia	Dizziness, sedation, edema, headache
Topiramate (Topamax)	50 mg qhs	200 mg bid	Na, Ca channels; enhances GABA action	Neuropathic pain, chronic lumbar pain	Sedation, weight loss
Skeletal Muscle Relaxants					
Cyclobenzaprine (Flexeril)	5 mg daily	5–30, divided	Central; unknown	Cervical/lumbar spinal pain, muscle spasm	Dry mouth, drowsiness, headache, confusion
Carisoprodol (Soma)	250–350 mg qid	1,000–1,400, divide qid	Central; likely interneuronal inhibition	Acute musculoskeletal pain (not for spasticity)	Dizziness, drowsiness, headache, ataxia, confusion, dependence*
Baclofen (Kemstro)	5 mg tid	30–80	Binds GABA-B, inhibits neurotransmitter release	Spasticity of spinal cord origin, upper motor neuron dz, acute back pain, trigeminal neuralgia	Drowsiness, dizziness, nausea, confusion
Antidepressants					
Amitriptyline (Elavil)	10–25 mg daily	75–300	Tricyclic SNRI	Tension headache, TMD, facial myofascial pain	Dry mouth, constipation, weight gain, drug interactions
Duloxetine (Cymbalta)	20–30 mg qhs	60–120	SNRI	Neuropathic pain, fibromyalgia	Nausea, somnolence, dry mouth, constipation
α2 Agonists					
Tizanidine (Zanaflex)	1–2 mg daily	2–36 divided tid	Presynaptic inhibition of motor neurons	Spasticity, paravertebral spasm	Dry mouth, somnolence, asthenia, dizziness

*Metabolized to barbiturate (meprobamate).
Source: Adapted from Benzon H, Srinivasa NR, Fishman SM, et al. *Essentials of Pain Medicine.* 3rd ed. Philadelphia, PA: Saunders Elsevier; 2011.

of ingestion. Some evidence suggests 2–3 g/d may be safe in chronic hepatic dz, use caution. Reduce dose with severe renal dz. Rectal absorption is slow and erratic. May be used in pregnancy.

Propionic Acid Derivatives: Ibuprofen, Naproxen, Ketoprofen, Diclofenac

Dosing of Commonly Used Propionic Acid NSAIDs			
Drug	Dose	Max Daily Dose	OTC
Ibuprofen (Advil, Motrin)	PO: 200–800 mg q6h IV: 400–800 mg q6h	3,200 mg	Yes
Naproxen (Aleve)	PO: 250 mg q6–8h or 500 mg q12	1,250 mg	Yes
Diclofenac (Voltaren)	PO: 25 mg q6h or 50 mg q12h	200 mg	No

Comments: See general NSAID comments. May exacerbate renal dz, especially in hypovolemia. Extensive protein binding may lead to adverse drug interaction. Ibuprofen has less protein binding than other propionic acids. Note that IV ibuprofen is now available.

Ketorolac (Toradol)
Dose: *Adult >50 kg and <65 y old:* 30 mg IV q6h, max 120 mg/d. ≥65 y old or <50 kg: 15 mg q6h, max 60 mg/d. **Max duration 5 d. Peds:** 2–16 y 0.5 mg/kg IV, then 0.25–0.5 mg/kg/dose q6h up to 48 h
Clearance: <50% hepatic metabolism, renal metabolism; 91% renal elimination
Comments: PO formulation available. Parenteral administration makes useful short-term adjunct to parenteral or epidural opioids for severe pain. When administered IV, analgesic > anti-inflammatory effect. Does not cause respiratory depression or biliary tract spasm. Routine doses may be equianalgesic to 10 mg morphine. Effect on platelet function and prolonging bleeding time is observed with spinal anesthesia but not with general anesthesia. Renal injury minimized with adequate hydration. Reduce dose or avoid in elderly and renal insufficiency.

Aspirin, Acetylsalicylic Acid
Dose: Analgesic/antipyretic: 325–650 mg PO q4–6h
Indications: Low-intensity pain, headache, musculoskeletal pain, antipyretic
Mechanism: Irreversibly acetylates COX
Comments: Typically stopped 5–10 d prior to surgery due to irreversible antiplatelet effect, which may be desirable for prevention of thrombosis, MI, CVA. Contraindicated in bleeding GI ulcers, hemorrhage, thrombocytopenia, hemophilia. Caution in uremia, von Willebrand's dz, asthma.

Pediatric Dosing of NSAIDs	
Drug	Dose
Acetaminophen	(PO) 10–15 mg/kg q4–6h; 40–60 mg/kg/d (divided) (PR) 30–40 mg/kg (one-time perioperative) (IV) 2–12 y (<50 kg) 12.5 mg/kg IV q4h OR 15 mg/kg IV q6h, not to exceed 75 mg/kg/d
Aspirin*	10–15 mg/kg q4h
Ibuprofen	4–10 mg/kg PO q6–8h
Ketorolac	0.5 mg/kg IV q6–8h, not for >5 d

*Risk for Reye's syndrome if concurrent influenza, viral illness.
Source: Adapted from Berde C, Masek B. Pain in children. In Wall PD, Melzack R, eds. *Textbook of Pain.* Edinburgh: Churchill Livingstone; 1999; and Ofirmev [package insert]. San Diego, CA: Cadence Pharmaceuticals Inc., 2010.

SELECTIVE COX-2 INHIBITORS

Celecoxib (Celebrex)
Indications: Osteo- and rheumatoid arthritis, juvenile arthritis, acute pain
Dose: *Adult:* 200 mg daily, may divide bid. *Peds:* 50 mg bid in pts 10–25 kg
Mechanism: Selective COX-2 inhibition
Comments: Potentially less GI adverse effects. Reduce dose by 50% in moderate hepatic impairment. May also be associated with CV thrombotic events, transaminitis, hypertension, fluid retention, renal injury, allergic or skin reactions (avoid in sulfa, aspirin allergy).

LOCAL ANESTHETICS

MEGAN GRAYBILL ANDERS

MECHANISM OF ACTION

- Local anesthetics (LAs) are weak bases, hydrophilic, tertiary amines
- Act by binding to Na^+ channel, thereby blocking depolarization-induced influx of Na^+ and blocking propagation of nerve impulse
- Differential blockade of nerve types depends on myelination, diameter, etc.; sensitivity of autonomic > sensory > motor fibers

STRUCTURE & CLASSIFICATION

LAs have a lipophilic benzene ring linked to an amine group by a hydrocarbon chain of amide or ester linkage.
- Esters
  - Rapidly hydrolyzed by plasma pseudocholinesterases (avoid in pts with deficiency)
  - A significant metabolite, para-amino benzoic acid (PABA), is a known allergen
- Amides
  - Metabolized by hepatic microsomal P450 enzymes
  - Rare allergic reactions may be from multidose vials containing a methylparaben preservative (structure similar to PABA)

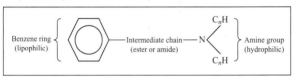

Benzene ring (lipophilic) — Intermediate chain (ester or amide) — N — Amine group (hydrophilic), with C_nH and C_nH

PHARMACODYNAMICS

- Ionization best correlates with onset of action. LAs exist in free equilibrium in both charged (ionized) and neutral (nonionized) forms:
  - The ionized form binds to the receptor and exerts the drug's action, but it is very hydrophilic and cannot penetrate the nerve membrane to exert its effect
  - The nonionized, lipid-soluble form allows the drug to penetrate nerve membrane
- Lipid solubility correlates with potency: higher solubility = greater potency
- Protein binding best correlates with duration of action
- The relative proportion of ionized and nonionized LA molecules is a function of the drug's pKa and the tissue pH
- pKa = pH at which the concentrations of ionized and nonionized forms are equal
- Clinical implications include slower onset in acidic (infected) tissue

Speed of LA onset affected by:
- pKa: Lower pKa of the anesthetic = greater the fraction of nonionized molecules at a given pH → easier membrane penetration → faster onset
- Bicarbonate (HCO_3) addition: Higher pH → more nonionized → quicker onset time
- Lipid solubility: Higher solubility generally = slower onset, may be due to sequestration in lipid membranes
- Higher concentration and total dose of local = faster onset due to diffusion gradient (↑ solution concentration explains ↑ onset of procaine and 2-chloroprocaine despite ↑ pKa)
- Site of injection and distance of diffusion to target nerve (presence of neural sheath delays onset)

Duration of LA action affected by:
- Protein binding: ↑ Protein binding → longer duration
- Site of local injection: More vascular sites have shorter duration (more systemic uptake)
- Degree of vasodilation (all locals except cocaine are vasodilators)
- Lipid solubility: ↑ Lipid solubility = ↑ duration
- Pseudocholinesterase deficiency: ↑ Duration of ester anesthetics
- Liver dz: ↑ Duration of amide anesthetics

SPECIFIC CONSIDERATIONS

Chloroprocaine
- Most rapid hydrolysis among ester class
- Increasing popularity for short-acting spinal; historical concern about neurotoxicity possibly related to bisulfite preservative
- Useful in obstetrics due to rapid onset, ↓ risk of systemic toxicity/fetal exposure (rapid hydrolysis in bloodstream)
- Useful in pts with significant liver dz, seizure hx

Lidocaine
- Versatile—used for topical, regional, intravenous, peripheral nerve block, and spinal/epidural anesthesia
- Transient neurologic symptoms (TNS) after spinal anesthesia (also reported with other LAs)
  - Pain/sensory Δ in lower back, buttocks, thighs—no motor or bowel/bladder dysfunction
  - Increased risk with lidocaine, lithotomy, ambulatory anesthetic; pregnancy may be protective
  - Symptoms occur within 2–24 h → complete resolution within 10 d (most in 2 d)
  - Tx with NSAIDs and opioids as needed

Bupivacaine
- Useful due to long duration in peripheral and epidural blocks, common in spinals
- High-quality sensory anesthesia relative to motor blockade
- Severe, refractory cardiovascular collapse with toxic intravascular doses

Liposomal Bupivacaine (Exparel®)
- Single-dose surgical site infiltration for postsurgical anesthesia; also approved for interscalene nerve block. Liposomal suspension promotes extended release (duration up to 72 h). May be diluted with up to 280 mL saline (max dose 266 mg).
- Nonbupivacaine-based LAs, including lidocaine, can cause immediate release of free bupivacaine if co-administered locally—wait at least 20 min after lidocaine, admixing with other LAs not recommended. ↓ Regular bupivacaine dose to ≤50% of mg dose of liposomal bupivacaine when using regular bupivacaine first. Avoid additional doses of bupivacaine within 96 h after dose.

Ropivacaine
- Greatest margin of safety among long-acting locals
- More vasoconstriction, less lipid solubility than bupivacaine → reduced systemic toxicity

Tetracaine
- Useful in spinals due to rapid onset, long duration (4–6 h with epi)
- Longer duration but possibly less adequate sensory blockade versus bupivacaine

Cocaine
- Vasoconstrictor property unique among LAs
- CNS stimulant through ↓ reuptake of norepi, dopamine, serotonin
- Used in 4% solution as topical anesthetic (sinus surgery, awake nasal fiberoptic) or 11.8% with tetracaine, epi (TAC) for ED wound repair
- Side effects: HTN, tachycardia, arrhythmias, coronary ischemia, stroke, cerebral & pulmonary edema, seizures

Topical Anesthesia for Minor Procedures (Pediatric IV Placement)
- EMLA cream: Eutectic Mixture of Local Anesthetics (Lidocaine 2.5%, Prilocaine 2.5%); onset ~45–60 min, duration ~2 h. Adult dose 2.5–10 g. Apply to intact skin using smallest amount necessary, cover with occlusive dressing.

EMLA Pediatric Dosing	
Age/Weight	**Max Dose (g)**
0–3 mo, <5 kg	1
3–12 mo, >5 kg	2
1–6 y, >10 kg	10
7–12 y, >20 kg	20

- Synera (lidocaine and tetrocaine): Heat activated patch, onset ~20 min. Do not cover patch.
- Avoid in G6PD deficiency; toxicity including methemoglobinemia possible. Caution in hepatic dz, pseudocholinesterase deficiency.

Commonly Used Ester Local Anesthetics (see also Chapter 6)

	pKa	Relative Potency—CNS Toxicity	Clinical Use	Concentration (%)	Onset	Duration (h)	Maximum Recommended Dose*
Chloroprocaine (Nesacaine)	8.7	0.3	Infiltration	1	Fast	0.5–1	800 mg; 1,030 mg + epi
			Epidural	2–3	Fast	0.5–1	800 mg; 1,030 mg + epi
			Periph. block	2	Fast	0.5–1	800 mg; 1,030 mg + epi
Cocaine	8.6	NA	Topical	2–12	Fast	0.5–1	150 mg
Procaine (Novocaine)	8.9	0.3	Spinal	10	Fast	0.5–1	7 mg/kg; 10 mg/kg (1,000 mg) + epi
Tetracaine (Pontocaine)	8.5	2.0	Topical	2	Fast	0.5–1	20 mg
			Spinal	0.5	Fast	2–6	20 mg

*Maximum dose may require modification with extremes of age, pregnancy, hepatic, renal, cardiac dysfunction.

Commonly Used Amide Local Anesthetics (see also Chapter 6)

	pKa	Relative Potency—CNS Toxicity	Clinical Use	Concentration (%)	Onset	Duration (h)	Maximum Recommended Dose*
Bupivacaine (Marcaine)	8.1	4	Infiltration	0.25	Fast	2–8	2.5 mg/kg (175 mg); 3 mg/kg + epi (225 mg)
			Epidural	0.03–0.75	Moderate	2–5	150 mg
			Spinal	0.5–0.75	Fast	1–4	20 mg
			Periph. block	0.25–0.5	Slow	4–12	150 mg
Etidocaine (Duranest)	7.7	2	Infiltration	0.5	Fast	1–4	300 mg; 400 mg + epi
			Epidural	1–1.5	Fast	2–4	300 mg; 400 mg + epi
			Periph. block	0.5–1	Fast	3–12	300 mg; 400 mg + epi
Lidocaine (Xylocaine)	7.9	1	Infiltration	0.5–1	Fast	1–4	4.5 mg/kg (300 mg); 7 mg/kg (500 mg) + epi
			Topical	4	Fast	0.5–1	300 mg
			Epidural	1.5–2	Fast	1–2	300 mg; 500 mg + epi
			Spinal	1.5–5	Fast	0.5–1	100 mg
			Periph. block	1–1.5	Fast	1–3	300 mg; 500 mg + epi
			IV regional	0.25–0.5	Fast	0.5–1	300 mg
Mepivacaine (Carbocaine)	7.6	1.4	Infiltration	0.5–1	Fast	1–4	400 mg; 500 mg + epi
			Epidural	1.5–2	Fast	1–3	400 mg; 500 mg + epi
			Spinal	2–4	Fast	1–2	100 mg
			Periph. block	1–1.5	Fast	2–4	400 mg; 500 mg + epi
Prilocaine (Citanest)	7.9	1.2	Infiltration	0.5–1	Fast	1–2	600 mg
			Epidural	2–3	Fast	1–3	600 mg
			Periph. block	1.5–2	Fast	1.5–3	600 mg
Ropivacaine (Naropin)	8.1	2.9	Infiltration	0.2–0.5	Fast	2–6	200 mg
			Epidural	0.05–1	Moderate	2–6	200 mg
			Periph. block	0.5–1	Slow	5–8	250 mg

*Maximum dose may require modification with extremes of age, pregnancy, hepatic, renal, cardiac dysfunction.

ADDITIVES TO ENHANCE LOCAL ANESTHETICS

- Vasoconstrictors (epinephrine, occasionally phenylephrine) → ↓ vascular uptake of drug, ↓ systemic absorption/toxicity, ↑ duration, and ↑ intensity of the block; little effect on onset time

Epinephrine Dilutions	
1:1,000	1 mg/1 mL (0.1%)
1:10,000	0.1 mg (or 100 mcg)/mL (0.01%)
1:100,000	10 mcg/mL
1:200,000	5 mcg/mL (commonly used)
1:400,000	2.5 mcg/mL

- Add to LA at time of use due to epi instability at higher pH
- Variable response between LA and the location of injection as to whether vasoconstrictors ↑ duration of action:
  - Infiltration, peripheral blockade: ↑ Duration of shorter (lidocaine) > longer-acting (bupivacaine) LA
  - Epidural blockade: Addition of epi to procaine, lidocaine, and bupivacaine → ↑ duration of block
  - Spinal blockade: Addition of epi (0.2–0.3 mg) to lidocaine, bupivacaine, tetracaine → sig. ↑ duration of block
- Epi may also ↑ quality of epidural/spinal due to α_2 adrenergic activation
- Bicarbonate–alkalinization of LA solution → ↑ percentage of nonionized form of the drug → ↑ membrane penetration, ↓ onset time; reduces pain during subcutaneous infiltration
- Opiates: ↑ Duration of neuraxial block, ↑ quality of surgical anesthesia, and postoperative analgesia
- Clonidine, dexmedetomidine: Useful in peripheral and neuraxial blocks, multiple sites of action; ↑ anesthesia and ↑ duration of block

LOCAL ANESTHETIC SYSTEMIC TOXICITY (LAST)

Systemic toxicity results from excessive plasma concentrations (due to absorption of LAs from tissue or inadvertent intravascular injection). Factors relating to rate of absorption:

- Dose of LA: A 1% solution of any drug contains 1,000 mg of drug per 100 mL of solution, or 10 mg/mL (note multiple doses of different LAs are additive)
- Rate of injection/infusion: Use incremental injection technique with intermittent aspiration
- Local vasodilation (epi vasoconstricts and reduces systemic absorption, some LAs are stronger vasodilators)
- Lipid solubility (potency) of LA, metabolism (plasma vs. liver), renal/hepatic dz, CHF
- Site of injection (based on vascularity of the tissue), with the greatest degree of absorption as follows:

  Intravascular > tracheal > intercostal > caudal > epidural > brachial plexus > subcutaneous

Toxicity mainly affects CV system and CNS. CNS is usually affected first. Progressive signs of LA toxicity:

  Lightheadedness → circumoral numbness/metallic taste → facial tingling → tinnitus → slurred speech → seizures → unconsciousness → respiratory arrest → cardiovascular depression → circulatory arrest

- "Test dose" of local with epi can indicate likely intravascular injection if associated with a significant and rapid ↑ HR, ↑ BP, or T-wave Δ; use caution as general anesthesia, active labor, β-blocker use can confound results
- CNS toxicity: ↑ With hypercarbia & acidosis (↓ seizure threshold, ↓ bound fraction of drug)
- CV toxicity:
  - May have transient ↑ in HR, BP due to CNS stimulation
  - Dose-dependent myocardial depression, hypotension, dysrhythmias (especially with bupivacaine)
  - ECG Δs: ↑ PR, ↑ QRS, ↑ QT intervals

LA Toxicity Treatment

- Stop injecting LA; get help; maintain airway (intubate if necessary); give 100% oxygen and consider hyperventilation in the presence of metabolic acidosis; treat seizures (benzodiazepines, propofol in small doses if hemodynamically stable)

- If cardiac arrest with LA toxicity: CPR, modified ALCS, and treatment of arrhythmias. Initiate lipid therapy. No role for propofol.
  - Lipid emulsion protocol: Rapid bolus 100 mL of 20% lipid emulsion if >70 kg; 1.5 mL/kg if <70 kg. Start infusion at 0.25 mL/kg/min (18 mL/min for 70-kg pt); if circulation not restored, can repeat initial bolus × 1–2 and ↑ infusion to 0.5 mL/kg/min. Dosing limit 12 mL/kg. (www.lipidrescue.org)
- ACLS modifications for LAST:
  - Reduce individual doses of epinephrine (<1 mcg/kg/dose)
  - Avoid β/calcium channel blockers, vasopressin, administration of additional LA
  - Recovery may be delayed (>1 h); continue high-quality CPR and consider ECMO/eCPR (or transfer to nearest cardiopulmonary bypass facility) for circulatory support

Methemoglobinemia (Normal Hemoglobin Oxidized to Methemoglobin)
- Causes: LAs (benzocaine, prilocaine), antibiotics (dapsone, trimethoprim), nitrates
- Symptoms and signs: SOB, cyanosis (traditional pulse ox unreliable), MS Δs, loss of consciousness; if >50% met-Hb → dysrhythmias, seizures, coma, and death
- Diagnosis: Blood is "chocolate-brown" color, ABG analysis will typically reveal normal pO_2 +/− metabolic acidosis, measure met-Hb level with co-oximetry
- Treatment: Supplemental O_2, 1% methylene blue 1–2 mg/kg IV (restores iron in Hb to its normal reduced O_2-carrying state), hyperbaric O_2.

NEUROMUSCULAR BLOCKING DRUGS AND REVERSAL AGENTS

MEGAN GRAYBILL ANDERS

MECHANISM

- Neuromuscular blocking drugs (NMBDs) work at the postsynaptic nicotinic acetylcholine (ACh) receptor of the neuromuscular junction (NMJ) → stop conduction of nerve impulses → leading to skeletal muscle paralysis
- Used to improve intubating conditions, facilitate mechanical ventilation, provide muscle relaxation for surgical manipulation
- **Nondepolarizing NMBDs**
  - Competitive ACh receptor antagonists: Bind receptor without depolarizing muscle membrane
  - Action of nondepolarizers can be overcome by increasing ACh in the synaptic cleft (the mechanism behind reversal of neuromuscular blockade with acetylcholinesterase inhibitors)
  - Conditions with upregulation of ACh receptors (burn, denervated muscle) show ↓ sensitivity, require ↑ dose
  - Nerve stimulation characteristics: Train-of-four (TOF) ratio <30%, fade of contraction with tetanic stimulation, post-tetanic facilitation of twitches
- **Depolarizing NMBDs**
  - Mimic ACh by binding to the α-subunit of the nicotinic cholinergic receptor, keeping the ion channel open
  - Cause prolonged depolarization which initially manifests as diffuse muscle contractions known as fasciculation
  - Activated, occupied receptors cannot react to further release of ACh, thereby causing muscle paralysis
  - Conditions with downregulation of ACh receptors (myasthenia gravis) show ↓ sensitivity, require ↑ dose
  - Nerve stimulation characteristics (Phase I/typical block): TOF ratio >70%, ↓ amplitude but sustained response to tetany, no post-tetanic facilitation of twitches

Nondepolarizing: Aminosteroids
- **Pancuronium**
  - Long acting, duration of action is ↑ in both liver and kidney failure
  - Slow onset limits' usefulness for intubation
  - Vagolytic, causes dose-dependent ↑ HR, ↑ BP, ↑ CO; no histamine release
- **Rocuronium**
  - Shorter onset than others, can be used in RSI instead of succinylcholine (SCh)
  - Intermediate duration at 0.6 mg/kg dose, can be prolonged when using 1.2 mg/kg RSI dose
  - Does not release histamine or cause cardiovascular effects
- **Vecuronium**
  - Intermediate acting, ↑ duration in hepatic dz, especially with repeated dosing
  - Does not release histamine or cause cardiovascular effects
  - Active metabolite; avoid long-duration infusions due to prolonged muscle weakness

Nondepolarizing: Benzylisoquinolines
- **Atracurium**
  - Cleared by hydrolysis via nonspecific plasma esterases and Hofmann elimination (nonenzymatic spontaneous degradation at normal pH and temperature); metabolism is independent of liver and kidney function
  - Metabolite laudanosine (hepatic metabolism, renal excretion) causes CNS stimulation/seizures at ↑↑ concentrations in animals
  - Use limited by dose-dependent release of histamine → hypotension, tachycardia, bronchospasm (modern practice favors cisatracurium)
- **Cisatracurium**
  - Metabolism primarily by Hofmann degradation (independent of liver, kidney, or plasma cholinesterase function, dependent on normal temperature and pH)
  - Does not cause histamine release at usual doses; minimal cardiovascular effects
  - Useful as infusion in ICU or OR since recovery is independent of infusion dose or duration

Depolarizing: Succinylcholine
- **Pharmacokinetics**
  - Only depolarizing drug available, used for its rapid onset and ultra-short duration
  - 1 mg/kg bolus produces optimal intubating conditions in most pts at 60 s; 90% strength recovered in ~10 min
  - Rapid hydrolysis in plasma by pseudocholinesterase (plasma cholinesterase); block duration determined by amount that reaches NMJ and rate of diffusion away from motor end plate
  - Succinylcholine (SCh) blockade may be prolonged with:
    - Atypical pseudocholinesterase: Genetic defect, diagnosed by dibucaine number (see Table—Characteristics of Altered Pseudocholinesterase Function)
    - Reduced pseudocholinesterase activity: Liver dz, pregnancy, uremia, extremes of age, burns, malnutrition, malignancy
    - Drug interactions (typically modest ↑ duration): Echothiophate (glaucoma eye drops), lithium, magnesium, pyridostigmine, oral contraceptives, esmolol, MAOIs, metoclopramide, some antibiotics, and antiarrhythmics
    - Organophosphate poisoning (irreversibly binds to cholinesterase)
    - Excessive dose (>6 mg/kg) or duration of use: Phase II block with characteristics of nondepolarizer blockade, e.g., tetanic fade, TOF ratio <30%
    - Hypothermia

Characteristics of Altered Pseudocholinesterase Function			
	Dibucaine #	SCh Duration of Action	Prevalence
Normal	80	5–10 min	NA
Heterozygous atypical	40–60	20–30 min	1 in 30–50
Homozygous atypical	20	3–6 h	1 in 2,000–3,000
↓ Plasma activity/level	80	<25 min	Variable

- **Clinical Considerations**
  - Indications: Bolus dosing used for rapid sequence induction when aspiration is a risk (i.e., full stomach, trauma, diabetes mellitus, hiatal hernia, obesity, pregnancy); infusion useful in very short surgical procedures requiring relaxation
  - Precautions
    - Known MH trigger—contraindicated in susceptible pts
    - Can ↑ intraocular and intracranial pressure (caution in eye and head injuries); however, intubation without adequate relaxation will also ↑ IOP/ICP
    - Avoid conditions with extrajunctional ACh receptor proliferation due to potential for ↑↑ potassium release, hyperkalemia (burn pts → probably safe if given <24 h or >6 mo of injury; spinal cord transection pts → probably safe if given <24 h of injury)
    - Avoid use in young male pts due to potential for undiagnosed muscular dystrophy and hyperkalemic arrest
- **Adverse Effects**
  - Cardiac: Sinus bradycardia, junctional rhythm, asystole due to stimulation of cardiac muscarinic receptors (especially in pts with ↑ vagal tone, e.g., children). More likely to occur when a 2nd dose of SCh is given within min. Pretreatment with atropine may prevent such responses. May also cause tachycardia via ↑ catecholamine release
  - Hyperkalemia: Serum K^+ transiently ↑ by 0.5–1.0 mEq/L, may be significant in pts with underlying hyperkalemia. As above, ↑↑ K^+ release may occur in pts with burns, trauma (especially crush), acidosis, severe infections, prolonged immobility, denervation, stroke, myotonia, muscular dystrophy, and spinal cord injuries
  - Allergic reactions: NMBDs are responsible for >50% of the anaphylactic reactions occurring during anesthesia; SCh is a common cause
  - Myalgias: Fasciculation caused by SCh may contribute to postoperative myalgias. Pretreatment with a low dose of a nondepolarizing NMBD (e.g., 0.05 mg/kg rocuronium) may ↓ the incidence and severity
  - Masseter spasm: Sustained contraction of masseter muscle may complicate intubation; can be an early sign of MH though not consistently related (see Appendix C for malignant hyperthermia)
  - Increased intragastric pressure: Lower esophageal sphincter tone also ↑, thus no apparent ↑ aspiration risk

Dosage, Onset, Duration of Action, and Metabolism of Common Neuromuscular Blockers

	Intubating Dose (mg/kg)[a]	Onset (min)[b]	Duration to Return ≥25% Twitch Height (min)	Duration to Return ≥0.9 TOF Ratio (min)	Continuous Infusion	Major Routes of Metabolism/Elimination
Depolarizing						
Succinylcholine (Anectine)	0.5–1 (RSI: 1–1.2)	0.5–1	6–8	(RSI: 10–12)	2–5 mg/min; limit dose, duration	Plasma cholinesterase
Nondepolarizing						
Pancuronium (Pavulon)	0.1	3–4	80–120	130–220		Renal (85%) Hepatic (15%)
Rocuronium (Zemuron)	0.6–1 (RSI: 0.9–1.2)	1–2	30–40 (RSI: 50–70)	55–80	5–10 mcg/kg/min	Hepatic (>70%) Renal (10–25%)
Vecuronium (Norcuron)	0.1	3–4	35–45	50–80	0.8–2 mcg/kg/min	Hepatic (50–90%) Renal (40–50%)
Atracurium (Tracrium)	0.5	3–4	30–45	55–80	4–12 mcg/kg/min	Hofmann and nonspecific esterases
Cisatracurium (Nimbex)	0.15	2–3	45–60	60–90	1–5 mcg/kg/min	Hofmann

[a]Calculate dose based on ideal body weight.
[b]For all NMBD, ↑ dose causes ↓ onset time.

Cholinesterase Inhibitors

- Inhibit acetylcholinesterase, thereby allowing ACh to build up at the NMJ and overcome competitive inhibition nondepolarizers
- Consider relative duration of action of NMBD and reversal agent; administration of reversal after some degree of spontaneous recovery helps prevent "recurarization" (increased weakness in PACU due to lasting effect of NMBD). Note that 70% of ACh receptors may still be blocked with apparently normal qualitative TOF

Anticholinesterases						
Agent	IV Dosage (mg/kg)	Peak Anta-gonism (min)	Duration of Anta-gonism[a] (min)	Atropine Dosage (mcg/kg)	Glycopyr-rolate Dosage (mcg/kg)	Meta-bolism
Edrophonium (Tensilon)	0.5–1.0	1–3	45–60	7–10	10[b]	30% hepatic
Neostigmine (Prostigmin)	0.03–0.07 (up to 5 mg)	7–10	55–75	15–30	10–15	50% hepatic
Pyridostigmine (Mestinon)	0.1–0.4	15–20	80–130	15–20	10	75% hepatic

[a]Duration of action for all agents ↑ in renal failure.

[b]Atropine preferred with edrophonium due to onset times; administer glycopyrrolate several min in advance.

- Common cholinergic side effects of anticholinesterases:
  - Cardiac muscarinic effects (bradycardia, sinus arrest). Minimized by concurrent dosing of an anticholinergic drug of similar onset time (glycopyrrolate with neostigmine, atropine with edrophonium; see Chapter 2H for more information on anticholinergics)
  - Bronchospasm, ↑ secretions, miosis, nausea, ↑ peristalsis
  - Nicotinic effects, especially paradoxical muscle weakness with large doses
  - Neostigmine may cross placenta and cause fetal bradycardia, consider concurrent administration of atropine (glycopyrrolate does not cross placenta)

Physostigmine

- Limited usefulness as reversal agent due to penetration of blood–brain barrier; may cause central cholinergic effects (delirium, seizures, impaired consciousness, respiratory depression)
- Used to treat central anticholinergic syndrome (see Chapter 2H)

Sensitivity of Muscles to Neuromuscular Blockade	
Most Sensitive	**Least Sensitive**
Extraocular > Pharyngeal > Masseter > Adductor pollicis > Abdominal rectus > Orbicularis oculi > Diaphragm > Larynx	

Speed of Onset & Recovery of Neuromuscular Blockade	
Fastest Onset	**Slowest Onset**
Larynx > Diaphragm > Orbicularis oculi > Adductor pollicis	
Fastest Recovery	**Slowest Recovery**
Larynx > Orbicularis oculi = Diaphragm > Adductor pollicis	

Sugammadex (Bridion®)

- Selective relaxant binding agent—cyclodextrin molecule encapsulates steroid NMBD, rendering it incapable of binding at the NMJ
- Strongest affinity for rocuronium, may be used for vecuronium reversal as well
- Can be given at any time after administration of rocuronium, thereby resulting in fast recovery of profound neuromuscular blockade (i.e., it cannot intubate, cannot ventilate situation)
- Associated rarely with bradycardia, hypersensitivity reactions
- Pts using hormonal contraceptives must use an additional, nonhormonal method for 7 d after dose; ideally discuss this preop
- Adult dosing (depends on level of neuromuscular blockade)
  - Routine reversal: 4 mg/kg after recovery to 1–2 post-tetanic twitches, 2 mg/kg after recovery to 2 TOF twitches
- Immediate reversal of induction bolus of rocuronium: 16 mg/kg

VASOACTIVE, AUTONOMIC, AND CARDIOVASCULAR DRUGS

MEGAN GRAYBILL ANDERS

INTRODUCTION

Adrenergic Receptor Sites and Action	
Receptor Site	**Action**
α_1	Vasoconstricts vascular smooth muscle, GU contraction, GI relaxation, gluconeogenesis, glycogenolysis
α_2	Decreased insulin secretion, causes platelet aggregation; decreased NE release, vasoconstriction of vascular smooth muscle
β_1	Increased cardiac contractility, heart rate, AV conduction; ↑ renin secretion; ↑ contractility and arrhythmias
β_2	Relaxation of vascular smooth muscle; bronchial relaxation. GI & GU relaxation, gluconeogenesis, glycogenolysis
D_1	Dilation of vascular smooth muscle (renal, mesentery, coronary; renal tubules, natriuresis, diuresis); juxtaglomerular cells (↑ renin release)
D_2	Inhibits NE release, may constrict renal and mesenteric smooth muscles

ADRENERGIC AGONISTS AND VASOPRESSORS

General comments: Act on α, β, or dopaminergic receptors (see Table—Dose-Dependent Actions of Adrenergic Agonists and Vasopressors). May cause tachycardia, hypertension, arrhythmias, myocardial ischemia, and tissue necrosis with extravasation (administer centrally, treat with phentolamine infiltration). Ensure adequate circulating volume; do not use vasopressors for treatment of hypovolemia.

Dobutamine (Dobutrex)
Indications: Heart failure
Dose: *Infusion prep:* 500 mg in 250 mL D5W or NS = 2,000 mcg/mL (2 mg/mL) *Adult:* 2 mcg/kg/min, titrate 2–20 mcg/kg/min, max 40 mcg/kg/min; *Peds:* 5–20 mcg/kg/min
Onset: 12 min
Duration: <10 min
Mechanism: Predominantly β_1-adrenergic agonist
Clearance: Hepatic metabolism, renal excretion
Comments: Strong inotrope, ↓ SVR especially at lower doses. BP effect is dependent on preload (volume status) and presence of "recruitable" inotropy (used for stress echo). Useful in cardiogenic shock and sepsis-induced myocardial dysfunction; ↓ tachyarrhythmias than dopamine. Can ↑ ventricular rate in atrial fibrillation. May develop tolerance after 3 d. Do not mix with sodium bicarbonate.

Dopamine (Intropin)
Indications: Hypotension, acute heart failure
Dose: *Infusion prep:* 400 mg in 250 mL D5W = 1,600 mcg/mL; *low dose* 2–5 mcg/kg/min, *medium dose* 5–15 mcg/kg/min, *high dose* 20–50 mcg/kg/min
Mechanism: Dose-dependent differential dopaminergic, α- and β-adrenergic agonist
Clearance: Monoamine oxidase (MAO)/catechol-*O*-methyltransferase (COMT) metabolism
Onset: 5 min
Duration: 10 min
Comments: Contraindicated in pheochromocytoma or ventricular fibrillation, caution with peripheral artery dz. Improved renal blood flow/GFR at lower doses but does not prevent renal dysfunction or death (*Ann Intern Med* 2005;142(7):510–524). β activity predominates at doses 3–10 mcg/kg/min and mixed α- and β-adrenergic effects at ≥10 mcg/kg/min, although traditional dose–response effects are not strongly reproducible. Do not mix with sodium bicarbonate.

Ephedrine (Generic)
Indications: Short-term treatment of hypotension, e.g., after induction in pt with normal catecholamine stores
Dose: *Bolus only*

Adult: 5–10 mg IV PRN, typically to max 50 mg or 0.1 mg/kg; 25–50 mg SC/IM q4–6h prn. *Peds:* 0.2–0.3 mg/kg/dose

Mechanism: Indirect α- and β-adrenergic stimulation via norepinephrine release at sympathetic nerve endings.

Clearance: Mostly renal elimination (unchanged)

Duration: 3–10 min

Comments: ↑ Blood pressure by ↑ cardiac output, peripheral vasoconstriction. Tachyphylaxis with repeat dosing due to norepinephrine depletion. May cause CNS stimulation, ↓ in uterine activity, and mild bronchodilation. Avoid in pts taking MAO inhibitors, closed-angle glaucoma.

Epinephrine (Adrenaline)

Indications: (1) Cardiac arrest, (2) bronchospasm, anaphylaxis, (3) heart failure, hypotension; (4) severe bradycardia

Dose: *Infusion prep:* 4 mg in 250 mL D5W or NS = 16 mcg/mL

Adult: (1) 1 mg IV/IO q3–5min during resuscitation, if no IV/IO consider endotracheal dose of 2 mg; infuse 0.1–0.5 mcg/kg/min for postarrest care; (2) 0.1–0.5 mg SC q10–15min, or 0.3 mg IM (1:1,000), or 0.1–0.25 mg IV slow bolus; (3) 5–10 mcg bolus; 0.02–0.3 mcg/kg/min; (4) bolus 10–20 mcg IV; infuse 1–4 mcg/min IV. *Peds:* (1) 1st dose 0.01 mg/kg IV/IO; subsequent doses 0.1–0.2 mg/kg IV/IO q3–5min; *intratracheal:* 0.1 mg/kg of 1:10,000 solution; (2) 0.01 mcg/kg SC (1:1,000 aqueous) q15min to q4h prn; for anaphylaxis give 0.01 mcg/kg q15min × 2 doses then q4h prn; (3) 0.1–1 mcg/kg/min, max 1.5 mcg/kg/min; (4) 0.01 mg/kg IV/IO or 0.1 mg/kg via ETT

Neonates: (1) 0.01–0.03 mcg/kg IV/IO q3–5min; *intratracheal:* 0.1 mg/kg of 1:10,000 solution

Mechanism: α_1- and nonselective β-adrenergic agonist

Clearance: MAO/COMT metabolism

Duration: 5–10 min

Comments: β-adrenergic effects predominate at lower doses (may cause paradoxical hypotension), ↑ in relative α_1 at higher doses. Cardiac dysrhythmias common, potentiated by halothane. May cause ↑ lipolysis, glycogenolysis, pulmonary edema, lactate, and hyperglycemia due to inhibition of insulin release. Reduces splanchnic circulation; high/prolonged doses may have cardiotoxic effect. Reserve 1 mg IV bolus for cardiac arrest to avoid significant hypertensive response.

Isoproterenol (Isuprel)

Indications: Indicated for heart block, shock, bronchospasm during anesthesia. Also used for ventricular arrhythmias with AV block, β-blocker overdose, 3rd-degree AV block awaiting pacemaker. No longer recommended for cardiac arrest.

Dose: *Infusion prep* 1 mg in 250 mL = 4 mcg/mL

Adult: AV nodal block: 5 mcg/min IV titrate up to 20 mcg/min (not weight based); *Shock:* 0.5–5 µg/min IV. *Peds:* Start 0.02–0.1 mcg/kg/min; titrate to effect 0.05–2 mcg/kg/min

Mechanism: Nonselective β-adrenergic agonist

Clearance: Hepatic and pulmonary metabolism via MAO/COMT; 40–50% renal excretion (unchanged)

Duration: 8–50 min

Comments: Potent positive chronotrope and inotrope; systemic > pulmonary vasodilation. ↑ Myocardial O_2 demand; causes less hyperglycemia than epinephrine. Useful in cardiac failure with bradycardia or asthma; caution in shock due to redistribution of perfusion to nonessential areas. Avoid in digitalis intoxication, pre-existing tachyarrhythmias; caution with MAOI/tricyclics. May cause hypotension with large doses, CNS excitation, pulmonary edema, dysrhythmias.

Phenylephrine (Neosynephrine)

Indication: Hypotension. Also used for SVT, tetralogy of Fallot "spells," hypotension induced by neuraxial block, outflow tract obstruction in obstructive hypertrophic cardiomyopathy.

Dose: *Bolus:* 50–100 mcg IV; 2–3 mg SC/IM q1–2h; *infusion prep* 40 mg in 250 mL = 160 mcg/mL; *infuse* 0.2–1 mcg/kg/min or 20–180 mcg/min. *Peds:* Bolus 0.5–10 mcg/kg IV *infuse* 0.1–0.5 mcg/kg/min

Mechanism: Potent direct α_1-adrenergic agonist

Duration: <5 min

Clearance: Hepatic and intestinal wall metabolism; renal elimination

Comments: Produces venous and arterial vasoconstriction, variable effect on CO (depends on preload/afterload and cause of hypotension). Bolus used for correction of sudden severe hypotension. May cause reflex bradycardia, microcirculatory constriction, uterine contraction or vasoconstriction, ↓ cardiac output in ischemic heart dz. Caution with MAOI/tricyclics; contraindicated in closed-angle glaucoma.

Dose-Dependent Actions of Adrenergic Agonists and Vasopressors

Drug	Receptor	Infusion Rate	CO	Inotropy	HR	MAP	Preload	SVR	RBF
Epinephrine	β₂	1–2 mcg/min	↑↑	↑↑	↑	↑,0,↓	↑	0,↓	↑
	β₁ + β₂	2–10 mcg/min	↑,0	↑↑	↑↑	↑↑	↑	↑,0,↓	↓,0
	α₁	>10 mcg/min	↑,0,↓	↑↑↑	↑↑	↑↑↑	↑↑	↑↑↑	↓↓
Norepinephrine	α₁, β₁ > β₂	4–12 mcg/min	↑,0,↓	↑	↑ or reflex ↓	↑↑↑	↑↑	↑↑↑	↑↑
Dopamine	Dopaminergic	<3 mcg/kg/min	↑	0	0	0,↓	(	0,↓	↑↑
	β	3–10 mcg/kg/min	↑,0,↓	↑	↑	↑	(	↓	↑
	α	>10 mcg/kg/min	↑,0,↓	↑↑	↑	↑↑	(	↑↑	↑
Dobutamine	β₁ >> β₂, α	2.5–10 mcg/kg/min	↑↑	↑↑↑	↑	↑,0,↓	↓	↓,↑	0,↑
Isoproterenol	β₁ > β₂	0.5–10 mcg/min	0/↑	↑↑↑	↑↑↑	↑,↓	↓	↓↓↓	0,↑
Ephedrine	α₁, β₁ > β₂	NA	↑↑	↑↑	↑	↑↑	↑↑	↑	↑,0,↓
Phenylephrine	α₁	0.15–0.75 mcg/kg/min	↓,0,↑	0,↑	↓ (reflex)	↑↑	↑↑	↑↑	0,↓
Vasopressin	V₁,V₂	0.02–0.1 units/min	↓,0	0,↑	0	↑↑	↑,0,↓	↑↑	↑
Angiotensin II (ATII)	ATII Type 1	2–80 ng/kg/min			0	↑↑↑		↑↑↑	

Source: Derived from Barash PG. *Clinical Anesthesia.* 6th ed. Philadelphia, PA: Lippincott Williams & Wilkins; 2006.

Norepinephrine (Levarterenol, Levophed)

Indications: Hypotension, especially in septic shock

Dose: *Infusion prep* 4 mg in 250 mL NS or D5W = 16 mcg/mL; *Adult:* Infuse 0.02–0.3 mcg/kg/min = 20–300 ng/kg/min or 4–12 mcg/min; *Peds:* 0.05–0.1 mcg/kg/min to max 2 mcg/kg/min

Mechanism: Synthetic preparation of naturally occurring neurotransmitter; precursor to epinephrine. Potent α-adrenergic, modest β-adrenergic agonist. Relative α-potency ↑ with doses >4–5 mcg/min.

Onset: 1–2 min

Duration: 1–2 min

Clearance: MAO/COMT metabolism

Comments: Peripheral vasoconstriction, ↑ systolic, diastolic, pulse pressure; positive inotropy; coronary vasodilation; minimal chronotropic effect; variable effect on splanchnic perfusion. May cause ↑ uterine contractility, constricted microcirculation, arrhythmias (especially with hypoxia, hypercarbia). 1st line in septic shock (ensure adequate blood volume); avoid in ischemic cardiogenic shock due to ↓ myocardial O_2 economy. Use extreme caution in MAOI/tricyclic antidepressants.

Vasopressin (Antidiuretic Hormone [ADH], Pitressin)

Indications: (1) Diabetes insipidus, abdominal distension, (2) postcardiotomy and septic vasodilatory/catecholamine-resistant shock, (3) pulseless ventricular tachycardia or ventricular fibrillation

Dose: *Infusion prep* 100 units in 100 mL NS = 1 unit/mL

Adult: (1) 5–10 units IM/SC or intranasal q6–12h prn; (2) IV infusion 0.03–0.1 units/min for postcardiotomy shock, 0.01–0.07 units/min for septic shock; (3) 40 unit IV/IO/ET bolus (single dose)

Mechanism: Synthetic analog of endogenous ADH; V1 receptors: Smooth muscle constriction; vasoconstriction of splanchnic, coronary, muscular, and cutaneous vasculature; V2 receptors: ↑ urine osmolality, ↓ urine volume

Clearance: Hepatic and renal metabolism; renal elimination

Duration: 10–20 min

Comments: Potential intestinal or skin ischemia. May cause oliguria, water intoxication, pulmonary edema; abdominal cramps (from ↑ peristalsis); anaphylaxis; contraction of gallbladder, urinary bladder, or uterus; vertigo or nausea. Pts with coronary artery dz are often treated with concurrent nitroglycerin. Do not abruptly discontinue IV infusion.

Angiotensin II (Giapreza)

Indications: Septic or other distributive shock

Dose: *Infusion prep* 1 mL into 500 mL NS = 5,000 ng/mL

Adult: Start 20 nanograms (ng)/kg/min, titrate up q5min by up to 15 ng/kg/min with max dose 80 ng/kg/min in 1st 3 h, max maintenance dose 40 ng/kg/min

Mechanism: Vasoconstriction (direct action on vessel wall via G-protein-coupled angiotensin II receptor type 1) and increased aldosterone release

Clearance: Metabolized by plasma/RBC/tissue enzymes; not renal/hepatic dependent

Duration: Plasma half-life <1 min

Comments: May ↑ thromboembolic events; use VTE prophylaxis. May interact with ACEI/ARBs

---

PHOSPHODIESTERASE INHIBITORS

General Comments: Improve myocardial contractility due to ↑ cyclic adenosine monophosphate, calcium flux, and calcium sensitivity of contractile proteins; cause systemic and pulmonary vasodilation. Inotropic effect does not rely on β-adrenergic stimulation and therefore not affected by β-blockade/downregulation.

Amrinone (Inocor, Inamrinone)

Indications: Low cardiac output states, heart failure, and as adjunct in pulmonary hypertension.

Dose: Adult/Peds: Load 0.75 mg/kg IV bolus over 2–3 min, then infuse 5–15 mcg/kg/min. *Infusion prep* 100 mg in 250 mL in crystalloid *without dextrose* = 0.4 mg/mL; max dose: 10 mg/kg/24 h. *Neonates:* Load 0.75 mg/kg IV bolus over 2–3 min, then infuse 3–5 mcg/kg/min

Onset: Immediate (peak at 5 min)

Duration: 0.5–2 h, 8 h with multiple doses

Mechanism: Inhibits myocardial cAMP phosphodiesterase (PDE III)

Clearance: Variable hepatic metabolism; renal/fecal excretion. Reduce dose 50–75% in ESRD

Comments: Mild inotropy with strong vasodilation. May cause hypotension, thrombocytopenia (long-term use), and anaphylaxis (contains sulfites)

Milrinone (Primacor)
Indications: Indicated for congestive heart failure
Dose: *Infusion prep* 20 mg in 100 mL = 200 mcg/mL. *Adult: Load:* 50–75 mcg/kg IV over 10 min; *infusion:* 0.375–0.75 mcg/kg/min titrate to effect. *Peds: Load:* 50 mcg/kg IV over 10 min, followed by infusion of 0.5–1 mcg/kg/min and titrate to effect
Onset: 5–15 min
Duration: 3–5 h
Mechanism: Inhibits myocardial cAMP phosphodiesterase (PDE III)
Clearance: Renal excretion (83%), hepatic metabolism (12%)
Comments: Amrinone derivative with 20× inotropic potency. May ↑ arrhythmias, outflow tract obstruction in IHSS. Associated with hypotension (caution with or avoid loading dose), headaches. Not recommended for acute MI. May improve diastolic relaxation (lusitropy).

ADRENERGIC ANTAGONISTS

α-Blockers
General comments: Cause peripheral vasodilation, used in the treatment of hypertension, pheochromocytoma, hypertrophic prostate. Associated with orthostatic and ↑ hypovolemic hypotension; treat overdoses with norepinephrine, not epinephrine ("epinephrine reversal" with ↑↑ hypotension due to unopposed β activity).

Phenoxybenzamine (Dibenzyline)
Indications: Preoperative "chemical sympathectomy" in pheochromocytoma
Dose: *Adult:* 10–40 mg/d PO (start at 10 mg/d and ↑ by 10 mg/d q4d prn). Usual dose 20–40 mg bid–tid. *Peds:* 0.2 mg/kg PO qd, max 10 mg; ↑ by 0.2 mg/kg to typical maintenance of 0.4–1.2 mg/kg/d q6–8h
Onset: Several h
Duration: Several d
Mechanism: Nonselective, noncompetitive, irreversible α-blockade; $\alpha_1 \gg \alpha_2$
Clearance: Hepatic metabolism, renal/biliary excretion
Comments: Long duration of action (may require ↑↑ doses of vasopressors after pheochromocytoma resection). May cause severe orthostatic hypotension and reflex tachycardia. Use largely replaced by phentolamine.

Phentolamine (Regitine, OraVerse)
Indications: (1) Hypertension from catecholamine excess in pheochromocytoma; (2) α-adrenergic drug extravasation. Also used for reversal of soft-tissue local (dental) anesthesia.
Dose: *Adult:* (1) 1–5 mg IV (5 mg for diagnosis); may be used as infusion during resection; (2) 5–10 mg in 10 mL of NS infiltrated into affected area; *Peds:* (1) 0.05–0.1 mg/kg/ dose IV/IM 1–2 h preprocedure q2–4h to max 5 mg; (0.05–0.1 mg/kg/dose IV/IM × 1 for diagnostic purposes); (2) 0.1–0.2 mg/kg diluted in 10 mL NS infiltrated into area of extravasation
Onset: 2 min (IV)
Duration: 10–15 min (IV)
Mechanism: Nonselective, competitive α-antagonist; relaxation of vascular smooth muscle
Clearance: Unknown metabolism, 13% excreted unchanged in urine
Comments: May cause marked hypotension, reflex tachycardia, cerebrovascular spasm, dysrhythmias, diarrhea

β-Blockers
General comments: Common in perioperative practice, do not hold home dose for surgery. Perioperative use (titration to HR 60–70, avoid hypotension) may ↓ MI in high-risk pts; starting on the d of surgery or use of fixed doses associated with ↑ stroke, death (*Circulation* 2014;130:2246–2264). Wide range of indications including HTN, arrhythmias, ischemic heart dz, chronic CHF, migraine prophylaxis. Vary in duration of action and receptor selectivity. May cause bradycardia, AV conduction delays, hypotension, bronchospasm; may mask symptoms of hypoglycemia. Contraindicated in uncompensated CHF, cardiogenic shock, severe bradycardia, heart block > 1st degree; caution in COPD/asthma. Abrupt withdrawal can precipitate rebound angina.

Comparative Effects of Common β-blockers				
Drug	Inotropy	HR	MAP	Receptor Antagonism
Esmolol	↓	↓↓	↓	β_1
Labetalol	↓	0/↓	↓↓	$\beta_1, \beta_2, \alpha_1$
Metoprolol	↓	↓	↓	β_1
Propranolol	↓	↓	↓	β_1, β_2

Labetalol (Normodyne, Trandate)
Indications: Hypertension, angina
Dose: *Adult:* IV: 5–20 mg increments or 1–2 mg/kg at 5–10 min intervals, to 40–80 mg/dose. Max total 300 mg; 200–400 mg PO q12h. *Infusion:* 2–150 mg/h, or 0.05 mcg/kg/min, titrate to effect. *Peds:* 0.12–1 mg/kg/dose q10min PRN to max 10 mg/dose, *infusion* 0.4–1 mg/kg/h, max 3 mg/kg/h
Mechanism: Selective α_1-adrenergic blockade with nonselective β-adrenergic blockade. Ratio of α/β-blockade 1:7 (IV), 1:3 (PO)
Clearance: Hepatic metabolism; renal elimination
Onset: 1–2 min
Duration: 2–8 h
Comments: Mixed antagonism unique among common IV drugs. Effective ↓ systemic blood pressure without reflex tachycardia. May cause orthostatic hypotension, skin tingling. Crosses placenta, no effect on uterine blood flow. Avoid in CHF.

Metoprolol (Lopressor, Toprol XL extended release)
Indications: Indicated for hypertension, acute MI, angina, stable CHF. Also used in tachyarrhythmias, hypertrophic cardiomyopathy, hyperthyroid
Dose: 2.5–5 mg IV boluses q2min, prn, up to 15 mg. 50–200 mg PO q8–24h
Onset: IV 1–5 min (peak at 20 min)
Duration: 5–8 h, dose dependent
Mechanism: β_1-adrenergic blockade (β_2-adrenergic antagonism at high doses)
Clearance: Hepatic metabolism (CYP2D6, absent in 8% Caucasians), renal elimination
Comments: May cause clinically significant bronchoconstriction (with doses >100 mg/d), dizziness, fatigue, insomnia. Crosses the placenta and blood–brain barrier.

Esmolol (Brevibloc)
Indications: (1) Supraventricular tachycardia, (2) intraoperative tachycardia and/or hypertension
Dose: *Infusion prep* 2,500 mg in 250 mL = 10 mg/mL; rate 25–300 mcg/kg/min. *Adult: Immediate control:* 80 mg (~1 mg/kg) over 30 s followed by 150 mcg/kg/min. *Gradual control:* 0.5 mg/kg load over 1 min followed by 50 mcg/kg/min; repeat load (max 3 doses) and titrate infusion q4min. *Peds:* Load 0.1–0.5 mg/kg IV over 1 min; *infusion* start at 50 mcg/kg/min, titrate to effect, max 300 mcg/kg/min
Onset: 1 min
Duration: 10–30 min after infusion
Mechanism: Selective β_1-blockade
Clearance: Degraded by RBC esterases; renal elimination of acid metabolite
Comments: Ultra-short acting, blunts response to intubation, may ↓ seizures in ECT

Propranolol (Inderal)
Indications: Hypertension, angina, migraine prophylaxis, pheochromocytoma, hypertrophic subaortic stenosis, supraventricular arrhythmia, portal hypertension, tremor. Also used for esophageal varices, tetralogy of Fallot cyanotic spells, thyrotoxicosis.
Dose: *Adult:* Test dose of 0.25–0.5 mg IV, then titrate up by 0.5 mg/min to effect. PO: 10–40 mg q6–8h, prn; 1–3 mg slow IV; 1 mg/dose IV q5min to max 5 mg. *Peds:* 0.15–0.25 mg/kg/d slow IV, repeat prn; 0.01–0.1 mg/kg slow IV
Onset: 2–10 min
Duration: 6–10 h
Mechanism: Nonspecific β-adrenergic blockade
Clearance: Hepatic metabolism; renal elimination
Comments: Effective dose highly variable. Membrane stabilizing/antiarrhythmic effect at ↑ doses. Crosses placenta and blood–brain barrier. Shifts oxyhemoglobin dissociation curve to the right.

α-AGONISTS

Clonidine (Catapres)

Indications: Hypertension. Multiple other uses including opiate and nicotine withdrawal, potentiation of local anesthetic analgesic effect.

Dose: 5–25 mcg/kg/d PO div q6h. Start: 5–10 mcg/kg/d div q6h; max: 0.9 mg/d; info: ↑ gradually q5–7d; transdermal: 1 patch/wk. Start: 0.1 mg/24 h patch, titrate q1–2wk; max: 0.6 mg/24 h (using two 0.3 mg/24 h patches). Info: If switching from PO, continue PO × 1–2 d

Onset: 30–60 min (PO), 2–3 d (transdermal)

Duration: 8 h (single PO dose)

Mechanism: α_2-adrenergic agonist (↓ central sympathetic outflow)

Clearance: Hepatic metabolism; excretion renal 65%, biliary 20%

Comments: May cause rebound hypertension (18–72 h after discontinuation), dry mouth, drowsiness, dizziness, constipation, sedation, weakness

Methyldopa (Aldomet)

Indications: Hypertension; used for hypertension in pregnancy

Dose: 250–500 mg PO bid (↑ q2d prn; max 3 g/d); 250–1,000 mg IV infused over 30–60 min q6h (max 4 g/d)

Onset: 3–6 h (PO), 4–6 h (IV)

Duration: 12–24 h (PO), 10–16 h (IV)

Mechanism: Stimulates α_2-adrenergic receptors (centrally acting antihypertensive) via active metabolites

Clearance: Metabolized by central adrenergic neurons and liver; primarily urine excretion

Comments: Other agents preferred due to slow onset; causes Na/H_2O retention, avoid in liver and end-stage renal dz, pheochromocytoma

CALCIUM CHANNEL BLOCKERS (CCB)

General Comments: Produce varying degrees of coronary and systemic vasodilation, ↓ HR (chronotropy), ↓ myocardial contractility (inotropy), ↓ cardiac conduction velocity (dromotropy). Co-administration with β-blockade ↑ risk of heart block. Contraindicated in sick sinus syndrome, 2nd- or 3rd-degree AV block (unless with functioning pacemaker).

Cardiovascular Effects of Common Calcium Channel Blockers					
	Diltiazem	Verapamil	Nicardipine	Nifedipine	Clevidipine
Inotropy	0/↓	↓	0/↓	↓	0/↓
Chronotropy	0/↓	↓	0	0	0
Dromotropy	↓↓↓	↓↓↓	0	0	0
Peripheral vasodilation	+	+	+++	+++	+++
Coronary vasodilation	++	++	+++	+++	+++
Reflex tachycardia	0	0	+	++	+

Diltiazem (Cardizem)

Indications: Supraventricular tachycardia, atrial fibrillation/flutter, angina

Dose: *Infusion prep* 100 mg in 100 mL = 1 mg/mL; *load* 2.5–25 mg (or 0.25 mg/kg) over 2 min, may rebolus 0.35 mg/kg in 15 min if no effect; infuse 2–15 mg/h for <24 h. PO: 30–120 mg PO q6–8h

Onset: 2–3 min

Duration: 1–3 h (bolus), up to 10 h (infusion)

Mechanism: Benzothiazepine CCB; prolongs AV nodal conduction, dilates coronary > peripheral arterioles

Clearance: Hepatic metabolism

Comments: Little effect on normal heart rates. Minimal inotropic effect. No effect on WPW accessory pathway. Caution with β-blockers and in wide QRS complex of unknown etiology, WPW, short PR interval. Rare LFT elevation.

Verapamil (Isoptin, Calan)

Indications: Angina, supraventricular tachycardia, atrial fibrillation or flutter, hypertension

Dose: *Adult:* 2.5–10 mg IV over ≥2 min. If no response in 30 min, repeat 5–10 mg (150 mcg/kg). *Peds:* 0–1 **y:** 0.1–0.2 mg/kg IV; 1–15 **y:** 0.1–0.3 mg/kg IV. Repeat once if no response in 30 min

Onset: 1–5 min (peak 10 min)

Duration: 0.5–6 h

Mechanism: Phenylalkylamine CCB, prolongs AV nodal conduction. Negative inotrope and chronotrope; systemic and coronary vasodilator

Clearance: Hepatic metabolism; renal elimination (active metabolite has 20% potency)

Comments: May ↑ ventricular response to atrial fibrillation or flutter in pts with accessory tracts. Associated with more hypotension than diltiazem, especially with volatile anesthetics. ↑ Digoxin levels, potentiates neuromuscular blockade (may make neostigmine reversal difficult).

Nicardipine (Cardene)

Indications: Short-term IV treatment of hypertension

Dose: *Infusion prep:* 20 mg in 200 mL = 0.1 mg/mL; 5–15 mg/h; start at 5 mg/h and titrate ↑ q5–10min

Onset: 1–3 min

Duration of action: 10–30 min after bolus dose

Mechanism: Dihydropyridine CCB, selective relaxation of arterial resistance vessels with minimal ↓ chronotropy/dromotropy

Clearance: Hepatic metabolism, renal/biliary excretion

Comments: Associated with headache, less reflex tachycardia than nifedipine. Contraindicated in advanced aortic stenosis, decompensated heart failure. Increased cost relative to other short-acting potent antihypertensives.

Nifedipine (Procardia)

Indications: Angina, hypertension. Also used for vascular spasm after SAH, preterm labor, Raynaud's

Dose: 10–30 mg PO tid–qid; 10 mg SL

Onset: 20 min PO, 2–3 min SL

Duration: 8 h

Mechanism: Dihydropyridine CCB, relaxes vascular smooth muscle causing systemic and coronary vasodilation; mild negative inotrope

Clearance: Hepatic metabolism (reduced efficacy with select CYP450 inhibitors)

Comments: Not available IV due to instability. Contraindicated in cardiogenic shock; caution in recent MI, CHF, unstable angina. May ↓ serum glucose in diabetics. More coronary vasodilation than nitroglycerin, antianginal effect also from ↓ myocardial oxygen demand.

Clevidipine (Cleviprex)

Indications: Short-term IV treatment of hypertension

Dose: *Adult:* Initiate infusion at 1–2 mg/h; ↑ q1.5–5min to 4–10 mg/h (max dose for short term is 32 mg/h, recommend avg dose <21 mg/h over 24 h)

Onset: 1–4 min

Duration: BP recovery in 5–15 min after discontinuation of infusion

Mechanism: Dihydropyridine CCB, ↓ SVR but not preload

Clearance: Ester hydrolysis in blood, tissue

Comments: Ultra-short acting. Prepared in lipid emulsion (supports bacterial growth, use within 12 h); highly protein bound. Avoid in egg, soy allergy. Associated with reflex tachycardia, atrial fibrillation, acute renal failure. Monitor for rebound hypertension after discontinuation. Contraindicated in severe aortic stenosis, heart failure. Increased cost relative to other short-acting potent antihypertensives.

VASODILATORS

Fenoldopam (Corlopam)

Indications: Short-term management (<48 h) of severe hypertension

Infusion: *Infusion prep:* 10 mg in 250 mL = 40 mcg/mL; 0.1–1.6 mcg/kg/min. Titrate q15min. Do not bolus.

Mechanism: Dopamine (D_1) receptor agonist causing rapid vasodilation of coronary, renal, mesenteric, and peripheral arteries

Clearance: Hepatic metabolism; 90% renal excretion

Onset: 5 min

Duration: 1–4 h after infusion

Comments: Promotes natriuresis and diuresis, maintains renal blood flow. Possible renal protective effect. May cause hypokalemia, dizziness, flushing, reflex tachycardia. Contains sulfites. Caution with glaucoma (may ↑ IOP).

Hydralazine (Apresoline)

Indications: Indicated for hypertension, pregnancy-induced hypertension, congestive heart failure

Dose: *Adult:* 5–20 mg IV q4h or prn. Max 40 mg/dose. PO available. *Pregnancy-induced hypertension* 5–10 mg IV q20–30min prn. *Peds:* 0.1–0.2 mg/kg/dose q4–6h, max 40 mg/dose

Mechanism: Unclear, causes direct ↓ vascular smooth muscle tone (arterial > venous)

Clearance: Extensive hepatic metabolism; renal elimination

Onset: 5–20 min (IV), peak ≥20 min

Duration: 2–6 h (IV)

Comments: May cause hypotension (diastolic > systolic), reflex tachycardia, systemic lupus erythematosus syndrome, thrombophlebitis. Potent cerebral vasodilator, maintains renal, splanchnic blood flow.

Isosorbide Dinitrate (Isordil)

Indications: Angina

Dose: 2.5–5 mg SL, may repeat q5–10min; not to exceed 3 doses in 15–30 min

Maintenance: 40–80 mg PO bid–tid

Onset: Slower than nitroglycerin (SL)

Duration: 4–6 h

Mechanism: Smooth muscle relaxation (NO donor)

Clearance: Nearly 100% hepatic metabolism; renal elimination

Comments: Reduces preload, afterload, myocardial O_2 demand. Tolerance may develop. May cause hypotension, tachycardia, occasional bradycardia, methemoglobinemia. Avoid within 24 h of phosphodiesterase inhibitors (e.g., sildenafil).

Nitroglycerin (Tridil, Glycerol Trinitrate, Nitrostat, Nitrol, Nitro-Bid, Nitrolingual)

Indications: Angina, myocardial ischemia or infarction. Also used for hypertension, congestive heart failure, esophageal spasm, induced intraoperative hypotension, transient uterine relaxation (bolus).

Dose: *Infusion prep:* 50 mg in 250 mL D5W or NS = 200 mcg/mL; IV infusion initially at 5 mcg/min. Titrate every 3–5 min by 10 mcg/min to max 200 mcg/min or 1–3 mcg/kg/min; SL: 0.15–0.6 mg/dose q5min to max 3 doses in 15 min. Topical: 2% ointment, 0.5–2.5 inches q6–8h, max 5 inches q4h

Mechanism: Metabolized to NO (similar to nitroprusside) → smooth muscle relaxation in venules >> arterioles, causing systemic, coronary, and pulmonary vasodilatation; bronchodilation; biliary, gastrointestinal, and genitourinary tract relaxation

Clearance: Nearly complete hepatic metabolism; renal elimination

Onset: 1–2 min

Duration: 3–5 min

Comments: Potent venodilator, causes ↑ venous capacitance, ↓ cardiac preload, ↓ myocardial O_2 demand. Causes coronary vasodilation, headache, absorption into IV tubing, potentiation of pancuronium. Tolerance may be avoided with 10–12 h nitrate-free period. May cause methemoglobinemia at very high doses. May diminish platelet aggregation, antagonize heparin. Avoid within 24 h of phosphodiesterase inhibitors (e.g., sildenafil).

Nitroprusside Sodium (Nipride, Nitropress)

Indications: Hypertension, induced intraoperative hypotension, acute congestive heart failure

Dose: *Infusion prep* 50 mg in 250 mL D5W or NS = 200 mcg/mL; *infusion* initially at 0.25–0.5 mcg/kg/min, then titrated to effect q3–5min (max 10 mcg/kg/min). Lower doses often adequate during general anesthesia

Onset: 30–60 s (peak 1–2 min)

Duration: 1–5 min

Mechanism: Direct NO donor → activates guanylyl cyclase → ↑cGMP → potent vascular smooth muscle relaxation (arterial > venous)

Clearance: RBC and tissue metabolism; renal elimination of thiocyanate metabolite

Comments: Useful for immediate onset, rapid titration. ↓ Preload and afterload. May cause reflex tachycardia, inhibition of hypoxic pulmonary vasoconstriction, excessive hypotension (especially with β-blockers); invasive BP monitoring recommended. **Cyanide toxicity** (product of initial degradation) is associated with tolerance of drug, ↑ mixed venous PaO_2, metabolic acidosis → rx with sodium nitrate, sodium thiosulfate, or amyl nitrate. **Thiocyanate toxicity** (accumulates in renal failure) is associated with nausea, hypoxia, psychosis, weakness, thyroid dysfunction.

Methemoglobinemia may require rx with methylene blue. Contraindicated with ↑ ICP (↑ CBP and abolishes autoregulation), hypovolemia, B_{12} deficiency. Avoid within 24 h of phosphodiesterase inhibitors (e.g., sildenafil). Protect from light.

ANTIARRHYTHMICS

Adenosine (Adenocard)

Indications: Paroxysmal supraventricular tachycardia. Also used in Wolff–Parkinson–White syndrome.

Dose: *Adult:* 6 mg rapid IV push, may repeat 12 mg × 2 within 1–2 min; *Peds:* 0.1–0.2 mg/kg rapid IV push, ↑ by 50 mcg/kg q2min to max 250 mcg/kg

Onset: 10–20 s

Duration: <10 s

Mechanism: Slows conduction through SA and AV node, interrupts AV re-entry pathways

Clearance: Metabolized in blood and tissue

Comments: Administer centrally if possible, follow dose with saline flush (ultra-rapid metabolism). Contraindicated in wide complex tachycardia, 2nd- and 3rd-degree AV blocks and sick sinus syndrome without pacing. Transient AV blockade may allow diagnosis of atrial fib/flutter underlying SVT. May accelerate rate in WPW, atrial fib/flutter. Significant adverse reactions: Hypotension, bronchoconstriction. 3–6 s asystole after administration common.

Amiodarone (Cordarone)

Indications: ACLS, malignant ventricular dysrhythmias. Also used for atrial fibrillation (especially acute onset), SVT.

Dose: *Infusion prep:* 1,200 mg in 250 mL D5W or NS = 4.8 mg/mL. PO available. *Adult: Pulseless arrhythmia:* 300 mg IVP, may repeat 150 mg IVP in 3–5 min to max 2.2 g/24 h; *arrhythmia:* load 150 mg IV over 10 min, may repeat 150 mg q10min if needed; *maintenance:* 1 mg/min × 6 h, then 0.5 mg/min × 18 h; may repeat bolus to max 15 mg/kg/d. *Peds:* 5 mg/kg IV/IO; load 5 mg/kg IV over 20–60 min; *maintenance* infuse 5–10 mcg/kg/min

Mechanism: Complex; prolongs action potential phase 3; α- and β-adrenergic blockade, ↓ AV conduction and sinus node function, prolongs PR, QRS, and QT intervals

Clearance: Hepatic metabolism, biliary excretion

Comments: Class III antiarrhythmic. Contraindicated in 2nd- and 3rd-degree heart blocks, severe sinus node dz or sinus bradycardia, cardiogenic shock, thyroid dz. May ↑ serum levels of digoxin, diltiazem, oral anticoagulants, phenytoin. May cause hypotension, bradycardia with rapid infusion. Long-term use associated with hepatic, pulmonary, thyroid toxicity.

Lidocaine (Xylocaine)

Indications: Ventricular tachycardia due to surgical manipulation, acute MI, digitalis toxicity

Dose: *Infusion prep:* 2 g in 250 mL D5W = 8 mg/mL. *Adult:* Load: 1–1.5 mg/kg IV over 2–3 min; 2nd dose 5–30 min after 1st dose, 0.5–1.5 mg/kg to total 3 mg/kg; *maintenance:* 15–30 mcg/kg/min IV (1–2 mg/min). *Peds:* Load: 0.5–1 mg/kg IV, may repeat ×2 doses; *maintenance:* 15–50 mcg/kg/min IV. 1 mg/kg IV

Onset: 45–90 s

Duration: 10–20 min

Mechanism: ↓ Conductance of sodium channels, ↓ ventricular excitability, ↑ stimulation threshold

Clearance: Hepatic metabolism to active/toxic metabolites; renal elimination (10% unchanged)

Comments: May cause dizziness, seizures, disorientation, heart block (with myocardial conduction defect), hypotension, asystole, tinnitus, unusual taste, vomiting. Crosses the placenta. Caution in pts with Wolff–Parkinson–White syndrome, intraventricular heart block, hypokalemia. No effect on SA node, generally no ↓ in arterial pressure or inotropy.

Procainamide (Pronestyl)

Indications: Life-threatening ventricular arrhythmia. Also used for atrial fibrillation/flutter.

Dose: *Adult:* Load 20 mg/min IV, up to 17 mg/kg, until toxicity or desired effect occurs; stop if ≥50% QRS widening or PR lengthening occurs; *maintenance:* 1–4 mg/min. *Peds:* Load: 3–6 mg/kg over 5 min, not to exceed 100 mg/dose; repeat q5–10min to maximum dose of 15 mg/kg; *maintenance:* 20–80 mcg/kg/min; max 2 g/24 h

Mechanism: Blocks sodium channels; ↓ excitability, conduction velocity, automaticity, and membrane responsiveness with prolonged refractory period

Clearance: Hepatic conversion of 25% to active metabolite N-acetylprocainamide (NAPA), a class III antidysrhythmic; renal elimination (50–60% unchanged)

Comments: Class I antiarrhythmic. May cause ↑ ventricular response with atrial tachydysrhythmias unless receiving digitalis; asystole (with AV block); myocardial depression; CNS excitement; blood dyscrasia; lupus syndrome with + ANA; liver damage. Intravenous administration can cause hypotension from vasodilation, accentuated by general anesthesia. Avoid in torsades de pointes, 2nd/3rd degree or complete heart block (unless pacemaker present), lupus, myasthenia gravis. ↓ Load by one-third in congestive heart failure or shock. Reduce doses in hepatic or renal impairment. Contains sulfite.

HEART FAILURE

Digoxin (Lanoxin)

Indications: Symptom improvement in heart failure, atrial fibrillation/flutter

Dose: *Adult: Load* 0.4–0.6 mg IV or 0.5–0.75 mg PO; *maintenance* 0.1–0.3 mg IV or 0.125–0.375 mg PO qd. *Peds: Load* (total daily doses usually divided into two or more doses); *Neonates:* 15–30 mcg/kg/d; *Infants: 1 mo–2 y:* 30–50/kg/d; *2–5 y:* 25–35 mcg/kg/d. *Peds: 5–10 y:* 15–30 mcg/kg/d; *>10 y:* 8–12 mcg/kg/d. *Maintenance:* 20–35% of loading dose (↓ in renal failure)

Mechanism: ↑ Myocardial contractility via inhibition of sodium/potassium ATPase leading to ↑ intracellular calcium; ↓ chronotropy via ↓ conduction in AV node and Purkinje fibers.

Onset: 30 min (peak 2–6 h)

Duration: 3–4 d

Clearance: Hepatic metabolism, renal excretion (50–70% unchanged)

Comments: Suppresses SA node, positive inotrope, ↑ peripheral vascular resistance. Narrow therapeutic range (therapeutic level: 0.8–2.0 ng/mL). May cause gastrointestinal intolerance, blurred vision, ECG changes, or dysrhythmias. Toxicity potentiated by hypokalemia, hypomagnesemia, hypercalcemia. Use cautiously in Wolff–Parkinson–White syndrome and with defibrillation. Heart block potentiated by β-blockade and calcium channel blockade. Symptoms of toxicity include CNS depression, confusion, headache, anorexia, nausea, vomiting, visual changes, arrhythmias, and seizures. Reduces hospitalization but not mortality in CHF (N Engl J Med 1997;336:525–533).

Nesiritide (B-Type Natriuretic Peptide, BNP, Natrecor)

Indications: Treatment of pts with acutely decompensated CHF with dyspnea at rest or minimal activity

Dose: *Infusion prep* 1.5 mg in 250 mL = 6 mcg/mL; *load* 2 mcg/kg over 1 min; *infuse* 0.01 mcg/kg/min. May ↑ no more often than q3h (max 0.03 mcg/kg/min), bolus 1 mcg/kg before changing rate

Mechanism: Binds to guanylate cyclase receptor; stimulates cGMP production, resulting in vascular smooth muscle relaxation (similar to nitric oxide)

Onset: 60% effect in <15 min, peak effect <1 h

Duration: 2–4 h (IV bolus)

Comments: ↓ Pulmonary capillary wedge pressure and systemic arterial pressure in heart failure pts; ↑ renal blood flow and GFR. No effect on cardiac contractility. Multiple chemical incompatibilities. May cause hypotension (especially with ACE inhibitors), ventricular and atrial dysrhythmias, angina, bradycardia, tachycardia, azotemia. Use caution in renal dz. Contraindicated in cardiogenic shock, SBP <90, valvular stenosis, restrictive/obstructive cardiomyopathy.

RAMSEY SABA • JESSE M. EHRENFELD • RICHARD D. URMAN

KEY POINTS

- *1st antibiotics* dose should begin within 60 min before incision (*Am J Surg* 2005;189(4): 395–404), ≤20 min before surgical incision for vancomycin and ciprofloxacin
- Cross-reactivity with cephalosporins (Cs) in pts with penicillin (PCN) allergy:
  - Supposed 10% cross-reactivity but may be overestimated because the existing PCN allergy was not routinely confirmed by skin testing, and some reactions were not immune mediated (*N Engl J Med* 2006;354:601–609)
  - The overall cross-reactivity rate is ~1% when using 1st-generation cephalosporins or cephalosporins with similar R1 side chains. For PCN-allergic pts, the use of 3rd- or 4th-generation cephalosporins or cephalosporins with dissimilar side chains than the offending PCN carries a negligible risk of cross allergy (*J Emerg Med* 2012;42(5):612–620)
- If pt is known to be colonized with MRSA, consider adding vancomycin to the recommended prophylaxis
- Consider redosing antibiotics during procedures with significant blood loss (i.e., >1,500 mL)
- *Note:* The following tables of spectra of activity for different antibiotics are generalizations. *Sensitivity data at your own institution* should be used to guide specific therapy.
- *Note:* Pts at extremes of weight and age and those with abnormal renal or hepatic function may require alterations of dose or frequency
- Infective endocarditis prophylaxis: See Chapter 1

ANTIBIOTICS FOR SURGICAL SITE INFECTION PROPHYLAXIS (PREINCISION DOSING)

Antibiotic	Adult Dose (IV)	Pediatric Dose (IV)	Infusion Duration (min)	Redosing Interval (h)[a]
Cefazolin (Ancef, Kefzol)	(Weight-based) ≤60 kg: 1 g; >60 kg: 2 g; ≥120 kg: 3 g	40 mg/kg	3–5	4
Cefotetan	2 g	40 mg/kg	3–5	6
Ceftriaxone	2 g	50–75 mg/kg	3–5	10
Ceftazidime	2 g	N/A	3–5	4
Cefoxitin	1–2 g	40 mg/kg	3–5	2
Cefuroxime (Ceftin)	1.5 g	25 mg/kg	3–5	4
Ciprofloxacin (Cipro)	400 mg	10 mg/kg (max 400 mg)[b]	60	6–8
Clindamycin[c]	600 mg	10 mg/kg	10–60 (<30 mg/min)	6
Ertapenem	1 g	15 mg/kg	30	24[d]
Fluconazole	400 mg	6 mg/kg	≤200 mg/h	Generally does NOT require redosing
Micafungin	100 mg	N/A	60	Generally does NOT require redosing
Gentamicin	5 mg/kg[e]	2.5 mg/kg (max 100 mg)	30–60	Generally does NOT require redosing
Metronidazole	500 mg	10 mg/kg	30–60	6–8
Vancomycin[c]	(Weight-based) <70 kg: 1 g; >70 kg: 1.25 g; ≥100 kg: 1.5 g	15 mg/kg	120 min if given by peripheral line, 60 min if given by central line	6–12

| Aztreonam | 1 g | 30 mg/kg | 30 | 4 |
| Ampicillin/ sulbactam | 3 g (ampicillin 2 g/sulbactam 1 g) | 50 mg/kg (of ampicillin component) | 30 | 2 |

[a]Re-administer at intervals of 1–2 times the half-life of the drug, adjust for renal dysfunction as needed. Some recommend redosing at termination of cardiopulmonary bypass.

[b]Caution due to ↑ adverse events in peds.

[c]Alternative for use in β-lactam allergy.

[d]Consider redose at 12 h in peds.

[e]If body weight >130% of ideal (IBW), use dosing weight = IBW + [0.4 × (total weight − IBW)].

Sources: Adapted from Bratzler DW, Dellinger EP, Olsen KM, et al. Clinical practice guidelines for antimicrobial prophylaxis in surgery. Am J Health Syst Pharm. 2013;70:195–283; and from Bratzler DW, Dellinger EP, Olsen KM, et al. Clinical practice guidelines for antimicrobial prophylaxis in surgery. Am J Surg. 2013;189(4):395–404; and Pediatric Affinity Group. How to guide Pediatric Supplement Surgical Site Infection.

PROCEDURE-SPECIFIC SURGICAL PROPHYLACTIC ANTIBIOTIC RECOMMENDATIONS

Procedure/Site	Preoperative Antibiotic	Severe β-Lactam Allergy
General and GI Surgery		
Esophageal	Ceftriaxone + metronidazole	Clindamycin + (ciprofloxacin or gentamicin)
Gastroduodenal surgery: percutaneous endoscopic gastrostomy (PEG), resection for gastric/duodenal ulcers, resection of gastric carcinoma, perforated ulcer procedures, bariatric surgery, pancreaticoduodenectomy (Whipple), Nissen	Ceftriaxone (outpatient PEG should receive cefazolin as prophylaxis)	Clindamycin + (ciprofloxacin or gentamicin)
Biliary tract surgery	**Low risk:** No prophylsis **High risk** (emergency, gallbladder rupture, open cholecystectomy, AGE >70, diabetes, immunosuppression, or insertion of prosthetic device): Ceftriaxone	Clindamycin + (ciprofloxacin or gentamicin)
Appendectomy (uncomplicated/non-perforated)	Ceftriaxone + metronidazole	Clindamycin + (ciprofloxacin or gentamicin)
Colon or rectal surgery	**Day prior to surgery:** For pts with a bowel prep, Neomycin 1 g PO and Erythromycin base 1 g PO at 5 PM and 10 PM **Day of surgery:** Ceftriaxone + metronidazole preoperatively	**Day prior to surgery:** For pts with a bowel prep, Neomycin 1 g PO and Erythromycin base 1 g PO at 5 PM and 10 PM **Day of surgery:** Clindamycin + (ciprofloxacin or gentamicin)
Head and Neck Surgery		
No involvement of mucosa and no implant	None	
No involvement of mucosa, but with placement of implant	Cefazolin	Clindamycin

Involves incision of oral, sinus, or pharyngeal mucosa, major neck dissection or parotid surgery, or ORIF Mandible Repair	Ceftriaxone + metronidazole	Clindamycin + (ciprofloxacin or gentamicin)
Abdominal Wall Hernia Repair		
Uncomplicated without mesh	None	
Uncomplicated with mesh	Cefazolin	Clindamycin
Complicated, recurrent, or emergent	Ceftriaxone + metronidazole	Clindamycin + (ciprofloxacin or gentamicin)
Obstetrical/Gynecologic		
Abdominal or Vaginal Hysterectomy	Cefotetan	Clindamycin + (Ciprofloxacin or gentamicin)
Pubovaginal sling procedure	Cefazolin or ciprofloxacin	Ciprofloxacin
Transvaginal oocyte retrieval	Cefotetan	Clindamycin + (ciprofloxacin or gentamicin)
Cesarean delivery	Cefazolin	Clindamycin + gentamicin (1.5 mg/kg; note different dosing)
Urologic Surgery		
Cystoscopy alone	**Low risk:** No prophylaxis **High risk** (urine culture positive or unavailable, preoperative catheter, or placement of prosthetic material): Ciprofloxacin	N/A
Cystoscopy with manipulation or upper tract instrumentation (including transurethral resection of bladder tumor or prostate and any biopsy, resection, fulguration, foreign body removal, or urethral/ureteral instrumentation including catheterization or stent placement/removal)	Ciprofloxacin	N/A
Transrectal prostate biopsy	Ciprofloxacin	N/A
Percutaneous renal surgery	Cefazolin	Ciprofloxacin
Open or Laparoscopic (for urologic procedures involving bowel manipulation, see Colon Surgery recommendations)	Cefazolin	Clindamycin + (ciprofloxacin or gentamicin)
Procedures involving implanted prosthesis (including penile prosthesis)	(Cefazolin or vancomycin) + (aztreonam or gentamicin)	Clindamycin + gentamicin
Shock-wave lithotripsy	Ciprofloxacin	N/A
Thoracic Surgery		
Any pneumonectomy (EPP/simple) and any implant	Vancomycin, ceftriaxone, and metronidazole	Vancomycin, levofloxacin, and metronidazole
Other nontransplant thoracic procedures (without esophageal involvement)	Cefazolin	Vancomycin
Other nontransplant thoracic procedures (with esophageal involvement)	Ceftriaxone + metronidazole	Clindamycin + (ciprofloxacin or gentamicin)

Lung transplantation	(Vancomycin, ciprofloxacin, metronidazole, and micafungin) or (vancomycin, ceftazidime, metronidazole, and micafungin) If cystic fibrosis, use pretransplant sputum cultures to guide recommendations	N/A
Cardiac Surgery		
Cardiac surgery	Vancomycin + cefazolin	Vancomycin + (ciprofloxacin or gentamicin)
Pacemaker/AICD insertion	Cefazolin	Clindamycin or vancomycin
LVAD/BIVAD placement	Vancomycin, ciprofloxacin, & fluconazole	N/A
Vascular Surgery		
Incisions involving the groin or lower extremities	Vancomycin + cefazolin	(Vancomycin or Clindamycin) + (ciprofloxacin or gentamicin)
All other vascular procedures	Cefazolin	Clindamycin
Neurosurgery		
Transsphenoidal surgery	Cefazolin	Vancomycin
Spine procedures not involving dura penetration or instrumentation	Cefazolin	Vancomycin
All other neurosurgery involving dura penetration and/or instrumentation	Vancomycin + ceftriaxone	Vancomycin + (ciprofloxacin or gentamycin)
Orthopedic		
Clean procedures on hand, knee, or foot, not involving implants	None	
Any orthopedic procedures involving prosthetic material (including THR, TKR, ORIF)	Vancomycin + cefazolin	Vancomycin
Laminectomy and spinal fusion	Vancomycin + cefazolin	Vancomycin
Plastic Surgery		
Minor clean procedures not involving implants	None	
All other procedures, including breast procedures	Cefazolin	Clindamycin + (ciprofloxacin or gentamicin)
Interventional Radiology		
Biliary/GI procedure (including chemo/radioablation, splenic embolization)	Ceftriaxone + metronidazole	Clindamycin + (ciprofloxacin or gentamicin)
Musculoskeletal, thoracic, and neuro procedures	Cefazolin	Clindamycin
Totally implantable venous access ports (e.g., Port-a-Cath)	Cefazolin	Clindamycin
Tunneled catheters	None	
Lymphangiogram, vascular malformation ablation, fibroid treatment	Cefazolin	Clindamycin

Interventional Pain		
Percutaneous-type spinal cord stimulators and intrathecal pumps	Cefazolin	Clindamycin
Paddle lead implantations	Vancomycin + ceftriaxone	Vancomycin + (ciprofloxacin or gentamicin)

**Adapted from Brigham and Women's Hospital perioperative antibiotics guideline with permission from Brigham and Women's Hospital Antimicrobial Subcommittee.

**List does not include recommended postoperative antibiotics which may be specific for certain procedures.

**Pts undergoing genitourinary procedures may require adjustment of antimicrobials for prophylaxis and treatment based on culture results and clinical situation.

Source: American Society of Health-System Pharmacists (ASHP), the Infectious Disease Society of America (IDSA), the Surgical Infection Society (SIS), and the Society of Healthcare Epidemiology of America (SHEA) Antimicrobial Prophylaxis Guidelines for Surgery. Am J Health Syst Pharm 2013;70(3):195–283.

HERBAL MEDICINES AND SIDE EFFECTS

Name of Herb	Common Uses	Possible Side Effects or Drug Interactions
Echinacea	Boosts the immune system and helps fight colds and flu, aids wound healing.	May cause inflammation of the liver if used with certain other medications such as anabolic steroids, methotrexate, or others.
Ephedra	Used in many over-the-counter diet aids as an appetite suppressant; also for asthma or bronchitis.	May interact with certain antidepressant medications or certain high blood pressure medications to cause dangerous elevations in blood pressure or heart rate. Could cause death in certain individuals.
Feverfew	Used to ward off migraine headaches and for arthritis, rheumatic dz, and allergies.	May ↑ bleeding, especially in pts already taking anticlotting medications.
GBL, BD, and GHB	Bodybuilding, weight loss aid, and sleep aid	These are abbreviations for illegally distributed, unapproved drugs (not supplements) that may cause death, seizures, or unconsciousness.
Garlic	For lowering cholesterol, triglyceride levels, and blood pressure	May ↑ bleeding, especially in pt already taking certain anticlotting medications. May ↓ effectiveness of certain AIDS-fighting drugs, e.g., saquinavir.
Ginkgo (also called ginkgo biloba)	For increasing blood circulation and oxygenation and for improving memory and mental alertness.	May ↑ bleeding, especially in pts already taking certain anticlotting medications.
Ginseng	Increased physical stamina and mental concentration	May ↑ bleeding, especially in pts already taking certain anticlotting medications. May see increased heart rate or high blood pressure. May cause bleeding in women after menopause.
Goldenseal	Used as a mild laxative and also reduces inflammation.	May worsen swelling and/or high blood pressure.

Kava-kava	For nervousness, anxiety, or restlessness; also a muscle relaxant	May ↑ the effects of certain antiseizure medications and/or prolong the effects of certain anesthetics. May cause serious liver injury. May worsen the symptoms of Parkinson's dz. Can enhance the effects of alcohol. May ↑ the risk of suicide for people with certain types of depressions.
Licorice	For treating stomach ulcers	Certain licorice compounds may cause high blood pressure, swelling, or electrolyte imbalances.
Saw palmetto	For enlarged prostate and urinary inflammation	May see effects with other hormone therapies.
St. John's wort	For mild-to-moderate depression or anxiety, and sleep d/o	May ↓ effectiveness of all currently marketed HIV protease inhibitors and nonnucleoside reverse transcriptase inhibitors (powerful AIDS-fighting drugs). May possibly prolong effects of anesthesia (not proven). May unknowingly ↓ levels of digoxin, a powerful heart medication.
Valerian	Mild sedative or sleep aid; also a muscle relaxant.	May ↑ the effects of certain antiseizure medications or prolong the effects of certain anesthetic agents.
Vitamin E	Used to prevent stroke and blood clots in the lungs. Also used to slow the aging process and for protection against environment pollution.	May ↑ bleeding, especially in pts already taking certain anticlotting medications. May affect thyroid gland function in otherwise healthy individuals. In doses higher than 400 IU/d, may cause problems with increased blood pressure in people who already have high blood pressure.

Source: American Society of Anesthesiologists. *What You Should Know About Herbal and Dietary Supplement Use and Anesthesia*; 2003.

MEGAN GRAYBILL ANDERS

5HT₃ ANTAGONISTS (ONDANSETRON, GRANISETRON, DOLASETRON)

Indication: Prevention, treatment of postoperative nausea and vomiting
Typical dose: Ondansetron (Zofran): *Adults:* 4 mg IV × 1; *Peds >1 mo:* 0.1 mg/kg IV × 1 (max 4 mg/dose)
Granisetron (Kytril): *Adults:* 1 mg IV; *Peds >2 y:* 0.01 mg/kg IV (max 1 mg/dose)
Dolasetron (Anzemet): *Adults:* 12.5 mg IV or 100 mg PO 2 h before surgery; *Peds:* 0.35 mg/kg (max 12.5 mg)
Mechanism: Antagonism of 5HT₃ receptors centrally (chemoreceptor trigger zone) and peripherally (abdominal vagal nerve terminals)
Clearance: Predominantly hepatic metabolism
Comments: Give prophylactic dose at the time of emergence. Postoperative redosing does not provide additional efficacy. All three appear equal in efficacy for PONV. Majority of studies in pediatric anesthesia use ondansetron. Decrease dose (max 8 mg/d ondansetron) in severe hepatic impairment. May be used in Parkinson's, does not antagonize dopamine receptors. Ondansetron also available as orally dissolving tablet. May cause headaches, transient transaminitis, QT prolongation (especially dolasetron). Risk of severe arrhythmias when administered with other drugs that prolong QT interval (see Droperidol).

AMISULPRIDE

Indication: Post-operative nausea and vomiting (PONV)
Typical dose: 5 mg, 10 mg IV
Mechanism: Dopamine D2/D3 receptor antagonist
Clearance: Hepatic metabolism; renal excretion
Comments: Not associated with sedation, extrapyramidal side effect or QTc segment prolongation; mild increase in prolactin level.

ABCIXIMAB (REOPRO)

Indication: Prevention of thrombus formation after percutaneous coronary intervention (PCI), unstable angina when PCI planned within 24 h, also used as adjunct in thrombolysis
Typical dose: 0.25 mg/kg IV 10–60 min prior to PCI, then 10 mcg/min IV infusion
Mechanism: Monoclonal antibody, inhibits platelet glycoprotein IIb/IIIa; prevents platelet adhesion and aggregation via inhibition of binding of fibrinogen, von Willebrand factor to platelet receptor sites
Clearance: Remains in circulation for ≥15 d in a platelet-bound state, but platelet function recovers in about 48 h
Comments: Intended for use with aspirin and heparin. Hypotension may occur with bolus dose. Bleeding complications, thrombocytopenia, & anaphylaxis are important side effects. Contraindicated with recent severe bleeding or bleeding d/o (specific contraindications similar to TPA).

ACARBOSE (PRECOSE)

See Antidiabetics table in Chapter 2H 63–64.

ACETAZOLAMIDE (DIAMOX)

See Diuretics table in Chapter 2H 54.

ALBUTEROL (PROVENTIL, VENTOLIN)

Indications: (1) Bronchospasm, also used for acute treatment of (2) hyperkalemia
Typical dose: *Adult:* (1) 2.5–5 mg nebulized or 2 puffs inhaled (90 mcg each, use spacer) q4–6h prn. May use continuous 10–15 mg/h nebulization if severe bronchospasm. (2) 10–20 mg nebulized. *Peds:* (1) <2 y: 0.2–0.6 mg/kg/d divided q4–6h (1 mg/kg is potentially toxic), 2–12 y: 0.63–2.5 mg q6–8h?

Mechanism: β_2-adrenergic agonist, has some β_1 activity. Stimulates adenyl cyclase → ↑ cAMP → bronchial smooth muscle relaxation. Promotes cellular reuptake of K^+

Onset: 2–5 min; **Peak:** 1 h; **Duration:** 3–6 h

Clearance: Hepatic metabolism, renal excretion

Comments: May cause tachycardia, tremor, hypokalemia. Use caution in cardiac dz, MAOI/tricyclic use. <20% of drug reaches respiratory tract, in OR nebulization vs. MDI appear to have equally poor delivery. Can administer MDI via anesthesia machine by placing canister into 60-mL syringe and connecting in place of gas sampling line (remove in-line humidifier, coordinate administration with hand ventilation, allow adequate time for exhalation between puffs, may require 6–8 actuations due to loss of drug to inside of ETT).

ALVIMOPAN (ENTEREG)

Indication: Accelerate return to GI function after bowel resection

Typical dose: 12 mg PO 30 min–5 h prior to surgery, then 12 mg bid starting postop day 1 until discharge (max 7 d)

Mechanism: Peripheral opioid antagonist, binds GI tract mu-opioid receptors

Clearance: Renal, biliary secretion

Comments: Short-term, inpatient use (≤15 doses) only. Contraindicated in pts taking therapeutic opioids for >7 d before surgery.

AMINOCAPROIC ACID (AMICAR)

Indication: Enhances hemostasis when fibrinolysis contributes to bleeding

Typical dose: *Adult:* 4–5 g (100–150 mcg/kg) IV load over 1 h, followed by 1 g/h infusion × 8 h or until bleeding is controlled

Mechanism: Stabilizes clot formation by inhibiting plasminogen activators and plasmin. Fibrinolysis inhibitor

Clearance: Primarily renal

Comments: Contraindicated in DIC. May cause hypotension, bradycardia, arrhythmias, thrombosis, LFT elevation, ↓ platelet function. ↓ dose in renal, cardiac, hepatic dz

ANDEXANET ALFA (ANDEXXA; RECOMBINANT FACTOR XA)

Indication: Reversal of anticoagulation when required due to life-threatening or uncontrolled bleeding in pts taking rivaroxaban or apixaban

Typical dose: *Low vs. high dose determined by anticoagulation drug/dose/interval since last taken; refer to package insert and use high dose if unknown.* Low dose: 400 mg at 30 mg/min, then 4 mg/min for up to 120 min. High dose: 800 mg at 30 mg/min, then 8 mg/min for up to 120 min.

Mechanism: Binds and sequesters Factor Xa inhibiting drugs and Tissue Factor Pathway Inhibitor

Comments: ↑ Risk of thromboembolic, ischemic, and cardiac events. Re-anticoagulation or incomplete reversal can occur. Do not inject diluent directly onto powder, swirl gently (do not shake), administer within 8 h at room temperature.

APIXABAN (ELIQUIS)

Indication: (1) Stroke prophylaxis with atrial fibrillation; (2) DVT or PE prophylaxis after knee or hip surgery; (3) DVT or PE treatment

Typical dose: (1) 5 mg PO bid; (2) 2.5 mg PO bid; (3) 10 mg PO bid × 7 d, then 5 mg bid

Mechanism: Factor Xa inhibitor; does not require cofactor (e.g., antithrombin III)

Clearance: Hepatic (CYP3A4), renal

Comments: Reduce dose in elderly and renal impairment. Not dialyzable. Reduce dose if taking concurrent CYP3A4 inhibitors. Hold at least 24 h before and 5 h after removal of epidural catheter; wait 48 h after traumatic neuraxial puncture before dosing. Can be reversed by andexanet alfa (Andexxa).

ARGATROBAN (ACOVA)

Indication: (1) Treatment or prophylaxis of thrombosis in heparin-induced thrombocytopenia; (2) PCI in pts with or at risk for heparin-induced thrombocytopenia

Typical dose: *Adult:* (1) 2 mcg/kg/min IV continuous infusion, max 10 mcg/kg/min, adjust until steady-state aPTT is 1.5–3 × initial baseline value (not to exceed 100 s).

(2) 350 mcg/kg IV over 3–5 min, then 25 mcg/kg/min IV continuous infusion, maintain ACT between 300 and 450 s. Check ACT 5–10 min after bolus; may rebolus 150 mcg/kg and ↑ infusion to 30 mcg/kg/min for ACT <300. For ACT >450 ↓ infusion to 15 mcg/kg/min and recheck ACT in 5–10 min. *Peds:* Safety and efficacy in children <18 have not been established; for seriously ill pediatric pts with HIT/HITTS start infusion at 0.75 mcg/kg/min (0.2 mcg/kg/min if hepatic impairment)

Mechanism: Direct, highly selective thrombin inhibitor. Inhibits fibrin formation; activation of factors V, VIII, and XIII; protein C; and platelet aggregation

Clearance: Hepatic metabolism with 22% renal excretion (16% unchanged)

Comments: Bleeding is the major adverse effect, may also cause hematuria or hypotension. Use ↓ starting dose in hepatic impairment. Not to be administered with other IV anticoagulants. Caution when switching to or from other anticoagulants. Prolongs aPTT and ACT, contribution to ↑ INR seen when initiating warfarin. Caution in pts with severe HTN, recent lumbar puncture, or major surgery. Reduce dose in hepatic dysfunction.

ATROPINE SULFATE

Indications: (1) Antisialogogue, (2) bradycardia/PEA/asystole, (3) adjunct with edrophonium in reversal of neuromuscular blockade, (4) antidote in organophosphate poisoning

Typical dose: *Adult:* (1) 0.2–0.4 mg IV, (2) 0.4–1.0 mg IV q3–5min, (3) 0.007 mg/kg, (4) 2–3 mg IV, repeat as needed, titrating to improvement of bronchospasm/airway secretions with adequate oxygenation (no max dose, may require massive dose). *Peds:* (1) 0.01 mg/kg/dose IV/IM (max 0.4 mg), (2) 0.02 mg/kg/dose IV q3–5min (max single dose, children: 1 mg; adolescents: 2 mg), (3) 0.015–0.03 mg/kg Minimum dose 0.1 mg IV (peds and adult)

Mechanism: Anticholinergic; competitive blockade of acetylcholine at muscarinic receptors

Clearance: 50–70% hepatic metabolism; renal elimination

Comments: Can be given via ETT (0.03 mg/kg diluted in NS). May cause tachydysrhythmias, AV dissociation, premature ventricular contractions, anti-parasympathetic/anti-muscarinic side effects (dilated pupils, dry mouth, urinary retention). Crosses blood–brain barrier and may exert CNS effects (delirium) in elderly or at high doses. Avoid in glaucoma, autonomic neuropathy, thyrotoxicosis, toxic megacolon, BPH. Ineffective in hypothermic bradycardia and 2nd-degree Type II AV block. Avoid in new-onset 3rd-degree AV block with wide QRS complexes.

BICARBONATE (SODIUM BICARBONATE)

Indication: (1) Metabolic acidosis, (2) hyperkalemia. Also used in alkalinization of urine to facilitate elimination of some compounds

Typical dose: (1) *Adult:* 2–3 mEq/kg over 4–8 h or 0.2 × kg × base deficit (mEq/L); titrate to response. *Peds:* 0.3 × kg × base deficit (mEq/L). (2) *Adult:* 50 mEq IV over 5 min

Mechanism: ↑ Plasma bicarbonate, buffers excess hydrogen ions ($Na^+ + HCO_3^- + H^+ \rightarrow H_2O + CO_2 + Na^+$)

Comments: 8.4% solution is ~1.0 mEq/mL. Does not correct respiratory acidosis; may ↑ pCO_2/ventilation requirements due to production of CO_2 in buffering process. Avoid in CHF, hypernatremia; caution in renal dysfunction due to large sodium load. Make ~isotonic infusion with 3 × 50 mEq vials in 1 L D5W. Infusion is incompatible with multiple meds. Extravasation causes tissue necrosis. Rapid dosing in children <2 y may cause intracranial hemorrhage. Controversy regarding role in prevention of contrast-induced nephropathy. Monitor ionized Ca^{2+}; may ↓, causing myocardial depression, impaired catecholamine response. In shock/lactic acidosis, continue to treat cause and reserve use for pH <7.15/serum bicarb <10–12 (even then, no convincing evidence for improved outcomes).

BICITRA (SODIUM CITRATE/CITRIC ACID)

Indication: Used for neutralization of stomach acid

Typical dose: *Adult:* 15–30 mL PO 15–30 min before induction; *Peds:* 5–15 mL PO 15–30 min before induction

Mechanism: Converted to active bicarbonate

Clearance: Renal (alkalinizes urine)

Comments: Nonparticulate antacid useful for preoperative administration. Inadvertent aspiration will cause ↓ chemical pneumonitis vs. conventional (aluminum, calcium, etc.) antacids. Avoid repeated dosing in severe renal dz, sodium restriction.

Do not combine with aluminum-containing antacids. May have laxative effect, cause hypocalcemia, metabolic acidosis. 10 mL bicitra is equivalent to 10 mEq bicarbonate

BIVALIRUDIN (ANGIOMAX)

Indication: Anticoagulation in pts with unstable angina or presence/risk of heparin-induced thrombocytopenia undergoing angioplasty or PCI
Typical dose: 0.75 mg/kg IV bolus, then 1.75 mg/kg/h for duration of procedure, 0.2 mg/kg/h up to 20 h. Perform ACT 5 min after bolus and rebolus 0.3 mg/kg if needed
Mechanism: Direct thrombin inhibitor
Clearance: Enzymatic degradation in plasma (slowed in hypothermia) and renal clearance
Comments: Useful due to short half-life (25 min with normal renal function, coag values return to baseline at 1 h), may be stopped shortly before procedures in critically ill pts with HIT/HITTS. Reports of successful use as heparin alternative (in patients with heparin antibodies) for anticoagulation during cardiopulmonary bypass. 1 mg/kg bivalirudin bolus followed by a 2.5 mg/kg/h, stop 15 min before discontinuing CPB. Use in this setting complicated by the fact that ACT/PTT are not suitable monitoring tests at CPB doses; maintain bivalirudin level 10–15 μg/mL. Clot may form in stagnant blood in surgical field, does not indicate insufficient level. In PCI indications, used with IIb/IIIa inhibitor and intended for use with full-strength aspirin. No known reversal agent. Clearance significantly impaired in renal dysfunction.

BOSENTAN (TRACLEER)

Indication: Treatment of pulmonary arterial hypertension
Typical dose: 62.5 mg bid × 4 wk, then ↑ to 125 mg bid if >40 kg
Mechanism: Competitive endothelin-1 antagonist; blocks receptors on vascular endothelium and smooth muscle, inhibiting vasoconstriction
Clearance: Hepatic CYP2C9, 3A4 metabolism, biliary excretion
Comments: Not for all pulmonary hypertension etiologies; avoid in pulmonary veno-occlusive dz as it may cause pulmonary edema. Adverse effects include teratogenicity, decline in hemoglobin, transaminitis, and liver failure. Alter dose with ↑ LFTs, ritonavir use. Avoid abrupt withdrawal.

BUMETANIDE (BUMEX)

See Diuretics table in Chapter 2H 54.

BUPRENORPHINE + NALOXONE (SUBOXONE)

Indication: Outpatient treatment of opioid dependence (opioid substitution therapy) by certified physicians
Typical dose: 12–16 mg (range 4–24 mg), sublingual
Mechanism: Combination tablet or film with buprenorphine (high-affinity partial mu-opioid agonist and kappa-opioid antagonist) and naloxone (potent mu-opioid antagonist)
Clearance: Hepatic metabolism, biliary/renal excretion
Comments: Produces opioid agonist effects (reducing withdrawal symptoms) with ceiling effect; naloxone component is poorly absorbed sublingually and deters abuse of tablets by intravenous injection. For elective procedures, coordinate with pain/addiction specialists; stopping therapy 3 d before surgery recommended to facilitate perioperative analgesia (pts may require substitution to avoid addiction relapse). Pts typically require ↑↑ opioid doses for adequate pain relief. Continuing therapy and allowing extra buprenorphine for acute pain may be an option for minor procedures.

CALCIUM CHLORIDE (CaCl₂); CALCIUM GLUCONATE (KALCINATE)

Indication: (1) Hypocalcemia, hyperkalemia; (2) hypermagnesemia, calcium channel blocker overdose. Not routinely used in ACLS
Typical dose: (1) 500–1,000 mg CaCl₂ IV over 5–10 min in emergency or infusion 1–5 mg/kg/h titrated to ionized calcium level, (2) 500 mg CaCl₂ IV or 500–800 mg gluconate, may repeat if CNS depression persists, (3) 1–2 g CaCl₂ IV, may repeat q20min up to 5 doses. Hypocalcemia secondary to citrated blood transfusion: 33 mg CaCl₂ or 100 mg Ca gluconate/100 mL blood transfused. *Peds:* 10–20 mg/kg/dose q10min prn. Calcium gluconate: 15–30 mg/kg IV prn

Mechanism: Cofactor in enzymatic reactions, essential for neurotransmission, muscle contraction, signal conduction pathways. Can ↑ peripheral vascular tone, cardiac contractility, potentiate effects of catecholamines in critical illness

Clearance: Incorporated into bone/tissues; renal excretion

Comments: $CaCl_2$ provides 1.36 mEq Ca^{2+} per mL of 10% solution (vs. gluconate, 0.45 mEq/mL), is preferred in emergencies. Administer via central line (especially $CaCl_2$) if possible due to vein irritation and necrosis associated with extravasation. May cause bradycardia or arrhythmia (especially with digoxin), ↑ risk of ventricular fibrillation.

CANAGLIFLOZIN (INVOKANA)

See Antidiabetics table on Chapter 2H 63–64.

CARBOPROST TROMETHAMINE (HEMABATE, 15-METHYL PROSTAGLANDIN F2α)

Indication: Refractory postpartum uterine bleeding

Typical dose: Not for IV use. 250 mcg IM, repeat q15min prn (max 2,000 mcg)

Mechanism: Prostaglandin with unclear mechanism. Stimulates uterine contractions, promotes hemostasis at site of placentation

Clearance: Primarily lung metabolism, renal excretion

Comments: Must be refrigerated. Stimulates GI smooth muscle and frequently causes diarrhea, nausea/vomiting. May cause temperature elevation, flushing, bronchoconstriction. Avoid in asthma, cardiac dz, pulmonary hypertension. Can be given intramyometrial during C-section.

CLOPIDOGREL (PLAVIX)

Indication: Acute coronary syndrome, prevention of coronary artery stent thrombosis, ischemic stroke, MI, peripheral arterial dz

Typical dose: 75 mg PO daily. 300 mg load used in ACS, PCI

Mechanism: Irreversible thienopyridine antiplatelet agent. ADP receptor blocker: Prevents fibrinogen binding, thus ↓ platelet adhesion/aggregation

Clearance: Hepatic CYP3A4, CYP2C19 metabolism. Requires metabolism to active metabolite, pts with some CYP450 variants are resistant to drug effect (genetic testing available)

Comments: Major side effect is bleeding—can be treated with platelet transfusion though ↓ efficacy of platelets within 2–4 h of dose. Concurrent use with heparin and aspirin is accepted, particularly in treatment of ACS. Potential ↓ efficacy when used with omeprazole may not be clinically meaningful. Recommend discontinuing 5–10 d before elective surgery (7 d before neuraxial anesthesia). Hold only for urgent/emergent surgery within 1 y of drug-eluting stent due to ↑ risk of fatal late stent thrombosis; consult with cardiologist 1st

CHLORAL HYDRATE (SOMNOTE)

Indication: Sedation, hypnosis. Used off-label for insomnia and procedural sedation, especially for pediatric pts by nonanesthetists.

Comments: Risk of respiratory/myocardial depression. No analgesic effect. Not currently manufactured in the US as of 2012.

CHLOROTHIAZIDE (DIURIL)

See Diuretics table in Chapter 2H 54.

DABIGATRAN (PRADAXA)

Indication: Anticoagulation in atrial fibrillation

Typical dose: 150 mg bid

Mechanism: Direct competitive thrombin inhibitor, prevents conversion of fibrinogen to fibrin, thrombus formation

Clearance: Renal elimination

Comments: Stop 1– 2 d (4–5 d in renal dysfunction) before surgery. Bleeding risk can be assessed with ecarin clotting time (ECT); a normal aPTT suggests little anticoagulant activity though even mild ↑ aPTT may be associated with clinically important drug levels. Does not reliably elevate INR. Reversed with idarucizumab. Blood products/clotting factors do not reverse effect. Hemodialysis may remove ~60%

DALTEPARIN (FRAGMIN)

Indication: (1) DVT prophylaxis, (2) systemic anticoagulation for DVT or PE treatment, (3) acute coronary syndrome

Typical Dose: (1) 2,500–5,000 units SC daily, (2) 100 units/kg SC bid, (3) 120 units/kg SC (max 10,000 units) q12h with aspirin

Mechanism: Low–molecular-weight heparin (LMWH) enhances inhibition of factor Xa and thrombin (IIa)

Clearance: Hepatic metabolism, renal excretion

Comments: More predictable dose–response relationship than heparin (see also Enoxaparin). Minimal effect on PTT. Rare thrombocytopenia. Caution with neuraxial anesthesia including indwelling catheters due to potential for spinal/epidural hematoma and neurologic complications. Available in multidose vials.

DANTROLENE (DANTRIUM)

Indication: Treatment of malignant hyperthermia

Typical dose: *Adult/Peds:* 2.5 mg/kg IV bolus (mix 20 mg/60 mL sterile water = 525 mL bolus for 70 kg pt). Repeat dose until symptoms improve up to max 10 mg/kg (although 30 mg/kg sometimes required). Postacute reaction 1 mg/kg q6h for 24–48 h, then taper or change to oral tx. For **RYANODEX** (Dantrolene Sodium), see Appendix C.

Mechanism: Direct-acting skeletal muscle relaxant, ↓ Ca^{2+} release from sarcoplasmic reticulum

Clearance: Hepatic metabolism with renal elimination

Comments: Powder dissolves slowly into solution—may require assistants to help prepare in clinical emergency. Note large volume to be administered. Potential hepatotoxicity. Tissue necrosis if extravasated. Prophylactic treatment not recommended. See also "Malignant Hyperthermia Protocol," Appendix C.

DESMOPRESSIN ACETATE (DDAVP)

Indication: (1) Hemophilia A, von Willebrand dz, uremic platelet dysfunction; (2) central diabetes insipidus

Typical dose: *Adult:* (1) 300 mcg intranasal, give 2 h before procedure or 0.3 mcg/kg IV over 15–30 min, give 30 min before procedure, (2) 5–40 mcg intranasal, may divide q8–12h. *Peds:* (1) 2–4 mcg/kg intranasal or 0.2–0.4 mcg/kg IV over 15–30 min, (2) 3 mo–12 y: 5–30 mcg/d intranasal, divided bid

Mechanism: Synthetic antidiuretic hormone; hemostatic mechanism unclear but involves release of factor VIII stores, possibly ↑ factor VIII concentration and ↑ von Willebrand factor activity. ↑ renal water reabsorption in collecting duct

Clearance: Renal excretion

Comments: Tachyphylaxis observed with multiple doses (at 12–24 h) for hemostasis. May cause headache, rare thrombotic events due to ↑ platelet adhesion. Rare risk of potentially fatal hyponatremia/seizures; consider ↓ fluid intake to minimize potential for water intoxication. May ↑ BP, use caution in cardiac and hypertensive dz.

DEXAMETHASONE (DECADRON)

Indication: (1) Cerebral edema from brain tumor; (2) airway edema; (3) prophylaxis of postoperative nausea and vomiting; (4) allergic reaction

Typical dose: *Adult:* (1) Load 10 mg IV, then 2 mg IV q8–12h, (2) 0.1 mg/kg IV q6h, (3) 4 mg IV, (4) 4–8 mg, taper off over 7 d. *Peds:* (1) 1–2 mg/kg IV load, then 1–1.5 mg/kg/d divided q4–6h IV (max 16 mg/d), (2) 0.5–2 mg/kg/d IV/IM divided q6, (3) 0.0625 mg/kg, (4) 0.15–0.6 mg/kg IV

Mechanism: Glucocorticosteroid; prevents/controls inflammation by controlling rate of inflammatory modulator protein synthesis, suppressing migration of inflammatory cells, reversing capillary permeability. Antiemetic mechanism unclear, likely central

Clearance: Hepatic metabolism, renal excretion

Comments: Potent glucocorticoid with almost no mineralocorticoid properties (see table "Relative Potencies of Commonly Administered Corticosteroids" under Hydrocortisone). Little or no benefit to higher doses for PONV though may ↑ side effects. Slow onset of action: Takes 4–6 h to ↓ airway edema; most effective for PONV prophylaxis when administered at induction. Causes perineal burning sensation with rapid IV injection. Risk of adrenocortical insufficiency if withdrawn abruptly after chronic use. Effects of chronic ↑ doses (hyperglycemia, delayed wound healing, immunosuppression) are relevant to surgical pts; however, no studies have identified complications associated with single antiemetic dose. Use lowest effective dose. Use with caution with ↑ doses in severe infection, latent TB. Like other steroids, may cause delirium or aggravate psychiatric d/o.

DIPHENHYDRAMINE (BENADRYL)

Indication: (1) Acute treatment of allergic reaction; (2) pruritus; (3) antiemetic, sedative, antitussive; (4) treatment of dystonic reaction/extrapyramidal symptoms

Typical dose: *Adult:* (1, 2) 10–50 mg IV q4–6h (max 100 mg/dose, 400 mg/d); (3) 25–50 mg PO/IM/IV q4–6h; (4) 50 mg IV/IM, may repeat in 20–30 min. *Peds:* (>10 kg) (1) 5 mg/kg/d IV div q6–8h (max 300 mg/d 75 mg/dose); (2) 0.5–1 mg/kg/dose PO/IV/IM q4–6h; (3) 1 mg/kg/dose PO/IV/IM

Mechanism: Antihistamine; histamine (H1) receptor antagonist; anticholinergic; CNS depressant

Clearance: Hepatic metabolism; renal excretion

Comments: Use as adjunct to epinephrine in anaphylaxis. May cause drowsiness, hypotension, tachycardia, dizziness, urinary retention, seizures, paradoxical excitation in children. Use caution in elderly patients (sedation, confusion). Additive sedation effect with other CNS depressants

DOLASETRON (ANZEMET)

See 5HT₃ Antagonists.

DROPERIDOL (INAPSINE)

Indication: (1) Prevention/treatment of postoperative nausea and vomiting. Also used for (2) sedation, GA adjunct, treatment of delirium although alternate drugs are preferred

Typical dose: *Adult:* (1) 0.625–1.25 mg IV (2) 2.5 mg is max recommended, additional 1.25 mg doses if benefit > risk. *Peds:* 2–12 y: 0.03–0.07 mg/kg (0.1 mg/kg max)

Mechanism: Butyrophenone neuroleptic, primarily anti-dopaminergic with some antagonism at NE, 5HT, GABA, α-adrenergic receptors

Clearance: Extensive hepatic metabolism, renal excretion

Comments: Potentiates other CNS depressants; may also cause anxiety, restlessness, dysphoria. Mild α-adrenergic blockade may cause hypotension via peripheral vasodilation, reflex tachycardia (especially in hypovolemia). Avoid in Parkinson's, pheochromocytoma (can precipitate catecholamine release). May cause extrapyramidal symptoms → rx with diphenhydramine. May prolong QT interval leading to serious arrhythmias including torsade de pointes, ventricular arrhythmias, cardiac arrest. Contraindicated in pre-existing prolonged interval (QTc >440 in males, >450 in females); use extreme caution if risk factors for QT prolongation including HR <50, cardiac dz, hypokalemia, hypomagnesemia, co-administration of other QT prolonging drugs (includes calcium channel blockers, ondansetron, antidepressants, fluoroquinolones, antiarrhythmics)

ENOXAPARIN (LOVENOX, LMWH)

Indication: (1) DVT prophylaxis, (2) treatment of acute DVT or PE, (3) acute coronary syndrome

Typical dose: (1) 40 mg SC daily or 30 mg SC q12h; (2) 1 mg/kg SC q12h (outpatient, with warfarin) or 1.5 mg/kg SC daily (inpatient, with warfarin); (3) 1 mg/kg SC bid with aspirin (30 mg IV bolus in STEMI). *Peds:* Safety/efficacy not established. (1) <2 mo: 0.75 mg/kg SC q12h; (2) 1.5 mg/kg SC q12h; >2 mo: (1) 0.5 mg/kg SC q12h; (2) 1 mg/kg SC q12h

Mechanism: LMWH, antithrombotic. Anti-factor Xa and antithrombin (anti-factor IIa) activity

Clearance: Hepatic metabolism, renal excretion

Comments: More predictable dose–response relationship and longer duration of action than unfractionated heparin. Preferred for DVT prophylaxis in arthroplasty, trauma. Unlike warfarin, may be used in pregnancy. Generally does not ↑ PT or PTT; monitor Factor Xa activity (4 h after dose) if needed (consider for dose adjustment in obesity, low body weight, pregnancy, renal impairment). Xa activity level not predictive of bleeding risk. Reduce dose for low body weight <45 kg, renal impairment with GFR <30. Rarely causes thrombocytopenia, contraindicated in major active bleeding. Incomplete reversal with protamine. Risk of spinal or epidural hematomas and neurologic damage with spinal puncture, neuraxial anesthesia including indwelling catheters (wait 12 h after prophylactic dose or 24 h after therapeutic dose before performing neuraxial block; ↑ risk with twice-daily vs. once-daily dosing; delay enoxaparin dose for 2 h after neuraxial catheter removal)

Clinical Characteristics of Commonly Encountered Diuretics

Drug	Typical Dose	Site of Action	Mechanism of Action	Comments
Acetazolamide (Diamox)	250–500 mg IV/PO q6 × 4 doses (max 100 mg/kg or 2 g per 24 h)	Proximal convoluted tubule (carbonic anhydrase inhibitor)	Inhibits H$^+$ excretion, causing ↑ Na$^+$, K$^+$, bicarb, H$_2$O excretion	Decreases ICP and IOP (via ↓ CSF, aqueous humor production). Used for respiratory alkalosis (altitude sickness) or metabolic alkalosis with respiratory acidosis
Bumetanide (Bumex)	0.5–2 mg IV (max 10 mg/d)	Na$^+$/K$^+$/2Cl$^-$ cotransporter in ascending loop of Henle (loop diuretic)	Inhibits reabsorption of Na$^+$/Cl$^-$, causing ↑ H$_2$O (also K$^+$, Ca^{2+}, phos) excretion	May cause hyponatremia, hypokalemia (potentiates digitalis arrhythmias), hypochloremia, dehydration, hyperuricemia. Useful for thiazide-refractory fluid retention and in renal impairment. Use caution in elderly pts, NSAIDs, ACE inhibitors. Bumetanide is very potent (1 mg = 40 mg furosemide)
Ethacrynic acid (Edecrin)	0.5–1 mg/kg IV (max 50 mg) or 25–100 PO q12–24h			
Furosemide[a] (Lasix)	10–40 mg IV or 20–80 mg PO q6–24h			May enhance loop diuretics and antihypertensives, can ↑ insulin requirements. Less effective in renal impairment. Net ↓ in calcium excretion
Chlorothiazide (Diuril)	0.5–1 g IV/PO q12–24h (max 2 g/d). Peds: 2–4 mg/kg IV, or 10 mg/kg PO q12h	Distal convoluted tubule (thiazide diuretic)	Inhibits Na$^+$ reabsorption, causing ↑ H$_2$O, Na$^+$ (also H$^+$, K$^+$, Mg^{2+}, phos) excretion	
Hydro-chlorothiazide (HCTZ, Microzide)	12.5–50 mg PO daily			
Mannitol[a]	0.25–0.5 g/kg q4–6h	Proximal descending tubule, (osmotic diuretic)	↑ osmolarity of urine, causes ↓ H$_2$O reabsorption	Filtered by glomerulus but cannot be reabsorbed
Spironolactone (Aldactone)	25–100 mg/d, Peds: 1–3 mg/kg/d q6–12h	Late distal tubule, cortical collecting duct (aldosterone antagonist)	↑ Na$^+$, Cl$^-$, H$_2$O excretion (preserves K$^+$, H$^+$)	"Potassium-sparing" diuretic, causes less hypokalemia than thiazides and loop diuretics. May cause severe hyperkalemia, antiandrogen effect (gynecomastia). Slow onset of action (d).

[a]See separate entries for furosemide, mannitol for additional information.

EPINEPHRINE, RACEMIC (VAPONEFRIN)

Indication: Croup (laryngotracheobronchitis), postextubation/traumatic airway edema; adjunct in bronchiolitis and bronchospasm

Typical dose: Inhaled via nebulizer. *Adult:* 0.5 mL of 2.25% solution in 3 mL NS q2–4h prn. *Peds:* <4 y: 0.05 mL/kg of 2.25% solution in 3 mL NS q2–4h prn; >4 y: 0.25–0.5 mL of 2.25% solution in 3 mL NS q2–4h prn

Mechanism: Mucosal vasoconstriction

Clearance: MAO/COMT metabolism

Comments: May cause tachycardia, arrhythmias. Rebound airway edema may occur up to 2 h after discontinuation

---

EPOPROSTENOL (FLOLAN, PROSTACYCLIN, PROSTAGLANDIN I_2 [PGI$_2$])

Indication: Pulmonary arterial hypertension

Typical dose: 2 ng/kg/min IV infusion, titrate by 1–2 ng/kg/min q15–30min. For short-term use in critical illness, may be inhaled via continuous nebulization (15–50 ng/kg/min doses studied, wean by 50%)

Mechanism: Pulmonary and systemic vasodilator; inhibits platelet aggregation

Clearance: Rapidly hydrolyzed in blood

Comments: Not for use in all types of pulmonary hypertension. Caution in pulmonary veno-occlusive dz or left ventricular systolic dysfunction; pulmonary edema may develop during initial IV dose titration. IV use cause brady- or tachycardia, hypotension, flu-like symptoms, nausea, vomiting, diarrhea. Avoid abrupt withdrawal or interruption of infusion (note half-life 2.7 min). Inhaled therapy offers potential benefit of minimal systemic hemodynamic effect, improvement of V/Q matching; use caution as "sticky" glycine preparation can clog ETT and cause ventilator malfunction. Potential uses for inhaled drug include acute pulmonary hypertension crisis, post-cardiac surgery, ARDS, neonates with congenital heart defects.

EPTIFIBATIDE (INTEGRILIN)

Indication: Prevention of thrombus formation after PCI, treatment of acute coronary syndrome

Typical Dose: Bolus 180 mcg/kg, then 2 mcg/kg/min infusion up to 72 h. Reduce infusion to 1 mcg/min in renal impairment with CrCl <50

Mechanism: Prevents platelet adhesion and aggregation by reversible inhibition of glycoprotein IIb/IIIa, fibrinogen, and von Willebrand factor

Clearance: Renal excretion, platelet function recovers within 4–8 h after discontinuation of infusion

Comments: Risk of bleeding complications including bleeding at sheath site (early removal encouraged, hold heparin first). May cause thrombocytopenia. Contraindicated with recent severe bleeding or bleeding d/o (specific contraindications similar to TPA)

ETHACRYNIC ACID (EDECRIN)

See Diuretics table in Chapter 2H 54.

EXENATIDE (BYETTA)

See Antidiabetics table in Chapter 2H 63–64.

FACTOR VIIA (NOVOSEVEN)

Indication: Bleeding episodes and (1) surgical intervention in hemophilia A or B, (2) congenital factor VII deficiency or acquired hemophilia. Also used for intracranial hemorrhage, diffuse alveolar hemorrhage, (3) coagulopathy associated with massive blood loss in trauma, cardiac surgery

Typical dose: (1) 90 mcg/kg IV before intervention, then q2h for duration of surgery × 2–5 d, then q2–6h until healing has occurred, (2) 70–90 mcg/kg IV q2–3h until hemostasis achieved (doses as low as 10 mcg/kg may be effective), (3) dosing is not standardized for these uses, ranges from 35–120 mcg/kg see hospital-based protocol

Mechanism: Promotes hemostasis through activation of extrinsic coagulation cascade; activates factors X, IX → converts prothrombin to thrombin → converts fibrinogen to fibrin, helps form hemostatic plug

Comments: Off-label use (trauma, complex or cardiac surgery, postpartum hemorrhage) is controversial due to concerns about safety, efficacy, very high cost. Limited available data does not conclusively demonstrate benefit, and may be associated with higher rate of arterial and venous thrombotic complications *(Cochrane Database Syst Rev. 2011;(2):CD005011)*. Consider risk/benefit for individual pts. Do not inject diluent directly onto powder, swirl gently (do not shake), administer within 3 h

FAMOTIDINE (PEPCID)

Indication: GERD, peptic ulcers
Typical dose: *Adult:* 10–20 mg IV q12h (dilute in 10 mL NS, administer <10 mg/min), 20–40 mg PO bid. *Peds:* 0.6–0.8 mg/kg/d IV, divide q8–12h (max 40 mg/d)
Mechanism: Competitive histamine (H_2) receptor antagonist, effect on gastric parietal cells ↓ gastric acid secretion
Clearance: 30–35% hepatic metabolism; 65–70% renal elimination
Comments: Given preoperatively for pulmonary aspiration prophylaxis (maximum effect within 30 min of IV dose), and for ulcer prophylaxis in selected critically ill pts. May cause confusion, dizziness, headache, diarrhea, thrombocytopenia. Reduce dose in renal impairment

FLUMAZENIL (MAZICON)

Indication: (1) Reversal of benzodiazepine sedation; (2) reversal of benzodiazepine overdose
Typical dose: *Adult:* (1) 0.2 mg IV over 15–30 s, if no response may redose q1min with 0.3–0.5 mg (max 3 mg/h), (2) as in (1); may ↑ to 5 mg, if still no response sedation unlikely to be benzodiazepine related. *Peds:* 0.01 mg/kg IV × 1 dose (max 0.2 mg/dose), subsequent doses 0.005–0.01 mg/kg IV q1min (max 1 mg)
Onset: 1–2 min, peak 6–10 min. **Duration:** 20–40 min, depends on doze of both benzodiazepine and flumazenil
Mechanism: Competitive antagonism of GABA receptor at benzodiazepine action site
Clearance: Extensive hepatic metabolism, renal excretion
Comments: May wear off before the effects of benzodiazepines; monitor for re-sedation and respiratory depression. Does not antagonize non-benzodiazepine CNS depression. May elicit withdrawal symptoms (including seizures) in chronic benzodiazepine users. Use lowest dose required. Avoid in unknown drug overdose, suspected tricyclic overdose; caution with ↑ ICP or seizure Hx (be prepared to manage seizures). Only partial reversal of respiratory depression

FUROSEMIDE (LASIX)

Indication: (1) Acute pulmonary edema/hypertensive crisis/elevated ICP, (2) symptomatic hyperkalemia, (3) chronic antihypertensive, (4) edema associated with CHF cirrhosis, renal dz
Typical dose: *Adult:* (1) 0.5–1 mg/kg (or 40 mg) IV over 2 min, (2) 40–80 mg IV, (3) up to 40 mg PO bid, (4) 10–40 mg IV, may ↑ by 20 mg q2h, refractory CHF may require large doses. Infusion: 0.1 mg/kg/h, titrate to effect (max 4 mg/min). *Peds:* 0.5–2 mg/kg/ dose IV (max 6 mg/kg/d). *Neonates:* 0.5–1 mg/kg/dose IV (max 2 mg/kg/d)
Onset: <5 min (IV), peak <30 min. **Duration:** 2 h
Mechanism: Loop diuretic; inhibits reabsorption of sodium and chloride at proximal/ distal tubules and loop of Henle
Clearance: Hepatic metabolism (10%), renal excretion
Comments: Oral dosing = ½ potency of IV. May cause hypovolemia and electrolyte imbalance (hypokalemia, hyponatremia, hypochloremic alkalosis). Caution in lupus, sulfa allergy. Do not use in anuria or worsening azotemia. Can ↓ CSF production but less effective than mannitol at ↓ ICP

GLIPIZIDE (GLUCOTROL)

See Antidiabetics table in Chapter 2H 63–64.

GLUCAGON (GLUCAGEN)

Indication: (1) Severe hypoglycemia, (2) GI diagnostics, also used for (3) refractory β-blocker/calcium channel blocker toxicity

Typical dose: *Adult:* (1) 1 mg IM/SC/IV, (2) 0.25–2 mg 1 min prior to procedure, repeat q20min, (3) 50–150 mcg/kg IV bolus, then 1–5 mg/h IV infusion. *Peds:* (1) 0.2–0.3 mg/kg (max 1 mg/dose). Repeat q20min prn. *Neonates:* 0.025–0.3 mg/kg/dose (max 1 mg/dose)

Mechanism: Stimulates adenylate cyclase → ↑ cAMP → promotes hepatic gluconeogenesis, glycogenolysis, catecholamine release. Insulin antagonist. Relaxes GI smooth muscle

Clearance: Hepatic and renal proteolysis

Comments: Positive inotrope and chronotrope (not blocked by b-blockade or catecholamine depletion), enhances AV nodal conduction in AV block. Use in cardiac (refractory low CO after bypass, low CO after MI, congestive heart failure, excessive b-blockade) limited by side effects (nausea and vomiting, hypokalemia, hypo- or hyperglycemia) and ↑ cost. Caution with insulinoma, pheochromocytoma. Give IV dextrose to replete glycogen stores.

GLYBURIDE (DIABETA)

See Antidiabetics table in Chapter 2H 63–64.

GLYCOPYRROLATE (ROBINUL)

Indication: (1) ↓ gastrointestinal motility, antisialogogue; (2) bradycardia; (3) adjunct to reversal of neuromuscular blockade

Typical dose: *Adult:* (1) 0.1–0.2 mg IV/IM/SC; 2.5–10 mcg/kg/dose IV/IM q3–4h; 1–2 mg PO; (2) 0.1–0.2 mg/dose IV; (3) 0.2 mg IV for each 1 mg neostigmine or 5 mg pyridostigmine or 0.01–0.02 mg/kg IV. *Peds:* (1) 4–10 mcg/kg/dose IV/IM q3–4h, max 0.2 mg/dose or 0.8 mg q24h; 40–100 mcg/kg/dose PO tid–qid. (2) 0.01–0.02 mg/kg IV. *Neonates/infants:* 4–10 mcg/kg/dose IV/IM q4–8h; 40–100 mcg/kg/dose PO q8–12h

Mechanism: Blocks acetylcholine action at smooth muscle parasympathetic sites, secretory glands, and CNS

Clearance: Renal elimination

Comments: Longer duration, better antisialagogue with less CNS and chronotropic effect than atropine. Does not cross blood–brain barrier or placenta. Unreliable oral absorption. May cause bronchospasm, blurred vision, constipation. Caution with asthma, ulcerative colitis, glaucoma, ileus, or urinary retention

	Clinical Characteristics of Commonly Used Anticholinergic Drugs			
Drug	Duration (min)	Effect on Heart Rate	Sedation	Effect on Secretions
Atropine	15–30	↑↑↑	+	↓
Glycopyrrolate	30–60	↑↑	0	↓↓

GRANISETRON (GRANISOL, KYTRIL)

See 5HT₃ Antagonists.

HALOPERIDOL (HALDOL)

Indication: Indicated for treatment of schizophrenia. Also used for agitation caused by delirium

Typical dose: *Adult:* (1) Mild agitation: 0.5–2 mg IV, moderate agitation: 5 mg IV, severe agitation: 10 mg IV. *Peds: 3–12 y and 15–40 kg,* 0.01–0.03 mg/kg/d div q8h (max 0.15 mg/kg/d). *Antiemetic:* 0.01 mg/kg/dose IV q8–12h

Mechanism: Butyrophenone neuroleptic; dopaminergic (D₁ and D₂) antagonist. Depresses reticular activating system

Clearance: Hepatic metabolism; renal/biliary elimination

Comments: Causes sedation, tranquility, immobility, antiemesis. IV use common in acute care but not FDA approved. Not for use with dementia-related psychosis. Avoid in Parkinson's, glaucoma, leukopenia. Associated with extrapyramidal symptoms (rarely including laryngospasm, rx with diphenhydramine) and arrhythmias (torsade de pointes), cardiac arrest at ↑ doses. Monitor ECG for prolonged QT interval. Associated with neuroleptic malignant syndrome (presentation similar to malignant hyperthermia). Lowers seizure threshold

HEPARIN, UNFRACTIONATED (UFH)

Indication: (1) DVT prophylaxis; systemic anticoagulation for (2) thromboembolism, DIC; (3) cardiopulmonary bypass. Unfrac used as (4) catheter lock to maintain patency

Typical dose: *Adult:* (1) 5,000 units SC q8h, (2) see hospital-specific protocols for infusion dosing and PTT goals, generally load 5,000 units IV, then 15–25 units/kg/h IV infusion, (3) 300 units/kg IV bolus, monitor and maintain ACT >400, (4) 100 units/mL, volume depends on catheter. *Peds:* (1) See hospital-specific protocols for infusion dosing and PTT goals, generally load 50 units/kg IV, then 20 units/kg/h IV infusion, titrate to goal PTT, (2) bypass: 400 units/kg, children: 300 units/kg, monitor and maintain ACT >400, (4) >10 kg: 100 units/mL; <10 kg: 10 units/mL; *premature infants:* 1 unit/mL, volume depends on catheter

Mechanism: Binds/activates antithrombin III → inactivates thrombin and other proteases (including IX, Xa, XI, XII, thrombin). Net effect prevents cleavage of prothrombin to active thrombin, inhibits conversion of fibrinogen to fibrin, inhibits activation of factor VIII

Clearance: Partial hepatic metabolism, renal excretion

Comments: Infusion requires PTT monitoring and dose titration. Prevents thrombus formation/extension but will not lyse existing clots. Requires ATIII, suspect deficiency and rx with FFP if unable to achieve therapeutic PTT. Enoxaparin is the preferred agent for DVT prophylaxis in arthroplasty, trauma. Contraindicated in severe thrombocytopenia, uncontrollable active bleeding (unless due to DIC). May cause hemorrhage; nonimmune (Type 1, within 2 d) and immune-mediated (Type 2, 4–10 d after initial exposure) thrombocytopenia (and thrombosis in Type 2) which can be life-threatening. Adjust dose in hepatic impairment. Reversed by protamine. Caution with lumbar puncture, neuraxial anesthesia including indwelling catheters due to risk of hematoma and neurologic impairment

HIGHLY ACTIVE ANTIRETROVIRAL THERAPY (HAART)

Indication: Treatment of infection by retroviruses, primarily HIV

Comments: Continue whenever possible in perioperative period to minimize ↑ in viral load and drug resistance. Evidence is sparse, though numerous potential interactions with anesthetic drugs including ↓ fentanyl clearance (ritonavir), ↑ level of meperidine active metabolite (ritonavir), ↑ duration of action of midazolam (saquinavir), prolonged neuromuscular blockade, altered pharmacokinetics of CYP/P450 metabolized drugs, and ↑ mitochondrial toxicity/lactic acidosis when nucleoside/nucleotide reverse transcriptase inhibitors (NRTIs) used with propofol. See www.hiv-druginteractions.org or hivinsite.ucsf.edu for more information

HYDROCHLOROTHIAZIDE (HCTZ, MICROZIDE)

See Diuretics table in Chapter 2H 54.

HYDROCORTISONE (SOLU-CORTEF)

Indication: (1) Severe acute adrenal insufficiency, (2) perioperative supplementation in pts taking chronic steroids, (3) status asthmaticus, (4) physiologic replacement in chronic adrenal insufficiency

Typical dose: *Adult:* (1) 100 mg IV, then 200–400 mg IV daily, divided q6h, (2) 25 mg IV at start of procedure, then 100 mg IV over 24 h, (3) 1–2 mg/kg q6h, 4 to 0.5–1 mg/kg when stable, (4) 20–30 mg PO daily. *Peds:* (1) 1–12 mo: 1–2 mg/kg bolus then 50 mg/m²/d infusion or 150–250 mg/d divided q6–8h, (3) 4–8 mg/kg IV × 1 (max 250 mg), then 2 mg/kg/d divided q6h, (4) 0.5–0.75 mg/kg/d PO divided q8h

Mechanism: Corticosteroid with glucocorticoid (prevents/controls inflammation by controlling rate of inflammatory modulator protein synthesis, suppressing migration of inflammatory cells, reversing capillary permeability) and mineralocorticoid (promotes Na⁺ and H₂O retention, K⁺ excretion) effects

Clearance: In tissues and liver to inactive metabolites, renal excretion

Comments: High doses are generally not recommended as they may cause hypernatremia, hypokalemia, hypertension (mineralocorticoid effect). Dose-dependent association with GI bleeding, secondary infection, psychosis, hyperglycemia, and delayed wound healing. Use lowest effective dose. Use with caution in severe infection, latent TB. With chronic (even topical) use, normal adrenal response can be suppressed as long as 9–12 mo. Consider "stress-dose" supplementation in adrenally suppressed pts undergoing major surgery (adequate dose is unclear, may vary, and may be lower than previously thought)

Relative Potencies of Commonly Administered Corticosteroids			
Drug	Glucocorticoid	Mineralocorticoid	Half-Life (h)
Dexamethasone	25	0	36–72
Hydrocortisone	1	1	8
Methylprednisolone	5	0.5	12–36

HYDROXYZINE (VISTARIL, ATARAX)

Indication: Anxiety, itching, nausea/vomiting
Typical dose: *Adults:* 25–100 mg IM **or** 50–100 mg PO q6. *Peds >6 y:* 50–100 mg PO daily (divided); *<6 y:* 50–100 mg PO daily (divided). Preoperative sedation: 0.5–1 mg/kg IM
Mechanism: H1 receptor antagonist; has muscle relaxant, analgesic, antihistaminic, antiemetic effects
Clearance: Hepatic (P450) metabolism; renal elimination
Comments: Not for IV use. Chemically unrelated to phenothiazines or benzodiazepines. May cause oversedation; potentiates CNS depressants including meperidine and barbiturates

IDARUCIZUMAB (PRAXBIND)

Indication: Reversal of dabigatran for emergency surgery or life-threatening/ uncontrolled bleeding
Typical dose: 5 g (adult). May consider additional 2nd dose of 5 g if coagulation not improved
Mechanism: Humanized monoclonal antibody fragment (Fab), targeting the direct thrombin inhibitor dabigatran
Clearance: Biodegradation, renal
Comments: May cause hypersensitivity reaction. Contains sorbitol; use caution in hereditary fructose intolerance. No effect on other anticoagulants.

INDIGO CARMINE

Indication: Evaluation of urine output and localization of ureteral orifices during urologic procedures
Typical dose: 40 mg IV slowly (5 mL of 0.8% solution), ↓ dose in infants/children to prevent skin discoloration
Mechanism: Rapid glomerular filtration produces blue urine; appears in urine in 10 min (average)
Clearance: Renal
Comments: May cause HTN from α-adrenergic stimulation, lasts 15–30 min after IV dose. Also causes transient false low pulse oximetry readings.

INDOCYANINE GREEN (CARDIO-GREEN)

Indication: Determining cardiac output, hepatic function, liver blood flow
Typical dose: *Adult:* 5 mg IV. *Children:* 2.5 mg IV. *Infants:* 1.25 mg IV. Max 2 mg/kg. Dilute with provided aqueous solvent to various concentrations (depends on application)
Mechanism: Binds to plasma proteins (albumin), distributes within plasma volume
Clearance: No metabolism, biliary excretion
Comments: Inject rapidly into central circulation for indicator-dilution curves. May cause anaphylaxis; use caution in pts with Hx of allergy to iodides. Absorption spectra (and therefore results) changed by heparin. Use within 6 h of reconstitution. May cause transient false low pulse oximetry readings

INSULIN, REGULAR

Indication: (1) Hyperglycemia; (2) diabetic ketoacidosis; (3) hyperkalemia
Typical dose: (1) Individualized; hospital-specific perioperative bolus and/or infusion protocols are generally available. 0.5–1 units/h (Type 1 diabetes) or 2–3 units/h

(Type 2 diabetes) is typical starting infusion rate. (2) 0.05–0.2 units/kg/h for severe hyperglycemia, ↓ when glucose is <300 mg/dL. Consider loading bolus 0.1 unit/kg. (3) 10 units IV (with 50 mL D5W if blood glucose is <250 mg/dL) over 5 min; consider dextrose infusion if dose is repeated

Mechanism: Protein hormone, stimulates glucose uptake by cells; shifts potassium into cells

Clearance: Liver >50%, kidney 30%, tissue/muscle 20%

Comments: Hypoglycemia is dangerous; symptoms of intraoperative hypoglycemia may be misinterpreted as "light" anesthesia or masked by β-blockers. Monitor blood glucose carefully. Mix 1 unit/mL normal saline for infusion. Glycemic goal for critically ill pts is 140–180 mg/dL, although lower range (110–140) may be beneficial if it can be achieved without hypoglycemia; IV infusion of insulin and dextrose is the preferred route in ICU (Standards of Medical Care in Diabetes—2019. *American Diabetes Association*). Infusion tubing absorbs insulin, priming may enhance delivery.

IPRATROPIUM BROMIDE (ATROVENT)

Indication: Bronchodilation, especially in chronic treatment of obstructive pulmonary dz

Typical dose: Adult: 500 mcg; Peds <12 y: 150–500 mcg nebulized, q20min up to 3 doses

Mechanism: Inhaled anticholinergic

Clearance: Hepatic, renal excretion

Comments: Combine with β2 agonist in acute bronchospasm (solution may be mixed with albuterol). Caution in glaucoma, BPH

LEVETIRACETAM (KEPPRA)

Indication: (1) Seizures, also used for (2) seizure prophylaxis in traumatic brain injury

Typical dose: (1) 500–1,000 mg IV/PO bid (max 3 g/d), (2) 20 mg/kg over 60 min then 1,000 mg q12 × 7 d

Mechanism: Unknown, may inhibit calcium channels or modulate neurotransmitter release

Clearance: Hepatic enzymatic hydrolysis, renal excretion

Comments: Adjust dose in renal dz. May cause somnolence. Avoid abrupt discontinuation

---

LEVOTHYROXINE (SYNTHROID, T4)

Indication: (1) Hypothyroidism, (2) myxedema coma, also used for (3) preservation of organ function in brain-dead donors

Typical dose: *Adult:* (1) 0.1–0.2 mg/d PO titrated to thyroid function tests; for IV use give 50–75% of daily oral dose, (2) 200–500 mcg IV ×1, then 100–300 mcg in 24 if needed, (3) 20 mcg IV ×1, then 10 mcg/h infusion. Peds: PO: 0–6 mo: 8–10 mcg/kg/d; 6–12 mo: 6–8 mcg/kg/d; 1–5 y: 5–6 mcg/kg/d; 6–12 y: 4–5 mcg/kg/d; >12 y: 150 mcg/d

Mechanism: Synthetic thyroxine hormone; ↑ basal metabolic rate, utilization of glycogen store, promotes gluconeogenesis

Clearance: Metabolized in the liver to triiodothyronine (T3, active); eliminated in feces and urine

Comments: Multiple drug interactions including phenytoin (may ↓ levothyroxine levels), warfarin (↑ effect), tricyclic antidepressants (may ↑ toxic potential of both drugs). May cause HTN, arrhythmias, diarrhea, weight loss. Contraindicated with recent myocardial infarction, thyrotoxicosis, or uncorrected adrenal insufficiency. Reduces vasopressor requirement in organ donors

---

LIRAGLUTIDE (VICTOZA)

See Antidiabetics table in Chapter 2H 63–64.

MAGNESIUM SULFATE (MgSO₄)

Indication: (1) Prevention and treatment of eclamptic seizures, (2) hypomagnesemia, (3) torsade de pointes. Also used for ventricular ectopy, preterm labor management, (4) pediatric asthma

Typical dose: *Adult:* (1) 4–5 g IV load (may give 8–10 mg IM simultaneously), then 1–3 g/h infusion titrated to serum level and avoidance of toxicity, (2) 1–2 g over

15 min, then 1 g/h until serum level normal (generally 2–6 g), (3) 1–2 g over 5–10 min. *Peds*: (1) 25–50 mg IV. (2) 25–50 mg IV over 10–15 min

Mechanism: Enzymatic cofactor, important role in neurotransmission and muscular excitability; bronchial smooth muscle relaxation

Clearance: Renal excretion

Comments: Causes CNS depression, anticonvulsant effect, blocks peripheral neuromuscular transmission (monitor deep tendon reflexes, respiratory rate, mental status in high-dose therapy). Rx overdose with calcium chloride or gluconate. Dose cautiously in renal impairment. May cause hypotension, particularly if infused rapidly. Potentiates neuromuscular blockade and predisposes to uterine atony

MANNITOL (OSMITROL)

Indication: Increased intracranial pressure, oliguric acute renal injury, promotion of urinary excretion of toxic materials

Typical dose: 0.25–2 g/kg over 30–60 min (in acutely elevated ICP can bolus 12.5–25 g over 5–10 min). Max 1–2 g/kg over 6 h

Mechanism: ↑ serum osmolarity, ↓ cerebral edema. Freely filtered by glomerulus, induces osmotic diuresis

Clearance: Rapid renal excretion

Comments: Avoid in anuria/severe renal dz, pulmonary edema, active intracranial bleeding, dehydration/hypovolemia. Causes transient expansion of intravascular volume; caution in hypertension or heart failure. Rapid administration may cause vasodilation, hypotension. Use filter on IV tubing, do not use solution if crystals are present

METFORMIN (GLUCOPHAGE)

See Antidiabetics table in Chapter 2H 63–64.

METHYLERGONOVINE (METHERGINE)

Indication: Uterine atony and postpartum hemorrhage

Typical dose: Not for IV use. 0.2 mg IM q15–20min (max 4 doses)

Mechanism: Synthetic ergot alkaloid, causes dose-dependent ↑ in uterine contraction/tone, likely through α-adrenergic receptors

Clearance: Hepatic metabolism

Comments: Must be refrigerated; administer only if clear/colorless. α-Adrenergic effect may cause peripheral vasoconstriction and potentially severe hypertension, especially when used with other vasopressor agents. Avoid in hypertension/preeclampsia, ischemic heart dz, pulmonary hypertension. May cause nausea

METHYLENE BLUE (METHYLTHIONINE CHLORIDE, UROLENE BLUE)

Indication: (1) Methemoglobinemia, also used for (2) vasoplegic syndrome post-cardiopulmonary bypass, refractory septic shock

Typical dose: (1) 1–2 mg/kg (0.1–0.2 mL) IV over 5 min, may repeat in 1 h. Give slowly to avoid local ↑ concentration and promotion of additional methemoglobin, (2) 1.5 mg/kg

Mechanism: ↑ erythrocyte reduction of methemoglobin to hemoglobin at low doses, may cause formation of methemoglobin at high doses. Potent reversible MAO-A inhibitor, inhibits MAO-B at high doses. Inhibits nitric oxide/cGMP pathway

Clearance: Tissue reduction; urinary and biliary elimination

Comments: Causes transient false low pulse oximeter readings and blue coloration of blood (alert surgeon/perfusionist of use in cardiac surgery), urine, skin. Contraindicated in G6PD deficiency; extreme caution in pulmonary hypertension and acute lung injury/ARDS. Avoid with concurrent use of pulmonary vasodilators, or nitrates for coronary vasodilation due to competing mechanism of action. Extravasation may cause necrosis. Risk of serotonin syndrome, avoid co-administration of serotonergic psychiatric drugs if possible. May cause nausea, diaphoresis, confusion. Facilitates pressor weaning and ↑ arterial pressure in septic shock, unknown effect on outcomes (2–3 h after bolus dose, some studies use continuous infusion). Sparsely studied but appears to improve vasoplegia and mortality after cardiac surgery, may have role in vasoplegic syndrome in anaphylaxis, liver transplant, other settings

METHYLPREDNISOLONE (SOLU-MEDROL)

Indication: (1) Allergic reactions, conditions treated with immunosuppression. Also used in (2) acute spinal cord injury, (3) induction of immunosuppression in solid organ transplant, (4) status asthmaticus

Typical dose: *Adult:* (1) 10–40 mg/d PO, may divide q6–12 or 10–250 mg IV/IM up to 6 doses/d, depending on condition treated, (2) 30 mg/kg over 15 min, then 5.4 mg/kg/h for 24–48 h. Must start within 8 h of injury, (3) 500–100 mg as directed by surgeon. *Peds:* Varies by indication: (1) 0.5–2 mg/kg/d, divide q12h IV/PO/IM, (2) 2 mg/kg/d load, then 2 mg/kg/d divided q6h IV/IM

Mechanism: See Hydrocortisone

Clearance: Hepatic metabolism; renal excretion

Comments: Potent glucocorticoid, relatively ↓ mineralocorticoid activity (see table "Relative Potencies of Commonly Administered Corticosteroids" under Hydrocortisone). As with other corticosteroids, dose-dependent association with GI bleeding, secondary infection, psychosis, hyperglycemia, and delayed wound healing. Use with caution with ↑ doses in severe infection, latent TB use the lowest effective dose

METHYLNALTREXONE (RELISTOR)

Indication: Indicated for treatment of opiate-induced constipation and failed laxative therapy

Dose: *<38 kg:* 0.15 mg/kg SC; *38–62 kg:* 8 mg (0.4 mL) SC; *62–114 kg:* 12 mg (0.6 mL) SC; *typical regimen:* Every other day but no more frequently than once/24 h

Mechanism: Peripherally acting mu opioid receptor antagonist. Does not cross blood–brain barrier

Clearance: Unknown metabolism. Excreted in urine/feces

Comments: Contraindicated in pts with known or suspected mechanical GI obstruction. In pts with severe renal impairment, ↓ dose by 50%. May cause diarrhea, abdominal pain, nausea, dizziness

METOCLOPRAMIDE (REGLAN)

Indication: Treatment of gastroparesis, antiemetic

Typical dose: *Adult:* 10–20 mg IV (near end of procedure for PONV prophylaxis) q6h. *Peds: 6–14 y:* 2.5–5 mg IV. *<6 y:* 0.1 mg/kg IV

Mechanism: Peripheral cholinomimetic, ↑ lower esophageal sphincter tone and upper GI motility/peristalsis without ↓ gastric pH. Dopamine antagonist in chemoreceptor trigger zone

Clearance: Hepatic metabolism, renal excretion

Comments: May cause extrapyramidal symptoms (i.e., acute dystonic reactions with involuntary muscle movement, potential laryngospasm) → rx with diphenhydramine. Rarely associated with neuroleptic malignant syndrome (presentation similar to malignant hyperthermia) and irreversible tardive dyskinesia. Rapid injection may cause anxiety. Avoid in intestinal obstruction, Parkinson's, pheochromocytoma; caution in hypertension, recent GI anastomoses, and with other drugs that can cause EPS. Transient ↑ in serum aldosterone → fluid retention (caution in CHF, cirrhotic pts). Prolongs QT interval

Naloxone (Narcan)

Indications: (1) Opiate overdose (severe/life threatening); (2) reversal of opiate respiratory depression; (3) treatment of opiate-induced pruritus

Dose: *Adult:* (1) 0.2–4 mg IV q2–3min prn (max 10 mg), then may infuse at 0.4 mg/h and titrate to effect; (2) 0.04–0.4 mg doses IV, titrated q2–3min. *Infusion:* Load 5 mcg/kg, infusion 2.5–160 mcg/kg/h; (3) 0.25 mcg/kg/h. *Peds:* (1) *Birth to 5 y:* <20 kg: 0.1 mg/kg IV q2–3min prn; *>5 y or >20 kg:* 2 mg/dose q2–3min prn; *infusion* same as adult. (2) 1–10 mcg/kg IV titrated q2–3min (up to 0.4 mg); (3) 0.25 mcg/kg/h

Onset: 1–2 min, **Duration:** 1–4 h, depends on route

Mechanism: Competitive inhibition of opioid receptors

Clearance: Hepatic metabolism (95%); primarily renal elimination

Comments: Precipitates opiate withdrawal in opioid-dependent pts; use smallest dose and titrate to desired respiratory rate and level of alertness. May cause hypertension, dysrhythmias, rare pulmonary edema, delirium, reversal of analgesia. "Re-narcotization" may occur because antagonist has short duration; monitor closely and redose as needed. Caution in hepatic failure and chronic cardiac dz

NITRIC OXIDE, INHALED (NO, iNO, INOMAX)

Indication: Neonatal hypoxic respiratory failure (congenital cardiac defects and pulmonary hypertension); also used for hypoxic respiratory failure, acute pulmonary hypertension and right heart failure in adults

Typical dose: *Adult:* 20–40 ppm (80 ppm also studied). *Peds:* 20 ppm. Wean slowly

Mechanism: Selective relaxation of pulmonary vasculature, improved arterial oxygenation

Clearance: Combines with oxyhemoglobin to produce methemoglobin and nitrate (nitrate quickly renally excreted)

Comments: Requires special equipment to administer. Do not discontinue abruptly. Little systemic hemodynamic effect. May cause ↑ bleeding by inhibition of platelet aggregation; dose-dependent methemoglobinemia especially with other nitrates (sodium nitroprusside, nitroglycerin). Caution in left ventricular dysfunction, may cause pulmonary edema. Expensive, adult clinical outcomes do not show clear benefit

---

OCTREOTIDE (SANDOSTATIN)

Indication: (1) Secretory neuroendocrine tumors (e.g., carcinoid), also used for (2) esophageal variceal and upper GI bleeding

Typical dose: (1) 100–600 mcg/d SC q6–12h, (2) 50 mcg IV bolus, then 25–50 mcg/h × 1–5 d

Mechanism: Somatostatin analogue (suppresses release of serotonin, gastrin, vasoactive intestinal peptide, insulin, glucagon, thyroid stimulating hormone, and secretin)

Clearance: Hepatic metabolism, renal excretion

Comments: May cause nausea, decreased GI motility, hypoglycemia or hyperglycemia, cholelithiasis, cholestatic hepatitis, hypothyroidism, arrhythmia including bradycardia, conduction abnormalities

---

OMEPRAZOLE (PRILOSEC)

Indication: GERD, GI ulcer, esophagitis, GI bleed prophylaxis

Typical dose: *Adults:* 20–40 mg PO daily. *Peds:* 0.6–0.7 mg/kg/d, max 3.3 mg/kg/d

Mechanism: Proton pump inhibitor, binds to H^+/K^+ ATPase (proton pump) in gastric parietal cells, blocking acid secretion

Clearance: Hepatic via P450 enzymes, renal elimination

Comments: Onset of action within 1 h, peak effect within 2 h. Inhibits some cytochrome P450 enzymes. For intravenous use, single enantiomer esomeprazole (Nexium) available in the United States.

ONDANSETRON (ZOFRAN)

See 5HT$_3$ Antagonists.

ANTIDIABETICS

Perioperative Considerations for Common Oral and Noninsulin Injectable Antidiabetic Medications				
Common Drugs	Class	Mechanism of Action	Hypo-glycemia	Comments
Metformin (Glucophage)	Biguanide	Improves insulin sensitivity, ↓ glucose production/ absorption	Rare	Rare ↑ lactic acidosis associated with renal dysfunction; avoid before/after IV contrast or in renal hypoperfusion
Sitagliptin (Januvia)	Dipeptidyl peptidase-4 (DPP-4) inhibitor	↑ Insulin secretion, ↓ glucagon secretion	Potential	May cause acute pancreatitis, angioedema, joint pain
Glyburide (DiaBeta) Glipizide (Glucotrol)	Sulfonylurea	↑ Insulin secretion, may ↓ gluconeogenesis	Potentially severe	Prolonged duration of action, unpredictable

Pioglitazone (Actos) Rosiglitazone (Avandia)	Thiazolidinedione	↑ Cell response to insulin, ↓ gluconeogenesis	Rare	May be associated with ↑ cardiac complications (especially rosiglitazone), fluid retention
Acarbose (Precose)	α-Glucosidase inhibitor	↓ GI absorption of carbohydrates		No benefit or effect on serum glucose if NPO.
Repaglinide (Prandin)	Glinide/ meglitinides	↑ Insulin secretion, especially early postprandial	Potential	
Exenatide (Byetta) Liraglutide (Victoza)	Glucagon-like peptide (GLP)-1 receptor agonist	↑ Insulin secretion, ↓ glucagon secretion	Rare	
Canagliflozin (Invokana)	Selective sodium-glucose transporter (SGLT)-2 inhibitor	↓ Glucose reabsorption in kidney		May cause polyuria, volume depletion

OXYTOCIN (PITOCIN)

Indication: (1) Treatment and (2) prophylaxis of postpartum hemorrhage, also used for labor induction
Typical dose: (1) 10–40 units IV in 1 L electrolyte solution, run at rate necessary to control atony, (2) 1–3 units IV bolus if low risk of uterine atony (e.g., elective caesarean delivery). Higher (5–10 units) or repeat doses may be required in prolonged or oxytocin augmented labor due to downregulation of receptors
Mechanism: Uterine stimulant, improves postpartum uterine atony
Clearance: Rapidly degraded in liver and kidneys
Comments: Structural similarity to antidiuretic hormone. May cause hypotension (caution in hypovolemia), tachycardia, nausea/vomiting, flushing, headache. Rarely, large doses may cause water retention, hyponatremia. In refractory atony with hemorrhage, consider other uterotonics: Methylergonovine, prostaglandins F2a (carboprost), and E$_1$ (misoprostol)

PHENYTOIN (DILANTIN)

Indication: (1) Status epilepticus; seizure prophylaxis, (2) arrhythmias (digoxin induced)
Typical dose: (1) *Adult:* Load 10–20 mg/kg IV at <50 mg/min (up to 1,000 mg cautiously, with ECG monitoring); maintenance: 300 mg/d or 5–6 mg/kg/d div q8h; for neurosurgical prophylaxis 100–200 mg IV q4h (at <50 mg/min). Use of prodrug fosphenytoin facilitates rapid loading in emergent situations (15–20 mg/kg IV at 100–150 mg/min). (2) 1.5 mg/kg or 50–100 mg IV at <50 mg/min q5–15min until dysrhythmia is abolished, side effects occur, or a maximal dose of 10–15 mg/kg is given. *Peds:* Load 15–20 mg/kg mg IV; maintenance: Age specific
Mechanism: Anticonvulsant effect via membrane stabilization, inhibiting depolarization. Antidysrhythmic effect, blocking calcium uptake during repolarization prolonging refractory period
Clearance: Hepatic metabolism; renal elimination (enhanced by alkaline urine)
Comments: Contraindicated in heart block, sinus bradycardia. May cause nystagmus, diplopia, ataxia, drowsiness, gingival hyperplasia, GI upset, hyperglycemia, or hepatic P450 enzyme induction. Asian pts with HLA-B*1502 have ↑ incidence severe dermatologic reaction (e.g., TEN, Stevens–Johnson syndrome). IV bolus may cause bradycardia, hypotension, cardiorespiratory arrest, or CNS depression. Venous irritant. Crosses the placenta. Significant variation in dose needed to achieve therapeutic concentration of 7.5–20.0 mcg/mL; measuring unbound levels may be helpful in pts with renal failure or hypoalbuminemia. Caution in renal and hepatic dz

PHOSPHORUS (PHOSPHO-SODA, NEUTRA-PHOS)

Indication: Hypophosphatemia
Typical Dose: 250–500 mg PO tid or 0.08–0.15 mmol/kg IV over 6–12 h

Mechanism: Electrolyte replacement
Clearance: Renal excretion (and reabsorption)
Comments: Risks of rapid IV infusion include hypocalcemia, hypotension, muscular irritability, calcium deposition, deteriorating renal function, hyperkalemia. Orders for IV phosphate preparations should be written in mmol (1 mmol = 31 mg). Use with caution in pts with cardiac dz and renal insufficiency. Do not give with magnesium- and aluminum-containing antacids or sucralfate, which can bind with phosphate. Causes osmotic diarrhea, may be used as bowel prep

PHYSOSTIGMINE (ANTILIRIUM)

Indication: Anticholinergic toxicity
Typical dose: *Adult:* 0.5–1 mg IV/IM (max rate 1 mg/min, max dose 2 mg). *Peds:* 0.02 mg/kg (max rate 0.5 mg/min, max dose 2 mg), repeat q5–10min if needed
Mechanism: Prolongs central and peripheral cholinergic effects; inhibits cholinesterase
Clearance: Plasma esterases
Comments: Crosses blood–brain barrier; therefore, useful for CNS anticholinergic toxicity (symptoms include delirium, somnolence, flushing, dry mouth, mydriasis, fever; occurs with administration of drugs including atropine and scopolamine, other tranquilizers and antihistamines). May cause bradycardia, tremor, convulsions, hallucinations, CNS depression, mild ganglionic blockade, or cholinergic crisis. Antagonized by atropine. Contains sulfite. Avoid in asthma, cardiovascular dz, intestinal/urologic obstruction

PIOGLITAZONE (ACTOS)

See Antidiabetics table on Chapter 2H 63–64.

POTASSIUM CHLORIDE (KCl, KDUR)

Indication: Hypokalemia
Typical dose: *Adult:* 20–40 mEq IV or PO q6–12, adjust dose to serum potassium levels. *Peds:* 0.5–2 mEq/kg PO q12h, 0.5 mEq/kg/h for 1–2 h (monitor closely)
Mechanism: Crucial for multiple physiologic processes including nerve conduction, myocardial contraction
Clearance: Renal
Comments: Indicated for hypokalemia, digoxin toxicity. IV bolus administration may cause cardiac arrest. Generally infuse at rate ≤10 mEq/h; may infuse 20 mEq/h with continuous ECG monitoring; can ↑ to max 40 mEq/h in urgent situations (serum level <2 mEq/L and/or ECG changes). Central line preferred route for concentrated solutions. May cause pain/phlebitis at injection site. Use potassium acetate instead in metabolic/hyperchloremic acidosis. PO administration may cause nausea, vomiting, delayed gastric emptying. Use caution in renal failure due to ↓ excretion capacity

PRASUGREL (EFFIENT)

Indication: Acute coronary syndrome, ↓ thrombotic cardiovascular events (including stent thrombosis)
Typical dose: 60 mg PO load, then 10 mg PO daily with aspirin
Mechanism: Thienopyridine, irreversible inhibition of platelet activation/aggregation through binding to ADP receptors
Clearance: Prodrug metabolized in intestine to active metabolite
Comments: Less inter-individual variability in effect than clopidogrel. Discontinuation is associated with ↑ cardiovascular events, especially with recent acute coronary syndrome. If possible, discontinue 7 d before surgery. Avoid neuraxial anesthesia for 7–10 d after discontinuation

PROCHLORPERAZINE (COMPAZINE)

Indication: (1) Severe nausea and vomiting, also used for psychosis
Typical dose: *Adults:* (1) 2.5–10 mg IV q3–4h or 5–10 mg PO q6–8h (max 40 mg/d). *Peds:* (1) 2.5 mg PO (max 7.5 mg/d if >2 y and 9–14 kg; max 10 mg/d if >2 y and 14–18 kg; max 15 mg/d if 18–39 kg; max 20 mg/d if >39 kg)
Mechanism: Phenothiazine with more antidopaminergic potency than promethazine
Clearance: Hepatic
Comments: May cause hypotension, excess sedation, extrapyramidal symptoms (acute dystonic reaction, rx with diphenhydramine); rarely associated with irreversible

tardive dyskinesia or neuroleptic malignant syndrome (presentation similar to malignant hyperthermia). Not for use in children <2 y, Parkinson's dz, or dementia-related psychosis

PROMETHAZINE (PHENERGAN)

Indication: (1) Rescue treatment in postoperative nausea and vomiting, (2) sedation, adjunct in anaphylaxis

Typical dose: *Adults:* (1) 6.25–12.5 mg IV/IM/PO, (2) 25–50 mg IV/IM/PO. *Peds:* 0.25–1 mg/kg PO/IV/IM q4–6h

Mechanism: Phenothiazine; potent antagonist of histamine (H1), also antagonizes dopaminergic, α-adrenergic, muscarinic receptors

Clearance: Hepatic

Comments: May cause sedation and respiratory depression, especially with use of narcotics or barbiturates (use lowest effective dose for PONV). Contraindicated in children <2 y due to risk of fatal respiratory depression. Avoid in Parkinson's, glaucoma, BPH. Caution in pulmonary dz, sleep apnea, seizures, bone marrow depression, sulfite allergy, elderly. Severe tissue damage/necrosis with extravasation or intra-arterial injection. May cause extrapyramidal symptoms (rx with diphenhydramine); rarely associated with neuroleptic malignant syndrome (presentation similar to malignant hyperthermia). Administer slowly to minimize risk of hypotension. Prolongs QT interval

PROSTAGLANDIN E₁ (ALPROSTADIL, PROSTIN VR)

Indication: Ductal-dependent and flow-restricting congenital cardiac defects (temporarily maintains patent ductus arteriosus until surgical correction)

Typical dose: Neonates: Starting dose 0.05–0.1 mcg/kg/min. Titrate to effect (typical 0.1–0.4 mcg/kg/min, max 0.6 mcg/kg/min). Usual dilution: 500 mcg/99 mL of NS or D5W = 5 mcg/mL

Mechanism: Vasodilation, inhibits platelet aggregation, vascular smooth muscle relaxation, and uterine and intestinal smooth muscle relaxation

Clearance: Rapid pulmonary metabolism; renal excretion

Comments: Used in pulmonary atresia/stenosis, tricuspid atresia, tetralogy of Fallot, coarct/interruption of aorta, transposition of great vessels. May cause hypotension, apnea (10–12%), flushing, and bradycardia. ↓ to lowest effective dose after observing ↑ in PaO₂ (in restricted pulmonary blood flow) or ↑ in pH, systemic blood pressure (in restricted systemic flow)

PROTAMINE SULFATE

Indication: (1) Heparin neutralization, (2) enoxaparin overdose

Typical dose: (1) Time elapsed since last heparin dose (see table—Dosing of Protamine for Heparin Reversal); based on ACT: 1.3 mg/100 U heparin calculated from ACT. Give via slow IV, <5 mg/min. (2) ~1 mg protamine/1 mg enoxaparin

Mechanism: Heparin antagonist. Polybasic compound combines with polyacidic heparin to form stable, inactive salt

Clearance: Fate of the heparin–protamine complex is unknown

Comments: May cause anaphylaxis, anaphylactoid reaction, severe pulmonary hypertension (particularly with rapid infusion after cardiopulmonary bypass), myocardial depression and peripheral vasodilation with sudden hypotension (secondary to histamine release) or bradycardia. Protamine–heparin complex antigenically active (particularly in pts receiving procaine and with fish allergy). Transient reversal of heparin may be followed by rebound heparinization. Can cause anticoagulation if given in excess relative to amount of circulating heparin (significance controversial). Monitor response with activated partial thromboplastin time or activated clotting time 5–15 min after dose. Only partially reverses enoxaparin

Dosing of Protamine for Heparin Reversal	
Time Elapsed (Since Last Heparin Dose)	**Protamine (mg) to Neutralize 100 U Heparin**
<30 min	1–1.5
30–60 min	0.5–0.75
60–120 min	0.375–0.5
>2 h	0.25–0.375

RECOMBINANT FACTOR VIIA (NOVOSEVEN)

See Factor VIIa.

REPAGLINIDE (PRANDIN)

See Antidiabetics table on Chapter 2H 63–64.

RIVAROXABAN (XARELTO)

Indication: (1) DVT prophylaxis after hip or knee replacement; (2) Stroke prophylaxis in atrial fibrillation; (3) DVT or PE treatment
Typical dose: (1) 10 mg PO daily; (2) 20 mg PO daily; (3) 15 mg PO q12h × 21 d, then 20 mg PO daily for 6 mo
Mechanism: Factor Xa inhibitor; does not require cofactor (e.g., antithrombin III)
Clearance: Hepatic (CYP3A4/5), renal
Comments: Adjust dose in renal dz. Hold at least 18 h before and 6 h after removal of epidural catheter; wait 24 h after traumatic neuraxial puncture before dosing. Not dialyzable. Can be reversed by andexanet alfa (Andexxa).

ROSIGLITAZONE (AVANDIA)

See Antidiabetics table on Chapter 2H 63–64.

SCOPOLAMINE PATCH (TRANSDERM SCÓP)

Indication: Prevention of postoperative nausea/vomiting
Typical dose: *Adult:* 1.5 mg/72 h. *Peds:* Not available. Patch cannot be cut. Apply to dry skin behind ear
Mechanism: Anticholinergic with peripheral and central muscarinic antagonism. May block transmission from vestibular nuclei to higher CNS centers and/or from reticular formation to vomiting center
Comments: Most effective for prophylactic use (instruct pts to apply night before and remove 24 h after surgery). Use care when handling patch: Contact with eyes may cause long-lasting mydriasis and cycloplegia. Common side effects include blurred vision, dizziness, dry mouth; may cause sedation, urinary retention, confusion. Avoid in glaucoma, seizures, intestinal obstruction; use with caution in elderly pts

---

SCOPOLAMINE INJECTION (HYOSCINE)

Indication: Pre-anesthetic sedation, antisialogogue, anesthetic adjunct
Comments: Previously used to provide amnesia during surgery in severe hypotension (i.e., exploratory trauma surgery with hemorrhagic shock). Sole US manufacturer discontinued production in 2015; no plans to resupply.

SILDENAFIL (VIAGRA, REVATIO)

Indication: (1) Pulmonary arterial hypertension. Also indicated in erectile dysfunction
Typical dose: 20 mg PO tid, 10 mg IV bolus tid
Mechanism: Inhibits phosphodiesterase Type 5, increasing cGMP to allow smooth muscle relaxation (pulmonary vasodilation)
Clearance: Hepatic metabolism (CYP3A4), biliary (83%) and renal (13%) excretion
Comments: Used in management of severe perioperative pulmonary hypertension and right ventricular dysfunction. Has both pulmonary and systemic vasodilatory effect. Avoid in hypotension, hypovolemia, autonomic dysfunction, pulmonary veno-occlusive dz. Potential for severe, refractory hypotension with organic nitrates (nitroglycerin, nitroprusside, isosorbide)

SITAGLIPTIN (JANUVIA)

See Antidiabetics table on Chapter 2H 63–64.

SPIRONOLACTONE (ALDACTONE)

See Diuretics table on Chapter 2H 54.

THAM

See Tromethamine.

TISSUE PLASMINOGEN ACTIVATOR (ALTEPLASE, ACTIVASE, TPA)

Indication: (1) Lysis of coronary arterial thrombi in hemodynamically unstable pts with acute MI, (2) management of acute massive PE in adults, (3) acute embolic stroke. Also used in (4) central venous catheter occlusion. *Typical dose:* (1) Load: 15 mg (30 mL of the infusion) IV over 1 min followed by 0.75 mg/kg (not to exceed 50 mg) given over 30 min. *Maintenance:* 0.5 mg/kg IV up to 35 mg/h for 1 h immediately following the loading dose. Total dose not to exceed 100 mg, (2) 100 mg IV continuous infusion over 2 h, (3) total dose of 0.9 mg/kg IV (maximum 90 mg); administer 10% as a bolus and the remainder over 60 min, (4) 2 mg in 2 mL instilled into occluded catheter, allow 30–120 min dwell time and may redose at 120 min. Remove via aspiration

Mechanism: Tissue plasminogen activator, generates plasmin and produces fibrinolysis

Clearance: Hepatic metabolism, renal excretion

Comments: Doses >150 mg have been associated with ↑ intracranial hemorrhage. Contraindicated with active internal bleeding, Hx of hemorrhagic stroke, intracranial neoplasm, aneurysm, or recent (within 2 mo) intracranial or intraspinal surgery, or trauma. Should be used with caution in pts who have received chest compressions or other anticoagulants and in hypertension, cerebrovascular dz, severe neurologic deficit, severe renal/hepatic dysfunction. Avoid IM injections, procedures involving arterial puncture (if possible) and central venous line placement at internal jugular/subclavian sites in pts who have recently received TPA

TRANEXAMIC ACID/TXA (CYKLOKAPRON)

Indication: (1) Hemophilia. Also used in cardiopulmonary bypass, spine surgery, liver transplant, (2) trauma

Typical dose: (1) 10 mg/kg q6–8h (up to 8 d postprocedure), (2) 1 g over 10 min, then 1 g over 8 h

Mechanism: Lysine analog. Inhibits fibrinolysis; competitive inhibitor of plasminogen inactivation, antiplasmin activity at high doses

Clearance: Renal excretion (>90% unchanged)

Comments: Mechanism similar to aminocaproic acid. May cause headache, visual changes, hypotension with rapid injection. May cause seizures. Reduce dose in renal failure. Associated with ↓ mortality in bleeding trauma pts when given within 3 h of injury (CRASH-2 trial, *Lancet* 2010;376(9734):23–32)

TROMETHAMINE (THAM ACETATE)

Indication: Metabolic acidosis associated with cardiac bypass surgery and cardiac arrest

Typical dose: mL of (0.3 M) solution = body weight (kg) × base deficit (mEq/L) × 1.1, given by IV infusion

Mechanism: Alkalinizing agent/organic buffer (pH 8.6). Actively binds H^+ ions. Binds not only cations of fixed and metabolic acids, but also hydrogen ions of carbonic acid, thus ↑ bicarbonate anion (HCO_3^-)

Clearance: Renal

Comments: Unlike bicarbonate, does not raise pCO_2. May be used in mixed respiratory/metabolic acidosis along with assisted ventilation. Also acts as an osmotic diuretic, increasing urine flow, urinary pH, and excretion of fixed acids, carbon dioxide and electrolytes. Avoid use in uremia, anuria (↓ excretion, potential hyperkalemia). Large doses may depress ventilation (↑ pH, ↓ CO_2). May cause severe tissue damage if extravasation occurs, hypoglycemia

VITAMIN K (PHYTONADIONE, AquaMEPHYTON)

Indication: Indicated for deficiency of vitamin K-dependent clotting factors, reversal of warfarin anticoagulation

Typical dose: See table below—"Guidelines on Treatment of Supratherapeutic Oral Anticoagulation," do not exceed 1 mg/min when giving IV infusion

Mechanism: Vitamin K is required for synthesis of clotting factors II, VII, IX, X

Clearance: Hepatic metabolism

Comments: INR may ↓ – within 4 h, effects peak at 24–48 h; high doses provide rapid reversal though make pt refractory to further oral anticoagulation (up to 7 d after 10 mg dose). May fail with hepatocellular dz. Rapid IV bolus can cause profound hypotension, fever, diaphoresis, bronchospasm, fatal anaphylaxis, and pain at injection site. Reserve IV administration for emergency use (serious or life-threatening bleeding, INR >20)

Guidelines on Treatment of Supratherapeutic Oral Anticoagulation	
INR <5 without significant bleeding	Lower or omit dose
INR 5–9 without significant bleeding	If rapid reversal required for urgent surgery, give ≤5 mg vitamin K PO, expect INR to be ↓ in 24 h. Can give additional 1–2 mg PO if needed
INR >9 without significant bleeding	Give 2.5–5 mg vitamin K PO, expect INR to be ↓ significantly in 24–48 h
Serious bleeding at any elevated INR	Give vitamin K 10 mg by slow IV infusion, supplement with FFP, PCC, or recombinant factor VIIa depending on urgency, vitamin K can be repeated q12h
Life-threatening bleeding	Give FFP, PCC, or recombinant factor VIIa with vitamin K, 10 mg by slow IV infusion. Repeat at 6–8 h if necessary

Source: Adapted from Ansell J, Hirsh J, Hylek E, et al. Pharmacology and management of the vitamin K antagonists: American College of Chest Physicians Evidence-Based Clinical Practice Guidelines. 8th ed. *Chest* 2008;133(6 Suppl): 160S–198S.

WARFARIN (COUMADIN)

Indication: Chronic anticoagulation in deep vein thrombosis, pulmonary embolism, atrial fibrillation, valve replacement

Typical dose: 2–15 mg/d (typically start 5 mg PO qd unless genotype available), individualize by monitoring INR (goal varies with indication)

Mechanism: Interferes with utilization of vitamin K by the liver and inhibits synthesis of factors II, VII, IX, X, proteins C & S, prothrombin

Clearance: Hepatic metabolism (influenced by P450 genetics, testing available); renal elimination

Comments: Narrow therapeutic range but varies required dose widely across pts, affected by many factors (diet, multiple drug interactions) within individuals. May cause fatal bleeding, skin necrosis. Contraindicated in severe renal or hepatic dz, GI ulcers, neurosurgical procedures, malignant HTN, pregnancy (teratogenic). Thrombostatic only, no lysis of existing thrombus

JESSE M. EHRENFELD • RICHARD D. URMAN

GAS SUPPLY

Oxygen: Path of Hospital Supply to Patient
Hospital supply to OR → O_2 pipeline supply inlet → anesthesia machine → O_2 pressure regulator → flowmeter → vaporizer → check valve → common gas outlet → fresh gas inlet → inspiratory one-way valve → breathing circuit inspiratory limb → Y-piece → endotracheal tube

Medical Gas Supply—Oxygen (O_2), Nitrous Oxide (N_2O), Air	
Central pipeline (wall source)	Linked to series or banks of high-capacity G- or H-size cylinders Diameter index safety system (DISS): ↓ Risk of incorrect tank–pipeline link
E-size cylinder (E-cylinder)	Portable source for transport; backup during pipeline failure Pin index safety system (PISS): ↓ Risk of improper E-cylinder–machine link

Properties of Compressed Gases and Color Coding of E-Cylinders (USA)			
Characteristic	Oxygen	Nitrous oxide	Air
Cylinder color	Green	Blue	Yellow
Physical state (at room temp)	Gas	Liquid and gas	Gas
Volume, full tank (L)	660	1,590	625
Pressure, full tank (psi)	2,200	750	1,800
Critical temp (°C)	–118	36.5	

Calculating remaining volume in E-cylinders (Boyle's law, $P_1V_1 = P_2V_2$ @ constant temp)
- **O_2 & Air:** *Pressure gauge reading reflects the volume of gas in the E-cylinder* Boyle's: O_2 gauge = 300 psi → liters O_2 left = 660 L × (300 psi/2,200 psi) = 90 L "Estimate:" [psi × 0.3]: O_2 gauge = 300 psi → liters O_2 left = (300 psi × 0.3) = 90 L
- **N_2O:** If liquid N_2O remains, pressure = 750 psi → *weigh tank to assess N_2O volume* Liters of N_2O in tank ~ (N_2O liquid weight in grams/44 g) × 0.5 L
  If only N_2O gas in tank (~25% N_2O left) → pressure falls <750 psi → calc per Boyle's

ANESTHESIA MACHINE
([1]SEE APPENDIX B FOR CHECKOUT RECOMMENDATIONS)

Flow Control in the Anesthesia Machine
Pressure Regulators • 1st-stage: Limit pipeline (50 psi) & cylinder (45 psi) pressures; pressure gradient ensures use of pipeline O_2 preferentially over cylinder O_2 when both are open • 2nd-stage: Maintains gas flow at a constant pressure to flowmeters (usu ~14 psi)
Flow Valves • Check valves: One-way valves (when present) stop retrograde flow into vaporizers   • If present, perform a negative pressure test to detect low-pressure circuit leaks • O_2 flush valve delivers high-flow (35–75 L/min) O_2 to common gas outlet, bypassing flowmeters & vaporizers → potential for barotrauma
Flowmeters • Hollow glass tubes with gradually ↑ inner diameter containing a "float" (e.g., ball) • Agent-specific per gas viscosity & density; calibrated individually to control flow rate • **O_2 flowmeter: Always placed downstream of other gas flow (closest to pt)** to minimize the risk of hypoxic delivery in case of an upstream flowmeter leak • At low flow rates, **laminar** gas flow: 3.14 × (radius)^4/(8 × length × **viscosity**) • At high flow rates, **turbulent** gas flow: Flow rate related to **density** (not viscosity)
Common Fresh Gas Outlet • Outflow from anesthesia machine: Blend of carrier gas and volatile anesthetic(s)

[1]See Appendix B for setting up the OR for an anesthesia case and other mnemonics.

Features to Prevent Delivery of Hypoxic Gas Mixtures	
O₂ supply pressure alarm	Alarms if O₂ supply pressure <30 psi
"Fail-safe" valve	Stop or ↓ N₂O flow in the event of low O₂ supply (<20 psi)
Mechanically coupled O₂ & N₂O flowmeters	Allows max 3:1 ratio of N₂O/O₂; maintains min FiO₂ of 0.25
Downstream O₂ flowmeter	Maintains delivery of O₂ despite a leak in an upstream flowmeter
O₂ analyzer	Important because it is the **only** machine monitor of low-pressure system integrity downstream from the flowmeters

Vaporizers

General Principles
- Agent-specific with regard to vapor pressure (VP), specific heat, & thermal conductivity
  - VP is determined by temp and physical properties of liquid
- Variable bypass—total gas flow is split into carrier & bypass gas flows
  - Concentration dial controls ratio of gas entering & bypassing vaporization chamber
  - Carrier gas: Flows over liquid agent in vaporizing chamber & saturates with agent; The carrier gas "carries" volatile agent to vaporizer outlet
  - Bypass gas: Exits vaporizer unchanged
  - Two flows mix at the vaporizer outlet & exit machine at common fresh gas outlet

Vaporizer Potential Hazards
- Agent with higher VP in a vaporizer designed for agent with lower VP → overdose
- Tipping of vaporizer: Liquid agent enters bypass chamber → ↑↑ output → overdose
- At very low (not pushing agent) or high (not saturated) flows: Output will be < dial setting
- "Pumping effect": Positive-pressure ventilation or use of O₂ flush valve → gas compressed by back pressure → gas released via bypass chamber → overdose

Desflurane Vaporizer (Tec 6)—Gas/vapor blender, not variable bypass
- Desflurane VP is high (~660 mmHg), almost boils at room temp
- Tec 6 maintains constant reservoir of 2 atm vapor regardless of ambient pressure
- Shut-off valve only opens when vaporizer is warmed up and conc. dial is on
- Higher altitudes = ↓ partial pressure, so ↑ conc. dial for same effect as at sea level

Ventilators

General Principles
- Most bellows ventilators are pneumatically driven by O₂ (double-circuit ventilators)
  - Driving gas circuit: Provides driving force for ventilator bellows & machine
  - Pt gas circuit: Gas supply to pt
- Inspiration: Pressurized O₂ from driving circuit fills space inside rigid container containing compressible bellows → bellows empty
  - Inspiratory time: Based on set tidal volume, inspiratory flow & respiratory rates
  - Termination of inhalation: Time-cycled and/or pressure limited
- Exhalation:
  - Ascending bellows: Rise during exhalation; will not rise if circuit disconnect/leak
  - Descending bellows: Hang during exhalation; fills by gravity even if leak/disconnect
- Fresh gas flow (FGF) decoupling (on most ventilators except older models):
  - Inspiration: FGF → reservoir bag
  - Exhalation: Bellows refill from reservoir & FGF
  - Therefore, FGF does not influence tidal volume delivered to pt

Ventilator Hazards
- Leaks & disconnects: Connection sites (esp. pt Y-connector), loose or cracked bellows, incompetent system components (e.g., scavenger system, pop-off valve)
  - Detection: **ETCO₂** monitor is most sensitive (↓ or no ETCO₂)
  - Also detected if set high/low values on adjustable pressure/resp. volume monitor
- Scenarios where **excessive positive pressure** leads to ↑ risk of barotrauma
  - Oxygen flush valve during inhalation: Scavenger spill valve is closed
  - Obstructed scavenger system: Kinked hose or stuck spill valve
  - Hole in bellows: Delivery of high driving gas pressures to pt
  - Ventilator stuck in inspiratory mode
- Excessive negative pressure:
  - Excessive suction on scavenging system
  - Naso- or orogastric suction catheter in trachea
  - Rapid descent of hanging bellows

- Causes of machine-set & delivered **tidal volume discrepancies**:
  - Leaks, breathing circuit compliance, gas compression, ventilator—FGF coupling
- No-flow states:
  - Disconnect (see above) or obstruction of ETT or circuit tubing
  - Loss of pipeline and cylinder gas sources
  - Misconnection of ventilator hose to nongas source
  - Ball-type positive end-expiratory pressure (PEEP) valve in inspiratory limb

Ventilator Alarms
- "Disconnect" alarms: Low peak insp. pressure (PIP), low tidal volume, low ETCO$_2$
- High PIP, high PEEP, sustained high airway pressure, negative pressure, & low O$_2$

BREATHING CIRCUIT: CONNECTS ANESTHESIA MACHINE TO PATIENT

Circle System Components—prevents rebreathing of exhaled CO$_2$ (Fig. 3-1)
- Reservoir bag: Reserve gas volume
- Oxygen analyzer: Measures inspired/expired O$_2$
- Adjustable pressure limiting valve (APL or pop-off valve):
  Can be adjusted to facilitate manual bag compression to assist ventilation of pt's lungs
  Allows venting of excess gas to waste scavenging system
- Bag/ventilator switch: Excludes or includes the reservoir bag & APL from system
- Inspiratory one-way valve:
  Open during **inspiration** & closed during expiration
  Prevents expiratory gas from mixing with fresh gas in inspiratory limb
- Expiratory one-way valve:
  Open during **expiration** & closed during inspiration
  Gas is then either vented through APL valve or passes to CO$_2$ absorber
- CO$_2$ absorbent: Removes CO$_2$ from breathing circuit (chemical neutralization)
  Soda lime is most common: Ca(OH)$_2$ (75%), H$_2$O (20%), NaOH (3%), KOH (1%)

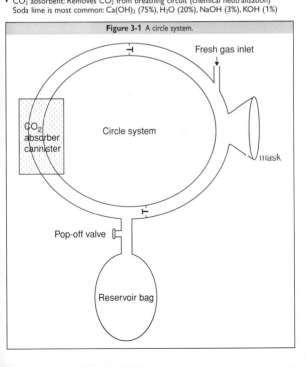

Figure 3-1 A circle system.

CO$_2$ Neutralization Reaction
CO$_2$ + H$_2$O → H$_2$CO$_3$
H$_2$CO$_3$ + 2NaOH → Na$_2$CO$_3$ + 2H$_2$O + heat
Na$_2$CO$_3$ + Ca(OH)$_2$ → CaCO$_3$ + 2NaOH

- Spirometer: Measures exhaled tidal volume & respiratory rate
- Circuit pressure gauge: Measures circuit airway pressure in cm H$_2$O

Waste Gas Scavenging System—Prevents OR Pollution	
Waste gas collecting assembly, transfer, & gas disposal tubing	
Waste gas scavenging interface	Closed to room: Requires pressure-relief valve
	Open: Does not require pressure-relief valve
Disposal assembly	Passive: Disposal tubing → outside ventilation duct
	Active: Disposal tubing → hospital vacuum system

U.S. National Institute of Occupational Safety and Health (NIOSH) Limits	
Agents	Parts per million (ppm) in ambient air
N$_2$O alone	25 ppm
Halogenated agents without N$_2$O	2 ppm
Halogenated agents with N$_2$O	0.5 ppm

Anesthesia Machine Leak Tests
Positive pressure test
Tests integrity of circuit from flowmeter to pt, unless check valves are present
1. Set all gas flows to zero (or minimum)
2. Close APL (pop-off valve) & occlude Y-connector
3. Pressurize breathing system to about 30 cm H$_2$O with O$_2$ flush
4. Ensure reservoir bag inflates and pressure stays constant for at least 10 s. If leak is present, check bellows, connections, etc. (see ventilator hazards, above)
5. Open APL (pop-off) valve & ensure pressure drops
Negative pressure test
Proper method to check for flowmeter leaks if check valves are present in the machine
1. Verify machine master switch & flow control valves are **off**
2. Attach suction bulb to common fresh gas outlet
3. Squeeze bulb until fully collapsed; verify bulb stays collapsed for >10 s
4. Open one vaporizer at a time & repeat step 3
5. Remove suction bulb & reconnect fresh gas hose; turn off open vaporizer

Closed-Circuit Anesthesia
- Use of FGFs exactly equal to the uptake of oxygen and anesthetic agents
- Requires (1) very low FGF, (2) total rebreathing of exhaled gases after absorption of carbon dioxide by CO$_2$ absorber, (3) closed APL or ventilator relief valve
- Advantages: ↑ Heat & humidification of gases; ↓ pollution & agent use; ↓ cost
- Disadvantages: ↓ Rate of agent concentration change; may cause hypoxic/hypercarbic mix; risk of excessive agent concentration

Airway Pressures
- Airway pressure = airway resistance + alveolar press. (i.e., chest & lung compliance)
- PIP = highest pressure in circuit during inspiration
- Plateau pressure = pressure during inspiratory pause (measures static compliance)

Some Causes of Increased Peak Inspiratory and Plateau Airway Pressures	
↑ PIP & ↑ Plateau Pressure	**↑ PIP & Unchanged Plateau Pressure**
1. ↑ Tidal volume	1. ↑ Inspiratory gas flow rate
2. ↓ **Chest/pulmonary compliance** (↑ static compliance)	2. ↑ **Airway resistance** (↓ dynamic compliance)
- *Above the diaphragm:*	- *Mechanical causes:*
• Pulmonary edema	• Kinked airway device (e.g., ETT)
• Pleural effusion	• Airway compression
• Tension pneumothorax	• Foreign body aspiration
• Endobronchial intubation	• Vocal cord paralysis
• Pneumonia	• Endotracheal/endobronchial mass

• Below the diaphragm:
  • Intra-abdominal packing/insufflation
  • Trendelenburg position
  • Ascites
	• *Physiologic causes:*
	  • Bronchospasm
	  • Secretions

Management of Increased Airway Pressures
- Inspiratory pressures >~40 cm H_2O should be treated as abnormal
- Check anesthetic equipment, airway device, & pt (see causes, above)

Systematic Approach to Troubleshooting Increased Airway Pressures
Anesthetic Equipment
• Check O_2 supply & all connections, including breathing circuit & Y-connector
• Hand-ventilate pt with self-inflating resuscitation bag
• If difficult, obstruction is at airway device &/or pt
Airway Device
• Assess whether airway device is kinked or obstructed
• Pass soft suction catheter down airway device to clear secretions
• Use fiberoptic bronchoscope with suction capability to assess ETT & clear secretions
Patient
• Lungs: Observe bilateral chest expansion, auscultate chest bilaterally
• Unilateral breath sounds may be due to endobronchial ETT or pneumothorax
• Wheezing or diminished breath sounds: Bronchospasm, aspiration, pulm edema
• Can use fiberoptic bronchoscope to assess airway for compression (e.g., masses)
• Check intra-abdominal gas insufflation pressure; communicate with surgeon

Open Breathing Systems (Historical, Not Typically Used in Modern Medicine)
- Insufflation: Blowing of anesthetic gas across pt's face
- Open-drop anesthesia: Volatile anesthetic dripped onto gauze mask on pt's face

Mapleson Breathing Circuits A to E: Five Systems Described in 1950s
- Differ in fresh gas tubing, mask, reservoir bag & tubing, & expiratory valve locations
- Characterized by (1) no valves directing gases to & from pt, (2) no CO_2 neutralization
- Mapleson **A** circuit = most efficient for spont**A**neous ventilation (Fig. 3-2)
  - FGF = minute ventilation, which is sufficient to prevent CO_2 rebreathing

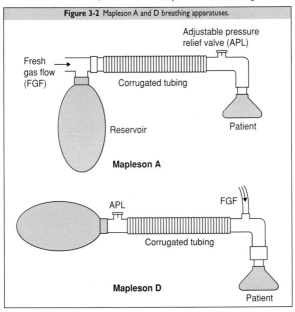

Figure 3-2 Mapleson A and D breathing apparatuses.

- Mapleson **D** circuit = most efficient for controlle **D** ventilation, most commonly used
  - FGF forces alveolar gas away from pt & toward pressure release valve

Bain Circuit: Modification of Mapleson D
- Fresh gas supply runs coaxially inside corrugated expiratory tubing
- Advantages: Compact, portable, easy scavenging, exhaled gases warm inhaled gases
- Disadvantages: Risk of kinking/disconnect of coaxial tubing (i.e., fresh gas inlet)

ELECTRICAL SAFETY IN THE OR

Electrosurgery
- Surgical diathermy: High-frequency alternating current to cut/cauterize blood vessels
  - Electrosurgical units (ESUs) generate high-frequency current; tip of small electrode
    → through pt → out large electrode (dispersion pad)
- Malfunction of dispersion pad: Inadequate contact/conducting gel/disconnect
  - Current will exit pt through alternate path (ECG pads, OR table) & may burn pt
- Bipolar electrodes limit current propagation to a few millimeters
- ESU may interfere with pacemaker & ECG recordings

Risk of Electrocution
- Contact with two conductive materials at different voltage potentials may complete
  circuit & result in electric shock
- Leakage current is present in all electrical equipment
  - Fibrillation threshold at skin is 100 mA
  - Current as low as 100 μA applied directly to heart may be fatal

Macroshock: Current applied at skin	Microshock: Current applied inside body
100 mA = cause V-fib	**100 μA** = cause V-fib
10 mA = painful, aversive stimulus	10 μA = max leakage of current
1 mA = perception of shock	

Ungrounded Power & Protection from Electric Shock
- Isolation transformer: Isolates OR power supply from ground potential (i.e., OR
  power supply is ungrounded)
  - If live wire contacts grounded pt, isolation transformer prevents current flow to pt
  - Building regulations may no longer require ORs to have isolated power systems
- Line isolation monitors (LIMs): Monitors the degree of isolation between the power
  lines and the ground
  - Alarm sounds if unacceptable current flow (≥5 mA) to ground becomes possible
    → unplug most recently plugged in piece of equipment
  - Alarm does *not* interrupt power unless ground leakage circuit breaker activated
  - **LIMs protect against macroshock but NOT *microshock*** (risk of microshock
    is decreased by grounded equipment, i.e., ground wire)

JESSE M. EHRENFELD • RICHARD D. URMAN

INTRODUCTION

Airway Anatomy	
Pharynx	Divided into nasopharynx, oropharynx, & laryngopharynx
Epiglottis	Separates laryngopharynx into hypopharynx (to esophagus) & larynx (to trachea)
Larynx	(C4–C6); laryngeal skeleton consists of 9 cartilages: 3 paired (corniculates, arytenoids, cuneiforms) & 3 unpaired (epiglottis, thyroid, cricoid); protects respiratory tract entrance & allows phonation
Thyroid cartilage	Largest & most prominent for lateral & anterior walls
Cricothyroid membrane	Connects thyroid & cricoid cartilage; ≈ 1–1.5 fb below laryngeal prominence; any incisions/needle punctures should be made in inferior 1/3 & directed posteriorly (due to cricothyroid arteries & vocal folds)
Cricoid cartilage	(C5–C6); shaped like signet ring, inferior to thyroid cartilage only, complete cartilaginous ring along laryngotracheal tree
Arytenoids	Originate on posterior aspect of larynx & posterior attachments of vocal cords May be the only visible structures in pts with an "anterior" airway
Laryngeal muscles	Lateral cricoarytenoid (adduction), posterior cricoarytenoid (abduction), transverse arytenoids → open/close the glottis, Cricothyroid, thyroarytenoid, vocalis → control vocal ligament tension

Airway Innervation—Sensory	
Glossopharyngeal nerve (CN IX)	Posterior third of tongue, oropharynx from nasopharyngeal surface to junction of pharynx & epiglottis, including vallecula; tonsillar area; gag reflex
Superior laryngeal nerve, internal branch (CN X/vagus)	Mucosa from epiglottis to vocal cords (sensory innervation of larynx above vocal cords), including base of tongue, supraglottic mucosa, cricothyroid joint
Superior laryngeal nerve, external branch (CN X/vagus)	Anterior subglottic mucosa
Recurrent laryngeal nerve (CN X/vagus)	Subglottic mucosa, muscle spindles
Trigeminal nerve (CN V)	Nares & nasopharynx

Airway Innervation—Motor	
Superior laryngeal nerve, external branch (CN X/vagus)	Cricothyroid muscles → tensing of vocal cords, inferior pharyngeal constrictors
Recurrent laryngeal nerve (CN X/vagus)	All other intrinsic muscles of larynx: Thyroarytenoid, lateral cricoarytenoid, interarytenoid, posterior cricoarytenoid
Glossopharyngeal (CN IX) & superior laryngeal, internal branch (CN X/vagus)	No motor innervational contribution

Note: All laryngeal innervation is by 2 branches of vagus: Superior laryngeal & recurrent laryngeal nerves.

- Injury of SLN (external branch) → hoarseness
- Injury of RLN → unilateral paralysis → paralysis of ipsilateral vocal cord → hoarse voice; bilateral paralysis → stridor & respiratory distress

AIRWAY ASSESSMENT

- Hx
  - Adverse events related to prior airway management
  - Radiation/surgical hx
  - Burns/swelling/tumor/masses
  - Obstructive sleep apnea (snoring)
  - Temporomandibular joint dysfunction
  - Dysphagia
  - Problems with phonation
  - C-spine dz (disk dz, osteoarthritis, rheumatoid arthritis, Down syndrome)
- Physical examination
  - Mallampati score (see also Chapter 1, Preoperative Patient Evaluation)
  - Symmetry of mouth opening
  - Loose/missing/cracked/implanted teeth
  - Macroglossia (associated with difficult laryngoscopy)
  - High-arched palate (associated with difficulty visualizing larynx)
  - Mandible size
    - Thyromental distance <3 fingerbreadths (fb) suggests poor laryngeal visualization
  - Neck examination
    - Prior surgeries/tracheostomy scars
    - Abnormal masses (hematoma, abscess, goiter, tumor) or tracheal deviation
    - Neck circumference & length
    - Range of motion (flexion/extension/rotation)

Signs of a Potentially Difficult Airway	
• Abnormal face shape	• Narrow mouth
• Sunken cheeks	• Obesity
• Edentulous	• Receding mandible
• "Buck teeth"	• Facial/neck pathology
• Mouth opening <3 fb	• Thyroid cartilage–mouth floor distance <2 fb
• Hyoid–chin distance <3 fb	
• Mallampati classes III & IV	
• Pathology around upper airway (peritonsillar abscess)	
• Limited range of motion	

Regional vs. General Anesthesia in Difficult Airway Patients	
Consider Regional	**Do Not Consider Regional**
Superficial surgery	Invasive surgery
Minimal sedation needed	Significant sedation required
Anesthetic may be provided with local	Extensive local will be required or risk of intravascular injection is high
Good airway access	Poor airway access
Surgery may be stopped at any time	Surgery cannot be stopped after start

Source: Adapted from Barash PG, Cullen BF, Stoelting RK, et al. *Clinical Anesthesia.* 5th ed. Philadelphia, PA: Lippincott Williams & Wilkins; 2005, with permission.

AIRWAY DEVICES

- Oral and nasal airways
  - Typically inserted secondary to loss of upper airway muscle tone in anesthetized pts → usu. caused by tongue/epiglottis falling against posterior pharyngeal wall
  - Length of nasal airway estimated by measuring from nares to meatus of ear
  - Use caution with insertion in pts on anticoagulation or with basilar skull fractures
- Mask airway
  - Facilitates O_2 delivery (denitrogenation) & anesthetic gas using airtight seal
  - Hold mask with left hand while right hand generates positive-pressure ventilation → (use <20 cm H_2O to avoid gastric inflation)
  - One-handed technique
    - Fit snugly around bridge of nose to below bottom lip
    - Downward pressure with left thumb & index finger, middle, & ring finger; grasp the mandible while pinky finger is placed under angle of jaw to thrust anteriorly

- Two-handed technique
  - Used in difficult ventilatory situations
  - Bilateral thumbs hold mask down while fingertips displace jaw anteriorly
- Edentulous pts may be a challenge to ventilate (difficult to create a mask seal)
  → consider leaving dentures in place, oral airway, buccal cavity gauze packing
- **Difficult mask ventilation: Maneuvers to maintain airway patency**
  - Call for additional help (have someone else squeeze bag)
  - Insert oral and/or nasal airways
  - Extend neck & rotate head
  - Perform jaw thrust

Independent Risk Factors for Difficult Mask Ventilation
• Presence of a beard
• Body mass index >26 kg/m^2
• Lack of teeth
• Age >55
• Hx of snoring

Source: Langeron O. Prediction of difficult mask ventilation. Anesthesiology 2000;92:1229.

- Supraglottic airways (laryngeal mask airways [LMAs])
  - Insertion technique
    - Pt placed in sniffing position
    - Deflated LMA cuff is lubricated & inserted blindly to hypopharynx
    - Cuff is inflated to create a seal around entrance to larynx
    - (Tip rests over upper esophageal sphincter, cuff upper border against base of tongue, sides lying over pyriform fossae)
  - Indications
    - Alternative to endotracheal intubation (not as a replacement) or mask ventilation
    - Rescue device in expected/unexpected difficult airway
    - Conduit for intubating stylet, flexible FOB, or small-diameter ET
  - Contraindications: Pharyngeal pathology, obstruction, high aspiration risk, low pulmonary compliance (need peak inspiratory pressures >20 cm H_2O), long surgeries
  - Disadvantages: Do not protect the airway, can become dislodged

Laryngeal Mask Airway Models		
Type	**Description**	**Advantage**
Disposable LMA	Most commonly used. Adults: Size #3–5	Alternative to ET intubation, useful in unexpectedly difficult airways
Flexible LMA	Thin-walled, small-diameter, wire-reinforced barrel that can be positioned out of midline	Kink-resistant
ProSeal LMA	Includes a gastric drain, posterior cuff to allow positive-pressure ventilation with 40 cm H_2O	Allows positive-pressure ventilation, protection from aspiration
Fastrach LMA	Cuff, epiglottic elevating bar, airway tube, handle, flexible endotracheal tube	Allows blind intubation in difficult airways ± fiberscope
i-gel LMA	Shape more accurately mirrors the perilaryngeal anatomy. No cuff.	Integrated bite block No cuff inflation required

- Endotracheal Tubes (ETTs)
  - Used to deliver anesthetic gas directly to trachea & provide controlled ventilation
  - Modified for a variety of specialized applications: Flexible, spiral-wound, wire-reinforced (armored), rubber, microlaryngeal, oral/nasal RAE (preformed), double-lumen tubes
  - Airflow resistance depends on tube diameter, curvature, length
  - All ETTs have an imprinted line that is opaque on radiographs

Oral Tracheal Tube Sizing		
Age	Internal Diameter (mm)	Tube Length at Lip (cm)
Full-term infant	3.5	12
Child	4 + age/4	14 + age/2
Adult		
Female	7.0–7.5	20
Male	7.5–8.5	22

- Rigid laryngoscopes: Used to examine larynx & facilitate tracheal intubation
  - Macintosh blade (curved): Tip inserted into vallecula; use size-3 blade for most adults
  - Miller blade (straight): Tip inserted beneath laryngeal surface of epiglottis; use size-2 blade for most adults
  - Modified laryngoscopes: Wu, Bullard, & Glidescope for use in difficult airways
- Flexible fiberoptic bronchoscopes
  - Indications: Potentially difficult laryngoscopy/mask ventilation, unstable cervical spines, poor cervical range of motion, TMJ dysfunction, congenital/acquired upper airway anomalies
- Light wand
  - Malleable stylet with light emanating from distal tip, over which ETT is inserted
  - Dim lights in OR & advanced wand blindly
    - Glow in lateral neck → tip in pyriform fossa
    - Glow in the anterior neck → correctly positioned in trachea
    - Glow diminishes significantly → tip likely in esophagus
- Retrograde tracheal intubation
  - Performed in awake & spontaneously ventilating pts
  - Puncture cricothyroid membrane with 18G needle
  - Introduce guidewire & advanced cephalad (use 80 cm, 0.025 in. wire)
  - Visualize wire with direct laryngoscopy & guide ETT through vocal cords
- Airway bougie
  - Solid or hollow, semimalleable stylets usually passed blindly into trachea
  - ETT is threaded over bougie into trachea; can feel "clicking" as passes over tracheal rings
  - May have internal lumen to allow for insufflation of O_2 & detection of CO_2
- Video laryngoscopes (Glidescope®, Storz® V-Mac™, and McGrath®)
  - Usually a MAC style blade with a camera at the distal tip attached to a mobile video screen
  - Assists with anterior airways, useful in obese pt; usually improves the view of the glottic opening; however, sometimes difficult to pass the ETT, unless a curved stylet is utilized

Required Equipment for Intubation
O_2, positive-pressure ventilation source (ventilator) & backups (bag–valve–mask/E-cylinder)
Face masks
Oropharyngeal & nasopharyngeal airways
Tracheal tubes & stylets
Syringe (10 mL) for inflation of tracheal tube cuff
Suction
Laryngoscope handles
Laryngoscope blades (Mac & Miller)
Flexible bougie
Pillow, towel, blanket for pt positioning
Stethoscope
Capnograph or end-tidal CO_2 detector

AIRWAY MANAGEMENT: OROTRACHEAL INTUBATION

- Elevate height of bed to laryngoscopist's xiphoid process
- Place pt in *sniffing position*: Neck flexion, head extension; aligns oral, pharyngeal, & laryngeal axes to provide the straightest view from lips to glottis
- Preoxygenate with 100% O_2
- Induce anesthesia

- Tape pt's eyes shut to prevent corneal abrasions
- Hold laryngoscope in left hand, scissoring mouth with right thumb & index finger
    - → Insert laryngoscope in the right side of mouth, sweeping tongue to the left
    - → Advance until glottis appears in view
    - → Never use laryngoscope as a lever in a pivoting motion (instead lift "up and away")
- Using the right hand, pass ETT tip through vocal cords under direct visualization
- Inflate ETT cuff with least amount of air necessary to create seal during positive-pressure ventilation
- Confirm correct placement of ETT with (1) chest auscultation, (2) $ETCO_2$, (3) ETT condensation, (4) palpation of ETT cuff in sternal notch
- *Earliest manifestation of bronchial intubation is ↑ peak pressure (right main stem bronchus common)*
- **Rapid sequence induction**
    - Indication: Pts at ↑ risk for aspiration (full stomach, pregnant, GERD, morbidly obese, bowel obstruction, delayed gastric emptying, pain, diabetic gastroparesis)
    - Use rapid paralyzing agent: Succinylcholine (1–1.5 mg/kg) or rocuronium (0.6–1.2 mg/kg)
    - Place cricoid pressure (Sellick maneuver) as pt is induced
        - Protect from regurgitation of gastric contents to oropharynx
        - Help visualize vocal cords during laryngoscopy
    - Intubate pt once paralytic takes effect (30–60 s); do **not** ventilate pt during this time
    - Proper cricoid pressure should be performed using "BURP" technique:
        - Displace larynx **(B)**ackward, **(U)**pward, **(R)**ight, with **(P)**ressure
- **"Modified" rapid sequence induction & intubation***
    - A variation of the standard RSI technique in which a mask airway is established **prior** to administration of a paralytic agent
    - May also include the use of nondepolarizing agent (pts with ↑ K^+)

AIRWAY MANAGEMENT: NASOTRACHEAL INTUBATION

- Indications: Intraoral, facial/mandibular procedures
- Contraindications: Basilar skull fractures, nasal fractures or polyps, underlying coagulopathies
- Preparation: Anesthetize & vasoconstrict mucosa with lidocaine/phenylephrine mix or cocaine → select nares that pt can breathe through most easily
- Lubricated ETT is advanced perpendicular to face below inferior turbinate via selected nares → direct bevel laterally away from turbinates
- Advance ETT until able to visualize tip in oropharynx under direct laryngoscopy → use Magill forceps with right hand to advance/direct through vocal cords

---

AIRWAY MANAGEMENT: AWAKE FLEXIBLE FIBEROPTIC INTUBATION

- Equipment: Ovassapian/Williams/Luomanen airway, topical anesthetics, vasoconstrictors, antisialogogues, suction, fiberoptic scope with lubricated ETT
- Indications: Cervical spine pathology, obesity, head & neck tumors, difficult airway hx
- Premedication: Sedation (midazolam, fentanyl, dexmedetomidine, ketamine)
- Technique:
    - **Take time to topicalize airway** (key to success; see Table—Nerve Blocks to Anesthetize the Airway)
    - Place special oral airway or grab tongue with gauze
    - Keep fiberoptic scope in midline while advancing until epiglottis appears
    - Advance scope beneath epiglottis using antero/retroflexion as needed
    - Once vocal cords are visualized, advanced off scope into trachea
    - Stabilized scope while ETT is advanced off scope into trachea → If resistance is encountered, rotate ETT tube 90°
    - After insertion, visualize carina with scope to avoid endobronchial intubation

---

*Ehrenfeld JM, Cassedy EA, Forbes VE, et al. Modified rapid sequence induction and intubation: a survey of United States current practice. Anesth Analg 2012 Jul; 115(1):95–101.

Nerve Blocks to Anesthetize the Airway

Topical anesthesia for tongue/oropharynx
- Cetacaine spray (tetracaine/benzocaine combination)
- → Benzocaine toxicity occurs at ≈100 mg; can lead to methemoglobinemia (tx with methylene blue)
- Viscous lidocaine: 2–4 mL, swish & swallow
- Nebulized lidocaine: 4%, 4 mL for 5–10 min (or atomizer)
- Lidocaine jelly: 2% on tongue blade, peaks in 5–10 min

Superior laryngeal nerve block (sensory innervation to epiglottis, arytenoids, & vocal cords)
- Laterally displace hyoid bone toward block side, direct 22G needle to lateral portion of hyoid bone
- Withdraw slightly & walk off bone inferiorly (below each greater cornu)
- Advance through thyrohyoid membrane (may feel loss of resistance)
- Aspirate & inject 2 mL of 2% lidocaine superficial & deep to membrane

Transtracheal block (recurrent laryngeal nerve)
- Penetrate cricothyroid membrane with 22-gauge plastic catheter, 10-mL syringe
- After aspirating air, remove needle & attach a syringe with 4 mL of 4% lidocaine
- Inject at end of expiration to anesthetize glottis & upper trachea

Recurrent laryngeal nerve block
- Aim for ipsilateral lesser cornu thyroid cartilage in tracheoesophageal groove
- Insert needle perpendicular to pt directing it medially, contacting lesser cornu of thyroid cartilage
- Once reached, withdraw needle slightly & inject

Glossopharyngeal nerve block (posterior third of tongue)
- Inject 2 mL 1–2% lidocaine in glossopharyngeal arch

	Practical Approach to Unanticipated Difficult Airway
Plan A	• Standard laryngoscopy with blade of choice • If unable to intubate → make 2nd attempt with a different blade • Make no more than 2 attempts (avoid ↑ risk of oral bleeding, secretions, & edema)
Plan B	• Direct laryngoscopy & insertion of bougie or intubating catheter • Confirm placement by (1) using hand on anterior neck to palpate catheter advancement through glottis; (2) after this, 40 cm of catheter should reach carina & provide resistance (no resistance will be encountered if in esophagus); (3) if using intubating catheter, may attach to ETCO₂ monitor
Plan C	• Insertion of LMA (disposable, Fastrach™, Proseal™) • 5.0 or 6.0 ETT will fit through disposable LMA (± fiberoptic assistance)
Plan D	• Terminate anesthetic & awaken pt • Emergency reversal of rocuronium with sugammadex = 16 mg/kg • Perform awake fiberoptic intubation • Perform surgical airway (i.e., tracheostomy)

Source: Adapted from Morgan GE, Mikhail MS, Murray MM. Clinical Anesthesiology. 4th ed. TBS Publishing; 2005: Chapter 19.

TRANSTRACHEAL PROCEDURES

- **Indications:** Emergency tracheal access when an airway cannot be secured via nasal/oral route
- **Percutaneous transtracheal jet ventilation**
  - Simple & relatively safe means to sustain a pt during a critical situation
  - Attach 12-, 14-, or 16G IV catheter to 10-mL syringe partially filled with saline
  - Advance needle through cricothyroid membrane with constant aspiration until you get air
  - Advance angiocatheter, disconnect syringe, attach oxygen source
    - High-pressure O_2 (25–30 psi), insufflation of 1–2 s, 12/min with 16-gauge needle → will deliver ~400–700 mL
    - Low-pressure O_2 (bag–valve–mask 6 psi, common gas outlet 20 psi)
- **Cricothyroidotomy**
  - Contraindications: Pts <6 y/o (upper part of trachea not fully developed) → incision through cricothyroid membrane ↑ risk of subglottic stenosis
  - Sterilize skin
  - Identify cricothyroid membrane

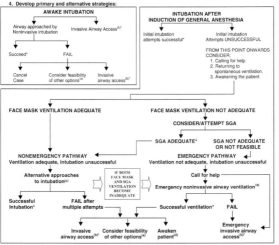

Figure 4-1 ASA difficult airway algorithm. (Note: 30% of anesthesia-related deaths stem from issues of airway management.)

(From Practice guidelines for management of the difficult airway: an updated report by the American Society of Anesthesiologists Task Force on Management of the Difficult Airway. *Anesthesiology* 2013;118(2):251–270. doi:10.1097/ALN.0b013e31827773b2. Reproduced with permission from The American Society of Anesthesiologists.)

- Transverse incision with #11 blade ≈1 cm on each side of midline
- Turn blade 90° to create space to pass ETT
- Insert ETT caudally, inflate cuff, confirm breaths sounds

TECHNIQUES OF EXTUBATION

- Extubation performed when pt either deeply anesthetized (stage 3) or awake (stage 1)
  - Extubation during light anesthesia (stage 2) may → laryngospasm/airway compromise
- Pt's airway should be aggressively suctioned while on 100% O_2 prior to extubation

- Prior to extubation, pt should be awake, following commands, neuromuscular blockade reversed
- Untape ETT, deflate cuff, remove ETT while providing small amount of positive pressure
  - Removes secretions at distal end of ETT
- Place mask on pt with 100% O_2 while verifying spontaneous & adequate ventilation
- Consider using 1.5 mg/kg of IV lidocaine 1–2 min before manipulation of airway & extubation (will blunt airway reflexes)
- Deep extubation
  - Indicated to prevent ↑ BP, ICP, IOP, or bronchospasm (in asthmatics)
  - Contraindicated in pts at ↑ risk for aspiration or who may have a difficult airway

---

DIFFICULT AIRWAY ALGORITHM

Originally published in March 1993 & revised in 2013, the ASA Difficult Airway Algorithm (Fig. 4-1) is designed to facilitate management of difficult airways & reduce adverse outcomes

ELISABETH M. HUGHES • KURT F. DITTRICH

INTRODUCTION

- Choice of anesthetic technique should be based on surgical factors such as the length of case, positioning of pt, and expected postop status; pt's comorbidities, and pt's desires and psychological state
- Communication with the pt and the surgical team is essential in determining an optimal plan

PATIENT INTERVIEW AND EVALUATION

- Discuss appropriate anesthetic options with the pt and assess their concerns
- Educating the pt may help alleviate misconceptions. Inquire about any procedures and experiences they may have had in the past and discuss differences between those and current anesthetic goals
- Answer all questions: Building patient report can reduce preop anxiety

PREMEDICATION

- Goals: ↓ Anxiety, provide analgesia for regional techniques/placement of invasive monitors/IV access, ↓ secretions (oral surgery/fiberoptic intubation), ↓ likelihood/risk of aspiration, control heart rate/bp
- Oral medication usually given 60–90 min and IM medication 30–60 min before arrival in OR

Class/Drug	Adult Dose (mg)	Onset/ Peak (min)	Notes
Benzodiazepines: Anxiolysis, sedation, & amnesia (no guarantee against recall, no analgesia)			
Diazepam (PO)	5–20 mg	30–60 in adults, 5–30 in children	Crosses placenta; highly protein-bound (↑ potency in pt with ↓ albumin)
Lorazepam (oral, IV)	0.5–4 mg	30–40	Among benzos, lorazepam has the most delayed onset & longest action (may cause prolonged sedation)
Midazolam (IM)	0.1–0.2 mg/kg	3–5; 10–20	Rapid onset & short duration; given within 1 h of surgery
Midazolam (IV)	Titrate 1–2.5 mg	Immediate, 3–5	
Opioids: Treat pain assoc with preop experience (regional anesthesia, central lines) provide little anxiolysis, may cause dysphoria; consider supplemental O_2			
Morphine (IM, IV)	1–2.5 mg	15–30; 45–90	Lasts 4 h
Fentanyl (IV)	Incremental titration of 25–50 mcg doses		
Antihistamines			
Diphenhydramine (PO, IM)	25–75 mg		Sedation; can use with cimetidine & steroids to protect against histamine release from allergic rxns
Anticholinergics: Useful for drying oral secretions (oral surgery/fiberoptic intubation)			
Atropine (IV)	0.2–0.4 mg		
Scopolamine (IV)	0.1–0.4 mg		Most sedating, no amnesia
Glycopyrrolate (IV)	0.1–0.2 mg		Least sedating agent (does not cross blood–brain barrier)

H_2 antagonists				
Cimetidine (PO, IM, IV)	300 mg			
Ranitidine (PO)	50–200 mg			
Famotidine (PO)	20–40 mg			
Antacids				
Sodium citrate (PO)	10–20 mL			
Gastric motility stimulator				
Metoclopramide (PO, IM, IV)	5–20 mg			
Antiemetics				
Ondansetron (IV)	4–8 mg			
Granisetron (IV)	10 mcg/kg			

Adapted from Hata TM, Hata JS. Chapter 22. Preoperative patient assessment and management. In: Barash PG, Cullen BF, Stoelting RK, eds. *Clinical Anesthesia.* 7th ed. Philadelphia, PA: Lippincott Williams & Wilkins; 2013:602–607.

Pediatric Premedication Dosing				
Medication	Route	Dose (mg/kg Except Where Noted)	Onset/ Duration (min)	Notes
Midazolam	PO/PR	0.25–0.75/0.5–1	20–30; 90	
	Nasal drop/ spray	0.2–0.5	10–20	May be preferred route for infants
	IV	0.5–5 y: 0.05–0.1 >5 y: 0.025–0.5	2–3; 45–60	
Diazepam	PO/PR	0.1–.05/1	60–90	Reliable GI absorption; prolonged action
Ketamine	PO/PR	3–6/6–10	20–25	
	Nasal	3	5; 45	
	IM	2–10 (suggest using high conc of 100 mg/mL to ↓ with injection)		This combo may prolong recovery
Clonidine	PO	2–4 mcg/kg	>90 min	
Fentanyl	PO/ transmucosal	10–15 mcg/kg/ 1–2 mcg/kg		Not as effective as midazolam; can cause facial pruritus, respiratory depression, & PONV

Adapted from Ghazal EA, Mason LJ, Cote CJ. Chapter 4. Preoperative evaluation, premedication, and induction of anesthesia. In: Cote CJ, Lerman J, Anderson BJ, eds. *A Practice of Anesthesia for Infants and Children.* 5th ed. Philadelphia, PA: Saunders; 2013:39–48.

ANESTHESIA TECHNIQUES: (GOALS)

- **Monitored anesthesia care (MAC):** Anxiolysis, sedation, analgesia, & monitoring by anesthesia personnel able to anticipate and react to changes in pt status & anesthetic state/requirements
- **General anesthesia:** Pt unresponsive to significant stimulation; often requires airway, ventilatory, and/or cardiovascular support
- **Neuraxial techniques:** Spinal/epidural alone or combined with above techniques for intraop & postop analgesia to chest, abdomen, & lower extremity
- **Peripheral nerve block:** Minimal physiologic effects make these techniques useful, especially in a pt with significant comorbidities

MONITORED ANESTHESIA CARE VS. GENERAL ANESTHESIA: ASA DEFINITIONS

- **MAC:** Anesthesia service that involves varying depths of sedation, analgesia, & anxiolysis but, most importantly, requires that provider is "prepared & qualified to convert to general anesthesia when necessary"

- **General anesthesia:** State when "pt loses consciousness & the ability to respond purposefully... irrespective of whether airway instrumentation is required"

Continuum of Depth of Sedation (ASA Definition)				
	Minimal Sedation	Moderate Sedation/ Analgesia	Deep Sedation/ Analgesia	General Anesthesia
Responsiveness	Normal response to verbal stimulation	Purposeful* response to verbal or tactile stimulation	Purposeful* response following repeated or painful stimulation	Unarousable even with painful stimulus
Airway	Unaffected	No intervention required	Intervention may be required	Intervention often required
Spontaneous ventilation	Unaffected	Adequate	May be inadequate	Frequently inadequate
Cardiovascular function	Unaffected	Usually maintained	Usually maintained	May be impaired

*Reflex withdrawal from a painful stimulus is **NOT** considered a purposeful response.

Commonly Used Drugs for Conscious Sedation			
Drug Name	**Induction Bolus Dose**	**Maintenance Infusion Rate**	**Maintenance Intermittent Boluses**
Benzodiazepines			
Midazolam	1–5 mg		1–2 mg
Rapid onset & short duration; often given alone or as anxiolytic adjuvant to opioid boluses, remifentanil infusion, and/or propofol infusion			
Opioid analgesics			
Alfentanil	5–20 mcg/kg	0.25–1 mcg/kg/min	3–5 mcg/kg q5–20min
Fentanyl	25–50 mcg		25–50 mcg
Remifentanil		0.025–0.1 mcg/kg/min	25 mcg
Avoid large boluses (risk of chest wall rigidity); ↓ dose when given with midazolam or propofol			
Hypnotics			
Propofol	0.25–0.5 mg/kg	2–4 mg/kg/h (30–70 mcg/kg/min)	0.3–0.5 mg/kg (300–500 mcg/kg)
Easily titratable, rapid recovery, antiemetic effects; pain on injection			
Dexmedetomidine	1 mcg/kg over 10 min	0.2–1 mcg/kg/h	—
Some analgesia with little respiratory depression; bradycardia & hypotension common side effects; may have prolonged sedation; small doses of midazolam & fentanyl initially may help reduce the initial bolus & prolonged sedation			
Ketamine	0.1 mg/kg	2–4 mcg/kg/min	
Maintenance of cardiovascular system & respiratory drive makes ketamine appealing; avoid in pt s with CAD, uncontrolled HTN, CHF, seizure Hx, and arterial aneurysms			

Adapted from Hillier SC. Chapter 29. Monitored anesthesia care. In: Barash PG, Cullen BF, Stoelting RK, eds. *Clinical Anesthesia.* 7th ed. Philadelphia, PA: Lippincott Williams & Wilkins; 2013:840.

FLUMAZENIL (FOR ANTAGONISM OF BENZODIAZEPINE EFFECTS)

- Initial recommended dose = 0.2 mg
- If desired level of consciousness not achieved in 45 s, repeat 0.2 mg dose
- 0.2 mg dose may need to be repeated q60s to max of 1 mg
- Note: Be aware of potential for resedation due to short half-life

---

INHALATIONAL INDUCTION

- Allows induction without IV access, as IV placement can be anxiety-provoking
- Onset of anesthesia faster in children than in adults (ratio of alveolar ventilation to FRC is in inverse proportion to body size; i.e., infants & children have increased ratio of alveolar ventilation to FRC)

Pediatric Technique

- For infants & children who tolerate a mask:
  - Start with 70% nitrous oxide in mask on pt
  - Introduce volatile agent only after 1–2 min of N_2O/O_2
  - Cut back N_2O and ↑ O_2 percentage as potent agent is added
- For anxious children—rapid induction (in as few as 4 breaths):
  - Often requires involvement of multiple personnel and/or parents
  - Prime circuit with 70% N_2O, O_2, & 8% sevoflurane
  - Place mask firmly on pt while monitoring airway throughout
  - With loss of consciousness, ↑ percentage of O_2 & ↓ N_2O
  - ↓ Sevoflurane conc over next few min as agent equilibrates
  - Support ventilation as needed
  - Place IV (often with an assistant to assure appropriate attention to airway)

Note: Sevoflurane induction has been assoc with bradycardia, especially in pts with Down syndrome (J Clin Anesth 2010;22:592–597)

Adult Inhalational Induction

- Consider for adults in whom IV placement is extremely anxiety-provoking/difficult
- Disadvantages: May cause ↑ cough, hiccups, & possibly ↑ risk of nausea/vomiting
- Prime circuit with 8% sevoflurane & 70% N_2O (usually requires 3 fill/empty cycles of an occluded anesthesia circuit)
- Instruct pt to exhale completely & then inhale from mask to vital capacity & hold
- If still conscious & unable to hold breath any longer, instruct pt to take additional deep breaths

---

INTRAMUSCULAR INDUCTION

- May be useful technique for:
  - Uncooperative pts in whom IV placement/inhalation induction impossible
  - Loss of control of pt and/or airway during attempted inhalation induction
  - Agitation/disinhibition with premedication
  - Need for rapid sequence induction without venous access
- Typical IM dosing:
  - Ketamine 3–12 mg/kg, 10% solution
  - Atropine 0.02 mg/kg, to reduce secretions
  - Succinylcholine 3–4 mg/kg, included for rapid sequence induction

Note: Atropine & succinylcholine may be combined in same syringe; administer midazolam after IV placement to prevent ketamine emergence delirium

---

RECTAL INDUCTION

Characteristics

- Convenient for healthy children old enough to have separation anxiety but still not mature enough to cooperate (8 mo–5 y/o)
- Parents & child familiar with rectal route for other medications (i.e., acetaminophen)
- Avoids needle for IM/IV induction & struggle involved with inhalational induction

Technique

- Cut 14-Fr suction catheter to 10 cm & lubricate
- Place catheter in pt's rectum & administer medication through syringe
- Follow medication with air bolus to purge remaining drug from catheter lumen
- Instruct parent/caregiver to hold buttocks together for at least 2 min
- Anticipate defecation & provide caregiver with waterproof mat
- Harmless hiccupping may occur
- Constant monitoring by anesthesia personnel required throughout
- Pt should be taken to procedure area as soon as sufficient sedation achieved
- Maintain primary attention on supporting pt's airway

Typical Agents and Dosing for Rectal Induction			
Medication	Dose (mg/kg)	Onset (min)	Comments
Midazolam	1		
Methohexital (1–10%)	25–30	5–15	Hiccups common; contraindicated in pts with seizure risk

Ketamine (5%)	4–8	7–15	Causes catecholamine release which ↑ intraocular & intracranial pressure; excess salivation can be treated with atropine; potential dysphoria treated with benzodiazepine

Adapted from Ghazal EA, Mason LJ, Cote CJ. Chapter 4. Preoperative evaluation, premedication, and induction of anesthesia. In: Cote CJ, Lerman J, Anderson BJ, eds. *A Practice of Anesthesia for Infants and Children.* 5th ed. Philadelphia, PA: Saunders; 2013:48–53.

Stages of Anesthesia		
Stage I	Amnesia	Time from induction of anesthesia to loss of consciousness
Stage II	Excitatory period	Irregular breathing, ↑ risk of laryngospasm, emesis, & arrhythmias
Stage III	Surgical anesthesia	Constricted pupils, regular breathing, no movement
Stage IV	Overdose	Hypotension, apnea, dilated/nonreactive pupils

COMPONENTS OF ANESTHESIA

- An anesthetic may contain any or all of the following components: **Anxiolysis, analgesia, hypnosis, amnesia, paralysis**
- Inhalational & IV agents provide anxiolysis & hypnosis, little or no analgesia (except for ketamine and nitrous oxide) *(Anesthesiology 2008;109(4):707–722)*

"BALANCED ANESTHETIC" TECHNIQUE

- A technique of general anesthesia based on the concept that administration of a mixture of small amounts of several neuronal depressants summates the advantages but not the disadvantages of the individual components of the mixture
- *A "balance" of virtues of different agents allows less of each to be used*
- Allows for faster emergence & less risk of cardiovascular collapse
- Use of muscle relaxants may ↑ risk of intraoperative awareness

MONITORING OF NEUROMUSCULAR BLOCKADE/PARALYSIS

Technique
Peripheral nerve stimulator (PNS) electrically stimulates motor nerve adductor pollicis (ulnar n.), orbicularis oculi (facial n.), posterior tibial n., peroneal n.

Train of Four
Four stimuli given at a frequency of 2 Hz every 5 s
→ Potentially eliciting 4 twitches (T1–T4)
→ TOF ratio T4:T1 indicates degree of neuromuscular block
→ Nondepolarizing agents:
  Produce progressive reduction in magnitude of T1–T4; the number of elicited twitches indicates degree of blockade with recovery, twitches appear in reverse order
→ Depolarizing agents (succinylcholine):
  Produce equal but reduced twitches (no fade)

Tetanic Stimulation
Tetanic stimulation: Concept that acetylcholine is depleted by successive stimulations; 50 Hz for 5 continuous s produces detectable fade in muscle contraction
→ The extent of fade is related to the degree of neuromuscular block
→ No fade = no neuromuscular block
→ Sustained response to tetanus present when TOF ratio is >0.7

Double-Burst Stimulation
- Two bursts of 3 stimuli at 50 Hz with each triple burst separated by 750 ms
- ↓ In the 2nd response indicates residual block
- Ratio is related to TOF ratio but easier to interpret reliably

Post-tetanic Count
- 50 Hz tetanic stimulus given for 5 s, followed by stimulus at 1.0 Hz 3 s later
- No. of responses detectable predicts time for spontaneous recovery

- Fade response appears earlier than train of 4
- Can be used under deep paralysis to estimate the time to recovery and potential for the use of reversal agents

Phase II Blockade with Succinylcholine
- Postjunctional membranes repolarized, but still not responding to acetylcholine
- Resembles blockade by nondepolarizing agents (get TOF fade, tetanic stim)
- Mechanism unknown, occurs when succinylcholine dose exceeds 3–5 mg/kg IV
- Reversal agents (neostigmine) may or may not antagonize phase II blockade

Clinical Assessment of Blockade	
Twitch Response	**Clinical Correlate**
95% suppression of single twitch at 0.15–0.1 Hz	Adequate intubating conditions
90% suppression of single twitch; train-of-four count of 1 twitch	Surgical relaxation with nitrous oxide–opioid anesthesia
75% suppression of single twitch; train-of-four count of 3 twitches	Adequate relaxation with inhalation agents
25% suppression of single twitch	Decreased vital capacity
Train-of-four ratio >0.75; sustained tetanus at 50 Hz for 5 s	Head lift for 5 s; vital capacity = 15–20 mL/kg; inspiratory force = −25 cm H_2O; effective cough
Train-of-four ratio >0.9	Sit up unassisted; intact carotid body response to hypoxemia; normal pharyngeal function
Train-of-four ratio = 1.0	Normal expiratory flow rate, vital capacity, and inspiratory force; Diplopia resolves

Source: Levine W, Allain RM, Alston TA, et al. *Clinical Procedures of the Massachusetts General Hospital.* 8th ed. Philadelphia, PA: Lippincott Williams & Wilkins; 2010, with permission.

AWARENESS

- Complication where pt regains consciousness during general anesthetic & can recall events afterward. Important to distinguish goals of general anesthesia from that of MAC.
- Pts experience ranges from benign recall of conversation to post-traumatic stress disorder (PTSD) involving disturbed sleep, nightmares, flashbacks, & general anxiety
- Negative psychological consequences can last for y after the event
- If awareness occurs, pts often respond favorably to a complete explanation, apology, & reassurance that they are not crazy. Psychology consult should be considered early if pt is in favor

Frequency of Awareness (from Prospective Study of 11,785 General Anesthetics)
- 0.15% of all cases
- 0.18% with paralysis
- 0.10% without paralysis

Patient Populations at Increased Risk of Awareness
- Trauma victims: 11–43%
- Cardiac surgery: 1.1–1.5%
- Obstetric cases under general anesthesia: 0.4%
- Hx of substance abuse
- Previous episode of intraoperative awareness
- Hx of difficult intubation or anticipated difficult intubation
- Chronic pain pts using high doses of opioids, anxiolytics, or psychostimulants
- ASA physical status IV or V
- Pts with limited hemodynamic reserve

From Sandin RH, Enlund G, Samuelsson P, et al. Awareness during anaesthesia: a prospective case study. *The Lancet* 2000;355:707–711.

Guidelines for Prevention and Management of Intraoperative Awareness	
Prevention	**Management**

• Check delivery of anesthetic agents to pt
• Consider premedication
• Give adequate dose of induction agents
• Avoid muscle paralysis unless it is needed, even then avoid total paralysis
• Supplement N_2O & opioid anesthesia with ≥0.6 MAC of volatile agent
• Administer ≥0.8 MAC when volatile agents are used alone
• Use amnesics when light anesthesia is only regimen tolerated by pt
• Inform pt about possibility of awareness
• Consider brain function monitoring (BIS)
	• Perform detailed interview with pt
	  Verify pt's account
	  Sympathize & apologize
	  Explain what happened
	  Reassure about nonrepetition in future
	  Offer psychological support
	• Record interview in pt's chart
	• Inform pt's surgeon, nurse, & hospital risk management office
	• Visit pt daily during hospital stay & keep in contact by telephone after
	• Do not delay referral to a psychologist or psychiatrist

From Ghoneim MM, Weiskopf RB. Awareness during anesthesia. *Anesthesiology* 2000;92:597–602, with permission.

BRAIN FUNCTION MONITORING, DEPTH OF ANESTHESIA, AND AWARENESS

- Brain function monitors analyze EEG signals & translate them into a number between 0 and 100 that corresponds to anesthetic depth
- Devices include BIS, SedLine, Entropy, and Narcotrend. ASA position: Brain function monitoring *not* routinely indicated & decision to use should be made on a case-by-case basis by individual practitioners
- BIS-guided anesthesia can reduce the risk of intraoperative awareness in surgical pts at risk for awareness in comparison to using clinical signs as a guide for anesthetic depth (*Cochrane Database Syst Rev* 2014;17:6:CD003843)

Interpretation of Brain Function Monitor Number During GA	
>60	Increased risk of awareness during GA
40–60	Appropriate anesthetic depth
<40	Excessive depth of anesthesia

BRAIN FUNCTION MONITORING & ANALGESIA

- Number correlates best with hypnotic component of anesthetic provided by benzodiazepines, propofol, & potent volatile agents
- N_2O, low-dose opioids, & neuraxial/peripheral nerve blocks have little effect on the number (*These agents do ↓ amount of additional hypnotic needed to keep the number constant when pts are exposed to noxious stimuli*)
- Ketamine confounds the number & care must be taken when BIS used during ketamine containing anesthetics. Use of nitrous oxide (alone) may result in inaccurate correlation of BIS and level of sedation and hypnosis (*A & A August 2006 vol. 103 no 2 485–9*).

Potential Advantages & Disadvantages of Brain Function Monitoring	
Advantages	**Disadvantages**

• May ↓ risk of awareness
• Prevents excessive anesthetic depth
  → Faster emergence & recovery
  → Reduction in drug costs
  → Possible lower long-term mortality
	• Cost of equipment
	• Provides false sense of security

From Sigl JC, Chamoun NG. An introduction to bispectral analysis for the electroencephalogram. *J Clin Mon Comput* 1994:392–404.

TOTAL INTRAVENOUS ANESTHESIA (TIVA)

- TIVA anesthetics usually include hypnotic (propofol) + analgesic (remifentanil)
- IV infusion drugs should be connected as closely as possible to pt's IV catheter (*minimize dead space where infusion medication can accumulate*)
- TIVA may be more susceptible to dosing errors
- Must always monitor for: IV lines that are infiltrated/kinked, disconnections & dosing errors

Advantages of TIVA Over inhalation Induction & Maintenance

- Smooth induction with minimal coughing/hiccupping
- Easier control of anesthetic depth
- More rapid, predictable emergence
- Lower incidence of PONV
- Ideal operating conditions for neurologic surgery with reduced cerebral blood flow & cerebral metabolic rate; allows intraoperative neuromonitoring
- ↓ Organ toxicity & atmospheric pollution
- Avoids N_2O side effects (expansion of closed airspaces & bone marrow suppression)

Common Indications for TIVA

- Anesthesia for airway endoscopies, laryngeal & tracheal surgeries
- Anesthesia in remote locations or during transport (i.e., GI lab)
- Malignant hyperthermia-susceptible pts
- Hx of significant PONV

Advantages of Continuous Infusions Compared with Intermittent Bolus Dosing

- Avoid oscillations in drug concentration
- Minimize relative over- or underdosing
- Provide stable depth of anesthesia
- Reduce incidence of side effects (hemodynamic instability)
- Shorten recovery times
- ↓ Total drug requirements by 25–30%

Typical Dosing Regimens for IV Agents Used for General Anesthetics

Drug	Induction Bolus	Maintenance Infusion Rate	Maintenance Intermittent Bolus
Etomidate	0.2–0.3 mg/kg	—	—
Propofol	2–3 mg/kg	6–10 mg/kg/h (100–180 mcg/kg/min)	—
Fentanyl	50–100 mcg	0.5–4 mcg/kg/h	25–50 mcg
Alfentanil	0.5–1.5 mg	1–3 mg/h	0.2–0.5 mg
Remifentanil	1–2 mcg/kg	0.1–0.25 mcg/kg/min	—
Sufentanil	0.2 mcg/kg	0.2–0.4 mcg/kg/h	—
Ketamine	0.1–0.2 mg/kg	5–10 mcg/kg/min	—

From Urman RD, Shapiro FE. Chapter 9. Anesthetic agents. Which one? In: *Manual of Office-Based Anesthesia Procedures.* Philadelphia, PA: Lippincott Williams & Wilkins; 2007:63.

Titration of Maintenance Infusions

- Titrate to anticipated intensity of observed responses to surgical stimulus
- Drug requirements are highest during endotracheal intubation
- Requirements ↓ during surgical prep & draping
- Infusion rates should be ↑'d a few min before skin incision
- Pt movement & changes in hemodynamics should guide infusions titration
- After start of surgery: If no response for 10–15 min, ↓ infusion rate by 20%. If response, administer bolus & ↑ infusion rate
- Opioid should be administered to achieve analgesia
- Hypnotic should be titrated to individual requirements & surgical stimulus
- Infusion rates need to be titrated down to restore spontaneous respiration at surgery's end

GUIDELINES FOR USING PROPOFOL

Induction of General Anesthesia
- 2–3 mg/kg IV (reduced in pts given opioids/other premeds, aged >50)

Maintenance of General Anesthesia
- 80–150 mcg/kg/min IV combined with N_2O or an opiate
- 120–200 mcg/kg/min IV if sole agent
- Consider reducing dose after 2 h (propofol accumulates)
- Turn off infusion 5–10 min prior to desired time of emergence (can give 1–2 mL boluses as needed to keep pt asleep until emergence)

Sedation
- 10–50 mcg/kg/min IV

EXTUBATION & EMERGENCE

Common Extubation Criteria

- Regular respiratory rate
- Stable SpO_2
- Adequate paralysis reversal (sustained head/leg lift for 5 s); able to protect airway
- Tidal volumes >4 mL/kg
- Return of consciousness (following commands)
- Stable end-tidal CO_2 at physiologic levels

Indications for Continued Postop Intubation

- Epiglottitis
- Localized upper airway edema secondary to surgery or trauma
- Surgery causing injury to recurrent laryngeal nerves
- Upper airway edema from massive intraop volume infusion (especially combined with prolonged Trendelenburg or prone positioning)
- Unstable hemodynamics or continued bleeding
- Neurologic compromise (GCS <8)

Deep Extubation

Indications	Asthma, ↑ risk of intracranial bleeding, delicate cosmetic sutures, compromised ocular globe, intravitreal gas
Contraindications	Full stomach, obstructive sleep apnea (relative), difficult airway
Advantages	↓ Coughing & bucking ↓ Strain on incision sutures ↓ Risk of ↑ intracranial and/or intraocular pressure
Disadvantages	Loss of stimulation leading to apnea Laryngospasm Aspiration

REGIONAL ANESTHESIA

ERIC R. BRIGGS

PERIPHERAL NERVE BLOCKS

Introduction
- Peripheral nerve blocks rely on local anesthetics injected around specific nerves/ nerve bundles to prevent transmission of impulses along those nerves
- Order of nerve blockade: Small sympathetic C fibers → small sensory (Aδ) fibers (pain & temp) → large sensory (Aβ) fibers (proprioception & touch) → large motor fibers (Aα)
- Uses include surgical anesthesia +/− general anesthesia, postop analgesia, or acute/ chronic pain management

Preparation and Materials
1. Standard pt monitors (SpO$_2$, ECG, blood pressure cuff)
2. Sedative medications & oxygen
3. Barrier equipment: Hat, mask, sterile gloves, +/− sterile gown
4. Block needle: Short, B-bevel (blunt), echogenic, or insulated needle
5. Infusion catheter (if performing continuous nerve block)
6. Local anesthetic (LA)
7. Method of nerve localization (i.e., nerve stimulator, ultrasound [US] machine, etc.)
8. Lipid emulsion agent to treat local anesthetic systemic toxicity (LAST), emergency airway equipment, & intubation medications

Nerve Localization Techniques	
US-guided	US probe used to visualize target nerve, block needle, & local anesthetic
Nerve stimulation	Insulated needle connected to nerve stimulator elicits muscle twitches in target nerve's pattern of innervation. Dial current down slowly from >1 mA–<0.5 mA while retaining muscle twitch
Paresthesia	Block needle used to elicit paresthesia when it contacts nerve. Injection should cause transient enhanced paresthesia; intense searing pain indicates intraneural injection (stop immediately, withdraw needle, reassess)
Infiltration/field blocks	Local anesthetic injected in close proximity to nerve to be blocked based on its constant relationship with anatomic landmarks

Contraindications—Similar to Those for Neuraxial Blockade
- **Absolute**
  Pt refusal, infection at site of needle puncture, true allergy to amide and ester LA
- **Relative**
  Severe anatomic abnormalities, uncooperative pt, neurologic dz or nerve injury, bacteremia, abnormal coagulation (endogenous or iatrogenic), anesthetized pt (except pediatric)

Complications—Common to All Nerve Blocks
- Nerve injury, local anesthetic systemic toxicity (LAST), infection, hematomas
- Sterile/aseptic technique should be used to reduce risk of infection
- Aspirate from syringe every 5–10 mL for blood/CSF to avoid intravascular/ intrathecal injection of local anesthetic

General Considerations for Quality Improvement and Safety without US
- Adequate knowledge of anatomy and equipment
- Pt positioning and monitoring
- Nerve stimulation used to confirm identity of targeted nerve; also used to ensure needle is not intraneural with no stim at low current
- Raj test to ensure needle not intraneural (after desired stimulation at desired MHz, inject 1 mL slowly and stimulation should stop unless needle is intraneural)
- Injection of the LA should be done slowly, following aspiration, and incrementally (usually 5 mL increments) with continuous assessment for intravascular injection
- Epinephrine should be added to LA as a vascular marker (e.g., 1:400,000 [2.5 mcg/mL])
- Accept only low injection pressures (<20 psi) to avoid intraneural injections

Ultrasound Basics

- US imaging based on transducer emitting sound waves (produced by piezoelectric crystal) into tissue and receiving sound reflected or scattered back to receiver
- US waves are high-frequency sound waves above 20 kHz
- Frequencies useful in regional anesthesia are in the 4–17 MHz range
- Tissues with different acoustic impedance interact with incident sound waves, causing attenuation, reflection, refraction, & scattering
- The greater the echogenicity of tissue, the brighter it is on sonogram
- Anechoic structures (e.g., blood vessels) appear black because US waves are transmitted through these structures with no reflection
- Hypoechoic structures (proximal nerves, adipose tissue) appear dark/near black because US waves are transmitted through these structures with little reflection
- Hyperechoic structures (e.g., bone, tendons) appear bright because US waves are blocked, and the strong signal returned to transducer gives these structures a white appearance

Transducer Selection

- Frequency determines image resolution and depth of tissue penetration
- Low-frequency transducers (2–7 MHz range) are best for deep structures (>4 cm): Low resolution, high penetration
- High-frequency transducers (10–15 MHz range) are best for superficial structures (0.5–4 cm): High resolution, low penetration

Imaging Plane

- Short axis (transverse/axial): Cylindrical structures are depicted in cross-section, producing a circular image
- Long-axis imaging: Shows object longitudinally, depicts course of cylindrical objects as linear
- In-plane (IP) needle technique (most common): Needle introduced within the plane of imaging shows needle as echogenic line. Only portion of needle within this very thin scan plane can be seen; possibility to advance needle further than intended when tip strays from scan plane
- Out-of-plane (OOP) needle technique: Needle introduced perpendicular to the plane of imaging and crosses scan plane, needle tip, or shaft shown as echogenic dot

Sonographic Appearance of Nerves

- Nerve fascicles appear hypoechoic, surrounded by hyperechoic epineurium and connective tissue
- Nerves change shape and echotexture along their course (e.g., proximal nerves, such as roots and trunks of brachial plexus, appear hypoechoic monofascicular but become hyperechoic and polyfascicular [honeycomb appearance] in periphery)
- Can appear round, oval, or triangular and may mimic other structures (e.g., vessels, tendons, fascia, muscle)

General Considerations for Quality Improvement and Safety

- Adequate knowledge of anatomy and equipment
- Pt positioning and monitoring as for conventional block techniques
- Avoid air trapping between the transducer and sterile cover; air pockets will result in dropout shadowing
- Remove air bubbles from syringe or tubing; air markedly degrades image quality after inadvertent injection
- Surface anatomy landmarks used in conventional, nonimage-guided techniques can be used to guide initial placement of US transducer; further adjustments made according to US image
- Advance needle only under real-time imaging and never if tip is not visualized
- Doppler function can be very useful to identify arteries and veins
- Approach nerves carefully and advance needle tangentially along perimeter of nerve and never directly into substance of nerve
- Nerve stimulation can be applied to confirm identity of targeted nerve or confirm needle is not intraneural but does not appear to improve block success rate
- Injection of the LA should be made incrementally, often in multiple sites, with continuous assessment of LA distribution
- If LA distribution cannot be visualized after test dose of 1–2 mL injection should be stopped. Aspirate and reassess needle tip placement to rule out intravascular injection
- Circumferential spread around nerves produces rapid and complete conduction block
- Injections should be made slowly with frequent aspiration and maintenance of low injection pressures (<20 psi) to avoid intravascular and intraneural injections

SUPERFICIAL CERVICAL PLEXUS (SCP) AND DEEP CERVICAL PLEXUS (DCP) BLOCKS

- *Indications*
  - Neck surgery including lymph node dissection, tracheostomy, carotid endarterectomy, thyroid surgery
- *Specific Considerations*
  - Phrenic nerve block will occur with DCP block; bilateral DCP blocks generally avoided
  - Significant concern for inadvertent intrathecal or epidural injection; avoid high volumes and high injection pressures
  - Intra-arterial injection into vertebral artery or carotid artery will cause seizure even with minimal volume
  - DCP block also covers SCP (no need to combine the two)
- *Important Landmarks/Anatomy*
  - *Mastoid process, C6 transverse process (TP) (Chassaignac tubercle)*
  - C2–4 anterior rami (divide into superficial & deep branches)
    - Superficial branches → cutaneous sensation of neck from jaw line to T2
    - Deep branches → ansa cervicalis; motor function muscles of ant neck and diaphragm (phrenic n.)
- *Superficial cervical plexus block*
  - Insert block needle at midpoint of posterior border of sternocleidomastoid (SCM)
  - Inject 10–15 mL of LA along posterior border of SCM, extending cranially & caudally 2–3 cm
  - Complications: Trapezius muscle paralysis can occur from blockade of CN XI
- *Deep cervical plexus block*
  - Line from mastoid process to TP of C6 (Chassaignac tubercle)
  - Along the line, mark off points that are 2, 4, & 6 cm from mastoid process, which correspond to C2, C3, & C4 TPs, respectively
  - At each point insert block needle at a slightly caudal angle until TP met, withdraw needle 2 mm and inject 5 mL of LA
  - Complications: Horner syndrome, phrenic & superior laryngeal nerve block, seizure, intrathecal/epidural/intravascular injection

BRACHIAL PLEXUS BLOCKS

- Brachial plexus: Nerve roots C5–8 and T1: <u>T</u>runks → <u>D</u>ivisions → <u>C</u>ords → <u>B</u>ranches (Fig. 6-1)

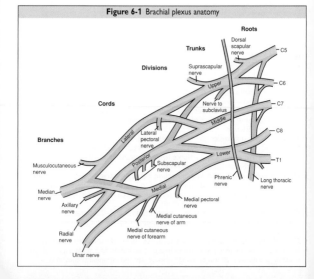

Figure 6-1 Brachial plexus anatomy

- Can block brachial plexus by injecting 25–40 mL of local anesthetic in certain areas along its path (interscalene, supraclavicular, infraclavicular, axillary)
- Can also perform individual nerve blocks distally for selective blockade or as rescue blocks (inject 3–5 mL of LA)
- Desired effect of electrostimulation in peripheral nerve distribution of UE:
  - Musculocutaneous n.—flexion at elbow
  - Median n.—flexion of fingers/wrist
  - Radial n.—extension of fingers/wrist
  - Ulnar n.—flexion of fingers/wrist with ulnar deviation

Interscalene Brachial Plexus Block
Consistently blocks C5–7; done at level of roots/trunks of plexus

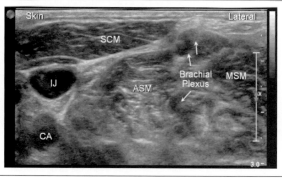

IJ, internal jugular vein; CA, carotid artery; SCM, sternocleidomastoid muscle; ASM, anterior scalene muscle; MSM, middle scalene muscle.

REGIONAL 6-4

Indications
- Shoulder, distal clavicle, and proximal humerus surgeries
- Poor choice for forearm/hand surgeries; does not cover C8 and T1 dermatomes
- *Specific Considerations*
  - Will affect phrenic nerve 100% of time, to varying degrees
  - Consider alternatives if pt has severe pulmonary dz or contralateral phrenic nerve or recurrent laryngeal nerve dysfunction
  - Horner syndrome (ptosis, miosis, anhidrosis) is common from blockade of stellate ganglion or a portion of the cervical sympathetic ganglion chain
- *Important Landmarks/Anatomy*
  - Sternocleidomastoid m. (SCM), cricoid cartilage, interscalene groove between anterior scalene muscle (ASM) and middle scalene muscles (MSM)
- *US-Guided Approach*
  - Position: Head up at 30°; head turned away
  - Small, high-frequency transducer ideal
  - Scan parallel to superior border of clavicle; identify subclavian artery and brachial plexus just lateral to it (supraclavicular block view)
  - Trace brachial plexus proximally until vertical, linear arrangement of roots/trunks observed between ASM and MSM
  - Typically, needle advanced in lateral-to-medial direction and IP just through MSM, resting needle tip between two most superficial hypoechoic targets (C5 and C6 roots)
  - Aspirate and inject 15–25 mL of LA in 5 mL increments; observe LA spreading along lateral border of plexus, pushing MSM posteriorly; can distribute LA anterior to plexus but may promote spread to phrenic nerve (anterior to ASM)
  - Can be done medial-to-lateral IP or OOP
- *Non-US Technique*
  - Palpate interscalene groove posterior to SCM; insert needle in this groove perpendicular to all planes at level of cricoid cartilage
  - Acceptable stimulation can involve pectorals, deltoid, triceps, biceps
  - If phrenic n. stimulated (diaphragm), needle is anterior to plexus; if accessory n. stimulated (trapezius m. twitch), needle is too posterior

Supraclavicular Brachial Plexus Block
"Spinal of the Arm"; done at level of trunks/divisions of plexus
- *Indications*
  - Surgery of upper extremity distal to shoulder
- *Specific Considerations*
  - Risk of pneumothorax
  - Can block phrenic nerve 50% of time (nerve stim study)
  - Consider alternatives if pt has severe pulmonary dz or contralateral phrenic nerve or recurrent laryngeal nerve dysfunction
  - Horner syndrome (ptosis, miosis, anhidrosis) is possible from blockade of stellate ganglion or a portion of the cervical sympathetic ganglion chain
- *Important Landmarks/Anatomy*
  - Clavicle, sternocleidomastoid m. (SCM), subclavian artery (SA), 1st rib, pleura
- *US-Guided Approach*
  - Position: Semi-sitting (head up at 30°), allowing shoulder to drop inferiorly; head turned away
  - Small, high-frequency transducer ideal
  - Scan parallel to superior border of clavicle; identify subclavian artery and brachial plexus just lateral to it; plexus resembles a "bundle of grapes"—multiple hypoechoic circles surrounded by hyperechoic connective tissue
  - Identify pleura and 1st rib; ideal image has plexus (bundle of grapes) sitting atop 1st rib (protects pleura)
  - Typically, needle advanced in lateral-to-medial direction IP through sheath surrounding plexus; 20–30 mL of LA injected incrementally and distributed throughout the nerve bundle; failure to inject LA into the deepest and most medial area (nerve pocket) of plexus next to SA risks sparing inferior trunk and its divisions (ulnar nerve)
- *Non-US Technique*
  - Insert needle 2.5 cm lateral to lateral border of clavicular head of SCM and 1 fb above clavicle; advance needle caudally and parallel to midline underneath clavicle; observe for desired stimulation; do not advance deeper than 2.5 cm if stimulation not elicited
  - Acceptable stimulation is motor response in the hand (radial/median/ulnar n.)

Infraclavicular Brachial Plexus Block
Done at cord level of plexus
- *Indications*
  - Surgery of upper extremity from elbow to finger tips
- *Specific Considerations*
  - Pneumothorax possible but much less likely vs. supraclavicular
  - Deeper block; may be difficult to visualize in obese pts
  - Ideal location for perineural catheter
- *Important Landmarks/Anatomy*
  - Clavicle, coracoid process, axillary artery (AA), deltopectoral groove, pectoralis major (PM) and pectoralis minor (Pm) m.
- *US-Guided Approach*
  - Position: Supine or semi-sitting; head turned away
  - Small, high-frequency or mid-range transducer
  - Place probe in deltopectoral groove; identify AA deep to pec major and minor; distinguish cords of plexus (will appear hyperechoic/honeycomb)
  - 4-in. needle likely required; needle advanced IP from lateral to medial (superior to inferior) to rest at 6 o'clock position of AA; needle trajectory can be superficial or deep to lateral cord
  - Typically, needle position maintained at 6 o'clock position throughout injection (immobile needle), observing for U-shaped spread around arterial wall medially and laterally; 30 mL of LA injected incrementally
- *Non-US Technique*
  - *Coracoid approach*: Needle inserted 2 cm medial & 2 cm inferior to coracoid process at an angle perpendicular to skin and advanced posteriorly
  - *Modified Raj approach*: Needle insertion point is 3 cm inferior from midpoint of clavicle; needle directed laterally toward AA as palpated in axilla
  - Acceptable stimulation is motor response in the hand

Axillary Brachial Plexus Block
Done at terminal branches of plexus (peripheral nerves)—median, radial, ulnar, & musculocutaneous nerves

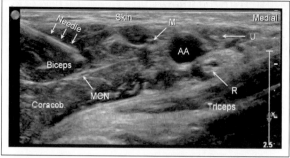

AA, axillary artery; M, median nerve; U, ulnar nerve; R, radial nerve; MCN, musculocutaneous nerve.

- **Indications**
  - Surgery of upper extremity from elbow to finger tips (same as infraclavicular)
- **Specific Considerations**
  - No risk of pneumothorax or phrenic nerve blockade
  - Nerves are very superficial
  - Allows targeting of individual nerves
  - Pt **must** be able to abduct arm; sometimes difficult following injury/surgery
  - Requires multiple needle passes to block nerves individually (mobile needle)
- **Important Landmarks/Anatomy**
  - Axilla, biceps m., triceps m., medial bicipital groove, axillary a. (AA)
- **US-Guided Approach**
  - Position: Supine; arm abducted 90° at shoulder; +/− flexed at elbow
  - Small, high-frequency transducer
  - Place probe in sagittal plane at proximal upper arm centered on groove between biceps and triceps m. (medial bicipital groove), identify AA
  - Trace AA proximally until probe makes contact with PM m., then slide probe distally along AA, identifying median, radial, ulnar, and musculocutaneous nerves (will appear hyperechoic/honeycomb)
  - Proximally, the median, radial, and ulnar n. should be in close proximity to AA; as the neurovascular bundle (NVB) is traced distally, the radial n. will dive deep to humerus, the median n. will remain in close proximity to AA, and ulnar n. will stay superficial but travel medially and away from AA
  - Musculocutaneous n. typically exits NVB very proximally, traveling laterally between biceps and coracobrachialis m.
  - Needle advanced lateral to medial IP; block nerves individually using 5–10 mL of LA (may require 30–40 mL of LA total); use intermittent injection technique
- **Non-US Techniques**
  - *Transarterial approach*: Palpate AA proximally in medial bicipital groove; fix AA between two fingers; while aspirating, advance short needle anterior to posterior through AA; once aspiration of blood stops, needle tip is just posterior to AA; inject 20 mL of LA in 5 cc increments after negative aspiration; slowly withdraw needle under continuous aspiration, once aspiration of blood stops, needle tip is just anterior to AA; inject 20 mL of LA in 5 mL increments after negative aspiration; alternatively, the total volume of LA can be deposited posterior to AA; will need to block musculocutaneous nerve separately
  - *Nerve stim techniques*: Single-injection vs. multiple-injection techniques; rely on typical configuration around AA; for single-injection, choose nerve with the most appropriate coverage for surgical site and incrementally inject entire volume of LA after appropriate stim; for multiple-injection (advanced technique), lower volumes (5–10 mL) injected around individual nerves after appropriate stim; median n. is lateral to AA, radial n. is medial and posterior to AA, ulnar n. is medial to AA and more superficial vs. radial n., and musculocutaneous n. deeper than median n.

Distal Blocks of Peripheral Nerves of Upper Extremity (see Figure 6-2 for anatomy)

- **Radial**
  - Elbow: Needle inserted lateral to biceps tendon until it makes contact with lateral epicondyle, withdraw 0.5 cm before injecting LA
  - Wrist: Subcutaneous injection of LA just proximal to radial styloid; ring extended both medially and laterally from radial styloid; 10 mL of LA total
  - US guided: Pt sitting with elbow flexed and forearm resting on lap; scan mid to distal humerus and identify hyperechoic radial nerve traveling away from humerus with distal scanning; inject 5–8 mL of LA around nerve
- **Median**
  - Elbow: Needle inserted medial to brachial artery pulsation 1–2 cm proximal to elbow crease
  - Wrist: Needle inserted between palmaris longus & flexor carpi radialis tendon until piercing the deep fascia
  - US guided at wrist: Identify nerve in carpal tunnel and scan proximally, differentiating nerve from tendon; inject 5 mL of LA around nerve proximal to carpal tunnel
  - US guided at elbow: Identify brachial artery at elbow; nerve is hyperechoic and very near artery; inject 5–8 mL of LA around nerve
- **Ulnar**
  - Elbow: Needle inserted in ulnar groove 1 cm proximal to medial epicondyle; with elbow flexed, direct needle distally toward hand and observe for stim.
  - Wrist: Insert needle medial and posterior to flexor carpi ulnaris tendon; advance 1 cm and inject 3–5 mL of LA; combine with subcutaneous injection over tendon for superficial cutaneous branches to hypothenar area
  - US guided at elbow: Arm abducted and elbow flexed; scan 5 cm proximally from medial epicondyle; identify hyperechoic ulnar nerve; inject 5–8 mL of LA
  - US guided at wrist: Identify ulnar artery; nerve will be next to artery; scan proximally 4 cm from wrist and inject 5 mL of LA around nerve
- **Musculocutaneous**
  - Proximal upper arm: Retract biceps m. laterally and inject 10 mL of LA into substance of coracobrachialis muscle
  - US guided: See axillary brachial plexus block above

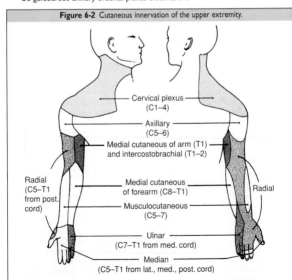

Figure 6-2 Cutaneous innervation of the upper extremity.

Cervical plexus (C1–4)

Axillary (C5–6)

Medial cutaneous of arm (T1) and intercostobrachial (T1–2)

Radial (C5–T1 from post. cord)

Medial cutaneous of forearm (C8–T1)

Musculocutaneous (C5–7)

Radial

Ulnar (C7–T1 from med. cord)

Median (C5–T1 from lat., med., post. cord)

(From Crawford LC, Warren L. Regional Anesthesia In: Pino RM, ed. *Clinical Anesthesia Procedures of the Massachusetts General Hospital.* 9th ed. Philadelphia, PA: Wolters Kluwer; 2016:263.)

DIGITAL NERVE BLOCK (UPPER EXTREMITY)

- Anatomy: Median & ulnar nerves → common digital nerves (located on bilateral ventrolateral aspect of each finger)
- Indications: Finger surgery (e.g., trauma, distal amputation)
- *Specific Considerations*
  - Local anesthetics (LA): Any plain local anesthetic (**no epinephrine**)
  - Complications: Hematoma, digit ischemia, nerve injury, infection, IV injection
- *Technique:*
  - Pronate hand, insert needle at dorsolateral aspect of base of finger; advance anteriorly toward base of phalanx
  - Stop when needle causing skin to bulge on palmar surface; aspirate, then inject 2–3 mL of LA; deposit some LA as withdrawing to cover dorsal nerves
  - Repeat on each side of base of finger

LOWER-EXTREMITY BLOCKS

- Lower extremity innervated by Lumbar (L1–4) & lumbosacral plexuses (L4–S3) (Fig. 6-3)
- **Lumbar plexus** gives rise to the femoral, obturator, & lateral femoral cutaneous (LFC) nerves; also gives rise to iliohypogastric, ilioinguinal, and genitofemoral nerves (covered in truncal blocks)
  - With the exception of the femoral nerve, individual nerve blocks are commonly performed by infiltration without nerve stimulation
  - The **psoas compartment/lumbar plexus block** achieves blockade of the entire lumbar plexus. Complications from block include epidural, subdural, or intrathecal injection, retroperitoneal hematoma, and/or visceral injury
- **Lumbosacral plexus** gives rise to sciatic nerve and posterior cutaneous nerve of the thigh
  - Sciatic nerve divides into tibial & common peroneal nerve at popliteal fossa
  - Tibial nerve gives rise to posterior tibial nerve & contributes to sural nerve
  - Common peroneal divides into superficial & deep peroneal nerves, contributes to sural nerve
- **Combination blocks**
  - 3-in-1 block was attempt to block femoral, LFC, and obturator nerves from femoral n. block site by holding distal compression and directing needle cranially in an attempt to promote proximal spread but does not block all 3 nerves reliably (<50% of the time)
  - Only reliable 3-in-1 block is lumbar plexus block

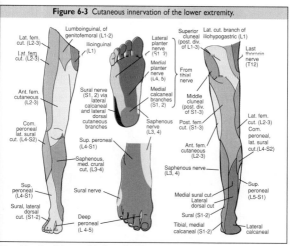

Figure 6-3 Cutaneous innervation of the lower extremity.

Adapted from Gray H. *Anatomy of the Human Body.* Philadelphia, PA: Lea & Febiger; 1918.)

- The lumbar plexus + sciatic block can provide anesthesia to essentially the entire lower extremity
- The knee joint is innervated by multiple nerves (femoral [anterior], obturator [medial], lat femoral cutaneous [lateral], and sciatic [posterior]) → a combination block would be needed to provide complete anesthesia for knee surgery
- Advantages over neuraxial blockade: Unilateral limb anesthesia, ↓ risk of sympathectomy (hypotension, urinary retention), & avoidance of neuraxial hematomas in pts on anticoagulation
- Disadvantage: Since anesthesia to the entire lower extremity usually requires >1 block, neuraxial anesthesia is a practical alternative

Lumbar Plexus Block
- *Indications*
  - Knee and hip surgeries and surgeries involving anterior, lateral, and medial thigh
- *Specific Considerations*
  - Deep block
  - Potential for epidural spread
  - Retroperitoneal hemorrhage possible; follow ASRA anticoagulation guidelines as for neuraxial procedures and deep blocks
  - Blocks femoral, obturator, and LFC nerves when LA injected into psoas muscle at level of iliac crest
  - Combine with sciatic n. block to anesthetize entire leg
- *Important Landmarks/Anatomy*
  - Midline and iliac crest; intercristal line (line drawn between bilateral iliac crests)
- *US-Guided Approach (advanced technique)*
  - Challenging due to depth of target; relies on same landmarks as non-US approach below
  - Position is lateral decubitus with hips and knees slightly bent
  - Low-frequency curvilinear transducer required
  - Identify spinous process (SP) just cephalad to intercristal line and scan laterally; locate TPs, psoas muscle will be located deep to TPs, ~4 cm lateral to midline
  - Probe can be held longitudinally or transversely and needle can be advanced IP or OOP
  - 10–20 mL of LA injected slowly and incrementally after negative aspiration; epinephrine as vascular marker should be used
- *Non-US Technique*
  - Position is lateral decubitus with hips and knees slightly flexed; ensure patella visible
  - Line A is drawn along midline of lumbar spine; Line B is drawn between iliac crests (intercristal line); needle is inserted 4 cm lateral to midline along intercristal line of side to be blocked and perpendicular to all planes
  - Desired stimulation is femoral nerve (patellar snap)
  - If bone contacted at 4–6 cm (TP), redirect slightly cranially or caudally; hamstring stim means needle too caudal and stimulating lumbosacral plexus (sciatic n.); withdraw and redirect if depth 8 cm and no stim

Femoral Nerve Block

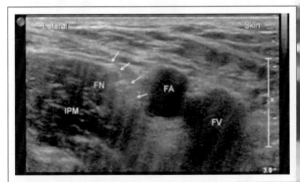

FA, femoral artery; FV, femoral vein; FN, femoral nerve; IPM, iliopsoas muscle.

- *Indications*
  - Surgeries involving femur, knee joint, anterior thigh, and medial leg below knee
- *Specific Considerations*
  - Superficial block at inguinal crease; obesity necessitates retraction of abdomen
  - Femoral n. has 2 main branches at this level; anterior branch supplies sartorius and pectineus m.; posterior branch is deeper, under fascia iliaca and supplies anterior thigh, quadriceps muscles, knee joint, medial lower leg (saphenous n.)
- *Important Landmarks/Anatomy*
  - Inguinal crease, femoral artery, fascia iliaca, fascia lata
  - Nerve lateral to artery and vein (NAVL)
- *US-Guided Approach*
  - Position is supine
  - High-frequency or mid-range transducer
  - Place probe in inguinal crease; obtain short axis view of femoral artery; nerve is hyperechoic structure just lateral to femoral a.; femoral n. sits atop iliopsoas m. and is covered by fascia iliaca
  - Needle advanced IP or OOP until it pierces fascia iliaca near femoral n.; inject 20–30 mL of LA incrementally and observe for spread deep to fascia iliaca, running deep to femoral a.
- *Non-US Technique*
  - Position is supine
  - Palpate femoral artery in inguinal crease; insert needle 1 cm lateral to fem A. pulse and slightly inferior to crease; direct needle slightly cephalad and advance until quadriceps muscles stimulated
  - Ensure quadriceps m. stimulated by observing for patellar twitches; if anterior thigh twitching but no patellar movement (sartorius m. stim from anterior br. of femoral n.), redirect needle slightly more lateral and advance deeper

Obturator Nerve Block
- *Indications*
  - Hip and knee joint surgeries (partial coverage), incisions involving medial thigh/knee
  - Suppression of obturator reflex: Sudden, forceful adduction of leg during TURBT can lead to bladder wall perforation from resector (spinal block does not abolish the reflex)
- *Specific Considerations*
  - Obturator n. divides into anterior and posterior branches; provides articular branches to hip joint (ant br) and knee joint (post br), innervates adductor muscles (ant and post br), and occasionally provides some cutaneous innervation to inferior medial thigh/knee (ant br)
  - Typically used in combination with other blocks to provide analgesia for the knee
  - Bladder is just deep to obturator foramen
- *Important Landmarks/Anatomy*
  - Pubic tubercle
- *US Guided Approach* (not useful for articular branch to hip joint)
  - Useful for blocking posterior branch for knee surgery
  - Position is supine with leg externally rotated
  - Mid-range or high-frequency transducer ideal
  - Probe parallel with inguinal crease and scan caudally; identify pectineus muscle medial to femoral artery; identify medial border of pectineus m. with its "fish mouth" appearance where it rests against adductor muscles (3 adductor muscles, stacked superficial to deep—longus, brevis, magnus)
  - Nerves are hyperechoic; identify anterior branch between adductor longus and brevis m.; posterior br between adductor brevis and magnus m.; needle directed IP or OOP and 5–10 mL of LA deposited around each nerve
- *Non-US Technique* (effective for hip analgesia)
  - Position is supine with leg abducted 30°
  - Needle insertion point is 1.5 cm lateral & 1.5 cm inferior to pubic tubercle; aim superiorly and advance until pubic ramus contacted; angle needle 45° laterally and walk off ramus inferiorly advancing slowly 2–3 cm until stimulation obtained (leg adduction)
  - May be helpful to start stimulation at higher current (2–3 mA)

Lateral Femoral Cutaneous Block
- *Indications*
  - Surgeries involving hip and lateral/anterior thigh incisions and skin grafts

- *Specific Considerations*
  - Cutaneous nerve only
  - Blind technique historically
  - Can use stim at higher current to elicit paresthesia
- *Important Landmarks/Anatomy*
  - Anterior superior iliac spine (ASIS), fascia lata
- *US-Guided Approach*
  - Position is supine
  - High-frequency transducer
  - Begin with probe in inguinal crease; identify fascia iliaca and fascia lata; trace facial layers laterally to a point just medial and inferior to ASIS; observe for hyperechoic structure deep to fascia lata and superficial to sartorius m. and inject 5–10 mL of LA around nerve
  - If nerve not identified, deposit LA deep and superficial to fascia lata
- *Non-US Technique*
  - Position is supine
  - Insert short beveled needle 2 cm medial and 2 cm inferior to ASIS; advance directly posterior, feeling for "pop" through fascia lata; distribute total of 10 mL of LA deep and superficial to fascia lata

Adductor Canal Block
- *Indications*
  - Analgesia of knee joint
  - Reliable block of saphenous nerve for analgesia of medial lower leg
- *Specific Considerations*
  - Comparable analgesia to femoral n. block for surgeries involving knee joint but with significantly less quadriceps weakness
  - Blocks only some branches of femoral nerve to quadriceps m.; blocks articular branches to knee and saphenous nerve
- *Important Landmarks/Anatomy*
  - Mid-thigh, femur, femoral artery, sartorius muscle
- *US-Guided Technique*
  - Position is supine with leg slightly externally rotated
  - High-frequency to mid-range transducer
  - Probe placed on mid-thigh in transverse plane; identify femur and scan medially to locate femoral artery; trace femoral a. proximally until it lies directly beneath sartorius m. and is more superficial
  - Nerves are hyperechoic structures lateral and medial to femoral a.; saphenous branch of femoral n. is typically located lateral to femoral a. when block performed proximal to mid-thigh
  - Needle advanced IP or OOP through sartorius m.; incrementally inject 10–20 mL of LA following aspiration, observing for periarterial spread deep to sartorius m. (within the adductor canal)

Sciatic Nerve Block (Classic, Anterior, Subgluteal)
- *Indications*
  - Surgeries of the lower extremity
- *Specific Considerations*
  - Typically deeper and more challenging block (4 or 6 in. needle required)
  - Can be blocked at multiple locations
  - Posterior cutaneous n. of the thigh is not branch of sciatic nerve but is often covered with proximal block of sciatic (classic); useful if incision involves posterior thigh
- *Important Landmarks/Anatomy*
  - Greater trochanter, posterior superior iliac spine (PSIS), sacral hiatus, ischial tuberosity, ASIS, pubic tubercle
- *US-Guided Approach* (Subgluteal)
  - Position: Lateral decubitus with hips and knees slightly flexed
  - Mid-range to low-frequency transducer for deeper target
  - Position probe between greater troch and ischial tuberosity; identify sciatic nerve as hyperechoic/honeycomb structure flattened out under gluteus muscle; trace nerve distally 4–7 cm for optimal view
  - Needle advanced IP or OOP and through tough common investing fascia; inject 20–30 mL of LA incrementally; observe LA spread between fascial layer and sciatic n., pushing nerve downward
- *Non-US Techniques*
  - *Classic Sciatic Block*: Position is lateral decubitus with hips and knees bent slightly; landmarks are PSIS and greater troch; Line A between greater troch and PSIS;

Line B at midpoint and perpendicular to Line A extending distally 4 cm; needle advanced perpendicular to all planes; acceptable stimulation is plantar or dorsiflexion and inversion or eversion of the foot
- *Modified Classic Sciatic Block*: Same as classic but adds a 3rd line; Line C from greater troch to sacral hiatus; needle insertion is intersection of Line B and Line C

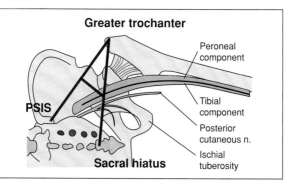

- *Anterior Approach*: Needs 6-in. needle; position is supine; Line A between ASIS and pubic tubercle; Line B perpendicular to Line A at point where medial one-third meets lateral two-thirds; Line C from greater troch, parallel to Line A; needle inserted where Line C meets Line B and advanced directly posterior; needle typically contacts femur and should be walked off femur medially, and advanced 4–5 cm past point of femur contact until twitch in foot detected
- *Subgluteal*: Position is lateral decubitus with hip and knee slightly flexed; Line A from greater troch to ischial tuberosity; Line B is the midpoint of Line A extending distally 4 cm, needle inserted perpendicular to all planes until twitch in foot detected; likely misses post cut n. of the thigh

Popliteal Block of Sciatic Nerve
- *Indications*
  - Surgery involving lower leg distal to knee
- *Specific Considerations*
  - Positioning concerns; may need leg elevated to allow access to popliteal fossa or prone position
  - Point at which sciatic nerve splits into tibial and common peroneal nerves
  - Combine with saphenous n. block for total anesthesia of lower leg
- *Important Landmarks/Anatomy*
  - Popliteal crease, tendon of biceps femoris muscle, tendons of semi-membranous (SM) and semitendinosus (ST) muscles, popliteal artery, femur
- *US-Guided Approach*
  - Position can be prone with leg extended or supine with leg elevated and slightly flexed
  - High-frequency to mid-range transducer
  - Probe in transverse plane at popliteal crease; identify popliteal artery and look for hyperechoic/honeycomb structure (tibial n.) superficial to popliteal a.
  - Trace tibial n. proximally, observing common peroneal n. travel lateral to medial to abut the tibial n., resembling a peanut shell when they touch; a common sheath covers the nerves here
  - Needle advanced IP or OOP and through the sheath between the two nerves; inject 20–30 mL of LA incrementally within the sheath, pushing the tibial and peroneal nerves apart
- *Non-US Techniques*
  - Stimulation desired: Plantar flexion or inversion of foot (tibial n.)
  - *Intertendinous Approach*: Prone position; 2-in. needle; Line A is popliteal crease; Lines B and C drawn along biceps femoris tendon and tendon of SM and ST muscles, extending 7 cm from popliteal crease; Line D connects Lines B and C 7 cm

proximal to popliteal crease. Insert needle at midpoint of Line D and advance posterior to anterior; if no stim, redirect laterally
  * *Lateral Approach:* Supine with leg straight; 4-in. needle; Line A is popliteal crease; Line B is anterior border of biceps femoris muscle; needle insertion is along Line B at a point 7 cm proximal from popliteal crease; needle advanced medially to make contact with femur, then withdrawn and advanced at a strict 30° angle posteriorly; nerve typically 1–2 cm deeper than femur depth

Saphenous Nerve Block
* *Indications*
  * Incisions on medial lower leg and foot
* *Specific Considerations*
  * Cutaneous nerve typically used with sciatic n. block for total anesthesia of lower leg
  * Can be blocked at multiple locations, including adductor canal (above) and medial malleolus with ankle block (below)
  * For foot surgery, most reliable location to block is malleolus
* *Important Landmarks/Anatomy*
  * Sartorius muscle, tibial tuberosity, saphenous vein
* *US-Guided Approach*
  * See adductor canal block above (greatest success)
  * Can facilitate transsartorial block (described below) by identifying sartorius m. and potentially saphenous n.
  * Can facilitate paravenous technique (described below) by identifying great saphenous vein
* *Non-US Techniques* (position is supine with leg externally rotated)
  * *At Tibial Tuberosity:* 5–10 mL of LA injected subcutaneously from medial tibial condyle posteriorly across proximal medial calf
  * *Paravenous:* Apply venous access tourniquet to aid identification of greater saphenous vein just inferior to patella; inject 5–10 mL of LA perivenously
  * *Transsartorial or subsartorial:* Palpate sartorius muscle just proximal to knee; using loss-of-resistance (LOR) technique, pass needle directly through belly of sartorius m. just proximal to patella; after LOR, aspirate and inject 10 mL of LA

Ankle Block (Fig. 6-4)
* *Indications*
  * Foot surgery
* *Specific Considerations*
  * 2 deep nerves (posterior tibial and deep peroneal nerves)
  * 3 superficial nerves (sural, saphenous, superficial peroneal nerves)
  * Block deep nerves 1st; subcutaneous injections for superficial nerves alter surface anatomy
* *Important Landmarks/Anatomy*
  * Lateral and medial malleoli, extensor hallucis longus (EHL) tendon, Achilles tendon
* *US-Guided Approach*
  * Useful for deep nerves
  * Position is supine with lower leg resting on a rolled blanket with foot suspended
  * High-frequency transducer
  * *Deep peroneal nerve:* Probe in transverse plane at or just below level of malleolus; identify dorsalis pedis artery; inject 5–8 mL of LA in tissue planes surrounding artery; nerve difficult to identify
  * *Posterior tibial nerve:* Probe in transverse plane just below medial malleolus; identify post tibial artery; post tibial nerve usually easy to identify as honeycomb structure just posterior to artery; trace nerve proximally above medial malleolus; needle advanced IP or OOP and 5–8 mL of LA injected around nerve
* *Non-US Technique* (must block all 5 nerves)
  * 3 superficial nerves (sural, saphenous, superficial peroneal): Subcutaneous injection of 15–20 mL of LA extending in a ring just proximal to malleoli; start at anterior surface (superficial peroneal), extending injection medially (saphenous) past med malleolus; then extend anterior injection laterally (sural) to Achilles tendon
  * Deep peroneal nerve: Identify EHL tendon just proximal to malleoli by having pt extend great toe; advance needle to bone (tibia) just lateral to EHL tendon; withdraw needle 2 mm and inject 5–8 mL of LA
  * Posterior tibial nerve (can add stim to better target nerve): Palpate post tibial artery posterior to medial malleolus, advance needle posterior and deep to artery; inject 5–8 mL of LA after negative aspiration; alternatively, insert needle half the distance between Achilles tendon and medial malleolus, advance needle to bone, withdraw 2 mm and inject LA after negative aspiration

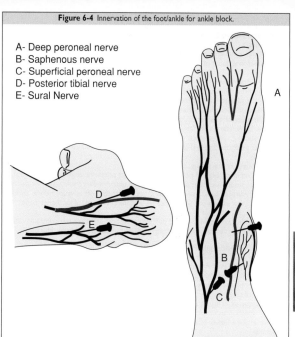

Figure 6-4 Innervation of the foot/ankle for ankle block.

A- Deep peroneal nerve
B- Saphenous nerve
C- Superficial peroneal nerve
D- Posterior tibial nerve
E- Sural Nerve

(Image courtesy of J. Ehernfeld.)

INTRAVENOUS REGIONAL ANESTHESIA (BIER BLOCK)

- *Indications*
  - Short procedures on extremities <1–1.5 h (e.g., carpal tunnel release)
- *Materials*
  - Double tourniquet
  - Esmarch bandage
  - Small (22–24 G) IV in arm to be blocked (to be removed following the block)
  - Additional IV access on nonoperative arm (for administration of other meds)
  - 40–50 mL of plain 0.5% lidocaine
- *Technique*
  - Elevate arm above body & exsanguinate arm (distal → proximal) using an Esmarch bandage
  - Inflate distal cuff 100 mmHg higher than systolic BP (or roughly 300 mmHg), then inflate proximal cuff to same pressure
  - Deflate distal cuff
  - Remove bandage, inject 40–50 mL of plain 0.5% lidocaine through the small-gauge IV & remove IV
  - Encourage surgeons to start operating as soon as possible
  - If tourniquet pain occurs, inflate distal cuff, & then release proximal cuff; this will provide additional 20–30 min of anesthesia. Inform surgeons of limited time left
- *Complications/problems*
  - Local anesthetic toxicity can occur if tourniquet is faulty/deflated too early
  - If surgery finishes in <20 min, keep tourniquet up for another 10 min; alternatively, release & reinflate tourniquet after 10 s
  - Be prepared to conduct a general anesthetic/MAC in the event surgery is prolonged or block insufficient

TRUNCAL BLOCKS OF PERIPHERAL NERVES

Intercostal Nerve Blocks
- *Indications*
  - Provides supplementary analgesia for rib fractures, thoracic procedures, mastectomy, upper abdominal procedures
- *Anatomy*
  - Intercostal nerves arise from ventral rami of T1–11
  - Each nerve sends off 5 branches, including gray and white communicantes, dorsal, lateral, and anterior cutaneous branches
  - Nerves run along inferior aspect of ribs in groove with intercostal artery & vein (from superior to inferior intercostal vein, artery, nerve)
  - Anterior & lateral cutaneous branches readily blocked at posterior angle of rib just lateral to paraspinous muscles
  - Blocks performed at mid-axillary line may miss lateral cutaneous branch
- *Technique*
  - Positioning: Prone, sitting, or lateral decubitus
  - Palpate inferior edge of rib to be blocked at its posterior angle (6–8 cm lateral to midline); insert needle at angle 20° cephalad until needle contacts inferior portion of rib; redirect caudally until needle slides underneath rib; advance needle another 3 mm (a fascial pop can sometimes be felt); inject 3–5 mL of local anesthetic
- *Complications*
  - Pneumothorax: Pts with limited pulmonary reserve are a relative contraindication
  - Local anesthetic toxicity: Risk greatly rises as the number of levels blocked ↑

Transversus Abdominis Plane Block (TAP Block)
- *Indications*
  - Incisions/pain involving abdominal wall; covers skin, muscle, and parietal peritoneum but does not cover visceral pain
  - Bilateral blocks required for midline incisions (do not exceed recommended safe doses of LA)
  - Controversy in literature regarding spread and level of block achieved with a single TAP injection esp cephalad to T10 but more cephalad injection site (subcostal) will help attain a higher block up to T7
- *Anatomy*
  - Innervation of anterior abdominal wall from spinal nerves T7–L1 (intercostal nerves T7–11; subcostal nerve T12; iliohypogastric & ilioinguinal nerves L1)
  - Anterior divisions of T7–11 travel anteriorly between internal oblique (IO) and transversus abdominis (TA) muscles, then perforate and supply rectus abdominis m. and terminate as anterior cutaneous branches
  - Anterior branch of T12 communicates with the iliohypogastric nerve
  - The iliohypogastric nerve (L1) divides between the IO and TA near the iliac crest into lateral and anterior cutaneous branches, the anterior branch supplies the hypogastric region
  - The ilioinguinal nerve (L1) supplies the upper & medial parts of the thigh & part of the skin covering the genitalia
- *Techniques*
  - Direct needle through external oblique (EO) and IO muscles and deposit LA in fascial plane between the IO and TA muscles in the TA plane (TAP)
  - *Conventional/non-US* site is the lumbar triangle of Petit between the lower costal margin and the iliac crest; borders: anterior—EO, posterior—latissimus dorsi m., inferior—iliac crest; relies on sensing two "pops" as needle traverses fascia above & below IO
    - Not recommended if US available due to proximity of peritoneum and subjective nature of sensing the "pops" with needle; improve sensitivity with blunt needle
  - *US-Guided Approach:* With pt in supine position, place high-frequency probe in a transverse plane on lateral abdominal wall between the lower costal margin and the iliac crest at anterior axillary line and identify 3 distinct muscle layers (EO, IO, and TA)
    - Advance needle (IP or OOP) through EO and IO muscles into plane between IO and TA muscles; aspirate and inject 20–30 mL of LA, observing that LA is deposited within the TAP and not into IO or TA muscles
    - Subcostal TAP block is modification of original technique in which US probe is placed just beneath and parallel to costal margin. The needle is introduced lateral to medial IP and 10 mL LA injected into TAP to extend analgesia above umbilicus

- Complications
  - Local anesthetic toxicity (bilateral injections), intraperitoneal injection, intravascular injection, bowel hematoma, intrahepatic injection, transient femoral nerve palsy
- Pectoralis Blocks (Pecs I and II)
  - Indications
    - Analgesia of anterolateral chest wall/breast and axilla resulting from blocking branches of intercostal and pectoral nerves
    - Surgeries involving breast, axilla, and lymph node explorations Less invasive alternative to brachial plexus and paravertebral blocks to cover same area
  - Anatomy
    - Interfacial injections; Pecs I between PM and Pm muscles; Pecs II is Pecs I plus between Pm and serratus anterior (SA)
    - Pecs I blocks the lateral (C5–7) and medial (C8&T1) pectoral nerves
    - Pecs II block adds the T2–6 intercostal nerves
  - Technique
    - With pt supine, position high frequency US probe near midaxillary line with inferolateral rotation; identify 3rd rib, PM, and Pm muscles
    - Advance needle through PM and Pm muscles; after negative aspiration, inject 10–15 mL of LA into the plane between Pm and SA muscles; withdraw needle and inject 15–20 mL LA into the plane between PM and Pm

Thoracic Paravertebral Block (PVB)

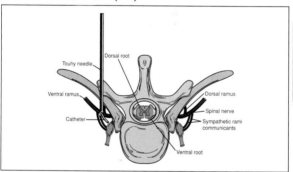

- Anatomy
  - Thoracic paravertebral space is a triangular space bordered medially by vertebral bodies, posteriorly by superior costotransverse ligament (CTL), and anterolaterally by parietal pleura; contains emerging spinal nerves with dorsal and ventral rami, rami communicantes, and the sympathetic chain (ventral ramus continues as intercostal nerve)
- Indications
  - Analgesia for rib fractures, thoracic surgery, breast surgery
  - Anesthesia for breast surgery or superficial chest wall surgery
  - Provides unilateral blockade of spinal nerves without sympathectomy
  - Multiple levels (one above and one below) can be covered with one injection site if higher volumes (10–15 mL) used
  - Catheter can be inserted for continuous infusion
- Techniques
  - Identify dermatomes/ribs needed to block, then identify SPs of corresponding thoracic vertebrae; needle will be advanced into the paravertebral space, just superficial to the pleura, where LA is deposited
  - Conventional/Non-US: With pt in sitting position, identify SP at level of spinal nerve needed to be blocked; needle insertion is 2.5 cm lateral to the SP; advance needle anteriorly and perpendicular to all planes until contact is made with TP; typical depth is 3–4 cm; attention to needle trajectory is critical (too medial risks epidural/spinal spread, too lateral risks pleural puncture)
  - Walk needle off TP caudally and 1–1.25 cm past depth at which TP contacted; a "pop" may be sensed as the CTL is penetrated; LOR can be applied to identify the paravertebral space as needle advanced through the CTL

- • *US Guided:* With pt in sitting position, place a high-frequency probe perpendicular or parallel to TP; identify CTL and pleura; advance needle IP or OOP through CTL, just superficial to pleura; aspirate and inject 5–15 mL of LA incrementally
- • *Complications*
  - • Epidural or spinal spread (high spinal), sympathectomy, pneumothorax

---

SPINAL/EPIDURAL ANESTHESIA

Neuraxial Anatomy (also see Figure 6-5)
- • Spinal cord extends from base of skull → L1–2 in adults/L3 in infants
- • Dural sac extends from base of skull → S2 in adults/S3–4 in infants
- • Anatomic landmarks: Tip of scapula (T7/8), iliac crest (L4 or L4/5), sacral cornu (S5)
- • Thoracic SPs: Angled caudally (in relation to vertebral bodies)
- • Lumbar SPs: Angled horizontally
- • "S-shape of spinal column": Thoracic kyphosis (convex) at T4; lumbar lordosis (concave) at L3
- • **Midline approach**—order of tissues encountered: Skin → subcutaneous tissue → supraspinous & interspinous ligaments → ligamentum flavum → epidural space → dura mater → subdural space → arachnoid mater → subarachnoid space (= intrathecal space) containing CSF
- • **Paramedian approach** (needle insertion 1 cm lateral to midline): Bypasses supraspinous & interspinous ligaments and SPs; needle walked up and over lamina; consider for narrowed intervertebral spaces, calcified ligaments, thoracic epidural (sharply angled, closely approximated overlapping SPs)

Figure 6-5 Dermatome map

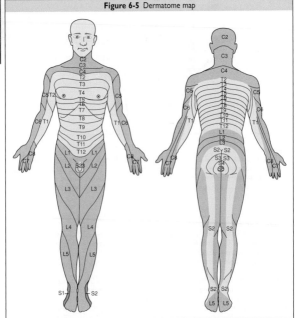

(From Overview and Basic Concepts. In: Moore KL, Dalley AF, Agur AM. *Clinically Oriented Anatomy.* 8th ed. Philadelphia, PA: Wolters Kluwer; 2018:51.)

Physiologic Effects

- **Neurologic:** Blockade of preganglionic sympathetic fibers exceeds sensory block (spinal > epidural), often by up to 2 dermatomes, with degree of blockade determined by block height
- **Cardiovascular**

  Sympathectomy (spinal > epidural) → loss of vascular tone → hypotension & reflex tachycardia

  Supra-T4 levels block cardioaccelerator fibers (T1–4) → paradoxical bradycardia → decreased CO & further hypotension

  Large volumes of local anesthetic used for epidurals → higher systemic absorption → direct cardiac depressant effects
- **Pulmonary**

  Impaired cough reflex, high blockade ↓ use of accessory resp muscles (intercostals, abdominals) → use caution in pts with limited pulmonary reserve

  Unchanged: Inspi fx (unless respiratory centers [C3–5] blocked), TV, MV, Vd

  PFT changes: ↓ Or unchanged VC, ↓ ERV, ↓ expiratory flow rate
- **GI**

  Sympathectomy → hyperperistalsis (unopposed parasympathetics) → N/V (prevented by tx of hypotension [fluids, vasoconstrictors], atropine if high thoracic block)
- **GU**

  Sacral blockade → atonic bladder (consider catheterization); renal blood flow usually maintained
- **Neuroendocrine**

  Avoid surgical stress response (incr catecholamines, vasopressin, GH, renin, angiotensin, cortisol, glucose, ADH, TSH) with adequate sensory blockade, nearly complete w surgery below umbilicus (possible cardioprotective effect of thoracic epidural/analg in pts with cardiovasc/cardiac dz)

Contraindications to Placing a Neuraxial Block

- **Absolute** (per NYSORA)

  Pt refusal/infection at site of needle puncture, bleeding diathesis (severe hypovolemia [uncorrected]), ↑ ICP, true allergy to amide and ester LA
- **Relative** (per NYSORA)

  Severe anatomic abnormalities or prior back surgery, uncooperative pt, neurologic dz (multiple sclerosis), infection distal to needle insertion site, and bacteremia (consider with prior antibiotic prophylaxis), severe cardiac dz (aortic/mitral stenosis), abnormal coagulation (endogenous or iatrogenic), anesthetized pt (cervical, thoracic)

ASRA Regional Anesthesia & Anticoagulation Guidelines (Summary)	
Medication Class	**Recommendation**
Antiplatelet agents	
Aspirin, other NSAIDs	No contraindications unless in pt with underlying coagulopathy or in combination with additional hemostasis-altering medications
Clopidogrel	Wait 5–7 d before needle insertion
Ticlopidine	Wait 10 d before needle insertion
GP IIb/IIIa inhibitors	Avoid neuraxial block until plt function has recovered
Abciximab	Wait 24–48 h before needle insertion
*Ticagrelor (Brilinta)	Wait 5–7 d before needle insertion
*Prasugrel (Effient)	Wait 7–10 d before needle insertion
Eptifibatide, Tirofiban	Wait 4–8 h before needle insertion
Low–molecular-weight heparin	
Prophylaxis	Wait 10–12 h (for low doses; <1 mg/kg bid, <1.5 mg/kg qd) or 24 h (for higher doses) before needle insertion
Therapeutic enoxaparin 1 mg/kg q12h or 1.5 mg/kg qd; dalteparin 120 U/kg q12h or 200 U/kg qd, tinzaparin 175/U/kg/d	bid and high-dose qd dosing: No regional anesthesia recommended. Remove catheter 2 h before the first dose, which should be no earlier than 24 h postop. Postop qd dosing: Remove catheter 10–12 h after the last dose & 4 h before the subsequent dose
Heparin and other medications	
Heparin	Assess platelet count prior to needle insertion and before removing catheter if pt on heparin >4 d

Subcutaneous (SQ)	No contraindication with bid and total daily dosing <10,000 units, wait 4–6 h before insertion; wait 12 h with total daily dosing >10,000 units and reduce heparin dose if indwelling catheter desired
Heparin intraop (vascular procedures)	Delay heparin 1 h after needle insertion, remove catheter 4 h after last dose and 1 h before subsequent dose; reheparinization possible 1 h after catheter removal
Full heparinization intraop (cardiac/bypass procedures)	Wait >1 h after needle insertion before full heparinization (delay surgery for 24 h after bloody tap)
Heparin IV pre-procedure	Discontinue 4–6 h before needle insertion and evaluate coagulation status
Warfarin	Discontinue 5 d prior to needle insertion Document normal INR prior to needle insertion & <1.5 prior to catheter removal
Thrombolytics (urokinase, streptokinase, alteplase, reteplase)	Absolute contraindication Wait at least 48 h and document normal clotting studies (include fibrinogen)
Direct thrombin inhibitors (desirudin, lepirudin, bivalirudin, argatroban)	Insufficient data suggest avoidance of neuraxial techniques
Oral direct thrombin and factor Xa inhibitors	Insufficient data and prolonged half-life suggest avoidance of neuraxial techniques
*Dabigatran (Pradaxa)	Wait 5 d (120 h) before needle insertion Can place sooner if no add. risk factors for bleeding and depending on CrCl: (CrCl 80 mL/min = 72 h; CrCl 50–79 = 96 h); no block if CrCl <30
Rivaroxaban (Xarelto)	Wait 3 d (72 h) before needle insertion
Apixaban (Eliquis)	Wait 3 d (72 h) before needle insertion
Fondaparinux (Arixtra)	Risk unknown; avoid indwelling catheters (long half-life: 21 h)
Herbal medication	No evidence for mandatory discontinuation before needle insertion; risk unknown, be aware of potential drug interactions

Please note that these recommendations now also include plexus and peripheral nerve blocks according to the last update

Adapted from *Reg Anesth Pain Med* 2018;43:263–309.

Patient Positioning for Block Placement
- Goal for optimal positioning: Widen intervertebral spaces
  → Knees flexed toward abdomen, chin flexed to chest, shoulders relaxed
- *Sitting position*: Easier to identify midline, can create saddle block if using hyperbaric solutions
- *Lateral decubitus position*: Use if pt unable to sit
  → Can preferentially block 1 side (if using hypo- or hyperbaric solutions)
- *Prone jackknife position*: Good for perirectal surgery (if using hypobaric solution)

Complications of Neuraxial Anesthesia
Common to both spinal and epidural anesthesia
• Backache
• Pruritus
• Hypotension
• Urinary retention
• Nerve injury
• Infection
• Hematoma
• Hypoventilation
Other spinal complications
• **Transient neurologic symptoms (TNS):** More common with ambulatory procedures, lithotomy position, lidocaine spinals. Symptoms: Delayed onset of pain and/or dysesthesia in lower back, buttocks, posterior thighs (can last up to 7 d)

- **Cauda equina syndrome:** Occurs with repeated admin of conc local anesthetic. Symptoms: Bowel/bladder dysfunction and/or neurologic impairment; seek immediate neurosurgical consult
- **Postspinal headache:** (See postdural puncture headache later)
- **High/total spinal:** Supracervical blockade can cause cardiovascular collapse, apnea, loss of consciousness; supportive treatment/intubation may be necessary

Other epidural complications
- **Postdural puncture headache (PDPH):** From inadvertent dural puncture (wet tap); usually self-limited (<7 d). Initial management: Hydration, caffeine (500 mg), NSAIDs, abdominal binders. Persistent or intolerable PDPH (>24 h): Epidural blood patches >90% effective
- **Spinal cord injury:** Can occur if wet tap occurs at level above where spinal cord ends
- **Local anesthetic toxicity:** Dizziness, tinnitus, CNS excitation, seizures, cardiac arrest can occur from systemic absorption or intravascular injection of local anesthetic. Treatment is supportive. Consider 20% intralipid emulsions for refractory cardiac arrest

SPINAL ANESTHESIA

- Rapid & reliable onset of lower body anesthesia by injecting local anesthetic into the intrathecal space
  - Blocks spinal cord fibers and nerve rootlets
  - Usually single-shot, although continuous catheters can be used
- Consider prior intravascular volume loading (500–1,000 mL fluid) to reduce effects of rapid sympathectomy
- Needles:
  - Small gauge (>24 G), pencil point needles (Sprotte, Whitacre) reduce risk of PDPH → Often require introducer (19 G) to penetrate superficial tissues
  - Large gauge (<22 G), cutting (Quincke, Greene) needles → Used in difficult spinals to penetrate fibrotic, calcified ligaments
- Introduce needle (midline or paramedian technique) at L2–5 interspaces until dural "pop" felt or if CSF flows freely when stylet removed

Factors Affecting Anesthetic Spread in Intrathecal Space	
Baricity	Local solution density in relation to CSF; mixing medication with dextrose or sterile water results in hyperbaric or hypobaric solutions (respectively) • Isobaric (density = CSF)—results in block at level where medication is injected • Hyperbaric (density > CSF)—results in spread of medication with gravity in intrathecal space • Hypobaric (density < CSF)—results in spread of medication against gravity in intrathecal space
Pt position	Gravity can help spread of medication within intrathecal space when hypo- or hyperbaric solutions used
Spinal curvature	Thoracic kyphosis at T4 prevents migration of medication toward cervical region when pt supine
Other factors: Dose, volume, temperature of medication injected, age, increased abdominal pressure, pregnancy, direction of needle bevel	
No effect: Weight, height, gender, barbotage	

- Duration of spinal anesthesia:
  - Dependent on type & dose of local anesthetic used
  - Duration can be prolonged with vasoconstrictors (phenylephrine/epinephrine)

Characteristics of Local Anesthetic for Spinal Anesthesia			
		Duration of block (min)	
Local Anesthetic	**Concentration (%)**	**Plain**	**w/Vasoconstrictors**
Procaine	10	30–50	50–75
Lidocaine	1–2, 5	45–60	75–90
Mepivacaine	2	50–70	80–120
Bupivacaine	0.5–0.75	90–120	140
Tetracaine	0.5	90–150	180–300
Ropivacaine	0.5–0.75	60–90	80–120
Chloroprocaine	2–3	30–60	

Level of Sensory Block and Dose Needed for Surgical Procedures

Sensory Level	Type of Surgery	Local Anesthetic and Dose
T4 (nipple)	Upper abdominal Surgery C-section	Tetracaine, bupivacaine, or ropivacaine **Dose:** 8–16 mg
T6–7 (xiphoid)	Lower abdominal surgery Appendectomy Herniorrhaphy	**Dose:** Lidocaine 75–100 mg, bupivacaine or ropivacaine 10–14 mg
T10 (umbilicus)	Hip surgery TURP Vaginal delivery	**Dose:** Lidocaine 50–75 mg, tetracaine 6–10 mg, bupivacaine or ropivacaine 8–12 mg
L1 (inguinal ligament)	Lower extremity	**Dose:** Tetracaine, bupivacaine, or ropivacaine, 6 mg
L2–3 (knee)	Foot surgery	**Dose:** Tetracaine, bupivacaine, or ropivacaine, 6 mg
S2–5	Hemorrhoidectomy	**Dose:** Lidocaine 30–50 mg

Table adapted from: Stoelting RK, Miller RD. *Basics of Anesthesia.* 5th ed. New York, NY: Churchill Livingstone; 2006.

Continuous Spinal Anesthesia (CSA)
- "Titratable spinal anesthesia" combining benefit of single-shot spinal (rapid onset) and epidural anesthesia (continuous technique) (maintain level and radid of block during surgery, titrate effect to pts response)
- Lower doses of LA for continuous technique can be used
- Useful in pts with severe systemic dz (e.g., severe aortic/mitral stenosis)
- Technique same as for single epidural anesthesia with intentional piercing of the dura mater and insertion of epidural catheter into intrathecal space (smaller gauge catheter, usually 22 G used to ↓ possibility of PDPH, microcatheters <24 G withdrawn from market)
- Controversy about increased risk of cauda equina syndrome (most reports on combination with microcatheters and use of hypobaric lidocaine)
- After confirmation of intrathecal catheter placement by aspiration of CSF slowly bolus with usual intrathecal dose for spinal anesthesia
- Mark catheter meticulously as spinal catheter to avoid wrong medication dosing
- Continuous management possible with intermittent bolus dosing and titration to effect or low-dose continuous infusion
- Spinal catheters are usually not left in place postoperatively

---

EPIDURAL ANESTHESIA

- Slower onset, more controlled segmental spread of anesthesia using larger quantities of medication (roughly 10 × more than spinal doses) injected into epidural space
- Usually a continuous catheter technique; can target select dermatomes (unlike spinal)
  - Thoracic epidurals → thoracic & upper abdominal surgeries
  - Lumbar epidurals → labor analgesia, lower abdominal, pelvic, lower-extremity surgeries

Identifying the Epidural Space

LOR technique	• Engage epidural needle in ligament • Attach low-friction syringe (filled with air/saline) to epidural needle • Apply constant/intermittent pressure to syringe as needle is slowly advanced • When needle passes through ligamentum flavum (into epidural space), plunger will be easily advanced (indicating an LOR)
Hanging-drop technique	• Drop of fluid placed on hub of epidural needle (once engaged in ligamentum flavum) • Advance needle until fluid sucked into needle hub (indicates epidural space)

- Catheter placement & epidural space verification:
  - Thread epidural catheter 3–5 cm into epidural space
  - Aspirate catheter to assess for intravascular/intrathecal insertion (look for blood/CSF)

- Consider epidural test dose (3 mL of 1.5% lidocaine with epinephrine 1:200,000) → shows if catheter intrathecal (dense spinal) or intravascular (tachycardia, tinnitus)
- *Medications*
  - Surgical anesthesia: High local anesthetic conc (2% lidocaine, 0.5% bupivacaine)
  - Postop pain/labor analgesia: Dilute local anesthetic conc. + opioid (0.1% bupivacaine + 0.005% fentanyl)
    (Combination provides synergy, and reduces side effects [motor block, pruritus])
  - Adjuvants can supplement block (clonidine, epinephrine, phenylephrine)

Characteristics of Local Anesthetics for Epidural Anesthesia				
Local Anesthetic	Concentration (%)	Onset (min)	Duration, Plain (min)	Duration, w/ Epinephrine (min)
Chloroprocaine	2–3	3–10	30–90	60–90
Lidocaine	1–2	5–15	60–120	90–180
Bupivacaine	0.25–0.5	10–20	120–240	150–240
Ropivacaine	0.2–0.5	10–20	120–240	150–200

From: Stoelting RK, Miller RD. *Basics of Anesthesia*. 5th ed. New York, NY: Churchill Livingstone; 2006.

- Factors affecting quality of epidural block
  - Volume injected, vasoconstrictors, site of injection, & parturients
  - Sodium bicarbonate can hasten block onset (↑ nonionized local → easier neuronal diffusion)
    - 1 mEq for each 10 mL lidocaine/chloroprocaine
    - 0.1 mEq for each 10 mL of bupivacaine (to avoid precipitation)
  - Pt position has no effect (unlike spinal anesthesia)
- Management
  - Continuous, bolus, or pt-controlled epidural analgesia (PCEA) techniques
  - Continuous infusion rate depends on pt characteristics & the type of solution used (continuous infusions often run at 4–10 mL/h with a bolus dose every 5–15 min)
- Epidural troubleshooting
  - One-sided block: Provide medication bolus, pull back or replace catheter
  - Patchy block assess for possible subdural block, replace catheter if necessary
  - Inability to thread catheter: Verify epidural space with LOR, then advance needle 1 mm & retry
  - Inability to remove catheter: Change pt position (flexing, extending, rotating spine); try carefully again later, NEVER pull using excessive force!

Doses of Epidural Opioids			
Drug	Dose (mg)	Onset (min)	Duration (h)
Alfentanil	2	5	1
Sufentanil	0.005–0.010	3–5	2–4
Fentanyl	0.05–0.10	5–20	3–5
Methadone	5–8	10–20	6–8
Hydromorphone	1	15–20	7–15
Meperidine	30–100	5–10	4–20
Morphine	3–5	30–60	12–24

COMBINED SPINAL–EPIDURAL (CSE) TECHNIQUE

- *Advantages*
  - Combines a rapid-onset block (spinal) with ability to provide continuous management (epidural)
- *Equipment*
  - Epidural tray with specifically designed Tuohy needle (has back hole for spinal needle insertion); alternatively, can use regular Tuohy needle with appropriately sized spinal needle
- *Dose of spinal medication*
  - Surgical anesthesia: Normal dose (see Table above)
  - Labor analgesia: Low-dose opioid + local anesthetic (fentanyl 25 mcg + bupivacaine 2.5 mg)

- *Technique*
  - Proceed as if placing an epidural
  - Place spinal needle through epidural needle past dura (once epidural space identified)
  - Once CSF is obtained, inject medication, remove spinal needle, & thread epidural catheter
- *Disadvantages*
  - Inability to test dose epidural catheter (no reassurance if epidural will work after spinal wears off)
  - Slightly ↑ incidence of pruritus, respiratory depression, or transient fetal bradycardia

---

CAUDAL ANESTHESIA

- Epidural anesthesia performed at sacral level close to where dural sac ends
- *Indications*
  - Commonly used in children for low superficial abdominal, perineal, or sacral anesthesia
  - Can be used for 2nd stage of labor, perineal, or sacral anesthesia in adults
  - More difficult in adults due to obscure anatomic landmarks
- *Anatomy*
  - *Sacral hiatus:* Posterior opening to sacral canal at S5 level (entrance identified by sacral cornua)
  - *Sacrococcygeal membrane:* Equivalent of ligamentum flavum (overlies entrance to sacral hiatus, can calcify in adults)
- *Positioning:* Lateral or prone
- *Technique*
  - Insert needle between sacral cornu at 45° angle until slight ↓ in resistance encountered (signifying penetration of sacrococcygeal membrane)
  - Redirect needle parallel to sacrum & insert another 1–1.5 cm
  - Syringe should be aspirated for CSF/blood & test dose should be given
  - Catheter may be threaded (similar to an epidural)
- *Medications*
  - Pediatric dose: 0.5–1 mL/kg of 0.125–0.25% bupivacaine +/– epinephrine
  - Adult dose: 15–20 mL of local anesthetic
- *Complications:* Similar to those for epidural anesthesia

JIMIN KIM • JASON BOUHENGUEL

POINT-OF-CARE ULTRASOUND (POCUS)

- POCUS has become an increasingly useful diagnostic and monitoring tool in the perioperative assessment of critically ill patient
- For basics of ultrasound, review Chapter 6

FOCUSED CARDIAC ULTRASOUND

- Used as an adjunct to the physical exam to recognize specific signs that represent a narrow list of potential diagnoses in certain clinical settings (*J Am Soc Echocardiogr* 2013;26:567–581)
- *Probe selection:* Phased array probe commonly used
- *Patient position:* Patients commonly evaluated in the supine position, slight left-side down (brings heart forward), left arm raised above/behind head (opens rib spaces)
- **4 basic views:**
  - Parasternal long axis
  - Parasternal short axis
  - Apical 4-chamber
  - Subcostal (2 views): Subcostal 4-chamber, subcostal IVC
- Online interactive learning modules offered by Toronto General Hospital, Department of Anesthesia: Virtual Transthoracic Echocardiography, http://pie.med. utoronto.ca/TTE/TTE_content/standardViews.html

Parasternal Long Axis (Fig. 7-1)
- *Transducer position:* 3rd or 4th intercostal space at left parasternal border; index marker toward patient's right shoulder (11 o'clock position)
- *Assessment:* LV size and function, LV outflow tract, mitral and aortic valves, LA size, RV size, aortic dissection, pericardial effusion, left pleural effusion

Parasternal Short Axis (Fig. 7-2)
- *Transducer position:* 3rd or 4th intercostal space at left parasternal border; index marker toward patient's left shoulder (2 o'clock position). Turn probe 90° clockwise from parasternal long-axis view to obtain view
- *Assessment:* LV size and function, RV size and function, pericardial effusion; can view at level of aortic valve, mitral valve, papillary muscle, and apex by tilting probe

Apical Four Chamber (Fig. 7-3)
- *Transducer position:* 4th or 5th intercostal space at midclavicular line or at point of apical pulsation; index marker toward patient's left side (3 o'clock position)
- *Assessment:* Global assessment, LV size and function, RV size and function, mitral valve, tricuspid valve, LA size, RA size, and pericardial effusion

Subcostal Views (2)
- **Subcostal Four Chamber (Fig. 7-4)**
  - *Transducer position:* Subxiphoid region of abdomen, slightly to right of midline; flatten transducer and push down; index marker toward patient's left side (3 o'clock position)
  - *Assessment:* Global assessment, LV size and function, RV size and function, mitral valve, tricuspid valve, LA size, RA size, and pericardial effusion; can also be used to detect cardiac motion during a code
- **Subcostal Inferior Vena Cava (Fig. 7-5)**
  - *Transducer position:* Subxiphoid region of abdomen; flatten transducer and pushdown; index marker toward patient's head (12 o'clock position). Turn probe 90° counter-clockwise from subcostal 4-chamber view to obtain view
  - *Assessment:* IVC size and variability (change in IVC size with respiration, use m-mode)

LUNG ULTRASOUND

- Useful in detecting several pathologic lung conditions
- Lung ultrasound often relies on interpretation of artifacts (reverberation of ultrasound signals)
- Large differences in acoustic impedances of soft tissues and air-filled alveoli present limitations in lung ultrasound; ultrasound energy is strongly reflected at the pleural interface
- *Patient position:* Patients commonly evaluated in the semirecumbent or supine position

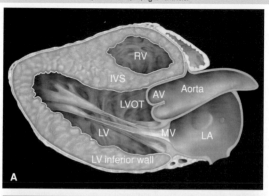

Figure 7-1 Parasternal Long Axis View. AV, aortic valve; IVS, interventricular septum; LA, left atrium; LV, left ventricle; LVOT, left ventricular outflow tract; MV, mitral valve; RV, right ventricle.

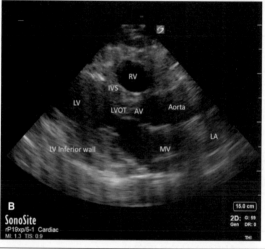

(Redrawn from Patrick J. Lynch; illustrator; C. Carl Jaffe; MD; cardiologist Yale University Center for Advanced Instructional Media. Medical Illustrations by Patrick Lynch (http://patricklynch.net), generated for multimedia teaching projects by the Yale University School of Medicine, Center for Advanced Instructional Media, 1987–2000. Creative Commons Attribution 2.5 License 2006.)

- *Probe:* Probe selection and position vary depending on evaluation of interest
  - *Linear probe:* Anterior chest; assessment of pneumothorax, pulmonary edema
  - *Phased array probe:* Posterior-lateral chest; assessment of pleural effusion

Ultrasound Artifact Analysis (and Pathology)
- A-lines
  - Normal, horizontal reverberation artifacts produced by sound waves reflecting off the pleural interface
  - Present any time a pleura–air interface is present (e.g., normal lungs or pneumothorax)
  - A-lines start from pleura and extend to bottom of image

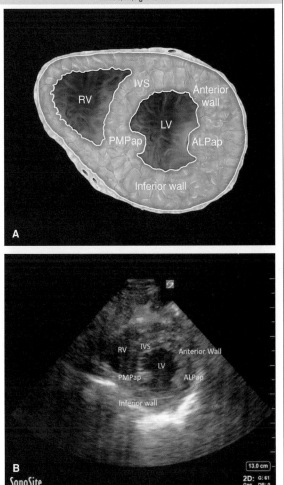

Figure 7-2 Parasternal Short Axis View. ALPap, anterolateral papillary muscle; IVS, interventricular septum; LV, left ventricle; PMPap, posteromedial papillary muscle; RV, right ventricle.

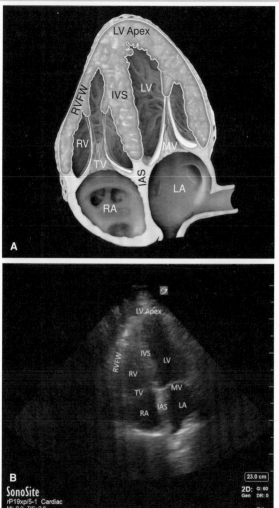

Figure 7-3 Apical Four Chamber View. IAS, interatrial septum; IVS, interventricular septum; LA, left atrium; LV, left ventricle; MV, mitral valve; RA, right atrium; RV, right ventricle; RVFW, RV free wall; TV, tricuspid valve.

Figure 7-4 Subcostal Four Chamber View. IVS, interventricular septum; LA, left atrium; LV, left ventricle; MV, mitral valve; RA, right atrium; RV, right ventricle; TV, tricuspid valve.

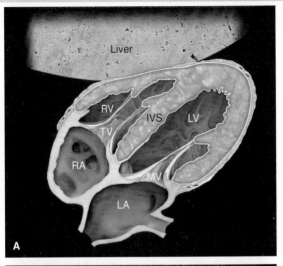

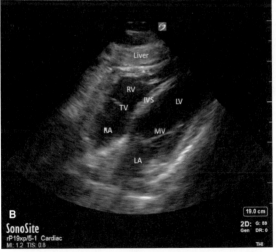

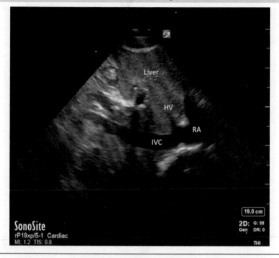

Figure 7-5 Subcostal Inferior Vena Cava View. HV, hepatic vein; IVC, inferior vena cava; RA, right atrium.

(labels on image: Liver, HV, RA, IVC; 19.0 cm; SonoSite; rP19xp/5-1 Cardiac; MI: 1.2 TIS: 0.8; 2D: G: 59 Gen DR: 0; THI)

Interstitial or Alveolar Disease (e.g., Pulmonary Edema, Consolidation, Contusion)
- B-lines
  - Vertical reverberation artifacts that produce hyperechoic lines ("comet tails") that originate from the pleural line and extend downward toward bottom of image
  - B-lines are often transient, move with lung sliding, and obliterate A-lines
  - Represents ↑ density/thickened interstitium from alveolar or interstitial edema
  - B-lines localized to 1 area of chest are suggestive of a consolidation (e.g., pneumonia, contusion), while B lines seen in multiple areas bilaterally may suggest pulmonary edema

Pneumothorax
- Lung sliding
  - Sliding movement of parietal and visceral pleura in apposition is a normal finding during respiration
  - Sliding artifact often described as "ants marching on a line"; absence of lung sliding would appear as a straight stationary line
  - In M-mode (time-lapse display of ultrasound waves over a single vertical line of interest), normal lung sliding yields the "sandy beach sign"; absence of lung sliding alternatively yields the "barcode sign" **Figure 7-6**
  - Presence of lung sliding rules out a pneumothorax in the location of lung being evaluation.
  - Absence of lung sliding does not absolutely imply pneumothorax as this can also be produced by other pathologic conditions (e.g., consolidation, atelectasis, mainstem intubation or occlusion, apnea, ARDS).
  - Ultrasound for detection of pneumothorax: sensitivity 86–98% and specificity 97–100% (trauma), sensitivity 95.3% and specificity 91.1% (ICU)
- Lung point
  - Transition point between normal lung sliding and absent sliding at the pneumothorax border
  - Highly specific (100%, presence of lung point rules in pneumothorax) but not sensitive for a pneumothorax (67%)
- Lung pulse
  - In M mode, periodic small vertical reverberation artifacts synchronous with the cardiac cycle caused by intra-thoracic pressure changes secondary to cardiac contractions transmitted throughout lung parenchyma
  - Presence of lung pulse rules out pneumothorax (suggests presence of lung parenchyma)

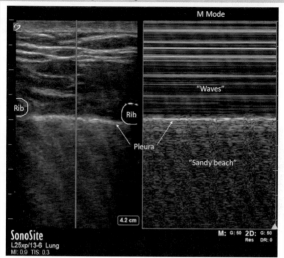

Figure 7-6 Lung ultrasound: M Mode

M Mode

"Waves"

"Sandy beach"

Rib

Rib

Pleura

SonoSite
L25xp/13-6 Lung
MI: 0.9 TIS: 0.3

4.2 cm

M: G: 50   2D: G: 50
Res   DR: 0

Pleural Effusion

- *Patient position:* Preferably seated upright or semirecumbent (pleural fluid typically localizes to most dependent regions of thorax). If supine, scan with ipsilateral arm adducted across chest to opposite side
- *Probe and transducer position:* Phased-array probe; along posterolateral aspect of chest at inferior costal border with index marker toward patient's head (12 o'clock position)
- Orient by identifying liver (right) or spleen (left), kidney, and spine (using the liver/spleen as acoustic window); scan cephalad to identify moving diaphragm. Lung starts where spine visualization ends (due to poor conduction through air-filled lung)
- In the presence of a pleural effusion or hemothorax, the thoracic spine will still be visible cephalad to the liver/diaphragm (due to improved conduction of sound waves through the pleural fluid); this is referred to as the "spine sign"
- Large effusions may be identified in the mid axillary line, while small effusions typically only identified posteriorly.

FOCUSED ASSESSMENT WITH SONOGRAPHY IN TRAUMA (FAST)

- See Trauma Chapter 17 for additional details
- 5 views: Evaluates pericardium and 3 potential peritoneal spaces for pathologic fluid (free fluid suggestive of injury in the peritoneal, pericardial, and pleural cavities)
- Provides a picture of a patient's condition at one moment in time; can repeat for reassessment of the patient's condition if patient is clinically decompensating
- *Probe selection:* Phased array probe or curvilinear probe (for abdominal portion)
- *Patient position:* Supine
- Traditional FAST exam views:
  - RUQ view: Perihepatic, Morison's pouch, or right flank view
    - Evaluates liver, hepatorenal space (Morison's pouch), right pleural space, inferior pole of right kidney, and right paracolic gutter
    - *Probe position:* 7–10th intercostal space, anterior to mid axillary line; index marker pointed toward patient's head (12 o'clock position)
  - LUQ view (perisplenic or left flank view)
    - Evaluates spleen, splenorenal recess, diaphragm, left pleural space, inferior pole of left kidney, and left paracolic gutter
    - *Probe position:* 7–10th intercostal space, posterior axillary line (pressing knuckles to bed in supine pt); index marker pointed toward patient's head (12 o'clock position)
  - Pelvic view (retrovesical, retrouterine, or pouch of Douglas view)

- Assesses most dependent space in peritoneum, most often posterior or superior to bladder and uterus
- Fluid-filled bladder may help analysis for pelvic fluid
- *Probe position:* Midline above pubic symphysis and angled caudal into pelvis; probe marker pointed toward patient's right (9 o'clock position) for suprapubic transverse view and toward patient's head (12 o'clock position) for suprapubic longitudinal view
- *Pericardial view:* Traditional subcostal 4-chamber view
- eFAST (extended FAST) exam: Traditional FAST exam + evaluation of pneumothorax

ULTRASOUND-GUIDED VASCULAR ACCESS

- Ultrasound guidance reduces number of access attempts (i.e., improves success rates), reduces time to venous cannulation, and reduces complications related to catheter placement.

Indications

Identification and evaluation of veins (vein diameter, patency, selection of appropriately sized catheter), central venous catheter placements, peripheral venous catheter placements (e.g., peripherally inserted central catheters), difficult peripheral intravenous access (e.g., obesity, pediatric, etc.), evaluation of catheter "tip navigation" (evaluates for proper direction of catheter tip), evaluation of puncture-related complications (e.g., local hematoma, pneumothorax)
- *Probe selection:* High-frequency linear probe

Ultrasound Views

- Transverse view (short axis, "out-of-plane" vein cannulation approach): Probe positioned at 90° angle to the course of the vein
  - Useful for vein identification and localization, allows for distinguishing vein from adjacent artery during cannulation
- Longitudinal view (long axis, "in-plane" vein cannulation approach): Identify transverse view, then rotate probe 90° so the long axis is parallel to the course of the vein
  - Useful for evaluating presence of valves, vein morphology
  - May be technically more difficult to maintain center of vessel in view and correct needle trajectory during needle insertion
- Central venous catheter placement
  - US-guided placement of central venous catheters has become standard of care
  - Be familiar with institutional-specific guidelines

AIRWAY ULTRASOUND (SEE FIG. 7-7)

- Can be used for assessment and prediction of difficult airway, prediction of size of ETT, preparation for airway-related nerve blocks, guidance for percutaneous tracheostomy
- Also used for confirmation of endotracheal intubation and correct placement of ETT

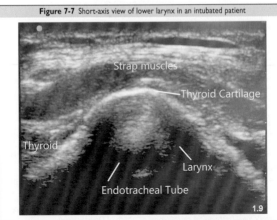

Figure 7-7 Short-axis view of lower larynx in an intubated patient

Strap muscles

Thyroid Cartilage

Thyroid

Larynx

Endotracheal Tube

1.9

FRANCIS X. DILLON

PULSE OXIMETRY

Basis: 2 wavelengths of light absorbed differently by Hb & Hb–O$_2$. Pulsating arteriolar flow subtracted from nonpulsatile venous blood → gives arterial saturation.

Hb–O$_2$ Dissociation Curve: Relates % of Hb saturation to PaO$_2$ (Fig. 8.1).

Right shift: Peripheral offloading of O$_2$ enhanced. Causes:
- ↑Temp, acidosis, ↑H$^+$ or pH↓ (Bohr effect), ↑CO$_2$, ↑2,3-diphosphoglycerate, adult Hb, myo-inositol trispyrophosphate (ITPP—experimental drug)

Left shift: Higher affinity Hb O$_2$ & offloading of O$_2$ inhibited. Causes:
- ↓Temp, alkalosis ↓H$^+$ or pH↑ (Bohr effect), ↓CO$_2$, ↓2,3-diphosphoglycerate, fetal Hb, carbon monoxide, methemoglobinemia (caused by aniline dyes, nitrates, nitrites, NO, sulfonamides, dapsone, phenacetin, phenazopyridine, nitroprusside, benzocaine, prilocaine, EMLA (topical anesthetics). Reversal by methemoglobin reductase (physiologic) or methylene blue (pharmacologic).

Information in Pulse Oximeter Waveform
- Pulsatile waves match heart rate
- Dicrotic notch = aortic valve closure (damped if cold, atherosclerotic, or on pressors)
- Envelope height varies with respiration if hypovolemic
- SpO$_2$ of 90% = PaO$_2$ 60 mmHg; SpO$_2$ of 98% = PaO$_2$ 90 mmHg (SpO$_2$ readings <90 are inaccurate)

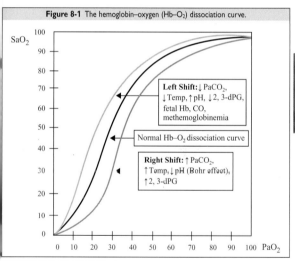

Figure 8-1 The hemoglobin–oxygen (Hb–O$_2$) dissociation curve.

SaO$_2$ (y-axis: 0–100)

Left Shift: ↓ PaCO$_2$, ↓Temp, ↑ pH, ↓2, 3-dPG, fetal Hb, CO, methemoglobinemia

Normal Hb–O$_2$ dissociation curve

Right Shift: ↑ PaCO$_2$, ↑Temp, ↓ pH (Bohr effect), ↑2, 3-dPG

PaO$_2$ (x-axis: 0–100)

(Courtesy of S. Shah, MD, with permission.)

Indications for Pulse Oximetry Monitoring
• Sedation for endoscopy, ECT, or TEE
• Weaning of low-flow O$_2$/ventilator support
• Monitoring during general anesthesia & in the PACU
• Monitoring following neuraxial blocks with opioids
• Sleep study documentation of apnea–hypopnea index (OSA)
• Ward observation following surgery in pts with OSA
• Ambulatory monitoring for pulmonary HTN or CHF

Hazards of Pulse Oximetry		
Hazard	**Predisposing Conditions**	
Finger or ear necrosis	Hypothermia	Tape/wrapping too tightly
	Ischemia	Edema
	↓ Cardiac output	Prolonged monitoring
	Use of pressors	Immaturity
	Ground fault/electrical failure	Prematurity
	MRI-induced currents	Sepsis

Pulse Oximetry Artifacts and Remedies		
Artifact	**SpO2 Reading**	**Remedy/Notes**
Low perfusion (hypothermia, pressors, atherosclerosis)	Lowers	Need to restore perfusion & pulsatile flow; can passively warm (do not actively warm, may cause burns)
Movement	Lowers/obliterates	Move probe from finger to ear
Nail polish	Lowers	Remove polish or turn probe 90°; black, purple, blue colors worst
Vasopressors	Lowers	Consider dobutamine (↑ extremity perfusion) or block between metacarpals
Carboxyhemoglobin (CO exposure)	Raises	↑ FiO2; hyperbaric O2; use orange color co-oximetry
Methemoglobinemia (benzocaine, etc.; see above)	Lowers	Administer methylene blue dye
Hemoglobinopathies	Lowers	Supportive care; transfusion
Anemia (severe)	Raises	Consider transfusion; in anemic pts, 100% SpO2 may still mean significantly ↓ O2 delivery; use supplemental O2
Acidosis	Lowers	Correct; shifts Hb–O2 curve to right
Alkalosis	Lowers	Correct; shifts Hb–O2 curve to left
Cardiopulmonary bypass	Lowers/obliterates	Restore pulsatile flow following CPB

NONINVASIVE SPECTROPHOTOMETRIC HEMOGLOBIN MONITORING (e.g., MASIMO® RADICAL-7®)

Basis: Pulse CO-oximetry uses multiple wavelengths of LED light in pulsatile bed; measures [Hb] via Hb extinction coefficients. SpO2, SpHb, metHb, COHb, pleth var index, O2 content. Compared to lab, correlation between the methods was Pearson $r = 0.72$, Bland–Altman: $0.1+/− 1.5$ SD. Noninvasive method overestimated HB slightly

- SpHb reduced frequency of transfusion from 4.5–0.6% in a prospective RCT (↓90%)
- SpHb reduced # of units transfused by 47%; and multiunit TF ↓ by 56% (a prosp cohort study). Also allowed for more rapid administration of Hb by 9 min.
- SpHb slightly underestimates Hb compared with point of care Hb (HemoCue®)

NEAR-INFRARED CORTICAL SPECTROPHOTOMETRY (e.g., MEDTRONIC INVOS™, CASMED FORE-SIGHT ELITE®, MASIMO-O3®)

Basis: Hb, HbO2, and oxidized cytochrome oxidase have different absorption spectra. Illuminating tissue with several wavelengths of near-infrared light will cause differential attenuation according to the relative amounts of Hb/HbO2 and oxidized brain cytochrome oxidase.

- Allows real time measurement of brain tissue oxygenation as deep as 2.5 cm
- Measures regional tissue oxygen saturation (rSO2) with a correlation coefficient $r = 0.90$ compared with estimation from jugular bulb and arterial sample O2 saturations
- In one study, rSO2-guided therapeutic interventions during cardiac surgery reversed ↓rSO2 and this correlated with improved neurocognitive outcomes

NONINVASIVE BLOOD PRESSURE MONITORING
(OSCILLOMETRIC SPHYGMOMANOMETRY)

Basis: Air cuff inflated around extremity, transducer reads oscillations from systolic pulsation
- Inflation pressure raised above systolic & then deflated until oscillations appear
- Max amplitude of oscillations = systolic; min amplitude of oscillations = diastolic
- Waveforms analyzed by software, not displayed (each device has its own algorithm)

Causes of Artifacts in NIBP Monitoring
- Movement, obesity, poor perfusion, hypotension, extreme hypertension, bradycardia
- Wrong cuff size: Too small cuff gives ↑ pressure reading
- Irregular pulse: A. fib, PVCs, *pulsus bisferiens* (hypertrophic cardiomyopathy), *pulsus alternans* (pericardial effusion), *pulsus paradoxus* (tamponade), *pulsus parvus et tardus* (aortic stenosis)

Complications
- Skin necrosis, soft tissue injury, phlebitis, neuropathy (peroneal, radial), compartment syndrome (biceps), petechiae, ecchymosis, IV line infiltration/occlusion, interference with pulse oximetry

NONINVASIVE CONTINUOUS BLOOD PRESSURE, SV, SVV, SVR, AND CARDIAC OUTPUT MONITORING (EDWARDS CLEARSIGHT™)

Basis: Air cuff inflated around finger, another transducer at heart level. "Volume clamp" method with counterpulsation designed to keep finger vessels isovolumic. 1 kHz sampling and digital signal processing (DSP) frequency for sensitivity and fidelity
- Validated against intermittent NIBP (see above) and continuous invasive (arterial line) monitoring. Less effectively validated (30% disparity) with thermodilution or TEE
- Bias for both conventional methods compared to this modality range from −1 to +4.5 mmHg with +/− SD of between 5 and 10 mmHg in several studies
- Waveforms analyzed by software, displayed in real time, displayed

Potential Causes of Artifacts in Noninvasive Continuous Monitoring
- Movement, obesity, poor perfusion, hypotension, extreme hypertension, bradycardia
- Poor fitting or too tight finger cuff size
- Irregular pulse: A. fib, PVCs, *pulsus bisferiens* (hypertrophic cardiomyopathy), *pulsus alternans* (pericardial effusion), *pulsus paradoxus* (tamponade), *pulsus parvus et tardus* (aortic stenosis)

Complications
- Pt injury from the device seems extremely unlikely and complications more likely related to overestimation of cardiac output or inaccurate SVV, SV, or SVR readings leading to inappropriate fluid or inotrope therapy

TEMPERATURE MONITORING

Basis: Thermistors (resistors with resistance inversely proportional to temperature) quantify temperature

Causes of Operative Temperature Loss	
Anesthesia factors:	↓ Hypothalamic set point (around 34.5°C)
	↓ Heat generation (anesthesia → metabolic slowdown)
	↓ Muscle thermogenesis from muscle relaxation
	Ventilation causes heat & moisture losses
OR heat losses:	Loss from convection, radiation, evaporation
	Loss from conduction (pt in contact with cold, wet surfaces)
	Irrigation of cavities (e.g., peritoneum) & viscera (e.g., bladder)

Complications of Hyperthermia
- More rapid and less predictable drug clearance
- Cellular & metabolic derangements (hypercarbia, acidosis)
- CNS more vulnerable to injury when warm as opposed to cool

Complications of Hypothermia (below 36°C)
- ↑ Length of stay, ↑ wound infections, coag. problems, ↑ shivering, ↑ dysrhythmias, ↑ morbid cardiac events, ↑ intraoperative blood loss, ↑ allogeneic transfusion requirement, ↑ norepinephrine, ↑ shivering, ↑ thermal discomfort, ↑ length of PACU stay

Artifacts
Related to probe placement (core temperature vs. peripheral)

Hazards
Trauma (from probe placement), infection, shock (from grounded equipment)

Placement
"Core temp" (esophageal, PA) more meaningful than "shell temp" (rectum, axilla)

Malignant Hyperthermia
- Temp ↑ of 0.5°C in 15 min is significant & concerning, also ↑ ing ETCO$_2$ production
- *Early* dantrolene administration is the only effective therapy (see Appendix C)

ARTERIAL BLOOD PRESSURE (ABP) MONITORING

Basis: Circulatory tree—intra-arterial catheter—fluid–transducer electromechanical system with characteristic frequency $f_0 = (1/2\pi)(\pi r^2 E/\rho L)^{1/2}$ optimal f_0 = 25–40 Hz
- Modeled by differential equation: Includes natural frequency & damping factor:
  - $DF = -\ln [\beta/\{\pi^2 + (\ln \beta)^2\}^{1/2}]$ where $\beta = A_1/A_2$, ratio of amplitudes of successive peaks after a high pressure flush of the arterial line
  - DF <0.4, underdamped, "ringing" waveform results, systolic overestimated
  - DF = 0.4–0.7 optimal fidelity; DF = 0.7–1.0 overdamped, low sensitivity, fidelity ↓
  - DF >1, very overdamped, lose high-freq waveform info (e.g., dicrotic notch)
- Short & rigid tubing, ↓ viscosity: All lead to ↓ resistance, ↑ f_0 & ringing with overshoot
- Arterial waveform from aorta to radial (slightly): MAP↓, DBP↓, and SBP↑ if no pressor medications used. Generally, femoral A-line better than radial for conveying all pressures. If pressor medications used; systolic difference can be 30 mmHg femoral–radial. If pressors used, NIBP may give more accurate pressures than radial.
- Mechanics of A-line transducer system (ideal system has freq response >25–40 Hz):
  - Short, rigid tubing with incompressible fluid (saline) typically used (↓ damping effect)
  - Piezoresistive quartz strain gauge attached to a diaphragm changes resistance with tension (minute variations in pressure from line)
  - Wheatstone bridge "amplifies" change in resistance & allows precise calibration
  - Higher f_0 electromechanical system → greater sensitivity especially at high HR
  - Dense fluid lowers f_0 of system → ↓ accuracy and ↓ sensitivity *(saline in art line better than blood for sensitivity and frequency response)*
- Sources of signal degradation:
  - Ringing/underdamping: Narrow rigid tubing of short length *(rapid frequency response & ↓ in damping ratio with ringing in arterial line)*; Overdamping on the other hand is from compliant system, wide soft short tubing, air bubbles
  - Transducer height can cause ↑/↓ in A-line reading: 12"-too-low transducer = 22.4 mmHg overestimate in pressure displayed *(Must avoid ↓ BP and ↓ CPP in sitting, chair procedures:* **SBP transducer should always be at level of the Circle of Willis.** *Significant clinical injuries have occurred in sitting position by incorrect transducer misplacement at heart level)*

SAFELY FLUSHING AN ARTERIAL LINE

- Turn stopcock (up usually) so that the transducer is opened to air
- Flush Luer-Lock to clear it of blood (hold gauze by stopcock to catch blood)
- Turn stopcock so that the handle is horizontal (i.e., in starting position)
- In short bursts of 2 s or less, pull rubber line or squeeze valve to flush line back toward pt
- Ensure that the entire line is eventually cleared of blood (no bubbles present)
  - *If line is flushed continuously (not in 2-s bursts), the brachial axillary and subclavian arteries may fill retrogradely with saline (transducer pressure head is 300 mmHg) to aortic arch & embolize (saline/air) to common carotid & brain*

HAZARDS OF ARTERIAL LINE MONITORING

- Embolization: From flush mechanism; limit flush <2 s to prevent retrograde flow
- Thrombosis: Risk ↑ with duration of placement; catastrophic if end artery (brachial)
- Nerve injury: Nerves closely related to arteries anatomically
- Vascular injury: AV fistula, hematoma, dissection, pseudoaneurysm, retained catheter or wire, femoral artery injury leading to hypotension and major morbidity
- Limb loss: Inadvertent drug injection (i.e., thiopental, phenergan) → severe vascular injury → amputation or chronic pain syndrome as sequelae

Indications for Arterial Blood Pressure Monitoring

- Surgical need for tight BP control (neurosurgical/vascular procedures)
- Measurement of mean arterial pressure crucial to derive cerebral perfusion pressure or coronary perfusion pressure (CPP): Neurosurgery, cardiac, beach-chair, semi-Fowler's ENT
- Measurement of oxygenation critical (e.g., pulmonary surgery with lung isolation, cardiac surgery, severe ARDS)
- Severe or labile hypertension, especially at emergence (CNS aneurysm coiling, carotid surg)
- Hypotension anticipated (sepsis, cardiogenic shock, hypovolemia, ENT, head and neck surg)
- Massive blood loss & need for transfusion anticipated (spine, craniofacial, major ortho surg)
- Need for frequent arterial blood sampling
  - Diagnosis & treatment of acidosis/alkalosis (intra-abdominal sepsis, organ transplantation)
  - Frequent lab values needed (blood glucose, K^+, hemoglobin, ACT, PTH)
- NIBP ineffective/impractical
  - Obese pts where NIBP cuff pressures are unreliable
  - Lengthy cases where cuff trauma may be significant or plt count ↓, INR↑
  - Cases where arm positioning make cuff potentially traumatic to med nerve (thoracotomy)
  - NIBP cuff subject to compression/motion artifact (cases with arms tucked)

Site of Arterial Cannulation	Disadvantage
Sup. temporal	Retrograde cerebral embolization possible
Radial	May be small, tortuous, or insufficiently anastomosed with ulnar artery
Ulnar	May be small, tortuous, or insufficiently anastomosed with radial artery
Brachial	An end artery: Risk of limb thrombosis; remove as soon as possible
Femoral	Atheromatous, deep, prone to massive blood loss, retroperitoneal hematoma, limb loss, infection, AV fistula, and aneurysm formation
Dorsalis pedis	Small & odd angle: Difficult to cannulate; waveforms often damped
Posterior tibialis	Tortuous & odd angle: Difficult to cannulate; waveforms often damped

CENTRAL VENOUS LINES & CENTRAL VENOUS PRESSURE (CVP) MONITORING

Uses: Monitoring (CVP & central blood O_2 saturation—surrogate for SvO_2, also jugular bulb venous SO_2 sampling). Central drug/fluid/blood product administration (may be safer route for vasoactives). Renal replacement therapy (CVVH/HD) & temporary pacemaker lead placement. Access for electrophysiology studies.

Hazards of Central Line Placement
- Pneumothorax, hemothorax, thrombus, thromboembolus
- Arterial puncture, hematoma, AV fistula formation
- Brachial plexus or nerve injury
- Infection including systemic sepsis, septic thrombus, endocarditis
- Knotting or breakage of catheter, retained wire, erosion through vessel, endocardium, myocardium
- Thoracic duct injury, chylothorax
- Microshock, dysrhythmias

Artifacts
- Positioning: (e.g., jackknife, Trendelenburg, semi-Fowler') may affect CVP
- Abdominal compression/retraction may impede CVP & blood return
- Insufflation of CO_2 in abdomen (laparoscopy) may artifactually raise CVP
- Rapid infusion through the same or nearby catheter may artifactually raise CVP
- AV fistula in the arm may cause artifactually high CVP ipsa/contralaterally

Indications for CVP Monitoring
• Monitoring central pressures (RA & CVP)
• Monitoring RV overload
• Treating RV infarction
• Vasoactive/chemo infusions (avoid venous & soft tissue ischemia/injury)
• Rapid infusion of fluid/transfusion
• Use of transvenous pacing electrodes or passage of a PA catheter

NORMAL CVP & CORRESPONDING ECG WAVEFORM (FIG. 8.2)

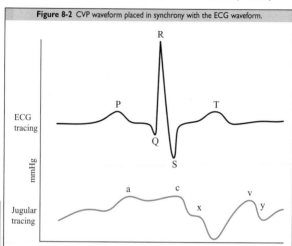

Figure 8-2 CVP waveform placed in synchrony with the ECG waveform.

Features of the CVP Waveform		
Waveform Feature	Results from	Remark
"a" wave	Venous distention from RA contraction	Biggest pulsation visible, especially during inspiration
"c" wave	Bulging of tricuspid valve into RA during RV isovolumic systole	Called the "c" wave because it coincides with (& is accentuated by) carotid pulse
"x" descent	(1) Atrial relaxation & (2) caudad displacement of tricuspid valve during RV systole	Occurs during systole, accentuated in constrictive pericarditis
"v" wave	Increasing volume of blood in the RA during ventricular systole when the TV is closed	Late systolic, accentuated with tricuspid regurgitation
"y" descent	Opening of tricuspid valve & subsequent rapid inflow of blood into RV	Rapid & deep with TR; slow with TS or atrial myxoma, both of which cause slowing of outflow from RA

CVP Waveform Abnormalities					
Abnormality	Absent "a" wave	Large "a" wave	Cannon "a" wave (occasional large pulsations at *irregular* intervals)	Ventricularized "c–v" waves (resemble cannon "a" waves but are frequent, and at *regular* intervals)	"M" or "W" waves (diminished x and prominent y descents)

Cause	No atrial contraction	Dyssynergic atrial contraction or obstruction of tricuspid valve	Atrial contraction against a closed tricuspid valve	Reflux of blood into right atrium in systole	Rapid flow out of atrium in diastole
Associated with	Atrial fibrillation	1st-degree AV block severe, tricuspid stenosis	PVC, vent. paced or junctional rhythm, AV dissoc., Complete HB, VT	Tricuspid regurgitation	Constrictive pericarditis

INTRAVASCULAR VOLUME MONITORING BY DYNAMIC RESPONSE OF PULSE PRESSURE VARIATION (PPV): PULSION™ PICCO®; AND STROKE VOLUME VARIATION (SVV): EDWARDS™ VIGILEO®, FLO-TRAC® (USING PERIPHERAL ARTERIAL CATHETER, OPTIONAL CENTRAL VENOUS CATHETER)

Basis: PP is proportional to SV. Hypovolemic pts have transient ↓ RVSV during inspiration. It translates to ↓↓LVSV after a few beats. SVV and PVV monitors quantitate this respiratory variation as a percentage by measuring variation of arterial pressure waveform.

- ≥13% PPV variation threshold of relative hypovolemia; <13% means euvolemia
- (PPV may require calibration with Li or thermodilution)
- ≥13% SVV variation threshold of relative hypovolemia; <10% means euvolemia
- (SVV only on ventilated pts, without dysrhythmia, but no calibration needed)
- ↑ SVV or ↑ PPV means fluid needed; if SVV ↓, PPV ↓ use inotropes instead to ↑ CO

MEASUREMENT OF CARDIAC OUTPUT (ALSO SEE APPENDIX A)

- Fick equation: $CO = VO_2 \div (CaO_2 - CvO_2)$ where:
  - VO_2 = oxygen consumption = uptake of O_2 from inspired gases in L/min
  - CaO_2 = content of O_2 in arterial blood in liters O_2/L blood
  - CvO_2 = content of O_2 in venous blood in liters O_2/L blood
- Mixed venous O_2 saturation (SvO_2):
  - Gives an indication of tissue oxygenation
  - Normal SvO_2 is 75% (range 60–80%); higher under anesthesia, up to 90%
  - CaO_2 (in mL/L blood) = [13.4 × Hb conc. (in mg/dL) × SaO_2/100] + [0.031 × PaO_2 (in mmHg)]
  - CvO_2 (in mL/L blood) = [13.4 × Hb conc. (in mg/dL) × SvO_2/100] + [0.031 × PvO_2 (in mmHg)]

Causes of Low Mixed Venous		Causes of High Mixed Venous	
Low O₂ Delivery	↑ O₂ Use	Low O₂ Use	Other
• Hypoxia • Anemia • ↓ Cardiac output • Alkalosis • Methemoglobinemia	• Fever • ↑ Metabolic states • Shivering	• CN poisoning • Hypothermia	• Impaired O₂ tissue delivery (sepsis, burns) • Mitral regurg

Note: If PA catheter is wedged (in contact with arterial blood), mixed venous will be high.

- PA Catheter Thermodilution technique measures CO via Stewart–Hamilton equation
  - Ensure tip of catheter is in main pulmonary artery
  - Quickly inject 10 mL of cold saline or 5% D5W into CVP port
  - Thermistor monitors temp change & reports area under curve in real time

Cardiac Output Erroneously Low	Cardiac Output Erroneously High
• Large volume injected • R-to-L shunt • Catheter tip too proximal	• Small volume injected • L-to-R shunt • Wedged catheter • Tricuspid regurgitation

CONSIDERATIONS FOR PA THERMODILUTION CATHETER INSERTION & MONITORING

- Decision for insertion: Many question utility of PA measurement, majority of clinicians untrained or uninformed about basic PA facts and measurements, TEE or TTE may be superior in demonstrating cardiac function, PA carries significant infectious risk
- Risk–benefit analysis critical: Must know what you are seeking to measure
  - **Filling pressures intraoperatively** → to determine exact amount of preload needed
    1. Useful in COPD (sensitive to excess fluid), large 3rd-space loss, pulm HTN, RV, or LV failure
    2. PA looks at LV-filling pressures (in addition to RV filling pressures, via CVP)
- **SVR**
    1. Liver transplantation where liver dz has caused chronic shunting, SVR ↓
    2. Sepsis, SVR may be too ↓ for adequate global perfusion
    3. Free flaps/plastic surgery where peripheral cold may make SVR ↑
    4. Pressors/inotropes infused where SVR may become too ↑
    5. CHF where SVR may be relatively ↑
- **Cardiac output** (cardiac, CHF, or large fluid cases)
    1. Frank–Starling curve (CO as a function of preload) shows if pt is in CHF or hypovolemic
      - Plot PA diastolic pressure (on x-axis) vs. CO (y-axis) on graph paper
    2. Titrate dopamine vs. dobutamine vs. amrinone to improve CO
    3. Provide real mixed venous O_2 blood sample for assessing O_2 saturation & delivery
- Insertion site (see Table—Percutaneous Access Sites for CVP or PA Catheter Placement)
  - Consider passing a PA sheath with obturator (plug) or CVP-inserted lumen
    - Allows later optional PA use if circumstances warrant it (e.g., oliguria, hypotension)

Percutaneous Access Sites for CVP or PA Catheter Placement					
Vein Location	Peripheral Arm (brachial or cephalic)	External Jugular Vein (EJV)	Internal Jugular Vein (IJV)	Subclavian	Femoral
Advantages	Easy to access; good for long-term access (PICC)	Easy to access	Easy to access	Most comfortable, best for long-term placement, pt may ambulate easily	No risk of hemothorax; easy to access during CPR
Disadvantages	Catheter may not pass through small vessel; may not give good CVP waveform	Catheter may not pass owing to angle of EJV as it joins the SCV; hard to do venipuncture into the EJV; may not give good CVP waveform, may injure brachial plexus	Near trachea and carotid; difficult to dress with bandage, uncomfortable for long-term access and hygiene	Clavicle may block access; subclavian artery near; pneumothorax or hemothorax possible	Risks of infection & thrombosis ↑; pt must be immobilized
Infection rate	NA	NA	↑ (1.5–1.8%)	↓ (0.45–0.61%)	↑ (1.3–1.8%)
Pneumothorax risk	Impossible	Low (0.3%)	Low (0.3%)	Possible (1.4%); obtain CXR after placement	Impossible

Lymphatic injury possible	No	No	No	Yes; thoracic duct may be lacerated if access L. subclavian vein	No
Thrombosis risk	NA	NA	↑ (5.4–7.0%)	↓ (2.0–2.1%)	↑ (5.2–5.4%)

- Tips for PA catheter placement (see Chapter 12, on Procedures in Anesthesia)
  - Calibrate carefully ("zeroing"): LV function decisions made on a few mmHg!
  - Check balloon & valve to ensure balloon holds air (1 cm) when valve is closed
  - Pass to 20 cm depth & assure CVP waveform before inflating (1 mL only) balloon
  - Be sure pt is flat, not with head down, when "floating" PA catheter
  - Know & anticipate waveforms & locations of distal tip
    - ≈20 cm is CVP, may inflate balloon with 1 cm air
    - ≈30 cm is RV, pressure much greater, no dicrotic notch
    - ≈40 is PA, diastolic c several mmHg ↑ & notch appears
    - ≈45 (near PCWP) some damping & ↑ in pressure will occur:
      - Let balloon tip occlude vessel while you very slowly advance catheter
      - When you get wedge waveform (Fig. 8.3), disconnect breathing circuit
      - Read mean PCWP (approximately equivalent to LVEDP; 4–15 mmHg normal)
      - Reconnect circuit, deflate balloon, and observe PA waveform return
      - Withdraw catheter 1–2 cm for safety & do not reinflate in situ
      - If you want another PCWP, the safest option is to withdraw to 20 cm & refloat
- **PA perforation:** Consider this if no wedge pattern seen even after deep insertion
  - Circumstances that predispose to PA perforation: Papillary muscle ischemia, mitral stenosis or regurgitation, pulm HTN or intrapulmonary shunting, LV failure. *Beware: After seeing no definitive wedge pattern, repeated attempts to advance catheter may perforate PA*
  - Many times PA catheter will give a good wedge pattern (the waveform continues to look like PA even though catheter is in PA & ought to have wedged). *Beware: Coiling or false negative wedging may occur, predisposing to PA rupture*

Common Reasons for PA Catheterization

- Assess RV pressure
- Diagnose & treat pulm HTN
- Assess hypotension: Sepsis vs. cardiogenic shock on the basis of CO & SVR
- Manage severe organ dysfunction/severe sepsis
- Administer fluids judiciously (COPD/pulm HTN/burns/renal failure)
- Diagnose & treat intraoperative oliguria
- Manage MI with shock
- Construct a Starling curve of CO vs. preload
- Manage valvular heart dz with appropriate preload & afterload adjustment
- Assess vasoactive therapy by serial CO & SVR measurements
- Manage pts with cerebral vasospasm after SAH (may involve induced hypertension, hemodilution, & hypervolemia under PA catheter monitoring)
- Manage cardiac pts after heart surgery

Possible (Relative) Contraindications to PA Catheterization

Previous/planned pneumonectomy (PA rupture would likely be fatal)	Existing pacemaker lead
Tricuspid prosthesis, pulmonic prosthesis, tricuspid stenosis, pulmonic stenosis	Warfarin, heparin, factor Xa inhibitors, antiplatelet drugs (e.g., clopidogrel, IIb/IIIa inhibitors, or high-dose aspirin), thrombin inhibitors, thrombolytics
R. atrial or ventricular masses; documented mural thrombi or valvular growth	Atrial dysrhythmias (consider echo to rule out atrial thrombus if suspected)
Cyanotic heart dz or R-to-L shunt	Floating during CPB
Latex allergy (if PA components are latex)	Tight AS (until chest is open, as floating → A. fib → loss of atrial kick → CV collapse)
Recent bifascicular block or LBBB Severe ventricular dysrhythmias	Mitral regurgitation/stenosis, which may make wedging impossible (predisposes to rupture)
Heparin-coated catheter in HIT+ pt	Sepsis or factors contributing to endocarditis

Figure 8-3 Typical waveform progression of PA catheter floating through the cardiac chambers.

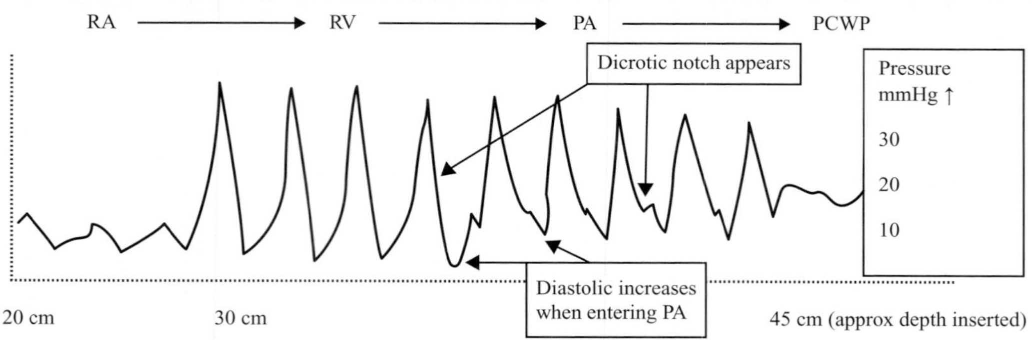

RA → RV → PA → PCWP

Dicrotic notch appears

Diastolic increases when entering PA

Pressure mmHg ↑

30

20

10

20 cm   30 cm   45 cm (approx depth inserted)

Normal PA Waveforms as Catheter Is Passed from CVP (RA) to RV to PA to PCWP

Hemodynamic Variables and Waveforms of the PA Catheter					
Distance (cm) Passed from Catheter Tip →					
PA catheter passage benchmark	0	20 or more	30 or more	40 or more	45 or more
Typical waveform	Damped CVP	Characteristic, undamped, CVP with a, c, x, v, y waves	RV wave with no dicrotic notch; low diastolic essentially equal to RA	PA wave with dicrotic notch and diastolic elevated over RVD value	Damped, decreased "wedge" waveform
Typical pressures (mmHg)	0 (catheter must read zero at LA level)	CVPm = RAM = 2–6	RVS = 15–25 RVD = 0–8 RVM = 5–14	PAS = 15–25 PAD = 8–15 PAM = 10–20	PAOP = PCWP ≈ LAM = 6–12
Typical difficulties encountered at this stage of passage	Tip bends or reflexes on itself, kinking, very high pressures eventually equilibrating with the max transducer pressure (300 mmHg)	Tip may traverse RA & continue down IVC (rather than entering the RA), giving a CVP waveform well beyond 20 cm	Catheter may coil in RV; giving an RV waveform well beyond 40 cm, beware knotting may occur in this setting	*Beware of pulmonary artery rupture!* Mitral insufficiency or intra-pulmonary shunting may make wedge impossible	*Beware of pulmonary infarction!* Catheter should not be left wedged; deflate balloon & restore PA waveform
Suggested remedy	Deflate, withdraw, refloat	Deflate, withdraw, refloat; consider fluoroscopic guidance	Deflate, withdraw, refloat; consider fluoroscopic guidance	Leave catheter in safe PA position if you believe it has been inserted far enough; use pulmonary diastolic as surrogate for PAOP	Deflate & withdraw PA catheter several centimeters if waveform remains or becomes wedged; be sure PA waveform returns

"v" Waves in a Wedge Tracing

Usually a sign of severe mitral regurgitation (get transmission of large pressure waves from LV, through incompetent mitral valve, into LA, and pulmonary vessels)

Complications of PA Catheter Placement		
Complication	**Consider**	**Remedy**
Ventricular dysrhythmias	Dysrhythmias may occur on PA catheter placement, usually self-limited	Lidocaine 50–100 mg IV during passage; check Mg, K levels, & pH
Pulmonary embolus	↑ Risk when PA catheters used compared with CVP	Take PA catheter out when no longer needed; heparin, aspirin, other anticoagulation for thromboprophylaxis as indicated

Catheter will not wedge; gives unchanged PA waveform even though inserted beyond 45–50 cm	Consider catheter coiling in RV; make sure pt is supine; consider possibility of intrapulmonary shunting, congestion, or MR (all of which may prevent wedge waveform even though catheter is properly placed)	Deflate, reinsert with pt supine; consider chest radiograph or using fluoroscopy; consider assistance from a colleague
During insertion, pressure climbs monotonically until off scale	Catheter may be catching on a central vein & kinking back on itself, blocking the lumen	Consider deflating, reinserting while pt is supine; consider radiography or fluoroscopy
Good CVP waveform, but catheter shows no RV waveform even though deeply inserted (30 cm)	Catheter may have traversed RA & be going down IVC; catheter may be having trouble getting through a small or stenotic tricuspid valve & kinking or coiling in RA	Consider deflating, reinserting while pt is supine; consider radiography or fluoroscopy; make sure balloon is not inflated with more than 1 mL of air (may prevent passage through valve)
Catheter will not pass after 20–25 cm, feels stuck or constrained; gives CVP waveform that is damped/goes off scale	Catheter may be going up arm or back up the IJV into the intracranial venous system	Deflate, withdraw carefully, reinsert with head or arm repositioned, or insert catheter into another vein
Catheter gives good RV waveform but will not pass into PA at or beyond expected length (40–45 cm)	RV may be abnormally large & catheter may not have reached pulmonic valve; pulmonic valve may be small or stenotic	Advance a few more centimeters carefully; do not overinflate balloon; consider fluoroscopic or radiographic guidance
Catheter wedges (morphology of waveform changes & envelope is smaller) but not convincingly	RV may be large & PA catheter may be coiling in RV; undiagnosed intracardiac R-to-L shunt should be considered. Consider intrapulmonary shunting, MS or MR; not uncommon in pts with systemic shunting (chronic liver failure)	Consider stopping attempts to wedge & try following PAD in lieu of PCWP. Consider using fluoroscopy to visualize and place
Catheter performs perfectly before & after wedging & deflation, but over time, appears to have wedged again on its own without being advanced manually	Catheter may have warmed & floated out distally (with balloon uninflated), thereby wedging tip into smaller pulmonary arteriole. (This is a setup for PA rupture!)	**DO NOT** *merely reinflate balloon!* First withdraw the catheter to 20 cm & if CVP waveform is good, refloat catheter to avoid PA rupture
PA waveform morphology cyclically changes or envelope varies with PEEP or during the respiratory cycle	Likely hypovolemia; when airway pressure ↑, PA compression occurs → waveform morphology & magnitude may change	Administer fluid, follow PAD, & observe waveform. Correlate with dynamic (SVV/PPV) data if available
Massive hemoptysis observed in tracheal tube or severe shock develops suddenly	**PA rupture**	Do not manipulate catheter; resuscitate as a team: Call for help (thoracic/cardiac surgeon); extubate & insert double lumen tube; stop bleeding from affected lung by inserting Fogarty catheter into lumen from which bleeding is seen; watch for compliance changes & obtain radiograph if shock occurs without hemoptysis; CPB may be needed during PA repair

PA catheter is fixed & cannot be withdrawn	Either knotting has occurred, some mechanical catch has occurred with the sheath, or catheter has been inadvertently sutured in place	Do not pull harder—this can be very hazardous. Consult interventional radiologist or surgeon for diagnosis & treatment
PCWP was damped appropriately when wedged, but with posteroinferior ischemic changes on ECG, large waves are seen in wedge position	Consider ischemia in posterior papillary muscle of mitral valve; this may have led to large "v" waves as the ischemic muscle caused sudden regurgitation in the formerly sound valve	Treat underlying ischemia or infarction as it becomes feasible; afterload reduction, aortic balloon counterpulsation, inotropic support, & diuresis may be necessary

Normal Values for Hemodynamic Variables

Variable	Value	Units
HR	60–100	beats/min
SBP	90–140	mmHg
DBP	60–90	mmHg
MAP	70–105	mmHg
RAP (= CVP)	2–6	mmHg
RVSP	15–25	mmHg
RVDP	0–8	mmHg
RVMP	5–14	mmHg
PASP	15–25	mmHg
PADP	8–15	mmHg
PAMP	10–20	mmHg
PAOP = PCWP	6–12	mmHg
PCWP ≈ LAP		

Summary of Derived Hemodynamic Variables

Variable	Formula	Approximate Value	Units
CO	CO = SV × HR	4.0–8.0	L/min
SV	SV = CO ÷ HR	60–100	mL/beat
SVI	SVI = CI ÷ HR	33–47	mL/m²-beat
BSA	BSA = $W^{0.425} \times H^{0.725} \times 0.007184$ (formula of Dubois and Dubois)	1.73	BSA in m²; W in kg; H in cm
CI	CI = CO ÷ BSA	2.31–4.62	L/min
SVR	SVR = (80 × [MAP − CVP]) ÷ CO	900–1,500	dyne-s/cm⁵
SVRI	SVRI = (80 × [MAP − CVP]) ÷ CI	1,600–2,400	dyne-s/cm⁵-m²
PVR	PVR = 80 × (MPAP − PAWP) ÷ CO	<250	dyne-s/cm⁵
PVRI	PVRI = 80 × (MPAP − PAWP) ÷ CI	255–285	dyne-s/cm⁵-m²

Summary of Advanced Derived Hemodynamic Values

Variable	Formula	Approximate Value	Units
LV stroke work = LVSW	SV × (MAP − PAWP) × 0.0136	58–104	g-m/beat
LV stroke work index = LVSWI	SVI × (MAP − PAWP) × 0.0136	50–62	g-m/m²-beat
RVSW	SV × (MPAP − RAP) × 0.0136	8–16	g-m/beat
RVSWI	SVI × (MPAP − RAP) × 0.0136	5–10	g-m/m²-beat
CPP	DBP − PAWP	60–80	mmHg
RVEDV	SV/EF	100–160	mL
RVESV	EDV − SV	50–100	mL
RVEF	SV/EDV	40–60	%

FRANCIS X. DILLON

INTRODUCTION AND OVERVIEW

Common Ventilation Modes: Continuous Mandatory Ventilation

- Volume control (VC): A set volume is delivered in a given interval cycled by time or pt
- Pressure control (PC): A set pressure is delivered in a given interval cycled by time or pt
- Main concerns with continuous mandatory ventilation (CMV) are diaphragmatic atrophy, asynchrony, need for sedation

MANY ADVANTAGES OF SPONTANEOUS BREATHING VS. POSITIVE-PRESSURE VENTILATION WHILE INTUBATED

- Coughing requires closure of glottis and forceful reopening by a rapid pressure wave from lungs; it is impossible when pt intubated, sedated. Lungs become atelectatic
  - Atelectasis occurs within min & secretions may accumulate, because they too are removed normally by coughing. V/Q mismatch and hypoxia occur
  - Presence of ETT or tracheostomy also obliterates intrinsic positive end-expiratory pressure (PEEP) (*pts cannot cough or even Valsalva effectively → this also predisposes to atelectasis, secretion retention, and pneumonia*)
  - Cumulative incidence of ventilator-associated pneumonia (VAP) is ~1–3% per d of intubation; about 15% of vented pts get VAP; 35% of ICU pts are vented
  - Diaphragmatic atrophy occurs within 24–48 h during CMV. Proteolysis plus ↓ synthesis in myocytes
  - Goals of liberating from ventilator: Diminish sedation and vent support (*both inspiratory pressure and PEEP are supportive*), restore oxygenation and ventilation (CO_2), strengthen breathing mechanics, ascertain upper airway cough and CNS coordination, and ↑ pt stamina to overcome deconditioning
- PEEP, allowing spontaneous breathing while ventilated, suctioning, turning and prone positioning, & alveolar recruitment maneuvers counteract atelectasis
- Extubation as soon as feasible allows cough & normal respirations to occur
- Use of supplemental oxygen:
  - FiO_2 ≤50% → usually nontoxic; pure O_2 must be given for >16 h for toxicity
  - Using supplemental O_2 postop may prevent wound infections, decreases pneumothoraces
  - COPD pts may tolerate supplemental O_2 without becoming apneic; consider noninvasive PEEP or CPAP upon extubation to allow lower FiO_2

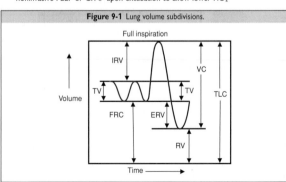

Figure 9-1 Lung volume subdivisions.

FRC, functional reserve capacity; IRV, inspiratory reserve volume; TV, tidal volume; ERV, expiratory reserve volume; RV, residual volume; VC, vital capacity; TLC, total lung capacity.

CAPNOGRAPHY

CO_2 identified in expired gas by spectrographic properties (using IR, Raman, or mass spectroscopy)

Uses and Indications for Capnography

- Detection of esophageal intubation: Must document CO_2 in exhaled gas with every intubation
- Detection of breathing circuit disconnection, inadvertent extubation, or insuff ventilation
- Detection of hyperventilation (leads to hypocarbia, cerebral EEG changes of ischemia)
- Detection of high metabolic rates (i.e., malignant hyperthermia or sepsis)
- Detection of low metabolic rates (i.e., hypothermia, lowered cardiac output states)
- Detection of pulmonary embolism (i.e., drop in $ETCO_2$ could be pulmonary embolus)
- Detection of bronchospasm/small airway obstruction (i.e., upward slant in $ETCO_2$ plateau)
- Calculation of V_D/V_T or dead-space ventilation (need $PaCO_2$ & $ETCO_2$)
  $V_D/V_T = ([PaCO_2 - P_{ET}CO_2]/PaCO_2)$; normal $V_D/V_T = 0.30$

Hazards of Capnography
- Old in-line IR detectors can heat up, causing facial thermal injury
- May fail to detect disconnection if machine disabled by secretions, or alarms disabled
- Adapters with excessive V_D (affect reliability of readings) or weight (cause extubation)
- ↑ Gas sampling rate may cause autotriggering of vent, affect delivered V_T (neonates)

CAPNOGRAPHS (FIG. 9-2)

FLOW–VOLUME LOOPS (FIG. 9-3)

MECHANICAL VENTILATION: PROTECTIVE STRATEGIES

Current Strategies to Prevent Volutrauma, Barotrauma, Atelectrauma, Tracheal Ischemia, & O_2 Toxicity
- Alveolar overdistention (volutrauma), rather than excessively ↑ airway pressure (barotrauma), may be more injurious to lung
- Smaller tidal volumes (6 mL/kg) are recommended with greater respiratory rate
- Higher $PaCO_2$ levels help survival (permissive hypercapnia) in treating ALI & ARDS
- "Noisy," proportional assist ventilation (PAV), neurally adjusted ventilator assistance (NAVA), (see below) PC, or pressure support (PS) ventilation may help reduce atelectrauma

Specific Settings
- TV 6 mL/kg (prevents volutrauma: Trauma from overdistention of alveoli)
- Plateau pressure <30 cm H_2O (prevents barotrauma: Trauma from excessive pressure)
- PEEP >6–10 cm H_2O (prevents atelectrauma: Repeated alveolar closure at end-expiration)
- FiO_2 <50% to prevent O_2 toxicity

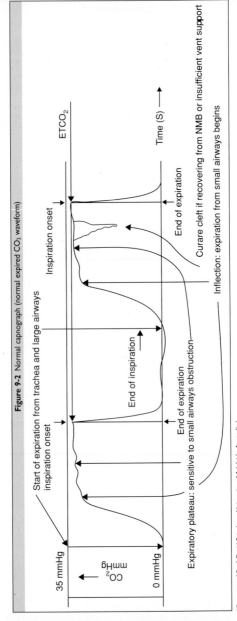

Figure 9-2 Normal capnograph (normal expired CO_2 waveform)

(Courtesy of Prof. David Sainsbury, University of Adelaide, Australia.)

Low-flow Supplemental O₂: Typical Means of Administration

Method of Administration	Device	O₂ Flow (L/min)	Estimated FiO₂*	Capnography Feasible	Humidified	Complications	Comment
Nasal cannula O₂	Nasal cannula attached to standardized flowmeter	0 1 2 3 4 5 6 7	0.21 0.25 0.29 0.33 0.37 0.41 0.45 0.49	Yes with specially designed cannulas; attach to sampling port of capnograph	No	Dried nasopharynx swallowing of air; bleeding, sinusitis; *Unlike HFNC, inspiration will dilure NCO₂ in nasopharynx, lowering actual FiC₂ delivered to lungs	Pts may mouth-breathe or have nasal constriction, sinusitis, packing, nasogastric tubes, etc. (add 4% FiO₂ for each L inc of O₂)
Venturi face mask	Venturi diluters attached to tubing	10+	0.30–0.50	No: Flow of gas too high	Yes	Highest FiO₂ only 0.50	Fixed FiO₂ dilutors entrain room air
Simple face mask		10+	0.55	Yes with sampling tube	No	Drying of mucosa	
Nonrebreather face mask with reservoir bag		10+	0.80	No: Flow too high	No	Drying of mucosa	
Ambu (bag-valve-mask)	Has 15-mm adapter to attach standard mask or ET tube	10+	1.0	No: Tight seal necessary if PPV planned	No	Spontaneous breaths difficult to see in semirigid Ambu bag	Spontaneous breathing or breaths from caretakers; PEEP feasible
Oxygen tent		10–15	0.50	Yes	Yes	Combustion risk	Used in pediatrics

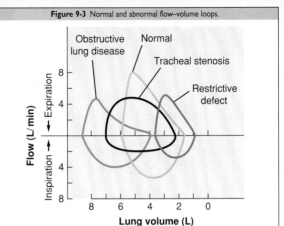

Figure 9-3 Normal and abnormal flow–volume loops.

(Adapted from Goudsouzian N, Karamanian A. *Physiology for the Anesthesiologist.* 2nd ed. Norwalk, CT: Appleton-Century-Crofts; 1984. In: Barash PG, Callan MK, Cullen BF, Stock MC, Stoelting RK, Ortega R, Sharar SR, Holt N, eds. *Clinical Anesthesia.* 8th ed. Philadelphia, PA: Wolters Kluwer; 2018:1003.)

Effects of Positive End-Expiratory Pressure (PEEP)	
Pulmonary System	
Advantages	*Remarks*
Improves hypoxemia	Hypoxemia caused by ARDS, pneumonia, pulm edema, drowning, atelectasis
Opens airways throughout resp cycle	By recruiting alveoli & larger lung segments
↑ FRC	Further improving oxygenation
Improves pulmonary compliance	Further ↓ risk of barotrauma & hypotension
↓ Inspiratory work of breathing	Further improving oxygenation, esp effective if pt is trapping air (auto-PEEP)
Prevents derecruitment	Protects against atelectasis esp during long surgeries
Treats auto-PEEP (airway trapping 2°↓ expiratory phase in asthma/COPD)	Diagnose this by looking at flow-time curve on ventilator (flow not returning to zero before inspiration = auto-PEEP)
Prevents atelectatic trauma (repetitive closure of alveoli at end-expiration)	Atelectatic trauma correlates with ↑ serum cytokines & markers of lung injury
Allows to ↓ FiO_2	May ↓ risk of O_2 toxicity
Disadvantages	*Remarks*
May cause barotrauma	Types of barotrauma include pneumoperitoneum, pneumomediastinum, pneumopericardium, pneumothorax, subcutaneous emphysema, tension pneumothorax, all of which may cause shock
May enlarge pneumothorax	PEEP contraindicated even if a small pneumothorax is present without chest catheter or tube
May worsen V/Q mismatching	Esp by enlarging West Zone 1 (apex of lung) where alveolar pressure > arterial pressure > venous pressure
↑ Dead-space ventilation (V_D/V_T)	Adds work without O_2 for pt
May worsen bronchopleural fistula leak	PEEP contraindicated in bronchopleural fistula
May cause significant leak following tracheal/pulm surgery (pneumonectomy)	PEEP contraindicated in recent tracheal surgery, lobectomy, lung transplant, or pneumonectomy unless chest tube present

| May lead to ↑ IV administration | PEEP may cause acute hypotension in the volume depleted |

Cardiovascular System

Advantages	Remarks
If successful, improves AaDO₂ & O₂ delivery to tissues & myocardium	Improved oxygenation decreases anaerobic lactatemia and acidosis
Treats airway obstruction (OSA)	OSA associated with hypoxemia, dysrhythmias, myocardial infarction, extreme sensitivity to opioids, death
↓ LV afterload	Opposite of its effect on RV afterload
Disadvantages	**Remarks**
↓ Left & right ventricular preload	Primary mechanism for reducing CO
↓ Venous return	Primary mechanism for reducing CO
↑ CVP	Makes it hard to assess fluid & preload status with CVP
↑ RV afterload	Worsens RV failure in certain individuals
↓ Ventricular compliance	Causes interventricular septum to bulge into LV (↓ CO)
Worsens hypotension in hypovolemia	As in hemorrhage, dehydration, sepsis

Central Nervous System

Advantages	Remarks
↑ O₂ delivery to CNS	If indeed PEEP is effective at treating hypoxemia
Treats OSA	OSA greatly ↑ risk of stroke, MI, dysrhythmias, death
Disadvantages	**Remarks**
↑ Intracranial pressure	By ↑ CVP & by directly ↑ CSF pressure
↓ Cerebral perfusion pressure	By ↓ MAP & ↑ CVP
↑ Risk of embolization into left circulation	May ↑ risk of opening an occult probe-patent foramen ovale (cause sudden R to L shunt, hypoxemia, embolization)

Hepatic, Renal, Neuroendocrine Systems

Advantages	Remarks
↓ Renal & hepatic blood flow (↓ CO)	May affect clearance of drugs or compound renal ischemia
Disadvantages	**Remarks**
↑ ADH secretion	Various effects but largely helps retain free water (preload) may make diuresis more difficult

PRONE VENTILATION FOR SEVERE ARDS

- VC mode with TV (6 mL/kg)
- NMB needed, use early, use standard rotation regimen
- Extensive padding, eye care important
- Increased risks of tube obstruction, disconnection, soft tissue ulcers
- Improves PaO₂/FiO₂ (P/F ratio, i.e., oxygenation) in a majority of pts
- Improves pulmonary hemodynamics without affecting systemic hemodynamics
- Apply within 36 h of intubation: Ind: P/F ratio <150, requiring ≥5 of PEEP, ≥0.6 FiO₂
- Improves effectiveness of pulmonary recruitment maneuvers
- Best used 18–23 h/d, as tolerated, until improvement or death of pt

Source: Guerin C, Reignier J, Richard J-C, et al. Prone positioning in severe acute respiratory distress syndrome. N Engl J 2013;368:2159–2168.

NONINVASIVE VENTILATION (NIV): CPAP vs. BiPAP vs. HIGH-FLOW NASAL CANNULA

- Helps avoid (re-)intubation, treats CHF, is a bridge to low-flow O₂ postextubation
- Risks: Aspiration, poor tolerance, mask trauma, mask leak entrains room air, and ↓ FiO₂

BiPAP vs. CPAP (both applied with specialized masks: Face, oral, nasal pillows; which seal and deliver positive airway pressure throughout respiratory cycle. Both effective)

- CPAP = delivery of continuous airway pressure (6–14 cm H₂O) throughout respiratory cycle

Overview of Modes of Ventilation

Simple Modes for Use in OR or in Cases of Brief Interval Intubation (ED, PACU)***

Mode of Ventilation	Advantage	Disadvantage	NMB Needed or Feasible?	Triggered by Breath?	Synchronized to Breath?	Spontaneous Breathing Allowed?
Volume control (VC)	Simple, delivers fixed TV & RR	May give excessive pressure if compliance decreases	Feasible	No: Breaths timed by ventilator	No	Yes, but pt may hyperventilate to hypocarbia
Pressure control (PC)	Simple, delivers fixed plateau pressure & RR	May give inadequate volume if compliance decreases	Feasible if ventilator is time-cycled	No	No	Yes, but pt may hyperventilate to hypocarbia

Simple Modes for Longer-term SUPPORT in ICU

Mode of Ventilation	Advantage	Disadvantage	NMB Needed or Feasible?	Triggered by Breath?	Synchronized to Breath?	Spontaneous Breathing Allowed?
Assist control (AC)	Delivers fixed minimum TV or pressure with each triggered breath	Each breath triggered means a ventilator breath delivered	Feasible & may be helpful to pt tolerating ventilator	Yes	Yes	Yes, but because every breath is supported by the ventilator, hyperventilation may occur
Intermittent mandatory ventilation (IMV)	Like AC but also allows periods of spontaneous ventilation	Spontaneous breathing periods not well tolerated without PS	Not if spontaneous respirations desired	No	No	Yes, stacking of breaths may occur and hyperventilation may occur

Modes Used (Usually in Combination) for Uncomplicated Weaning in ICU or PACU

Mode of Ventilation	Advantage	Disadvantage	NMB Needed or Feasible?	Triggered by Breath?	Synchronized to Breath?	Spontaneous Breathing Allowed?
Pressure support (PS)	Augments spontaneous breathing; good for weaning	Suboptimal if no reliable respiratory drive; TV changes with lung compliance	Neither	Yes	Yes	Yes, it must occur or there will be no PS (used with SIMV)
Synchronized mandatory ventilation (SIMV)	Synchronized to breath	None	Feasible—but without spontaneous RR, this is just AC	No	Yes	Yes (used with PS)

Modes Used to Treat Severe Hypoxemia or Lung Injury in ICU or for Difficult Weaning

Mode of Ventilation	Advantage	Disadvantage	NMB Needed or Feasible?	Triggered by Breath?	Synchronized to Breath?	Spontaneous Breathing Allowed?
Inverse ratio (IR): I:E ratio inverted, ≥1	For severe hypoxemia; may be used in either PC or VC setting	Poorly tolerated in awake pts; barotrauma possible if they cough	May be needed if heavy sedation is insufficient	No	No	No

			beneficial if there is no spontaneous breathing		Respiratory failure
Volume control (PRVC), also known as Volume control plus (VC+)	upper inspiratory pressure limit; ventilator adjusts pressure to compliance; less barotrauma				
Airway pressure-release ventilation (APRV)	Allows spontaneous respiration and reduced risk of barotrauma	As in PC, TV may vary depending on compliance	Neither	No	Yes: This mode is like CPAP at a high level, allowing spontaneous breaths with intermittent release of CPAP
Continuous positive airway pressure (CPAP) or positive end-expiratory pressure (PEEP)	↑ oxygenation without active support; demonstrates weaning	Requires good respiratory drive and effort	Neither	No	Yes. PEEP and CPAP are similar; CPAP occurs during spontaneous breathing; PEEP occurs during positive-pressure ventilation
Bilevel positive airway pressure (BIPAP) or BIVENT	Allows spontaneous respiration in hypoxemic pts	↓ mean airway pressure than APR; less barotrauma	Neither	No	Yes: This is like APRV but with a longer expiratory phase. Useful in severe hypoxemia
Modes Used to ↑ Resp Variation, Compensate for ET Tube, ↓ Lung Injury, ↓ Vent Asynchrony					
Proportional assist ventilation (PAV, PAV+)	↓ ventilator asynchrony; fewer vent and sedative changes	Better sleep quality but no better survival or weaning outcomes	Neither	Yes	Yes: Ventilator assists more strongly with more pt effort
Neurally adjusted ventilator assistance (NAVA)	Coordinates ventilation and pt effort; less asynchrony, ↑ weaning outcomes	Requires esophageal sensor to measure intensity of electrical impulse	Neither	Yes	Like PAV; reduces asynchrony and vent, sedative changes
Noisy ventilation (PSV with Gaussian- or other-distributed pressures)	↑ recruitment of atelectatic alveoli and decreased closure of airways	Noninferior to nonnoisy PS ventilation	Neither	Yes	No but, synchrony with ventilator better with noisy PSV than plain PSV
Automatic tube compensation (ATC)	Adjusts for resistance of ET tube, used with PS, PAV	Not widely available; not much studied; used with other vent modes	Neither	Yes	Yes
High-frequency ventilation (HFV) 1–2 mL/kg TV with RR up to 12 Hz	Higher average AW pressure; reduced PAW pressure	Not widely available or commonly used. Does not improve survival in ARDS	Feasible and may be necessary	No	No. Usually used with NMB or heavy sedation

PRVC, HFV, APRV, & BIPAP ventilation, allow significant ↑ in avg airway pressure (recruit more alveoli & improve AaDO₂) & allow pt to breathe spontaneously; advantage = less sedation & muscle relaxation required.

Treatment Modalities that Improve Oxygenation, ICU Course and Mortality in Patients with ARDS

Intervention	Improves Oxygenation	Improves Mortality	Shortens ICU or Ventilator Course	Quality of Evidence	Study Acronym or Review Reference
Protective ventilation (TV 6 vs. 12 mL/kg)	Yes	Yes	Yes	Good	ARDSnet or ARMA; VALI/VILI Trial
Higher vs. Lower PEEP ARDSnet bracket	No	No	No	Good	ALVEOLI Trial
Permissive hypercapnia	Yes	No	No	Poor	Crit Care 2010;14:237
Prone positioning	Yes	Yes	Yes	Good	PROSEVA Trial
Neuromuscular blockade early	Yes	Yes	Yes	Good	ACURACYS Trial; also Crit Care Med 2004;32:113–9
Early mobilization of ICU pts including those on mechanical ventilation	No	Yes	Yes	Early but promising	Am J Med Sci 2011;341:373–7
Diuresis or HF/UF (target CVP <4)	Yes	Yes	No	Good	FACTT Trial
Inhaled NO	Yes	No	No	Good	Crit Care Med 2014;42:404–12
Inhaled epoprostenol	Yes	No	No	Poor	Chest 2015;147:1510–22
APRV	Yes	Yes	Yes	Early but promising	Resp Care 2016;61:761–73; Int Care Med 2017;43:1648–9
VV ECMO	Yes	Yes	No	Good	CESAR Trial; ELSO Guidelines; N Engl J Med 2018;378:1965–75

Abbreviations: ARDS, adult respiratory distress syndrome; CVP, central venous pressure; PEEP, positive end-expiratory pressure; HF, hemofiltration; UF, ultrafiltration; APRV, airway pressure release ventilation; ECMO, extracorporeal membrane oxygenation; TV, tidal volume; VV, venovenous; ICU, intensive care unit; NO, nitric oxide; ELSO, Extracorporeal Life Support Organization.

References for study trials: ARDSnet or ARMA: The ARDS Network. N Engl J Med 2000;342:1301–8; ALVEOLI: The NHLBI ARDS Clinical Trials Network. N Engl J Med 2004;351:327–36; PROSEVA: The PROSEVA Study Group. N Engl J Med 2013;368:2159–68; ACURACYS: The ACURACYS Study Investigators. N Engl J Med 2010;363:1107–16; FACTT: The NHLBI ARDS Clinical Trials Network. N Engl J Med 2006;354:2564–75; CESAR: The Lancet 2009;374(9698):1351–63; ELSO Guidelines: Guidelines for Cardiopulmonary Extracorporeal Life Support, Version 1.4 August 2017, Ann Arbor, MI, USA, www.elso.org

- BiPAP = two levels of positive air pressure, inspiratory (triggered by insp flow) & expiratory (present throughout the rest of the respiratory cycle) *(expiratory pressure is lower to facilitate exhalation)*, typical values expressed in insp/exp cm H_2O, e.g., 10/6 cm

High-flow Nasal Cannula Therapy Is an Alternative to NIV with Mask. Used in nonhypercarbic hypoxemia. Warmed humidified high-flow nasal cannula at 50 L/m, FiO_2 start at 1.0, titrate to keep SpO_2 90–92%. Causes mild positive pressure in airway (like PEEP) and decreases work of breathing. Better tolerated than mask NIV in many pts especially claustrophobic ones. Wean this to low-flow NC, NIV, or low-flow or Venturi mask when improved

Approach to Patients with Berlin Definition Moderate (PaO_2/FiO_2 <200) to Severe (PaO_2/FiO_2 <100) ARDS		
Intervention	**Adjustment**	**Watch For:**
Set TV to 5–8 mL/kg predicted BW	Volume (VC or SIMV) or pressure control (PC) modes will work; Keep initial plateau pressure <30 cm H_2O	Hypotension, optimize SVV (= 13%) to avoid excessive fluid administration, maintain perfusion, O_2 delivery
Set PEEP to 10–12 cm H_2O	Less PEEP than 10–12 cm H_2O may not recruit enough to improve hypoxemia	Barotrauma especially pneumothorax
Optimize PEEP by increments of 2–3 cm H_2O	Keep Plateau Pressure below 30 cm H_2O; it will rise in tandem with PEEP	Failure to improve oxygenation: Consider the next steps

Salvage Therapy for Patients Who Fail to Improve or Who Develop Berlin Definition Severe ARDS (PaO_2/FiO_2 <100)		
Neuromuscular blockade for 48 h early in course of ARDS	Document TOF depth of blockade, keep at 2/4 or less	Discontinue when feasible; limit duration; Use a protocol
Prone positioning	16-h sessions optimal; most effective early (<48 h) in course of ARDS	Positioning eye and soft tissue trauma, airway movement or dislodgment, right main stem intubation
Furosemide or hemofiltration/ultrafiltration (HF/UF): A fluid restrictive strategy is thought to improve oxygenation and survival in ARDS	40 mg bolus then 19 mg/h infusion. Consider HF/UF via nephrology consultation	Electrolyte losses; hypovolemia; HF involves risks of access, etc.
Inhaled nitric oxide or inhaled epoprostenol	NO dosage range 5–80 PPM Epoprostenol dosage range 10–50 ng/kg/min	Too rapid NO or epoprostenol weaning may result in rebound hypoxemia or pulmonary hypertension
Seek and empirically treat for presumed infections, as cause of ARDS, especially VAP	Consider BAL or biopsy. Consider CT of body to look for infections in abdomen, etc. Consider atypical, viral, fungal pathogens.	Narrow antibiotic choices when culture, biopsy, or antigen results become available
Alternative mode: APRV is gaining widest acceptance in treating ARDS and hypoxemic respiratory failure (See Ref. 1 below)	(1) Set Phigh <30 cm H_2O, and equal to previous Pplat (VC) or previous Ppeak (PC) (2) Plow 0 or 5 cm H_2O (3) Set RR 10–14 BPM (4) Set Tlow/Thigh at 9:1 and adjust Tlow for mean airway pressure <30 (5) Adjust Tlow so that EEFR/PEFR is 75%	APRV works by high pressure in inspiration; lungs' elasticity helps decrease WOB by recoiling in expiration Contraindicated in severe obstructive pulmonary dz; Barotrauma; hypercapnia are possible. If Tlow is too short: Ventilator is not supporting pt enough. Expiration too short to help WOB If Tlow is too long: Atelectrauma, not protecting lung

| Venovenous ECMO (See Ref. 2 below) Cannulae in internal jugular veins, femoral veins, or right atrium. Supports lung but not heart function. | For approximately total CO_2 removal and oxygenation in adult, two things to vary: (1) ECMO blood flow rate (~3 L/min = about 2/3 of the pt's CO) and (2) O_2 membrane sweep rate (~6 L/min); sweep is ~twice the ECMO blood flow rate | Vascular access complications; hemorrhage, hemolysis, embolism Utility as a life-saving measure still in question No proven demonstration of increased survival with ECMO in any study |

Abbreviations: ARDS, adult respiratory distress syndrome; HF, hemofiltration; UF, ultrafiltration; APRV, airway pressure release ventilation; BAL, bronchoalveolar lavage; BPM, breaths per minute; CO, cardiac output; CT, computed tomography; ECMO, extracorporeal membrane oxygenation; EEFR, in APRV: End-expiratory flow rate; PC, pressure control; PEEP, positive end-expiratory pressure; PEFR, in APRV: Peak expiratory flow rate; PPM, parts per million; RR, respiratory rate; SIMV, synchronized intermittent mandatory ventilation; TV, tidal volume; VC, volume control; VV, venovenous; TOF, train-of-four; Phigh, APRV high level pressure; Plow, APRV low level pressure; Pplat, SIMV plateau pressure; Ppeak, SIMV peak pressure; Thigh, APRV time interval for high level (inspiration) pressure application; Tlow, APRV time interval for low pressure (expiration) application; WOB, work of breathing; ICU, intensive care unit; NO, nitric oxide; ELSO, Extracorporeal Life Support Organization.
1. Reference for initiating APRV: Zhou Y, et al. *Intensive Care Med* 2017;43:1648–59.
2. Reference for Venovenous ECMO: ELSO Guidelines: Guidelines for Adult Respiratory Failure. ELSO Guidelines for Cardiopulmonary Extracorporeal Life Support, Version 1.4 August 2017, Ann Arbor, MI, USA, www.elso.org

DISCONTINUING MECHANICAL VENTILATION (ALSO CALLED WEANING OR LIBERATING FROM MV)

SIMV Plus PS is a Common Weaning Mode in Many ICUs
- Start with full support (IMV ≈ 10), plus PS 10–15 cm H_2O, PEEP 5–10, FiO_2 ≤60
- ↓ by 1–2 breaths/min over h to d until IMV = 0
- Now wean PS 1–2 cm H_2O at a time until PS/PEEP is 10/5 or 5/5 cm H_2O or lower (for more deconditioned pts, you may need to go as low as PS/PEEP = 2/5)
- At the same time gradually reduce FiO_2 according to SaO_2 or PaO_2 (more sensitive to oxygenation changes). Assess P/F ratio = PaO_2/FiO_2. It should be >120
- Order rapid shallow breathing index (RSBI) trial to assess possibility of extubation. RSBI equals (RR [breaths per min]/TV [liters]). Criterion for extubation is RSBI <100, e.g., 25 breaths/min RR divided by 0.250-L TV = RSBI of 100 breath/l-min. Other criteria are listed below.
- Have a postextubation plan: Extubate to CPAP or NC or FM. Survey P/F, RR, work of breathing. Anticipate stridor or resp failure soon after extubation. Be available and nearby

Criteria for Extubation Used in Many ICUs (Pts Should Meet Each of Them)	
Criterion	Remarks
5-sec head lift (correlates with NIP of 50 cm H_2O): Best indicator of upper airway strength	Conscious head lift to command, not from coughing, is optimal. The pt cannot be in steep semi-Fowler's (too easy)
PaO_2/FiO_2 >120 or equivalently, PaO_2 >60 on FiO_2 of 0.50	O_2 requirement should be 50% or lower before extubation is considered; FiO_2 40% is better
PEEP support <6 cm with adequate oxygenation	Sudden withdrawal of PEEP may cause fall in PaO_2 and sudden ↑ in work of breathing requiring reintubation
CNS intact (ideally GCS ≥12)	See GCS Scale, Chapter 22
Ability to maintain $PaCO_2$ <50 mmHg and 7.30 < pH < 7.50	Sepsis, hyperthermia, hyperalimentation, ↑ CO_2 production; these causes may be addressed; metabolic alkalosis from GI losses or diuretics may cause CO_2 retention; treat alkalosis with NaCl & KCl in IV fluid or other measures

Ability to breathe without tiring, splinting, diaphoresis, tachypnea, tachycardia, bradycardia, anxiety. RSBI <100 breaths/l-min	Extubation of chronic pts from PS of ≥5 cm H_2O may cause them to tire after extubation. Consider extubating to NIV RSBI = breathing frequency (RR)/tidal volume in liters (see above for example calculation)
Ability to clear secretions without plugging bronchioles	Assess secretions prior to extubation, remember anticholinergic side effects of opioids. Consider mucolytics and bronchoscopy
No overt risk of pulm aspiration (no bowel obstruction or high NG/OG output), GCS ≥12	Aspiration may occur even with intact airway reflexes if bowel obstruction is severe or GI bleeding is brisk
Adequate Hb, cardiac output, & cardiovascular stability	Hg ≥8.0–10 allows adequate O_2-carrying capacity (for $AaDO_2$) & viscosity (for maintaining SVR & therefore BP)
Pain is controlled adequately to allow spontaneous breathing without excessive splinting	Consider intercostal, intervertebral, epidural, or intrapleural local anesthetics or subarachnoid block to allow deep breathing and cough and prevent atelectasis

FLUIDS, ELECTROLYTES, & TRANSFUSION THERAPY

ALYSSA K. STREFF • MICHAEL N. SINGLETON

FLUID MANAGEMENT

Fluid Compartments
- *Total body water (TBW)* ≈ 60% body weight in males; 50% in females (TBW inversely proportional to amount of adipose tissue in body)
  - *Intracellular fluid (ICF)* ≈ 2/3 of TBW
  - *Extracellular fluid (ECF)* ≈ 1/3 of TBW
    - *Interstitial fluid volume* ≈ 2/3 of ECF, *Plasma volume* ≈ 1/3 of ECF

Assessing Volume Status
- Accurate assessment of volume status is challenging; consider entire clinical picture
- A systematic approach to estimating blood status is shown in Figure 10-1

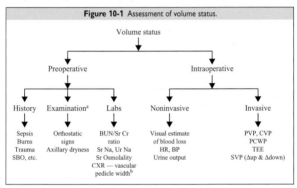

Figure 10-1 Assessment of volume status.

[a]Only orthostatic signs (postural Δ in HR >30 bpm, postural dizziness) & axillary dryness are predictive of hypovolemia due to blood loss (*JAMA* 1999;281:1022). Skin turgor, capillary refill time, oliguria not helpful.
[b]Vascular pedicle width on CXR correlates well with volume status (*Chest* 2002;121:942).
SBO, sm bowel obstruction; PVP, peripheral venous press; TEE, transesophageal echo; SVP, systolic pressure variation on A-line trace in mechanically ventilated pts.

Volume Deficits
- *ICF deficits (free water losses)*: Insensible losses from skin & resp system, free water loss by kidneys (diabetes insipidus, central, or nephrogenic)
  - Characterized by cellular dehydration, ↑ plasma osmolality, & ↑ Na
  - Will not present as acute circulatory collapse; gradually correct with free water
- *ECF deficits*: Blood loss, GI losses (vomiting, diarrhea), & distributional changes (ascites, burns, "3rd spacing")—of much greater concern in perioperative period
  - *Labs*: ↑ BUN/Cr ratio, ↓ urine Na excretion (<20 mEq/L, FENa <1%), & conc urine
  - Can cause rapid circulatory instability; treat expeditiously with isotonic crystalloids, colloids, or blood

Volume Replacement
- Traditional approaches to fluid replacement (using isotonic crystalloids):
  Fluid replacement = maintenance + deficit + insensible losses + surgical losses
  - *Maintenance* (mL/h): 4–2–1 formula (4 mL/kg/h for 1st 10 kg; 2 mL/kg/h for next 10 kg; 1 mL/kg/h beyond that)
  - *Deficit* (mL): Maintenance × h NPO; 50% replaced in 1st h, & 25% in 2nd & 3rd h
  - *Insensible losses* (mL/h): Depending on magnitude of surgical insult—4 mL/kg/h (mild), 6 mL/kg/h (moderate), 8 mL/kg/h (severe)
  - *Losses*: Blood loss replaced with 1:3 crystalloid, or 1:1 colloid; other losses (ascitic fluid) replaced according to estimated electrolyte composition

- Traditional approach criticized:
  - Data have shown that blood volume is normal even after a perioperative fast, and the assumption of a large fluid deficit requiring replacement may be incorrect (*Acta Anaes Scand* 2008;52(4):522).
  - Fluids are not benign. Excessive fluid administration results in increased morbidity and mortality. There is a movement to consider IV fluids as medications; judicious use and context is critical (*Curr Opin Crit Care* 2013;19:290).
  - Fluid administration has been shown to disrupt the endothelial glycocalyx, resulting in worse vascular permeability (*Best Pract Res Clin Anaes* 2014;28:227)
  - Goal-directed fluid therapy (GDFT) using hemodynamic parameters and the assessment of fluid bolus responsiveness have been suggested to guide fluid delivery, as opposed to empiric administration. GDFT has not yet been shown to ↓ mortality, but may reduce complications and LOS (*Brit J Anaes* 2013;111:535)
  - In one study, a "restrictive" fluid regimen was not associated with a higher rate of disability-free survival than a "liberal" fluid regimen but associated with a higher rate of acute kidney injury (*N Engl J Med* 2018;378(24):2263–2274)
  - Lung U/S may be used for early visualization of extravascular lung water to prevent over resuscitation (*J Crit Care* 2016;31(1):96–100)
  - Approach to perioperative fluid management (*Anesthesiology* 2008;109(4):723–740):
    - ECF deficit after usual overnight fasting is low
    - Clear fluids PO should be encouraged until 2 h prior to surgery
    - Insensible fluid loss via perspiration/evaporation is a max of 1 mL/kg/h, even during major abdominal surgery
    - A fluid-consuming 3rd space does not exist
    - Low maintenance IVF rate (2–3 mL/kg/h) plus goal-directed boluses to optimize stroke volume or replace acute losses is recommended

Crystalloids & Colloids
- Crystalloids are predominately solutions of sterile water with added electrolytes. Colloids also contain water and electrolytes, but have an added colloid substance (albumin, hetastarch, dextran protein, gelatin) that does not freely cross a semipermeable membrane.
- The theoretical advantage of colloids is the ability to maintain or improve plasma oncotic pressure. However, there is no evidence for superiority of either colloids or crystalloids (*may be some advantages in using each in specific subgroups of pts*).
  - SAFE trial: Compared 4% albumin vs. NS in 7,000 critically ill pts. No overall difference in mortality, length of stay, or need for mechanical ventilation. Subgroup analysis showed higher mortality with albumin in trauma pts, predominately head injury.
  - CRISTAL trial: Compared colloids vs. crystalloids for resuscitation in ICU hypovolemic shock. No improvement in 28-d all-cause mortality with colloids.
- Hetastarch solutions appear more efficacious for restoration of intravascular volume, especially regarding the microcirculation in sepsis. However, VISEP, 6S, and CHEST trials have shown increased risk of kidney injury and mortality, resulting in black box warnings from the FDA.

	Na (mEq/L)	Cl (mEq/L)	K (mEq/L)	Ca (mEq/L)	Mg (mEq/L)	Buffers/other (mEq/L)	pH	Osmolarity (mOsm/L)
Normal ECF	140	103	4	5	2	Bicarbonate (25)	7.4	290
Plasmalyte	140	98	5	—	3	Acetate (27); Gluconate (23)	7.4	295
Lactated Ringer's	130	109	4	3	—	Lactate (28)	6.4	273
Normal Saline	154	154	—	—	—	—	5.7	308
1/2 Normal Saline	77	77	—	—	—	—	4.5	143
3% Saline	513	513	—	—	—	—	5.6	1025
Albumin 5%	145	145	<2	—	—	50 g/L albumin	7.4	310
Hetastarch 6%	154	154	—	—	—	60 g/L starch	5.9	310

Notes on Specific Fluids
- 5% *dextrose*—used to replace free water; isotonic to plasma but rapidly becomes free water (dextrose is metabolized); used to treat dehydration losses

- *Balanced crystalloid or 0.9% saline*—SMART-MED, SMART-SURG, SALT-ED trials showed a reduction in major adverse kidney events at 30 d w/ balanced solutions
- *0.9% saline* or "normal" saline (NS)—the chloride content is significantly higher than plasma (154 vs. 102 mEq, respectively). Large volume administration may result in hyperchloremic metabolic acidosis. Usage should be limited.
- *Plasma-lyte*—major advantage is the buffer capacity, giving a pH equivalent to plasma. Contains magnesium; caution in renal insufficiency
- *Lactated Ringer* (LR)—contains calcium and potassium that approximate plasma concentration; lactate added to buffer metabolic acidosis
  - Unsuitable for pts with end-stage liver dz: Lactate requires metabolism in liver to CO_2 & water. Plasma-lyte possibly better in major hepatectomy (*Acta Anaesth Scand* 2011;55(5):558–564)
  - Contraindicated as a diluent for blood transfusions: Calcium binds to the citrate anticoagulant in blood products
- *Hypertonic saline* (3%, 7.5%, and 23.4%)—higher osmolality is used to reduce cerebral edema & ICP. Current evidence suggests that hypertonic saline is more effective than mannitol in reducing ICP in TBI (*Crit Care Med* 2011;39:554–559).
- *Albumin*—5% & 25% conc. available; 5% albumin = isotonic with plasma; circulatory half-life normally 16 h (as short as 2–3 h in pathophysiologic conditions); made from pooled human blood; minimal/no risk of transmitting infections. Although the physiologic rationale is unclear, albumin should be **avoided in pts with severe TBI** (see SAFE trial comments above). There is some data that supports the combination of 25% albumin boluses and furosemide infusions in hypoproteinemic pts with acute lung injury in an attempt to ↑ osmotic pressure and improve oxygenation (*Crit Care Med* 2005;33:1681–1687).
- *Hydroxyethyl starch* (hetastarch)—high-molecular-weight synthetic colloid, ↑ plasma oncotic pressure up to 2 d; available as 6% solution in NS or LR; renally excreted; should be avoided in pts with sepsis as they may be associated with a significantly increased risk of renal dysfunction in this setting (*N Engl J Med* 2008;358:125–139)
  - Side effects → elevates serum amylase, anaphylactoid rxns, coagulopathy (inhibits platelets, ↓ factor VIII and vWF); restrict dose to 20 mL/kg in order to minimize plt inhibition
- *Dextran*—dextran 40 & dextran 70 (numbers refer to average molecular mass of solution); side effects include anaphylactoid rxn, ↑ bleeding time, interference with blood cross-matching, rare cases of noncardiogenic pulmonary edema, renal obstruction/acute renal failure
  - Dextran 40 → used in vascular surgery to prevent thrombosis/stroke; however, there is no evidence of this, and it likely harms pts through more perioperative MI/CHF (*J Vasc Surg* 2013;57(3):635–641)
  - Dextran 70 → used for same indications as 5% albumin
- *Voluven* (HES 130/0.5)—Hetastarch with a low molecular weight and a low degree of substitution that may be associated with a smaller bleeding risk compared to older starches. However, some of the studies reporting a lower bleeding risk have been retracted due to scientific misconduct, and a recent in vitro study did not find a significantly lower bleeding risk (*Intensive Care Med* 2011;37:1725–1737). In light of 6S and VISEP trials, the use of hydroxyethyl starch solutions should be considered contraindicated in pts with sepsis (*N Engl J Med* 2012. DOI: 10.1056/NEJMoa1204242).

APPROACH TO ACID–BASE ANALYSIS

Check arterial pH:
pH <7.40 (acidic)
- *PCO_2 >40 respiratory acidosis:*
  Hypoventilation/decreased respiratory drive (e.g., overdose/drugs), Obstruction (COPD), Neuromuscular dz, Increased carbon dioxide production (malignant hyperthermia)
- *PCO_2 <40 metabolic acidosis*
  → Check gap: Na^- (bicarb + Cl)
- Normal gap (12 ± 2)
  Decreased bicarb, diarrhea, renal tubular acidosis
- Increased gap (>12)
  Methanol
  Uremia
  DKA (diabetic ketoacidosis)
  Paraldehyde

INH (isoniazid)
Lactic acidosis
Ethylene glycol (antifreeze)
Salicylates

- **BICAR-ICU Trial:** Treatment with sodium bicarbonate did not improve organ failure at 7-d or all-cause mortality at 28 d in ICU pts with severe metabolic acidemia (pH <7.2), with the exception being those pts with acute kidney injury

pH >7.40 (alkalemic)
- $PCO_2 < 40$ respiratory alkalosis
  Hyperventilation
- $PCO_2 > 40$ metabolic alkalosis
  Vomiting, diuretics, antacid abuse, increased aldosterone

Primary Acid-Base Disorders				
1° Disorder	**Problem**	**pH**	**PaCO₂**	**HCO₃**
Metabolic acidosis	Gain of H^+ or loss of HCO_3	↓	↓	↓
Metabolic alkalosis	Gain of HCO_3 or loss of H^+	↑	↑	↑
Resp acidosis	Hypoventilation	↓	↑	↑
Resp alkalosis	Hyperventilation	↑	↓	↓

Acid-Base: Rules of Compensation	
1° Disorder	**Formula**
Metabolic acidosis	$\downarrow PaCO_2 = 1.25 \times \Delta HCO_3$ (also, $PaCO_2$ = last 2 digits of pH)
Metabolic alkalosis	$\uparrow PaCO_2 = 0.75 \times \Delta HCO_3$
Acute resp acidosis	$\uparrow HCO_3 = 0.1 \times \Delta PaCO_2$ (also, $\downarrow$ pH = $0.008 \times \Delta PaCO_2$)
Chronic resp acidosis	$\uparrow HCO_3 = 0.4 \times \Delta PaCO_2$ (also, $\downarrow$ pH = $0.003 \times \Delta PaCO_2$)
Acute resp alkalosis	$\downarrow HCO_3 = 0.2 \times \Delta PaCO_2$
Chronic resp alkalosis	$\downarrow HCO_3 = 0.4 \times \Delta PaCO_2$

Source: Adapted from Sabatine MS. *Pocket Medicine*. 7th ed. Philadelphia, PA: Wolters Kluwer; 2020.

Strong Ion Difference (Stewart Acid/Base)
- Strong Ion Difference (SID) = Strong Cations (Na, K, Ca, Mg) − Strong Anions (Cl)
  - Abbreviated SID = (Na − Cl)
  - Normal SID ~42, ↑ SID = ↑ alkalosis, ↓ SID = ↑ acidosis

ELECTROLYTES

Hyponatremia (Na⁺ <135 mEq/L)
- *Etiology* (Fig. 10-2) *and Outcomes*
  - Preoperative hyponatremia associated with increased mortality and LOS (Arch Intern Med 2012;172(19):1474–1481)
- *Symptoms*—nausea, vomiting, weakness, muscle cramps, visual disturbances, ↓ level of consciousness, agitation, seizures, coma
  - Cerebral edema → when Na⁺ <123 mEq/L
  - Cardiac symptoms → when Na⁺ <100 mEq/L
- *Treatment*
  - Mild hyponatremia: Free water restriction ± loop diuretics
  - Severe hyponatremia with neurologic symptoms: 3% hypertonic saline
  - Urgent intervention for seizures or impending herniation: 100 mL of 3% NaCl infused intravenously over 10 min × 3 prn. Raises Na concentration 1.5 mEq/L in men, 2.0 mEq/L in women.
  - Intervention for lethargy, dizziness, gait disturbances, etc.: 3% NaCl infused at 0.5–2 mL/kg/h (too rapid correction → central pontine myelinolysis. Maximum correction of 10 mmol/L in the first 24 h, 18 mmol/L in 48 h)
- *SIADH treatment*
  - Free water restriction; demeclocycline used for chronic cases
  - Loop diuretic + fluid replacement with hypertonic saline

Guide to Using Hypertonic Saline
1. Calculate Na deficit that needs to be repleted Sodium deficit = body weight × 0.6 × (desired serum Na⁻ actual serum Na)
2. Calculate infusion rate to raise serum Na by 1–2 mEq/L/h 3% NaCl infusion rate = sodium deficit/12.312 = cc/h infusion rate over 24 h

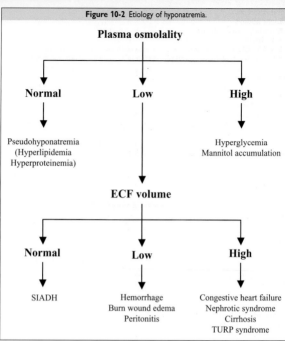

Figure 10-2 Etiology of hyponatremia.

(Modified from Braunwald E, Fauci AS, Kasper DL, et al., eds. *Harrison's Principles of Internal Medicine.* 15th ed. New York, NY: McGraw-Hill; 2001.)

Hypernatremia (Na⁺ >145 mEq/L)

- *Etiology* (Fig. 10-3) *and Outcomes*
  - Preoperative hypernatremia associated with increased 30-d morbidity and mortality *(Am J Med 2013;126(10):877–886)*

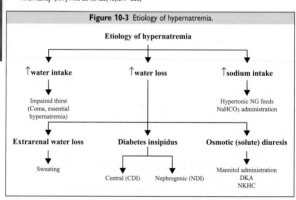

Figure 10-3 Etiology of hypernatremia.

DKA, diabetic ketoacidosis; NKHC, nonketotic hyperosmolar coma; NDI, nephrogenic diabetes insipidus.

- *Symptoms*—thirst, lethargy, mental status changes, coma/convulsions
  - Slowly developing hypernatremia is usually well tolerated
  - Acute severe hypernatremia → cellular dehydration → brain shrinkage → meningeal vessels tear → intracranial hemorrhage
- *Treatment*—restore normal osmolality & volume by correcting water deficit; water can be replaced PO (safest) or by IV infusion of free water or hypotonic crystalloids

$$\text{Free water deficit (L)} = [([Na^+] - 140)/140] \times \text{TBW (L)}$$

Lower plasma Na by 0.5 mEq/L/h; no more than 12 mEq/L/24 h (too rapid correction → acute brain swelling)
  - Central diabetes insipidus—treated with intranasal DDAVP
  - Nephrogenic diabetes insipidus—may be reversible if cause identified
  - Symptomatic polyuria—treated with Na restriction & thiazide diuretics

Hypokalemia (K <3.5 mEq/L)

Major Causes of Hypokalemia	
Mechanisms	**Causes**
Inadequate intake	Alcoholism, hyperaldosteronism, starvation, anorexia nervosa
Renal losses	Diuretics, chronic metabolic alkalosis, ↓ Mg^{2+}, renal tubular acidosis
GI losses	Vomiting, diarrhea, villous adenoma
ECF to ICF shift of K^+	β_2 agonists, insulin, acute alk, vit B_{12} therapy, lithium overdose

Source: From Kaye AD, Kucera IJ. Intravascular fluid & electrolyte physiology. In Miller RD, ed. *Miller's Anesthesia*. 6th ed. Philadelphia, PA: Elsevier; 2005.

- *Symptoms*—fatigue, muscle cramps, progressive weakness leading to paralysis; ↑ risk of arrhythmias; can enhance digitalis toxicity; cause hepatic encephalopathy
  - *ECG*—U waves, ventricular ectopy ± prolonged QT
  - Preop hypokalemia assocd. w/ adverse cardiac events (*JAMA* 1999;281(23):2203–2210)
- *Treatment*—IV K^+ (up to 40 mEq/L via peripheral IV; 100 mEq/L via central line) infusion at 20 mEq/h unless paralysis/ventricular arrhythmias present, treat underlying cause; avoid dextrose solutions (↑ insulin response → further ↓ K^+)

Hyperkalemia (K^+ >5.5 mEq/L)
- *Etiology* (see Table—Etiology of Hyperkalemia)

Etiology of Hyperkalemia	
Mechanisms	**Causes**
Pseudohyperkalemia	Sample lysis, marked leukocytosis, or megakaryocytosis
Altered internal K^+ balance	Acidosis, hypoaldosteronism, malignant hyperthermia
Altered external K^+ balance	Renal failure, drugs (ACEi, ARB, NSAIDs, K^+-sparing diuretics)
Miscellaneous iatrogenic	Succinylcholine-induced hyper K^+, ischemia–reperfusion

Source: From Kaye AD, Kucera IJ. Intravascular fluid & electrolyte physiology. In Miller RD, ed. *Miller's Anesthesia*. 6th ed. Philadelphia, PA: Elsevier; 2005.

- *Symptoms*—cardiac toxicity most serious
  - *ECG changes*—peaked T waves → prolonged PR interval & QRS duration → loss of P waves → widening of QRS complex → sine waves (merged QRS & T waves) → V fib/asystole
- *Treatment* (see Table—Treatment of Hyperkalemia)

Treatment of Hyperkalemia			
Intervention	**Dose**	**Onset**	**Comment**
Ca+ gluconate Ca+ chloride	1–2 amps IV	s to min	Stabilizes cell membrane Transient effect
Hyper-ventilation	↑ minute ventilation >3× baseline	s to min	Transient effect Drives K+ into cells
Insulin	Reg. insulin 10 U IV 1–2 amps D50W	15–30 min	Transient effect Drives K+ into cells
Bicarbonate (NaHCO₃)	1–3 amps IV	15–30 min	Transient effect Drives K+ into cells in exchange for H+

β_2 agonists	Albuterol 10–20 mg inh or 0.5 mg IV	30–90 min	Transient effect Drives K+ into cells
Kayexalate	30–90 g PO/PR	1–2 h	↓ total body K+ Exchanges Na+ for K+ in gut
Diuretics	Furosemide ≥40 mg IV	30 min	↓ total body K+
Hemodialysis	For renal failure/life-threatening ↑ K+		↓ total body K+

Source: Adapted from Sabatine MS. *Pocket Medicine*. 7th ed. Philadelphia, PA: Wolters Kluwer; 2020.

Hypocalcemia (Ca^{2+} <8.4 mg/dL)
- Ca^{2+} levels must be corrected for serum albumin conc (or use ionized calcium)

$$\text{Corrected } [Ca^{2+}] = [Ca^{2+}] + \{0.8 \times (4.0 - [\text{albumin}])\}$$

- *Etiology*—hypoparathyroidism, pseudohypoparathyroidism, hypomagnesemia, low vitamin D levels, hyperphosphatemia (seen in tumor lysis syndrome or rhabdomyolysis), presence of calcium chelating agents
  - Common OR causes: (1) Hyperventilation, (2) blood transfusion >1.5 mL/kg/min
- *Symptoms*—acute hypocalcemia → ↑ nerve/muscle excitability → paresthesia/tetany (Chvostek & Trousseau signs), laryngospasm, hypotension, & dysrhythmias
- *Treatment:* Treat hypomagnesemia (if present) first
  - Ca^{2+} gluconate infusion (2 g in 50–100 mL saline) over 10–15 min
    → Followed by calcium chloride or calcium gluconate infusion (0.5–1.5 mg/kg/h of **elemental** calcium)
  - 1 g of calcium gluconate = 93 mg elemental calcium; 1 g calcium chloride = 272 mg elemental calcium

Hypercalcemia (Ca^{2+} >10.3 mg/dL)
- *Etiology*—1° hyperparathyroidism, malignancy, vit D or A intoxication, immobilization, drugs (thiazides)
- *Symptoms*—mild to moderate hypercalcemia often asymptomatic; osteopenia with pathologic fractures, nephrolithiasis, GI, & neurologic symptoms (weakness, confusion, stupor, coma). *If weakness is present, use decreased doses of muscle relaxants.*

"stones, bones, abdominal groans and psychic overtones"

- *Treatment*—1st-line treatment = correction of hypovolemia with normal saline. May also use bisphosphonates, calcitonin & Ca^{2+} ↓ agents (mithramycin & steroids)

Hypomagnesemia (Mg^{2+} <1.3 mEq/L)
- *Etiology*—nutritional (inadequate intake, TPN, chronic alcoholism), ↑ renal excretion (hypercalcemia, osmotic diuresis, drugs (diuretics, aminoglycosides, amphotericin B); common in critically ill pts
- *Symptoms*—resp muscle weakness, arrhythmias (torsades de pointes)
- *Treatment:* 1–2 g of $MgSO_4$ in 15 min, followed by 24-h infusion (6 g in 1 L). Always monitor pts receiving IV magnesium for signs of acute hypermagnesemia, including respiratory depression & areflexia. Use ↓ doses for pts with renal insufficiency.
- *Pain*—magnesium supplementation assocd. with improved pain control (*Eur J Anaesthesiol* 2002;19(1): 52–56)

Hypermagnesemia (Mg^{2+} >2.5 mEq/L)
- *Etiology*—usually iatrogenic, seen during treatment of pre-eclampsia, pts taking Mg^{2+} containing antacids/laxatives; renal insufficiency ↑ risk
- *Symptoms*—abnl EKG (prolonged PR, ↑ QRS) (5–10 mEq/L), lower DTRs (10 mEq/L), lethargy, weakness, resp. failure (10–15 mEq/L), hypotension, brady, cardiac arrest (>20–25 mEq/L)
- *Treatment*—IV calcium (1–2 g calcium gluconate over 10 min); mech ventilation for resp failure; temporary pacing for significant bradyarrhythmias; dialysis may be required if renal insufficiency is present.

Hypophosphatemia (PO_4^{3-} 2.8 mg/dL)
- *Etiology*—malabsorption (vit D deficiency, chronic alcoholism), ↑ renal excretion (hyperparathyroidism, osmotic diuresis, postrenal transplant), transcellular shifts (insulin admin, resp alkalosis, malnutrition treatment)
- *Symptoms*—muscular abnl (weakness, impaired diaphragmatic fx, rhabdomyolysis), neurologic abnl (paresthesias, dysarthria, confusion, seizures, coma), hematologic abnl (hemolysis & platelet dysfx)
- *Treatment*—IV phosphate for severe/acute dz
  - Na- or K-phos 0.08–0.16 mmol/kg in 500 m: 0.45% saline over 6 h, serum phosphate, calcium & potassium monitored q8h, STOP IV repletion when oral therapy possible, MUST avoid hyperphosphatemia (can lead to hypocalcemia)

Hyperphosphatemia (PO₄³⁻ >4.5 mg/dL)

- *Etiology*—usu 2° to ↓ renal excretion (renal failure, hypoparathyroidism, bisphosphonate therapy), transcellular shifts (rhabdomyolysis, hemolysis, tumor lysis syndrome), & ↑ intake (vit D intoxication, phosphorus cathartics)
- *Symptoms*—attributable to hypocalcemia (see above) & metastatic calcification of soft tissues (when calcium–phosphorus product >70)
- *Treatment*—correct renal insufficiency, dialysis if in renal failure, phosphorus-binding antacids

TRANSFUSION THERAPY

Blood Typing Tests

- ABO incompatibility → most common reason for transfusion reactions (>99%)
- *ABO, Rh typing*
  - Rh-negative pts produce anti-Rh Ab's *only* after being exposed to Rh antigen
  - 0.2% chance of transfusion reaction after this test
- *T/S (type & screen)*
  - Recipient's plasma (may contain antibodies) + stock RBC soln (known antigen's) → watch for rxn (testing recipient for presence of Ab's)
  - 0.06% chance of transfusion reaction after this test
- *T/C (type & cross)*
  - Recipient's plasma (may contain antibodies) + donor RBCs → watch for agglutination (suggests incompatibility)
  - Can detect M, N, P, Lewis, Rh, Kell, Kidd, Duffy antibodies
  - 0.05% chance of transfusion reaction after this test

Emergency Transfusion

- Give **type-specific** or **type O** blood
- Rh-negative pts should receive anti-Rh globulin if given Rh-positive blood
- After 8–10 units type O whole blood, **do not** switch to type-specific blood (A, B, or AB): Hemolytic rxn possible (due to anti-A & anti-B Ab's in type O transfused blood)

Recipient's Blood			Reactions with Donor's RBCs			
ABO "Blood Type"	RBC Antigens	Plasma Antibodies	Donor is Type O	Donor is Type A	Donor is Type B	Donor is Type AB
O	—	Anti-A; Anti-B	C	I	I	I
A	A	Anti-B	C	C	I	I
B	B	Anti-A	C	I	C	I
AB	A&B	—	C	C	C	C

C, compatible; I, incompatible

COMMON BLOOD PRODUCTS

Red Blood Cells (RBC)

1 unit ≈ 300 mL: 180 mL RBC, 130 mL storage solution (Hct ~ 55%); ↑ pt's Hct 3%/unit
Indications (practice guidelines, few RCTs):
The American Society of Anesthesiology states that "red blood cell transfusion should not be in indicated by a single hemoglobin trigger, but instead should be based upon the pt's risks of developing complications of inadequate oxygenation" (*Anesthesiology* 1996;84(3):732).

- RBCs should be administered unit by unit with interval re-evaluation (*Anesthesiology* 2015;122:241–275).
- Pts without active bleeding or ongoing cardiac ischemia: Transfusion generally not required at hct's >21% (*The TRICC Study, NEJM* 1999;340:409–417)
- Restrictive transfusion strategies shown to be noninferior in terms of mortality to liberal strategies in septic shock and mod-high risk cardiac surgery pts (*TRISS Study, NEJM* 2014;371(15):1381–1391; *TRICS III Study, NEJM* 2017;377(22):2133–2144)

Packed Red Blood Cells (PRBC)

- PRBCs must be ABO & Rh-compatible
- Used to ↑ O₂-carrying capacity of blood
- 1 unit of PRBCs can ↑ hematocrit by 2–3%, Hct of PRBC is 55–60%
- *Leukocyte reduced* → to prevent nonhemolytic febrile transfusion rxns
  - Indicated for transplant pts
  - Prevention of CMV transmission (CMV resides in WBC)
  - Pts with Hx of nonfebrile hemolytic transfusion rxns

- *Washed* → removes plasma from RBC products to prevent allergic transfusion rxn mediated by recipient Ab's. Significantly alters the integrity of the RBCs.
  - Indicated for pts with IgA deficiency
  - Consider washing if previous severe allergic transfusion reactions despite no allergen/antigen identified
- *Irradiation* → to prevent transfusion associated graft vs. host dz, where transfused lymphocytes attack incompatible HLA of host tissue
  - Indicated for severely immunocompromised pts (not HIV), Premature infants <1,200 g, and stem cell/bone marrow transplant pts

Equation for Arterial O$_2$ Content in Blood

$$CaO_2 = (1.36 \times Hemoglobin \times SpO_2) + (PaO_2 \times 0.003)$$

Significance:
1. As hemoglobin drops, O$_2$ content drops
2. Hgb makes the largest contribution to O$_2$ content in blood
   → Transfusion may be of greater benefit than slight rise in PaO$_2$ for chronically hypoxemic pts

Calculating Allowable Blood Loss
Estimated allowable blood loss = EBV $\times$ (Hct$_{initial}$ − Hct$_{low}$)/Hct$_{initial}$
Estimated blood volume (EBV) = weight (kg) $\times$ average blood volume

Average Blood Volume	
Premature neonates	95 mL/kg
Full-term neonates	85 mL/kg
Infants	80 mL/kg
Adult men	75 mL/kg
Adult women	65 mL/kg

Estimating Blood Loss in Surgical Sponges	
Sponge Type	**Fluid Capacity**
4 × 4 sponge	10 mL
Ray-tech sponge	10–20 mL
Lap sponge	100 mL

Available Blood Components				
Component	**Content**	**Indications**	**Volume**	**Shelf Life**
RBCs Whole	RBCs and WBCs, platelet debris, plasma, fibrinogen	Red cell volume and plasma volume replacement	450 ± 50 mL	Heparin 48 h ADSOL 42 d ACD 21 d CPD 28 d CPDA–1 35 d
Packed RBCs	RBCs, WBCs, plasma, platelet debris	Red cell volume replacement	200 mL	Same as whole blood
Frozen RBCs	No plasma, minimal WBCs, & platelet debris	Red cell volume replacement in special circumstances	160–190 mL	Frozen: 3 y Thawed: 24 h
Platelets	Platelets, low WBCs, some plasma	Platelet count <50,000–100,000, clinical signs of dilutional thrombocytopenia, and/or platelet dysfunction	30–50 mL/unit	Pheresis: 24 h Room temperature: 5 d Frozen with DMSO: 3 y
Fresh frozen plasma	Plasma proteins, all coagulation factors	Bleeding from factor deficiencies, anti-thrombin III deficiency, massive transfusions, coumadin reversal	200–250 mL	Thawed: 6–24 h Frozen: 1 y

Cryo-precipitate	Factors VIII, XIII, fibrinogen, fibronectin, von Willebrand factor (vWF)	Hemophilia A, von Willebrand dz (vWD), fibrinogen deficiency	25 mL/unit	Thawed: 4–6 h Frozen: 1 y
Factor VIII concentrate	Factor VIII, fibrinogen, vWF	Hemophilia A (classic hemophilia)	Lyophilized (requires reconstitution)	2–8°C: 1 y Room temp: 3 mo
Factor IX concentrates (Konyne, Proplex)	Factor II, VII IX, X	Hemophilia B (Christmas dz)	Lyophilized (requires reconstitution)	2–8°C: 1 y Room temp: 1 mo
Albumin 25% (5%)	Albumin	Volume expansion, maintenance of intravascular oncotic pressure	250 or 500 mL, (50 mL)	3–5 y
Plasma protein fraction	Albumin, alpha globulin, beta globulin	Volume expansion, maintenance of intravascular oncotic pressure	250 mL	3–5 y

Source: From Ritter DF, Sarsnic MA. Transfusion therapy, part I. *Prog Anesthesiol* 1989;3:1–14.

Whole Blood
- Largely replaced by component therapy (more efficient use) outside of complex pediatric cardiac surgery & military hospitals in war zones *(J Trauma 2006;60(6):S59)*

Platelets
- A single 6 pack of platelets ≈ 300 mL; usually ↑ platelet count by ≈ 30,000
- Pooled & single-donor units have equal hemostatic effectiveness
- Stored at room temp for up to 5 d (↑ risk of bacterial infection after 5 d)
- Contains all plasma coagulation factors (except factors V & VIII → found in FFP)
- No need for ABO compatibility
  - Rh-negative women of childbearing age should receive Rh-negative platelets
- Contraindications: TTP/HUS & HIT

Suggested Platelet Transfusion Thresholds	
<10,000	Prophylaxis (based on studies in cancer pts; N Engl J Med 337(26):1870–1875)
<20,000	Any bleeding or preprocedure; pts with concurrent coagulation d/o/infection
<50,000	Major bleeding or during surgery; prior to CNS or major eye surgery; bleeding with trauma; pretracheal bleeding; after prolonged cardiopulmonary bypass
Give platelets for ITP with life-threatening bleeding from GI/GU tracts or from CNS; mucous membrane bleeding usually precedes fatal hemorrhage	

Platelet refractoriness:
- *Definition*—platelets ↑ <7,000/μL when measured 15–60 min after 2 separate platelet transfusions
- *Causes*—nonimmune (drugs, infection, splenomegaly), anti-HLA or antiplatelet Ab's
- *Treatment*—request ABO-matched platelets, check post-transfusion increment, check HLA percent reactive antibodies (**PRA**), perform HLA typing, & consult transfusion medicine; if diffuse mucosal bleeding → consider aminocaproic acid (Amicar)

Fresh Frozen Plasma (FFP)
- Contains all plasma coagulation factors (factor 8 diminished 40% with thawing)
- INR of FFP is ~1.6
- Duration of effect <7 h (half-life of factor VII ≈ 7 h)
- Transfusion of FFP is indicated in the setting of:
  - Correction of microvascular bleeding in the presence of INR >2.0
  - Massive transfusion (>1 blood volume in 24 h)
  - Urgent reversal of warfarin-induced anticoagulation (5–8 mL/kg)
- FFP must be ABO-compatible; volume expansion is *not* an appropriate use of FFP
- Higher risk of transfusion-related acute lung injury (TRALI) than RBC or platelets
- Contraindications: Known anaphylactoid reactions to plasma products (pts with anti-IgA antibodies)

Indications for FFP Transfusion	
INR >2.0	Prophylactic transfusion prior to invasive procedures or actively bleeding pts
INR 1.5–2.0	FFP *may* be of value in actively bleeding pts; uncertain benefit as pre-procedure prophylaxis; unlikely to correct INR value without massive no. of units of FFP *(Transfusion 2006;46:1279)*
INR <1.5	FFP *not* indicated

Cryoprecipitate
- Contains vWF, factor VIII, fibrinogen, factor XIII; usual dose = 8–10 units
- 6 bags (1 pool) of cryo raises Fibrinogen 45 mg/dL
- ABO compatibility *preferred*, not required
- *Indications:*
  - Hypofibrinogenemia (<80–100 mg/dL in presence of bleeding)
  - vWD (unresponsive to DDAVP)
- *Contraindications:* Pts with hypofibrinogenemia (<100 mg/dL) from generalized coagulopathies likely other deficits as well, should receive FFP instead

Factor VII (NovoSeven, eptacog alfa)
- Used in uncontrollable bleeding in surgical and hemophilia pts
- Initiates coagulation in only those sites where tissue factor (TF) is also present (TF is exposed to the blood in vessel injury)
- May ↑ risk of DVT, PE, MI
- May improve outcomes in acute intracerebral hemorrhage

DDAVP
- Release of endothelial stores of factor VIII and ↑VIII:vWF
- Useful in vWD (types 1 & 2a) and some cases of hemophilia A

4-Factor Prothrombin Complex Concentrates
- Contains Factors II, VII, IX, X, Protein C&S, Antithrombin III
- Becoming favored over FFP for reversal of warfarin and Factor Xa inhibitors *(Thromb Haemost 2016;116(5):879–890; Am J Hematol 2019;94(6):697–709)*

TRANSFUSION COMPLICATIONS

Complications of Massive Transfusion
- ↑ K^+, ↓ Ca^{2+} (citrate preservative binds Ca^{2+})
- Dilutional coagulopathy thrombocytopenia
- Metabolic alkalosis (due to citrate-forming HCO_3)
- Hypothermia

Transfusion Complications: Estimated Risk			
Noninfectious	**Risk (Per Unit)**	**Infectious**	**Risk (Per Unit)**
Febrile	1:100	CMV	Common
Allergic	1:100	Hepatitis B	1:220,000
Delayed hemolytic	1:1,000	Hepatitis C	1:1,600,000
Acute hemolytic	<1:100,000	HIV	1:1,800,000
Fatal hemolytic	<1:250,000	Bacteria (PRBCs)	1:500,000
TRALI	1:5,000	Bacteria (platelets)	1:12,000

Source: Goodnough LT, Brecher ME, Kanter MH, et al. *N Engl J Med* 1999;340:438; Busch MP, Kleinman SH, Nemo GJ. *JAMA* 2003;289:959–962.

Infectious Complications
- *Hepatitis B:* ≈ 35% of infected individuals demonstrate acute dz ≈ 1–10% become chronically infected
- *Hepatitis C:* Up to 85% of infected pts suffer chronic infection → 20% develop cirrhosis, 1–5% develop hepatocellular carcinoma
- *Bacterial infx:* Most common causes of transfusion-related deaths (1 in 2,000 platelet recipients gets an infection → 10–25% of these develop severe sepsis; mortality for transfusion-assoc sepsis ≈ 60%)
- *Other infx:* Viral (cytomegalovirus, West Nile virus), protozoan (malaria, toxoplasmosis), bacterial (Lyme), and prion (Creutzfeldt–Jakob) dz

Coagulopathic Complications

Typically seen in the setting of massive blood transfusions
- *Dilutional thrombocytopenia* → treat with platelets if microvascular bleeding occurs
- *Disseminated intravascular coagulation (DIC)* (see below)
- *Low factor V & VIII levels* → ↓ to 15% & 30% of normal values, respectively, in stored blood; contribute to inadequate hemostasis after massive transfusion; give FFP in the setting of bleeding with prolonged APTT & normal platelet count

Transfusion Reactions

- *Acute hemolytic transfusion reaction*
  - Due to ABO or major antigen incompatibility
  - Usually due to clerical errors, incidence of 1:250,000 transfusions
  - Symptoms—Chills, fever, chest, flank pain → often masked by anesthesia; may only see hypotension, unexplained bleeding, & hemoglobinuria

Treatment of a Suspected Hemolytic Transfusion Reaction

1. Stop transfusion
2. Treat hypotension with fluids and/or vasopressors
3. Maintain urine output (75–100 mL/h) with fluids, mannitol, & furosemide
4. Alkalinize urine (give 40–70 mEq bicarb per 70 kg body wt) to prevent precipitation
5. Send unused blood & fresh pt sample to blood bank (for re-cross match)
6. Send blood sample to lab for free Hb, haptoglobin, Coombs test, DIC screen
7. Consider corticosteroids

- *Nonhemolytic transfusion reactions*
  - Etiology—Usually febrile or allergic in nature; caused by antibodies against donor WBCs or plasma proteins
  - Signs—Fever, hives, tachycardia, & mild hypotension
  - Treatment—Rule out hemolytic transfusion rxn & bacterial contamination, symptomatic treatment/support
  - Prevention—Leukocyte-reduced PRBCs & washed PRBCs may ↓ incidence
- *Transfusion-Related Acute Lung Injury (TRALI)*
  - Noncardiogenic pulmonary edema occurring within 4 h of blood product *(most commonly with FFP administration)*
  - Mechanism—rxn between donor anti-HLA or antileukocyte Ab's & recipient leukocytes
  - Treatment—stop transfusion, supportive care
  - Outcomes—mortality ≈ 5–10%, most pts recover within 96 h
- *Transfusion-Associated Circulatory Overload (TACO)*
  - The circulatory system becomes overwhelmed with additional volume of blood products
  - Symptoms—tachycardia, HTN, dyspnea, or pulm. edema within 6 h of transfusion
  - Treatment—reduced transfusion rate, diuresis, oxygen

Metabolic Complications

- *Citrate intoxication*—uncommon unless blood transfused >150 mL/70 kg/min
  - Hypothermia, liver dz, liver transplantation, & hyperventilation ↑ risk
  - Monitor ionized calcium during rapid transfusions
  - Treat hypocalcemia with Ca gluconate (30 mg/kg) or Ca carbonate (10 mg/kg)
- *Hyperkalemia* unlikely at transfusion rates <120 mL/min
  - Rarely of clinical significance
  - Treat with calcium gluconate to stabilize the cardiac membranes, beta agonists, insulin along with glucose, and furosemide

Immune Complications—Transfusion-Related Immunomodulation (TRIM)

- Immune suppression, which may be reflected in beneficial effects (improved renal allograft survival postrenal transplant) or harmful effects (increased rate of oncologic recurrence)
- Mechanisms are unclear but may include clonal deletion of alloreactive lymphocytes, induction of anergy, and soluble HLA peptides directed against adaptive immunity
  (Blood Rev 2007;21:327–348)

Diagnosis and Management of Transfusion Reactions

Type	Notes	Symptoms	Cause	Treatment
Febrile nonhemolytic transfusion reaction	• Most common (1:200–500) • 15% will have a 2nd reaction	Fever (1°C above pretransfusion), chills ± mild dyspnea within 1–6 h after transfusion	RBCs: Class I HLA Ab against donor leukocytes Plts: Storage-dependent cytokines	• Stop transfusion and rule out hemolytic reaction, severe infection • Give antipyretics, IM *meperidine* in pts with chills and rigors • Use leuko-reduced blood products in the future
Simple allergic reaction	• 1:333–500	Hives ± itching	Transfused allergens in plasma cause mast cell degranulation	• Pause transfusion • If only hives ± itching, may continue same unit • Give antihistamines if pt symptomatic • Unlikely to recur in future, consider premedication with antihistamines and use washed cells if repeated reactions
Transfusion-related acute lung injury	• 1:5,000 • 1–6 h after onset of transfusion • CVP is normal • Looks like ARDS • Death ≈ 10%	Acute respiratory distress, hypoxemia, hypotension, fever, pulmonary edema	Donor antibodies agglutinate host neutrophils to cause lung injury	• Stop transfusion • ABCs, O₂, mechanical ventilation, diuresis, steroids • If recovers, not at increased risk for recurrent episodes following transfusions from other donors
Acute hemolytic transfusion reaction	• 1:15,000, fatal in 1:250,000 to 1:600,000 • Results in DIC, shock, acute renal failure	Fever, chills, N/V, pink plasma, flank pain, pink, red or pink urine, or any combination of the above symptoms	Destruction of donor RBC by preformed recipient Abs. Usually secondary to ABO incompatibility	• Stop transfusion, leave IV attached for treatment • Start NS at 100–200 mL/h • Lasix 40–80 mg IV initially, then titrate to UO >100 mL/h for 24 h • From other arm obtain direct antiglobulin test (will be positive), CBC, lytes, new blood bank sample • May require pressors; watch for hyperkalemia
Anaphylactic transfusion reaction	• 1:20,000–1:50,000 • Rapid onset	Rapid anaphylaxis including hypotension angioedema, respiratory distress	Due to presence of specific anti-IgA Abs in small subset of IgA deficient pts	• Immediately stop transfusion • ABCs, vasopressors may be necessary • Epinephrine 0.3 mL of 1:1,000 solution SQ • Methylprednisolone • Prevent by using IgA-deficient blood, ultra-washed or deglycerolized RBCs

	Incidence/Notes	Etiology	Signs/Symptoms	Management
Sepsis	• 1:500,000 for PRBCs • 1:12,000 for platelets	Due to bacterial contamination of product (longer storage increases risk)	High fevers, rigors, nausea without diarrhea, and hypotension	• Stop transfusion • Send bag, tubing, remaining product to blood transfusion service • Draw blood cultures • Start broad-spectrum antibiotics
Delayed hemolytic transfusion reaction	• 1:2,000 • Seen after multiple transfusions, transplantation, pregnancy • 2–10 d posttransfusion	Amnestic Ab response from re-exposure to foreign red cell Ag including Rh antigens	Slow drop, slight fever, ↑ in unconjugated bilirubin, spherocytes	• None in absence of brisk hemolysis • Inform pt and blood transfusion service so that future transfusions avoid implicated antigens
Posttransfusion purpura	• Uncommon • Mostly in multiparous women • 5–10 d after transfusion of platelet-containing products	Amnestic antibody response from re-exposure to PlA-1 antigen	Severe thrombocytopenia lasting d to wk	• Preferred therapy is IVIG in high doses 1.0 g/kg/d × 2 d • Only washed cells or PlA-l–negative cells in future in consultation with blood transfusion service
Transfusion-associated graft-versus-host dz (GVHD)	• Rare and almost always fatal • Occurs in pts with immunodeficiency or in cases of homozygous host and heterozygous donor • Develops 4 d to 1 mo after transfusion • Not induced by FFP, cryo, or deglycerolized red cells	Allogeneic attack of host tissue by activated donor lymphocytes Difference from post-BMT GVHD is high incidence of pancytopenia Most die from infection	Fever, rash (maculopapular), RUQ pain, >LFTs, diarrhea anorexia pancytopenia Dx: 1. Biopsy 2. HLA typing of circulating lymphocytes	• No real therapy • Majority of cases (>90%) are fatal • Anecdotal success with several agents (Br J Haematol 117(2):275) • Prevent by using irradiated products

COAGULATION

Disorders of Coagulation

Exposure of blood to damaged endothelium results in activation of platelets and simultaneous production of fibrin through the coagulation cascade.

Primary Hemostasis	Secondary Hemostasis
• Constriction of injured vessels • Exposure of subendothelial collagen • Adhesion & aggregation of blood platelets on damaged surface • Formation of 1° hemostatic plug	• Formation of thrombin catalyzed by surface of activated platelets • Formation of thrombin via activation of factor VII by tissue factor • Conversion of fibrinogen → fibrin catalyzed by thrombin • Formation of fibrin clot & its stabilization

Extrinsic versus intrinsic coagulation pathways:
- Accessory (intrinsic) pathway: Factors VIII, IX, XI, XII
- Extrinsic pathway: Factors III (tissue factor), VII
- Common pathway: Factors V, X, thrombin (2), fibrin (1)

Coagulation Studies

Thorough Hx = best tool to detect presence of a coagulation d/o
- *Prothrombin Time (PT)*—measure of extrinsic and common coag pathway (factors I, II, V, VII, X)
  - Sensitive to factor VII deficiency
  - International normalized ratio (INR) standardizes PT value for interlab comparison
  - Normal PT values ≈ 11.0–13.2 s
- *Partial Thromboplastin Time (PTT)*—test of intrinsic and common coag pathway (factors I, II, V, VIII, IX, X, XI, & XII)
  - Notably, will not detect deficiencies in factor VII or XIII
  - Elevated in pts on heparin & pts with other circulating anticoagulants (factor VII antibodies, lupus anticoagulant)
  - Normal PTT values ≈ 25–37 s
- *Activated clotting time (ACT)*—modified clotting time of blood, Normal ≈ 110–130 s
  - Accessory (intrinsic) pathway activated by adding kaolin or diatomaceous earth
  - Can be performed in OR (point-of-care test)
- *Bleeding time*—crude assay of platelet function; poorly reproducible, rarely used
- *Fibrinogen*—normal level ≈ 170–410 mg/dL
  - May be depleted in massive hemorrhage or DIC
  - An acute phase reactant; can be elevated following trauma or inflammation
  - Goal fibrinogen level >100 mg/dL for pts with severe bleeding/massive transfusion
- *Fibrin degradation products (FDP)*—made by action of plasmin on fibrinogen
  - ↑ In DIC, 1° fibrinolysis, & severe liver dz (due to impaired clearance)
  - Influence clotting by interfering with fibrin monomer polymerization & by impairing platelet function
- *D-dimer*—specific fragment produced when plasmin digests cross-linked fibrin
  - ↑ In DIC, pulmonary embolism & in the immediate postop period
- *Thromboelastogram (TEG)*
  - Viscoelastic assay measuring the viscosity of blood as it clots under physiologic conditions. Demonstrates when the clotting cascade begins, how quickly in proliferates, how firm the clot becomes, and how quickly it breaks down.
  - Trauma pts requiring MTP saw improved 28-d mortality when hemostatic resuscitation guided by TEG over conventional assays (*Ann Surg* 2016;263:1051–1059).

Screening Test Abnormalities in Inherited and Acquired Coagulopathies			
PT	PTT	Inherited	Acquired
↑	↔	Factor VII deficiency	Vit K deficiency; Liver dz; factor VII inhibitors
↔	↑	Hemophilia, vWD	Factor inhibitors; antiphospholipid Ab
↑	↑	Deficiency: Fibrinogen, factor II, factor V	DIC; liver dz; inhibition of fibrinogen, factor II, V, or X

Source: Adapted from Sabatine MS. *Pocket Medicine.* 7th ed. Philadelphia, PA: Wolters Kluwer; 2020.

Effects of Some Commonly Used Agents on Coagulation Parameters

Agent	Bleeding Time	PT	PTT	ACT	Time to Peak Effect	Time to Normal Hemostasis Posttherapy	Comments
Aspirin	↑↑↑	—	—	—	h	1 wk	Platelet function not accurately predicted by bleeding time
Other NSAIDs	↑↑↑	—	—	—	h	3–5 d	Platelet function not accurately predicted by bleeding time
Heparin, regular intravenous	↑	↑	↑↑↑	↑↑↑	min	4–6 h	Monitor activated clotting time or activated thromboplastin time
Heparin, regular subcutaneous	↑	↑	↑↑	↑↑	1 h	4–6 h	Activated thromboplastin time may remain normal: monitor anti-Xa activity
Heparin, low molecular weight subcutaneous	—	—	—/↑	—/↑	12 h	1–2 d	Activated thromboplastin time may remain normal: monitor anti-Xa activity
Thrombolytic agents	↑↑↑	↑	↑	—	min	1–2 d	Frequently administered along with intravenous heparin

↑, clinically insignificant increase; ↑↑, possibly clinically significant increase; ↑↑↑, clinically significant increase.

Characteristics of Common Anticoagulants

	Warfarin	Unfractionated Heparin	Low–Molecular-Weight Heparin	Direct Thrombin Inhibitors
No. of cascade targets	Many	Many	Few	Few
Activity specificity	Nonspecific	Nonspecific	Specific	Specific
No. of daily doses	1	2–3	1–2	1–2
Route	PO	IV, SC	SC	IV, PO, SC
Monitoring	INR	aPTT, plt count	Plt count, anti-Xa	aPTT, liver fx
Variability in response	High	High	Low	Low
Risk of HIT	None	2–5%	1–2%	None
Other notes	Inhibits factors II, VII, IX, X, protein C	Binds antithrombin III	Inhibits factor Xa	

Source: Adapted from Nutescu EA, Shapiro NL, Chevalier A, et al. Cleve Clin J Med 2005;72(suppl 1):S2–S6.

Properties and Antidotes for Anticoagulants & Fibrinolytics

Anticoag	$t_{1/2}$	Labs	Rx for overdose w/o serious bleeding*
UFH	60–90' RES	↑ PTT	Protamine IV 1 mg/100 U unfractionated heparin (UFH) (max 50 mg). For infusions, dose to reverse = 2× rate of UFH given per h
Bivalirudin	25', K	↑ PTT	Dialysis
Lepirudin	80', K	↑ PTT	Dialysis
Argatroban	45', L	↑ PTT	? Dialysis
Dabigatran	12–17', K	dTT/↑ PTT	Idarucizumab (Praxbind) or PCC if bleeding
Enoxaparin	8°, K	(anti-Xa)	? Protamine (reversal incomplete)
Fondaparinux	24°, K	(anti-Xa)	? Dialysis
Rivaroxaban	7–11°, K	(anti-Xa)	Andexanet alfa or PCC if serious bleeding
Apixaban	9–14°, L	(anti-Xa)	Andexanet alfa or PCC if serious bleeding
Warfarin	36°, L	↑ PT	*No bleeding:* INR >5: vit K 1–2.5 mg by mouth INR >10: vit K 2.5–5.0 mg by mouth *Bleeding:* Vit K 10 mg IV + FFP or PCC
Fibrinolytic	20–90' LK	↓ fbgn ↑ FDP	Cryoprecipitate, FFP, ± aminocaproic acid

*Initial step should be immediate d/c of anticoag. Decision to dialyze should take into account time for anticoag to be metabolized (noting renal/liver insufficiency) w/o dialysis versus. Potential sequelae of bleeding while waiting. K, kidney; L, liver; RES, reticuloendothelial system.

Platelet Inhibitors

Aspirin
- *Irreversibly* inactivates cyclooxygenase (COX) enzyme
- Suppresses prostaglandin & thromboxane production
- Effects of aspirin last for the lifespan of the platelets, 7–10 d

Ibuprofen
- NSAID that *reversibly* inhibits COX

Clopidogrel (Plavix), Prasugrel, Ticagrelor – P2Y 12 Antagonists
- Blockade of adenosine diphosphate (ADP) receptor on platelet cell membranes

Abciximab, Eptifibatide, Tirofiban
- Platelet aggregation inhibitors (inhibits glycoprotein IIb/IIIa)

Dipyridamole (Persantine)
- Inhibits platelet adhesion by preventing phosphodiesterase enzymes (PDE) from breaking down cAMP (cAMP blocks the platelet aggregation response to ADP)
- Vasodilating properties from inhibiting PDE

Bleeding Disorders (Coagulopathies)
- *Classic hemophilia (hemophilia A, factor VIII deficiency)*
  - X-linked recessive trait, 1:5,000 live male births
  - Prolonged PTT but normal PT & normal platelet function
  - Bleeding episodes related to level of factor VIII activity
    - <1% factor VIII activity: spontaneous bleeds
    - 1–5% factor VIII activity: bleeding after minor trauma
    - >5% factor VIII activity: infrequent bleeding
  - Treatment: Factor VIII replacement (cryo, lyophilized/recombinant factor VIII)
    - Activity levels of 20–40% recommended prior to surgery
    - Half-life of factor VIII ≈ 8–12 h
    - 20% of pts will eventually develop factor VIII antibodies
  - High incidence of hepatitis & HIV (given exposure to blood products)
- *Christmas dz (hemophilia B, factor IX deficiency)*
  - Sex-linked, occurring almost exclusively in males, incidence 1:100,000
  - Presentation similar to hemophilia A
  - Treatment: Factor IX concentrates, rFVIIIa, or FFP
  - For surgical hemostasis → factor IX activity levels of 50–80% required
  - Half-life of factor IX ≈ 24 h
- *vWD*
  - Abnormalities of vWF
    - Glycoprotein produced by megakaryocytes & endothelial cells
    - vWF stabilizes factor VIII & forms cross-links between platelets & endothelial cells

- vWD classification:
  - As type 1 (classic), type 2 (variant), & type 3 (severe)
  - Type 1 vWD = most common, accounts for 75% of cases. Autosomal dominant inherited. Decreased levels vWF
  - Type 2 vWD = 25% of cases. Typically quality defects of vWF
  - Type 3 vWD = complete deficiency of vWF
- Most common inherited bleeding d/o, prevalence = 1%
- Pts present with variable bleeding tendency; epistaxis often presenting feature
- Most common laboratory finding = prolonged bleeding time
- Treatment—Desmopressin (0.2 mcg/kg in 50 mL saline over 30 min) or cryoprecipitate; desmopressin has half-life ≈ 8–12 h

Hyperfibrinolysis
- Markedly enhanced fibrinolytic activity (trauma, surgery, liver dz)
- Diagnosis: TEG (preferred), D-Dimer, fibrinogen-split products
- Treatment: Lysine analogues (tranexamic acid [TXA], aminocaproic acid)
- TXA has been shown to safely reduce mortality and transfusions in many bleeding populations, especially if given early. (MATTERs, CRASH-2, WOMAN trials)

Heparin-Induced Thrombocytopenia (HIT)

Overview of Heparin-Induced Thrombocytopenia		
Feature	Type I	Type II
Mechanism	Direct effect of heparin	Immune (Ab) mediated
Incidence	20%	1–3%
Onset	After 1–4 d of heparin	After 4–10 d; can occur early (<24 h) if prior exposure in last 100 d; can occur after heparin is stopped
Platelet nadir	>100,000/μL	30–70,000/μL or 50% ↓ from baseline
Sequelae	None	Thrombotic events (HITT) in 30–50%
Management	Continue heparin; observe	**Stop heparin;** start alternative anticoagulation therapy

Source: Adapted from Sabatine MS. *Pocket Medicine.* 7th ed. Philadelphia, PA: Wolters Kluwer; 2020.

- Type II HIT = immune-mediated thrombocytopenia triggered by IgG antibodies against heparin platelet factor 4 (PF4) complexes (PF4 antibodies)
- Bound antibody → stimulates platelet activation → thrombocytopenia, platelet aggregation, & thrombosis
- Many pts develop the antibody but not the clinical syndrome
  - 50% of cardiac surgery pts exposed to heparin developed PF 4 Ab's, 1% got HIT
- Risk *reduced* with use of low–molecular-weight heparin
- Risk *eliminated* with use of fondaparinux or direct thrombin inhibitors
- Type II HIT treatment:
  - Stop all heparin exposure, including heparin flushes
  - Start alternative anticoagulation with direct thrombin inhibitors
    - Argatroban (1–2 mcg/kg/min), Lepirudin (0.4 mg/kg bolus, then 0.15 mg/kg/hr)
  - Oral anticoagulation: Do not start until platelet count is >100,000/μL
    - Warfarin should overlap direct thrombin inhibitors (as warfarin reduces protein C levels before prothrombin, causing transient hypercoagulable state)
    - Optimal duration of therapy unknown, consider >6 wk

Disseminated Intravascular Coagulation (DIC)
DIC: Consequence of abnormal, diffuse activation of the coagulation, & fibrinolytic systems

Causes of DIC	
Acute	Chronic
- Sepsis, ARDS	- Malignancy
- Shock	- Liver dz
- Trauma	- Retained dead fetus
- Obstetric (e.g., amniotic fluid embolism)	- Intra-aortic balloon pump
- Hemolytic transfusion reaction	- Peritoneovenous shunt
- Extensive burns	- Aortic dissection/aneurysm

- *Pathogenesis*
  - Excessive deposition of fibrin throughout microvasculature & consumption of coagulation factors and widespread platelet activation & fibrinolysis
- *Clinical features*
  - Petechiae, ecchymoses, oozing from surgical or IV sites
  - Diffuse thrombosis → life-threatening ischemia of vital organs
- *Laboratory features*
  - Elevated D-dimers, PT, & PTT levels
  - Serial measurements reveal a falling fibrinogen level & platelet count
  - FDPs elevated (but nonspecific)
  - Peripheral blood smears → schistocytes (from microvascular RBC trauma)
- *Treatment*
  - Recognition & treatment of underlying cause of DIC
  - FFP or cryoprecipitate to keep fibrinogen >50 mg/dL & replace clotting factors
  - Platelets should be kept >25,000–50,000/μL
  - Consider heparin for pts with predominantly thrombotic DIC
  - Inhibitors of fibrinolysis (aminocaproic acid, aprotinin) **NOT** recommended

Vitamin K Deficiency
- Vitamin K is needed by the liver to make prothrombin (factor II); factors VII, IX, X; protein C; protein S. Deficiency can lead to coagulopathy and ↑ PT/INR
- Treatment: Vitamin K 2.5–10 mg SC/IM/PO or 1–10 mg IV at ≤1 mg/min
- **Sickle Cell dz** (also see Chapter 32, Chronic Pain Management)
- Abnl hemoglobin (HbS) results in sickling → chronic hemolysis, vaso-occlusive crises
- End-organ effects: Renal & pulm infarction, liver cirrhosis, CVAs, bone ischemia

Perioperative Management of Sickle Cell Disease
• Ensure adequate hydration
• Avoid factors that cause sickling (hypoxia, hypothermia, dehydration, acidosis, polycythemia, infection)
• Consider preop simple transfusion to HCT ≈ 30%
• Consider exchange transfusion to keep HbS <40% (can also ↓ blood viscosity)

JONATHAN P. WANDERER

HYPOXIA

Unexplained oxygen desaturation

Actions (Fig. 11-1)
- Call for help and a code cart
  - Ask: "Who will be the crisis manager?"
- Turn FiO_2 to 100% at high gas flows
  - Confirm inspired $FiO_2 = 100\%$ on gas analyzer
  - Confirm the presence of end-tidal CO_2 and changes in capnogram morphology
- Hand-ventilate to assess compliance
  - Listen to breath sounds
- Check:
  - Blood pressure, PIP, pulse
  - ET tube position
  - Pulse oximeter placement
  - Circuit integrity: Look for disconnection, kinks, holes
- Consider actions to assess possible breathing issue:
  - Draw blood gas
  - Suction (to clear secretions, mucus plug)
  - Remove circuit and use ambu-bag
  - Bronchoscopy
- Consider causes:
  - Is airway/breathing issue suspected?
- NO airway issue suspected
  - Circulation
    - Embolism
      - Pulmonary embolus
      - Air embolism—venous
      - Other emboli (fat, septic, CO_2, amniotic fluid)
    - Heart dz
      - Congestive heart failure
      - Coronary heart dz
      - Myocardial ischemia
      - Cardiac tamponade
      - Congenital/anatomical defect
        - Severe sepsis
        - If hypoxia associated with hypotension
    - Drugs/allergy
      - Recent drugs given
      - Dose error/allergy/anaphylaxis
      - Dyes and abnormal hemoglobin (e.g., methemoglobinemia, methylene blue)
  - YES airway issue suspected
    - Aspiration
    - Atelectasis
    - Bronchospasm
    - Hypoventilation
    - Obesity/positioning
    - Pneumothorax
    - Pulmonary edema
    - Right mainstem intubation
    - Ventilator settings, leading to auto-PEEP

Additional Diagnostic Tests
- Fiberoptic bronchoscope
- Chest x-ray
- Electrocardiogram
- Transesophageal echocardiogram

INTRAOP 11-1

BRONCHOSPASM

Causes
- Pre-existing reactive airway dz (asthma)
- Manipulation of upper airway (oral endoscopy)
- ETT with inadequate anesthesia
- ETT causing carinal or bronchial stimulation (endobronchial intubation)
- Excessive histamine release (morphine, atracurium) or β-blockade
- Anaphylaxis
- Pulmonary edema

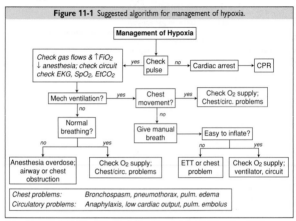

Figure 11-1 Suggested algorithm for management of hypoxia.

(Adapted from Murphy PG, Fale A. *A Pocket Reference to Anaesthesia*, 2nd ed., Science Press; 2002.)

Investigations
- Examine ETT for patency (secretions, kinks) & proper position
- Examine for wheezing, air movement
- Capnograph → shows expiratory upsloping
- High-peak airway pressures, hypoxia, & hypercarbia
- **Rule out:** Pneumothorax, pulmonary embolism, & pulmonary edema

Management
- ↑ FiO_2
- ↑ Anesthetic depth (inhalational agents are bronchodilators)
- ↑ Expiratory time, ↓ RR as this helps ↓ gas trapping
- Give nebulized albuterol via ETT (not effective in severe bronchospasm/lost airway)
- Epinephrine IV/SC (esp for anaphylaxis) → titrate to effect
- Aminophylline (2nd-line treatment—6 mg/kg bolus, then 0.5 mg/kg/h)
- Hydrocortisone (long term)

HYPOTENSION

MAP <60 mmHg or 20–25% reduction from baseline

Differential Diagnosis
- Decreased preload
  - ↓ Blood volume (hemorrhage, inadequate fluid replacement, 3rd spacing)
  - ↓ Venous return (change in pt position, i.e., Trendelenburg)
  - Pericardial tamponade, pneumothorax, surgical compression of venous structures, pneumoperitoneum from laparoscopy, excessive PEEP
- Decreased afterload
  - Sepsis, vasodilating drugs (anesthetics), anaphylactic reaction, neurologic injury
- Decreased contractility
  - MI, arrhythmias, CHF, anesthetic effect, electrolyte imbalances

Investigations
- Examine BP cuff for fit
- Examine preoperative BP trends
- Calculate fluid balance (including blood loss)
- Ensure that the IV site is intact & not infiltrated
- Examine arterial line waveform for respiratory variation

Treatment Options
- Administer fluid bolus
- ↓ Anesthetic agents
- Administer vasopressors (phenylephrine 40–100 mcg/ephedrine 5–10 mg)
- Administer other vasoactives/inotropes (norepinephrine, dobutamine, milrinone, dopamine)
- Consider invasive monitoring (CVP, arterial line, PA catheter, echocardiogram)

HYPERTENSION

BP >140/90 mmHg or MAP >20–25% baseline value

Differential Diagnosis
- Primary HTN
  - HTN with no known cause (70–95% of hypertension)
- Secondary HTN
  - Pain/surgical stimuli (inadequate anesthesia, tourniquet pain), ETT stimulation, bladder distention
  - Hypercarbia, hypoxia, hypervolemia, hyperthermia
  - Intracranial pathology (↑ ICP, herniation, hemorrhage)
  - Endocrine problems (pheochromocytoma, Cushing syndrome, hyperthyroidism, hyperparathyroidism)
  - Alcohol withdrawal
  - Malignant hyperthermia
  - Inadvertent vasoactive drug administration
  - Antihypertensive medication withdrawal
- Consider timing of HTN with case events:
  → HTN prior to induction
- Withdrawal from antihypertensive medications, essential hypertension, pain
  → HTN postinduction
- Laryngoscopy effect, improper ETT placement, hypercarbia from esophageal intubation, misplacement of gastrostomy tube into trachea, pain, hypoxia
  → HTN during the case
- Inadequate pain control, hypercarbia, pneumoperitoneum, fluid overload, drugs (vasopressors), bladder distention, tourniquet pain

Investigations/Treatment Options
- Examine BP cuff size & placement, arterial line waveform
- Review anesthetic/surgical events of the case
- Check for hypoxia/hypercarbia
- Check vaporizer agent level
- Administer antihypertensives (β-blockers/vasodilators)

HYPERCARBIA

↑ CO_2 levels (as measured by blood gas or end-tidal gas analysis) (normal values 38–42 mmHg)

Differential Diagnosis
- ↑ CO_2 production
  - Malignant hyperthermia
  - Sepsis
  - Fever/shivering
  - Thyrotoxicosis
- ↓ CO_2 elimination
  - Reduced minute ventilation
    Altered lung mechanics (atelectasis, pneumoperitoneum with CO_2, surgical retractors preventing lung expansion)
    Airway obstruction (secretions, mucous plugging)
    Inadequate ventilator settings (↓ volumes, ↓ fresh gas flows)
    Oversedation

- Increased dead space
  ETT malfunction (kinks, endobronchial intubation)
  Exhausted CO_2 absorber
- Drug effects (muscle relaxants/narcotics/benzodiazepines)
- Consider timing of $\uparrow CO_2$ with case events:
  $\rightarrow \uparrow CO_2$ at the start of a case
- Improper ETT placement, inadequate ventilator settings, oversedation of spontaneously breathing pt
  $\rightarrow \uparrow CO_2$ postinduction/during case
- MH, neuroleptic malignant syndrome (NMS), improper vent settings, thyrotoxicosis, release of tourniquet, exhausted CO_2 absorber
  $\rightarrow \uparrow CO_2$ during emergence
- Inadequate reversal of muscle relaxants, residual narcotic/anesthetic effects, neurologic causes, electrolyte disturbances, hypoglycemia

Investigations/Treatment Options
- Examine pulse oximeter
- Ensure appropriate ventilator settings
- Examine CO_2 absorber for exhaustion
- Consider ABG
- If spontaneously breathing: Assist breathing, lighten sedation
- If mechanically ventilated: $\uparrow$ Minute ventilation

HYPOCARBIA

$\downarrow CO_2$ levels (as measured by blood gas or end-tidal gas analysis)

Differential Diagnosis
- Hyperventilation
- $\downarrow$ Metabolic rate (hypothermia, hypothyroidism)
- Pulmonary embolism
- Air embolus
- Cardiac arrest (hypoperfusion)
- ETT dislodgement/circuit disconnect

Investigations/Treatment Options
- Check breathing circuit
- Check blood pressure, heart rate, SpO_2
- Check/modify ventilator settings
- Treat underlying cause

$\uparrow$ PEAK AIRWAY PRESSURES

Differential Diagnosis
- Circuit problem (stuck valve, PEEP valve on wrong, kinked hose)
- ETT problem (kinked/bitten, plugged with mucus, bad positioning)
- Drug induced (opiate chest wall rigidity, inadequate paralysis/anesthesia, MH)
- $\downarrow$ Pulmonary compliance (asthma, insufflation, pneumothorax, aspiration)

Treatment
- Check tubes, hand ventilate, 100% FiO_2
- Listen to lungs, suction ETT, add bite block, consider paralysis

---

OLIGURIA

Urine production <0.5 mL/kg/h (also see Chapter 25, Renal System and Anesthesia for Urologic Surgery)

Differential Diagnosis
- Prerenal: Intravascular fluid depletion
- Renal origin: Lack of renal perfusion (hypotension, cross clamping, renal artery stenosis), intrinsic renal damage (nephrotoxic drugs/vasculitis)
- Postrenal: Ureteral obstruction/disruption, obstruction of Foley catheter

Investigations/Treatment Options
- Examine vital sign monitors to establish hemodynamic stability
- Examine/irrigate Foley catheter for obstruction/improper placement
- Review possible nephrotoxic drugs & withdraw
- Examine fluid administration/blood loss/surgical manipulation

- Consider fluid challenge to treat prerenal oliguria
- Treat underlying cause

MYOCARDIAL ISCHEMIA/INFARCTION

Damage to heart muscle from imbalance between myocardial O_2 supply & demand

Etiology
- Atherosclerosis (accounts for 90% of MIs)
- Coronary aneurysms
- Coronary artery spasm
- O_2 demand outweighs supply (e.g., aortic stenosis)
- Blood viscosity changes (polycythemia)
- Embolic sources (endocarditic vegetations)

Investigations
- Lead II—best for arrhythmia detection (RCA association & nodal system)
- Lead V5—best for ischemia detection (LAD & anterior/lateral areas of heart)
- Both lead II & V5 will detect >90% of ischemic events
- ST-segment depression ≥0.1 mV (usually subendocardial pattern → due to partially obstructed coronary)
- ST-segment elevation ≥0.2 mV (usually transmural pattern → due to thrombosed coronary)
- T-wave inversions & Q-waves
- Dysrhythmias
- Hypotension
- TEE (most sensitive method for determining early ischemia)
- CK, CK-MB, troponins, cardiac consult (for possible coronary intervention)

Treatment Options
Goal: Maintain acceptable balance of myocardial O_2 supply & demand (Note: If ↑ afterload, preload, contractility, & heart rate → ↑ myocardial O_2 demand)
- Maintain BP within 20% of preoperative levels
- Confirm correct placement of ECG leads, consider 5- or 12-lead ECG
- Notify surgeon of ischemia & coordinate completion of surgical procedure
- Place pt on 100% FiO_2 & ensure adequate ventilation
- Consider reducing anesthetic agents
- Consider β-blocker administration if tachycardic
- Evaluate BP stability & consider invasive monitoring (arterial line/CVP/PA)
- If hypotensive with ischemic ECG changes ↑ BP with pressors to ↑ myocardial perfusion pressure
- Consider fluid therapy & inotropic agents to support myocardial contractility
- Consider anticoagulation (aspirin, heparin)
- Obtain intraoperative cardiology consult to coordinate care

---

MALIGNANT HYPERTHERMIA

In the presence of triggering agent: Unexpected, unexplained ↑ in end-tidal CO_2, unexplained tachycardia/tachypnea, prolonged masseter muscle spasm after succinylcholine. Hyperthermia is a late sign.

See Appendix C.

BRADYCARDIA

Heart rate <60 bpm

Differential Diagnosis
- Altered impulse formation (↑ vagal tone or ↓ SA node automaticity)
- Pharmacologic agents (β-blockers, Ca-channel blockers, cholinergics, narcotics, anticholinesterases, α_2-agonists)
- Pathologic causes (hypothermia, hypothyroidism, sick sinus syndrome, hypoxemia)
- Myocardial ischemia
- Surgical/anesthesia stimuli (traction on eye, neuraxial anesthesia, laryngoscopy)
- Reflex bradycardia

Investigations/Treatment
- Confirm correct ECG lead placement
- Check vital signs for hemodynamic stability
  → If stable, consider anticholinergics/ephedrine

→ If unstable, ↑ FiO₂ to 100%, abort anesthetic, administer epinephrine/atropine/ CPR, consider placement of pacing device
- Treat underlying cause

TACHYCARDIA

Heart rate >100 bpm

Differential Diagnosis

Tachycardia + Hypertension
- Pain/light anesthesia/anxiety
- Hypovolemia, hypercapnia, hypoxia, acidosis
- Drugs: Vagolytic drugs (pancuronium, meperidine), ketamine, ephedrine, epinephrine, anticholinergic drugs (atropine/glycopyrrolate), desflurane, isoflurane, β-agonists, vasodilators → reflexive tachycardia (hydralazine), caffeine
- Electrolyte abnormalities: Hypomagnesemia, hypokalemia, hypoglycemia
- Myocardial ischemia
- Endocrine abnormalities: Pheochromocytoma, hyperthyroidism, carcinoid, adrenal crisis
- Bladder distension

Tachycardia + Hypotension
- Anemia
- Congestive heart failure
- Valvular heart dz
- Pneumothorax
- Immune-mediated problems (anaphylaxis, transfusion reactions)
- Myocardial ischemia
- Sepsis
- Pulmonary embolism

Treatment Options
- Ensure adequate oxygenation and ventilation
- Verify ECG leads' placement
- Assess BP & prepare to treat depending on scenario
- Consider arterial line placement
- Assess volume status if hypotension exists and treat accordingly
- Assess depth of anesthesia
- Treat underlying cause

DELAYED EMERGENCE

Differential Diagnosis
- Residual drug effects (volatile agents, narcotics, muscle relaxants)
- Neurologic complications (seizure with postictal state, CVA, infection, tumor effect)
- Metabolic (electrolyte abnormalities, hypoglycemia, hyperglycemia, adrenal failure)
- Respiratory failure (due to hypercarbia/hypoxia)
- Cardiovascular collapse
- Hypothermia
- Sepsis

Investigations/Treatment Options
- Check for residual neuromuscular paralysis with train-of-four monitor and ensure that muscle relaxants have been reversed
- Ensure hypoxia & hypercarbia do not exist (check arterial blood gas)
- Check glucose/electrolytes & replace accordingly (rule out hypoglycemia and hypo/ hypernatremia)
- Consider narcotic reversal with Naloxone 40 mcg IV and repeat every 2 min up to 0.2 mg
- Consider benzodiazepine reversal with Flumazenil 0.2 mg IV every 1 min up to 1 mg
- Check for hypothermia and warm if body temperature is <34°C
- Consider neurologic imaging if neurologic examination warrants
- Supportive care

ANAPHYLAXIS

Severe type 1 hypersensitivity allergic reaction (IgE) with degranulation of mast cells/ basophils

Differential Diagnosis
- Anaphylactoid—not IgE-mediated, no prior sensitization to antigen required
- Vasovagal reactions generalized urticaria/angioedema, asthma exacerbations
- Myocardial infarction, stroke

Clinical Manifestations
- Cardiovascular collapse, tachycardia, dysrhythmias
- Bronchospasm, pulmonary & laryngeal edema, hypoxemia
- Rash, skin flushing, peripheral/facial edema

Treatment Options
- Remove stimulus (if known)
- Oxygen, consider intubation
- Give volume if hypotensive
- Hydrocortisone 250 mg to 1.0 g IV or methylprednisolone 1–2 mg/kg IV
- For rapidly decompensating situations give epinephrine 20–100 mcg IV bolus followed by infusion if necessary (can give 0.5–1.0 mg IV for cardiovascular collapse)
- Diphenhydramine 50 mg IV/ranitidine 50 mg IV
- Norepinephrine 4–8 mcg/min
- Sodium bicarbonate 0.5–1 mEq/kg for persistent acidosis
- Consider intubation (if pt not intubated)
- Evaluate airway for edema prior to extubation

Prevention
- Premedicate with diphenhydramine (H_1-blocker), ranitidine (H_2-blocker), prednisone

---

LATEX ALLERGY

Incidence/Risk Factors
- Pts with spina bifida & congenital genitourinary abnormalities
- Health care workers (housekeepers, lab workers, dentists, nurses, physicians)
- Rubber industry workers
- Atopic pts (asthma, rhinitis, eczema)
- Pts who have undergone multiple procedures

Mechanism
- IgE-mediated immune response

Preoperative Evaluation
- No routine diagnostic testing indicated (RAST & skin tests used occasionally)

Equipment/Drug Considerations
- Routine preop administration of H_1- & H_2-blockers **not** usually recommended

Anesthetic Considerations
- Avoid products that may contain latex (*gloves, tourniquets, blood pressure cuffs, face masks, ETT tubes, PA catheters, IV tubing with latex injection ports, rubber stoppers in medication vials*)
- Notify entire OR team (nurses, surgeon) & place large sign on OR door

Treatment
- Latex reaction may present as anaphylaxis (>20 min after exposure)
- Symptoms include hypotension, bronchospasm, rash
- Treatment similar to anaphylaxis treatment (see above) (*remove offending agent, give 100% O_2, fluid resuscitation, epinephrine, corticosteroids, diphenhydramine, aminophylline*)

GASTRIC ACID ASPIRATION OR VOMITING UPON INDUCTION OF ANESTHESIA

- Can cause chemical pneumonitis

Clinical Manifestations
- Early signs: Coughing, shortness of breath, wheezing, hypoxia, & cyanosis
- Late signs: Fever, metabolic acidosis, RML, & RLL infiltrate on CXR

Management
- If possible, place pt in head-down position
- Turn the pt's head to the side if actively vomiting while unconscious and aggressively suction
- Administer 100% O_2
- Consider placement of a suction catheter into the trachea to remove large particulate matter

- Perform rigid bronchoscopy (but no lavage)
- Obtain chest x-ray
- Antibiotics (staph, pseudomonas coverage) & steroids generally not recommended

COMPLICATIONS OF LARYNGOSCOPY AND INTUBATION

Causes
- Inexperienced use of laryngoscope
- Difficulty in placing ETT
- Poor existing dentition

General Complications
- Physiologic stimulation, hypercarbia, hypoxia, dental damage (#1 cause of malpractice claims)
- Airway trauma, vocal cord paralysis, arytenoid dislocation, ulceration/edema of glottic mucosa
- Tube malfunction and/or malposition

Specific Complications
- Postintubation croup in children secondary to tracheal/laryngeal edema
- Recurrent laryngeal nerve damage from ETT cuff compression → vocal cord paralysis
- Laryngospasm from stimulation of superior laryngeal nerve
- Involuntary/uncontrolled muscular contraction of laryngeal cords
- Caused by pharyngeal secretions or direct stimulation of ETT during extubation
- Treatment: (1) Gentle positive pressure ventilation, (2) succinylcholine (0.25–1 mg/kg to relax laryngeal muscles)
- Negative-pressure pulmonary edema
- Can occur during strong inspiratory effort caused by large negative intrathoracic pressure gradient against closed vocal cords
- Prevention: Place bite block prior to emergence
- Treatment: Maintain airway, provide O_2, consider PEEP/reintubation

JESSE M. EHRENFELD

PERIPHERAL VENOUS ACCESS

Indications
- IV administration of drugs & fluids

Technique
- Apply tourniquet to extremity (proximal to access site)
  - Alternatively can use BP cuff—inflate between systolic & diastolic pressures
- Choice of vein
  - Straight vein, ideally at a bifurcation
  - Antecubital veins provide better flow than peripheral veins
    - Irritating drugs (e.g., propofol) are less painful on injection
    - Flow may become interrupted if arm is flexed (positional/emergence)
    - Accidental brachial artery puncture possible due to close proximity
  - Cannulation attempts should be from distal to proximal veins
    - Avoid infiltrate from previous attempt at proximal site
- Skin disinfection: Alcohol (enhances visibility of vein due to vasodilating effect)
- Local anesthesia: Skin infiltration with lidocaine, local anesthetic cream/tape for kids
- Vein fixation: Apply tension on skin with your nondominant hand
- Vein puncture: 20–30° angle to penetrate skin, 0–10° angle to advance catheter
- Flash in IV chamber signals needle tip in vessel (will occur before catheter is in vein)
  - Advance entire device 2–3 mm, then advance plastic catheter alone into vessel
- Remove & secure disposal of metal needle
- Fix plastic catheter with clear adhesive tape on access site, date, & time IV
- Assess catheter position by fluid challenge to test for potential infiltration

Complications
- Fluid/drug infiltration (signs include swelling, paresthesia, or pain)
  - Immediately disconnect IV line
  - Evaluate for possible tissue necrosis/compartment syndrome
- Intra-arterial injection
  - Immediately disconnect IV line
  - Goal: Enhance vasodilation & prevent vasoconstriction
    - Inject 10 mL saline 0.9%, 10 mL lidocaine 1% with 5,000 units heparin
    - Consider stellate ganglion block, use of arterial vasodilators (Ca^{2+} channel blockers)

RAPID INFUSION CATHETER (RIC LINE)

Indications
- Rapid infusion of blood and IV fluids

Technique
- Insert a 20 g or 18 g (preferred) standard IV cannula (usu. in the antecubital fossa)
- Insert RIC guidewire through the IV cannula
- Remove IV cannula, dilate and insert RIC line using the Seldinger technique

ARTERIAL ACCESS (ALSO SEE CHAPTER 8, ON PERIOPERATIVE MONITORING)

Indications
- Need for continuous BP monitoring
- Surgery on pts with significant comorbidities (ASA III–V)
- Procedures with significant blood loss
- Need for frequent arterial blood gas samples

Technique: Radial Artery
- Allen test to assess collateral flow of ulnar artery is unreliable
- Choose nondominant pt hand unless surgical contraindication
- Fixate hand on wrist board
- Skin disinfection: Alcohol or chlorhexidine
- Pulse localization: Palpate (1–2 cm from wrist between bony head of radius & flexor carpi radialis tendon); can also use ultrasound to localize artery
- Local anesthesia: Infiltrate with lidocaine medial & lateral to the artery
- Artery fixation: Apply tension on the skin toward the periphery

- Arterial puncture: 30–45° angle to penetrate skin (Fig. 12-1)
- Flash in chamber signals intra-arterial location of needle tip
  - Transfixation technique:
    - Advance entire needle 2–3 mm further
    - Remove & secure needle for disposal
    - Slowly withdraw plastic catheter maintaining a shallow angle to skin until pulsatile flow occurs
    - Insert guidewire and advance catheter over-the-wire (Seldinger technique)
  - Over-the-needle technique:
    - Advance catheter by itself once flash is obtained
    - Remove & secure needle for disposal
- Fix plastic catheter with clear adhesive tape on access site
- Assess arterial flow by connection to transducer
- Note: If cannulation attempt unsuccessful, **do not** attempt ipsilateral ulnar artery cannulation; instead, find alternative extremity (risk of hand necrosis)

Technique: Brachial Artery
- Palpate brachial artery at ventral side of upper arm between biceps & triceps (close to antecubital fossa)
- Perform the same cannulation technique described for radial artery above
- Complications include ischemia of upper extremity, brachial plexus injury

Technique: Axillary Artery
- Palpate axillary artery in the groove between biceps & triceps lateral to pectoralis minor
- Perform the same cannulation technique described for radial artery above
- Complications include ischemia of upper extremity, brachial plexus injury

Contraindications
- Local infection
- Diminished peripheral blood flow
- Insufficient collateral blood flow

Complications
- Bleeding, blood clot, arterial spasm or laceration, peripheral ischemia, or hand necrosis

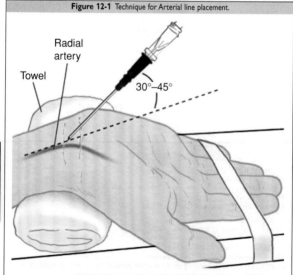

Figure 12-1 Technique for Arterial line placement.

Radial artery

Towel

30°–45°

Redrawn from Reichman EF. Chapter 57, Arterial Puncture and Cannulation. *Emergency Medicine Procedures.* 2nd ed. New York: McGraw-Hill, Inc.; 2013; Figure 57-5.

CENTRAL VENOUS ACCESS (ALSO SEE CHAPTER 8, ON PERIOPERATIVE MONITORING)

Indications
- Total parenteral nutrition (TPN)
- Administration of hyperosmolar or irritating drugs
- Administration of vasopressors
- Requirement of CVP, PA, SvO_2, CO measurements
- Limited peripheral vascular access
- Hemodialysis
- Need for transvenous pacing

Contraindications
- Internal jugular vein
  - Infected site, carotid artery stenosis, ↑ ICP, access site in surgical field
- Subclavian vein
  - Infected site, contralateral pneumo- or hemothorax, contralateral thoracic intervention
  - Contralateral attempts to cannulate subclavian vein, ↓ pulm fx of contralateral lung
  - Coagulopathy, emphysema (relative)

Technique: Internal Jugular Vein (IJ)
- Positioning: Trendelenburg (provides venous distention to prevent air embolism)
- Aseptic technique: Sterile gown, face mask, gloves, skin disinfection, & whole-body drape
- Localization: Ultrasound to locate carotid artery & IJ (or palpation if US unavailable)
- Local: Infiltrate skin with local anesthetic (e.g., lidocaine) if pt awake
- Cannulation
  - Ultrasound technique—18G needle under direct visualization
  - Palpation technique
  - Place 24G finder needle 8–10 mm lateral to carotid pulse at bifurcation of medial & lateral head of sternocleidomastoid muscle with needle aimed at ipsilateral nipple and angle 30–45° to skin
  - Once venous blood aspirated, puncture IJ with 18G needle at the same site, angle, & depth
- Aspirate venous blood, disconnect syringe, & assess for nonarterial venous blood flow
  - Some providers will transduce catheter to ensure nonarterial placement
- Advance guidewire through 18G needle (never lose control of guidewire)
- Withdraw 18G needle keeping guidewire in place
  - Some providers will verify guidewire location by observation with TEE or US
- Perform 8–10 mm skin incision parallel to guidewire
  - Sharp side of scalpel points up toward 2 o'clock (RIJ) or 10 o'clock (LIJ)
- Insert dilator over guidewire & then remove dilator
- Insert catheter over guidewire (Seldinger technique) into vein
- Aspirate & flush all catheter lumens
- Assess for venous blood flow by connecting to transducer
- Obtain CXR if possible to exclude procedure-related complications (e.g., pneumothorax)

Technique: Subclavian Vein (SC)
- Subclavian vein not collapsed in hypovolemic state (suspended to clavicula & pectoralis)
- Positioning: Trendelenburg (provides venous distention to prevent air embolism)
- Aseptic technique: Sterile gown, face mask, gloves, skin disinfection, & whole-body drape
- Local: Infiltrate skin with local anesthetic (e.g., lidocaine) if pt awake
- Puncture: 18G needle in midclavicular line (30–45° angle to skin) until hit clavicle (Fig. 12-2)
  - Once contact bone, advance needle underneath clavicle toward the sternoclavicular joint
  - Aspirate venous blood, advance guidewire
- Continue insertion of central line as described for IJ above

Technique: Femoral Vein (Fem)
- Aseptic technique: Sterile gown, face mask, gloves, skin disinfection, & whole-body drape
- Local: Infiltrate skin with local anesthetic (e.g., lidocaine) if pt awake
- Localization: Palpate femoral artery (Fem medial to artery)

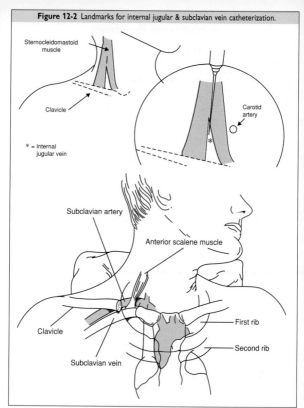

Figure 12-2 Landmarks for internal jugular & subclavian vein catheterization.

Sternocleidomastoid muscle

Clavicle

* = Internal jugular vein

Carotid artery

Subclavian artery

Anterior scalene muscle

Clavicle

Subclavian vein

First rib

Second rib

(Reproduced with permission from Wachter RM, Goldman L, Hollander H. *Hospital Medicine*. Philadelphia, PA: Lippincott Williams & Wilkins; 2005; Figures 27.16 & 27.18.)

- Puncture: 24G finder needle (30–45° angle to skin) 1–2 cm below inguinal ligament
  - Aspirate venous blood, insert 18G needle using the same position & angle
  - Advance guidewire
- Continue insertion of central line as described for IJ above

Complications
- Arterial cannulation, hematoma, pneumothorax (SC > IJ), chylothorax (LIJ or LSC)
- Hemothorax, infection, sepsis (Fem > SC > IJ), thrombophlebitis (Fem > SC > IJ)
- Nerve injury (Horner syndrome, brachial plexus lesions), air embolism

Ultrasound-Guided Central Line Placement
Insertion of central lines with US guidance has been proven to enhance safety:
- Fewer needle passes with increased success rate
- Reduced time for catheterization
- Fewer complications
- Benefit is most evident for IJ rather than SC or Fem, and for inexperienced operators

One-look technique
- Doppler US to locate artery and vein
- Confirm vessel location and patency, mark the skin, and then perform catheterization in the usual fashion

Real-Time Visualization of IJ
- Two-dimensional ultrasound guidance for IJ with a 7.5–10 MHz transducer protected by a sterile sheath
- US probe in nondominant hand to obtain a view of the target vessel
- Vein identified by anatomic location and by its compressibility. Artery appears mildly pulsatile
- US guidance with either transverse (short axis) or longitudinal (long axis) views
- *Transverse view:* Easier to learn, simultaneous identification of the artery and vein
- *Longitudinal view:* Visualization of the needle tip at all times, may reduce perforation of the posterior wall of the vein
- Transducer with sterile sleeve is held perpendicular to skin surface with the vein in the center of the US screen
- Vessel is punctured under direct vision with an 18G needle placed at the center of the transducer (transverse view) precisely over the vein (skin indentation from the needle tip is visible before puncturing the skin, then needle pass can be visualized as it enters the vein)
- In pediatric pts, a 20- to 24G needle may be used for the first cannulation and then exchanged with a larger gauge over a guidewire
- Proceed as described in the standard landmark technique above, but confirmation of the intravenous location of the guidewire with longitudinal view before vessel dilation

Real-Time Visualization of SC
- Transducer is placed in the infraclavicular groove at the level of the middle or lateral third of the clavicle
- Axillary vein and artery are imaged as they exit the bony canal formed by the clavicle and the first rib
- Artery is most commonly cephalad to the vein and noncompressible, and does not vary in diameter with respiration
- Either transverse or longitudinal view for guide needle insertion as described above
- Proceed as described with landmark technique followed by confirmation of guidewire location in vein

---

INSERTION OF A PULMONARY ARTERY CATHETER (PAC)
(ALSO SEE CHAPTER 8, ON PERIOPERATIVE MONITORING)

Indications
- Management of complicated myocardial infarction (ventricular failure, cardiogenic shock)
- Assessment of resp distress (cardiogenic vs. noncardiogenic pulm edema, 1° vs. 2° pulm HTN)
- Assessment of shock
- Assessment of fluid requirements in critically ill (hemorrhage, sepsis, acute renal failure, burns)
- Postop management of cardiac pts
- Need for heart rate pacing

Contraindications
- Tricuspid or pulmonary valve mechanical prosthesis
- Right heart mass (thrombus and/or tumor)
- Tricuspid or pulmonary valve endocarditis

Technique
- Central venous access as described above
- Positioning: Floating PA catheter easier in flat or slightly reverse Trendelenburg *in contrast to central line placement (Trendelenburg)*
- Aseptic technique: Sterile gown, face mask, gloves, skin disinfection, & whole-body drape
- PAC setup
- Calibrate ("zero") PAC, check PAC for damage, test balloon inflation/deflation
  - Connect all lumens to stopcocks, flush to eliminate air bubbles
  - Check PAC tip frequency response by touching tip
  - PAC threaded through sterile sleeve prior to insertion into cannula
- PAC inserted percutaneously into major vein (IJ, SC, femoral) via an introducer sheath
  - RIJ: Shortest & straightest path
  - LSC: Acute angle to enter SVC (compared to RSC or LIJ)
  - Fem: Distant sites, difficult if R-sided cardiac chambers enlarged (*often fluoroscopic guidance necessary*)

- Insert into introducer maintaining preformed curve (*RIJ approach: Concave-cephalad*)
- Once PAC enters RV, a clockwise quarter turn moves tip anteriorly (*allows easier passage past in PA*)
- After inserting PAC to 20 cm mark (30 cm mark if femoral route used), inflate balloon with air (1–1.5 mL)
- **Always inflate balloon before advancing & always deflate balloon before withdrawal**
- While advancing, waveforms will be observed (distal lumen pressure monitoring):
  - RA ≈ 25 cm (RIJ)
  - RV ≈ 30 cm (↑ systolic pressure than RA, absence of dicrotic notch)
  - PA ≈ 40 cm (↑ diastolic pressure, ↓ systolic pressure)
  - PCWP ≈ 45 cm (some damping & ↓ pressure with occlusion of PA)
- Obtaining pulmonary capillary wedge pressure
  - Disconnect breathing circuit
  - Determine volume of air in balloon required to obtain a PCWP waveform (*volume < half balloon max may indicate tip too far distal*)
  - Read PCWP (correlates with LVEDP ≈ 4–15 mmHg is normal)
  - Reconnect breathing circuit, deflate balloon, observe PA waveform return
  - PA diastolic pressure usually correlates well with PCWP pressure (*should be used as parameter to assess left ventricular filling*)
  - Withdraw PAC slightly (1–2 cm) to prevent PA rupture from distal tip migration
  - Secure catheter sleeve once PCWP is obtained (*assure that PCWP pattern is reproducible before removing sterile field*)
- Troubleshooting a coiled/knotted catheter:
  - Prevention: Withdraw PAC slowly to ↓ risk of knotting catheter upon itself
  - Use fluoroscopy if necessary to remove a knot
  - Remove PAC & introducer as one unit if unable to release a knot
  - Obtain a CXR to check PAC position

Complication: PA Perforation
- Predisposed when **no wedge pattern evident after deep insertion**
  - Circumstances that predispose to PA perforation: *Papillary muscle ischemia, mitral stenosis or regurgitation, pulm HTN, intrapulmonary shunting, LV failure*
  - Caution if no definitive wedge pattern is observed (*repeated attempts to advance PAC may lead to PA perforation*)
  - Coiling or actual false-negative wedging may occur & predispose to PA rupture

DECOMPRESSION OF A PNEUMOTHORAX (NEEDLE THORACOSTOMY)

Indication
- Tension pneumothorax (symptoms: Hypotension, ↓ SpO₂, ↓ breath sounds, & tympanic to percussion on affected site; deviated trachea; & mediastinum on CXR)

Technique (Fig. 12-3)
- Insert large bore cannula or needle (14G) into the 2nd intercostal space on midclavicular line
- Release pressure in pleural cavity (*converts tension pneumothorax → simple pneumothorax*)
- Subsequent chest tube insertion usually required to treat pneumothorax

Complications
- Lung laceration (esp if no tension pneumothorax present)
- Reaccumulation of air in pleural space (*may be undetected if needle thoracostomy becomes dislodged*)

INSERTION OF A NASOGASTRIC TUBE (NGT)

Indication
- Decompression & emptying of stomach (after RSI, prior to laparoscopy, GI surgery)
- Aspiration of gastric fluid (lavage to detect intragastric blood in the setting of GI bleed)
- Tube feeding
- Drug administration

Contraindications
- Base of skull fractures, severe facial fractures (esp to nasal bones)
- Obstructed esophagus or airway

Figure 12-3 Landmarks for a needle thoracostomy.

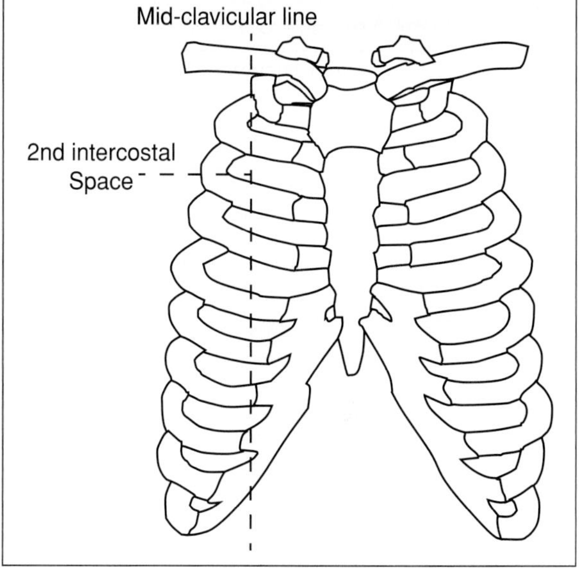

Mid-clavicular line

2nd intercostal Space

Technique
- Measure tube length (tip of pt's nose to ear & down to xiphoid process)
- Lubricate end of plastic tube being inserted into anterior nares
- Advance tube through nasal cavity & into throat
- Pass pharynx rapidly with gentle continuous pressure to go into stomach (if pt awake, encourage pt swallowing)
  (if pt asleep, consider use of laryngoscope to visualize entry into esophagus)
- Confirm placement by CXR (safest), aspiration, or injecting air (stomach auscultation)

Complications
- Malplacement (endotracheal, intracranial)
- Esophageal perforation
- Pulmonary aspiration, pneumothorax
- Nose erosion/bleeding, sinusitis, sore throat

DAVID A. EDWARDS • JENNA WALTERS

INTRODUCTION

- Acute pain is undertreated (Anesth Analg 2007;105:205–221)
- Undertreated acute pain can become chronic pain
- Adequate pain control is considered a human right (Anesth Analg 2007;105:205–221)

DEFINITIONS

Pain Durations		
Acute pain	0–6 wk	New onset or exacerbation, normal healing period
Subacute pain	1–3 mo	Prolonged, transitional (acute to chronic)
Chronic pain	>3 mo	Persistent, pathologic, or continuous stimulus induced

Pain Terms	
Pain	"An unpleasant sensory or emotional experience associated with actual or potential tissue damage, or described in terms of such damage" (IASP)
Dysesthesia	Unpleasant abnormal sensation (spontaneous or evoked)
Paresthesia	Abnormal sensation (spontaneous or evoked)
Hyperesthesia	↑ Sensitivity to any stimulus
Hyperpathia	Painful syndrome of ↑ pain in response to a stimulus (especially repetitive stimulus)
Hyperalgesia	Painful stimulus is more painful than expected (pinprick hurts even more) • *Primary hyperalgesia*—painful zone innervated by nerves in region of the lesion • *Secondary hyperalgesia*—expanded area that becomes painful as a result of becoming sensitized • *Opioid-induced hyperalgesia*—acute opioid exposure paradoxically ↑ pain, acute opioid withdrawal ↑ pain sensitivity, or chronic opioid exposure ↑ pain sensitivity
Allodynia	Painful response to nonpainful stimulus (e.g., light touch skin causes pain)
Hypoesthesia	↓ Sensitivity to nonpainful stimulus
Hypoalgesia	↓ Pain in response to normally painful stimulus
Anesthesia	Absence of sensation to painful or nonpainful stimulus
Analgesia	Absence of pain to painful stimulus
Anesthesia dolorosa	Painful sensation in anesthetic area
Meralgia paresthetica	Numbness/pain from lateral femoral cutaneous n. compression
Multimodal analgesia	Principle of combining analgesic modalities (meds, procedures, techniques) at lower individual doses to improve pain tx while decreasing risks/side effects (as opposed to polypharmacy, combining meds at higher doses resulting in increased risks/side effects)
Opioid tolerant	An increased dose of opioid is required for the same effect (NIH definition of opioid tolerant pt = taking 60 mg morphine PO in 24 h ×7 d)
Dependence	A state of normal function in the presence of drug, but a withdrawal syndrome when the drug is removed
Addiction	Compulsive substance use despite negative life interference

NORMAL PAIN MECHANISMS & PAIN PATHWAYS

Pain Pathways
- Pain transmission:
- 1st-order neurons → spinal cord 2nd-order neurons → brainstem 3rd-order neurons → thalamic 4th-order neurons → association areas, frontal, and somatosensory cortex

Nerve Fiber Types				
Aα	Myelinated	Large	Fast (~100 m/s)	Motor, proprioception
Aβ	Myelinated	Large	Fast (~50 m/s)	Light touch, pressure
Aγ	Myelinated	Large	Fast (~50 m/s)	Muscle spindle motor, proprioception
Aδ	Thinly myelinated	Medium	Fast (~20 m/s)	Cold temp, supramaximal heat pain, pressure pain (single stim)
B	Thinly myelinated	Medium	Moderate (~14 m/s)	Autonomic, preganglionic sympathetic
C	Unmyelinated	Small	Slow (~1 m/s)	Warm temp, heat pain, pressure pain (repetitive), postganglionic sympathetic

PAIN ASSESSMENT & MEASUREMENT

History & Physical Exam (see also Fig. 32-1)
• STEP 1: Identify what type of pain the pt has (*J Clin Investig* 2010;120:3742–3744)
• STEP 2: Quantify pain severity
• STEP 3: Choose medication and nonmedication options to treat specific pain type

Types of Pain		
Nociceptive	An adaptive (protective) pain; pain sensed by pain receptors (nociceptors) that sense thermal, mechanical, or chemical stimuli • *Somatic pain*—musculoskeletal pain (broken bones, unhealed wounds, surgical) • *Visceral pain*—pain from organs (bladder, bowel, ovaries)	Superficial somatic: Sharp, easily localized (burns) Deep somatic: Throbbing, aching, worse with movement, poorly localized (broken bones) Visceral: Pressure, deep, dull, diffuse, poorly localized, referred
Inflammatory	An adaptive (protective) pain; results from local inflammation (arthritis, infection, tissue injury)	Throbbing Ache
Pathologic	A maladaptive pain; damage/dysfunction of nervous system (diabetes, surgical transection, nerve injury) • *Neuropathic pain*—diabetic neuropathy • *Dysfunctional pain*—central sensitization, fibromyalgia, tension type headache	Electric, burning, stabbing, cutting, pins and needles, tingling, shooting

Pain Measurement
Quantify pain severity using a scale and/or pt reported questionnaire
• *Numeric Rating Scale (NRS)*: 1–10 point line intensity of pain (0 = no pain, 10 = worst pain imaginable)
• *Visual Analog Scale (VAS)*: A continuous scale represented by a 100-mm line with "no pain" at one end, and "pain as bad as it could be" at the other end. Pts are asked to draw a line through where their pain is on that scale.
• *Faces Pain Scale, FLACC scale* (face legs arms cry consolability): A scale used for pediatrics
• *Multidimensional Pain Scales*: They assess effect of pain on mood & daily function; Examples are Brief Pain Inventory (BPI) and McGill Pain Questionnaire (MPQ).
• *Opioid Consumption*: 24-h opioid consumption is often used as a measure of pain control

Figure 13-1 Wong–Baker faces pain rating scale.

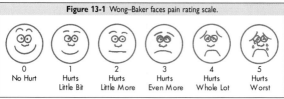

0	1	2	3	4	5
No Hurt	Hurts Little Bit	Hurts Little More	Hurts Even More	Hurts Whole Lot	Hurts Worst

ACUTE PAIN MANAGEMENT

Adverse Physiologic Effects of Uncontrolled Acute Pain	
Cardiac	HTN, tachycardia, dysrhythmias, MI
Pulmonary	Atelectasis, mismatch, pneumonia
Endocrine	Protein catabolism, hyperglycemia, fluid retention
Immune	Immune function impairment
Coagulation	Hypercoagulation, ↑ platelet adhesion
GI	Ileus
GU	Urinary retention

Treatment

Summary of Options for Postop Pain Management (see also Chapter 2c, Analgesics)		
Route	Therapy Class	Medication/Dose
IV/IM	Opioids	Fentanyl 25–100 mcg q30–60min Hydromorphone 0.2–2 mg q4–6h Meperidine 25–50 mg q3–4h Morphine 1–10 mg q2–6h Codeine 15–30 mg q2h
	NSAIDs	Ketorolac 30 mg q6h, Ibuprofen 200–800 mg q6h Diclofenac 50–100 mg
	Mixed agonists/antagonists	Butorphanol 1 mg q3–4h IV Nalbuphine 10 mg q3–6h IV
	Other	Acetaminophen 1,000 mg IV q6h (total 4 g/d) Ketamine 0.2–0.8 mg/kg IV, 2–6 mg/kg IM
PO	NSAIDs	Ibuprofen 400–800 mg q4–6h Ketorolac 10–20 mg q4–6h Naproxen 250 mg q6–8h or 500 mg q12h Diclofenac 50 mg TID
	COX-2 inhibitors	Celecoxib 200–400 mg q12h
	Opioid/nonopioid combinations	Acetaminophen/propoxyphene napsylate (Darvocet) q4–6h Acetaminophen/oxycodone (Percocet) q4–6h Acetaminophen/codeine (Tylenol with codeine) q4–6h Acetaminophen/hydrocodone (Vicodin) q4–6h
	Opioids	Hydrocodone 5–10 mg q4–6h Morphine 10–30 mg q3–4h Hydromorphone 2–4 mg q4–6h Meperidine 50–150 mg q3–4h Oxycodone 5 mg q3–6h Codeine 15–60 mg q4–6h Propoxyphene 65 mg q4h Tramadol 50–100 mg q4–6h
	Calcium channel antagonists/anticonvulsants	Pregabalin 150 mg pre- or postoperatively Gabapentin 300–1,200 mg pre- or postoperatively
	Others	Acetaminophen 650 mg q4–6h Ketamine 6–10 mg/kg
Transdermal		Fentanyl patch 25–100 mcg/h q72h Diclofenac 1% patch or topical gel
Intranasal	Opioids	Fentanyl 1.5 mcg/kg Meperidine 162 mg Butorphanol 1–2 mg Ketamine 6–10 mg/kg Ketorolac 31.5 mg
Local anesthetics		Neuraxial anesthesia Regional nerve block Local infiltration by surgeon Continuous subcutaneous catheter
Nonpharmacologic methods		Heat/cold therapy, massage, TENS relaxation, hypnosis, acupuncture, biofeedback

Common Oral Opioids: Adult Dosages	
Drug	Starting Dose
Morphine immediate release	15 mg PO q4–6h prn
Morphine extended release (MS Contin)	15 mg PO q8–12h
Codeine/acetaminophen*	
Tylenol #2 (15 mg/300 mg)	1–2 tab q4–6h
Tylenol #3 (30 mg/300 mg)	1–2 tab q4–6h
Tylenol #5 (60 mg/300 mg)	1–2 tab q4–6h
Hydrocodone/acetaminophen*	
Norco (5/325, 7.5/325, 10/325)	1–2 tab q4–6h
Vicodin (5/300, 7.5/300, 10/300)	1–2 tab q4–6h
Methadone	2.5–5 mg PO q8h
Oxycodone/acetaminophen*	
Percocet (2.5/325, 5/325, 7.5/325, 10/325)	1–2 tab PO q4–6h prn
Oxycodone	5–15 mg PO q4–6h prn
Oxycodone extended release (OxyContin)	10–20 mg PO q12h
Tramadol (Ultram)	50–100 mg PO q4–6h prn

*Max acetaminophen dose = 4 g/d in adults. Large percentage of population lack enzyme to convert codeine → morphine (accounts for variability in analgesic effects).

Equianalgesic Opioid Dosage Table for Adult Patients					
Drug	Conversion factor to morphine	Onset (min)	Peak (h)	Half-life (h)	Duration (h)
Morphine	×1	15	1	2–4	3–6
Hydrocodone	×1	60	2	3–4	4–8
Tramadol	×0.1	60	2	6	6
Oxycodone	×1.5	15	1	3	4–6
Hydromorphone	×5	15–30	1	2	4–5
Meperidine	×0.1	10–15	1	4	2–4
Codeine	×0.15	30	1.5	3–4	4–8
Oxymorphone	×3	30	0.5	7	3–6
Levorphanol	×8–11	15	0.5–1	12–15	6–15
Tapentadol	×0.3	30	1.5	4	4
Buprenorphine	×40	45	1–3	24–60	15–30
Fentanyl IV (mcg)	×75–100	4		4	2–4

Fentanyl patch (mcg/h)
  12.5 mcg/h = 30 MEDD
  25 mcg/h = 60 MEDD
  50 mcg/h = 120 MEDD
  75 mcg/h = 180 MEDD
  100 mcg/h = 240 MEDD
	×2.4	12–24 h		7	60–72 h

Methadone
  PO (acute)
  IV (acute)
  PO (chronic)
    1–20 mg/d
    21–40 mg/d
    41–50 mg/d
    51–80 mg/d
	
	3
	×6
	
	×4
	×8
	×10
	×12
		
		30
		8
			
			0.5–1.5
			(3–5 d
			for
			steady
			state)
				
				24–36
				8–60
					
					4–8 (24–48
					with
					repeated
					dosing)

*There is a nonlinear relationship for methadone equianalgesic dosing. Caution must be used, especially in chronic opioid users. The more opioid a pt is on, the more sensitive they will be to methadone. MEDD, morphine equivalent daily dose.

Common Nonopioid Adjuvant Dosage for Adult Patients				
Group	Drug	Route	Dose	Side Effects
COX-1, 2 Inhibitors	Aspirin	PO	325–650 mg	Urticaria, angioedema, Reye syndrome (avoid in children <12 y)
	Ibuprofen	PO, IV	PO: 200–800 mg TID IV: 400–800 mg TID	GI pain, dyspepsia, bone fracture
	Ketorolac	IV/IM	15–30 mg q6h (max 120 mg daily)	GI pain, dyspepsia Caution in elderly and with renal impairment
	Diclofenac	IV, IM, PO, topical	50–100 mg	GI pain, dyspepsia
	Meloxicam	PO	7.5–15 mg q24h	GI pain, dyspepsia
	Naproxen	PO	250–500 mg q6–8h (max 1,000 mg daily)	GI pain, dyspepsia
	Celecoxib	PO	100–200 mg daily	Reduced GI side effects (short-term)
	Acetaminophen (CNS COX-1,2)	PO, PR, IV	PO: 500–1,000 mg IV: 500–1,000 mg q4–6h; max 4 g/d	Hepatotoxicity, GI upset
Anticonvulsants	Gabapentin	PO	300 mg PO TID titrated to range of 600–1,200 mg TID	Sleepiness, confusion, bloating, leukopenia, thrombocytopenia, depression
	Pregabalin	PO	25–150 mg PO daily, titrate to TID as tolerated	Sleepiness, confusion, bloating, depression
NMDA antagonist	Ketamine	IV, IM, PO	IV: 0.2–0.8 mg/kg IV infusion: 3–5 mcg/kg/min IM: 2–6 mg/kg PO: 6–10 mg/kg	Myocardial depressant, cerebral vasodilator, sympathetic nervous system (↑ HR & CO), hallucinations
α2 Agonists	Tizanidine	PO	2–4 mg qhs, titrate to 2–12 mg TID as tolerated	Hypotension, bradycardia, sleepiness, dizziness, nausea, dry mouth, anxiety, blurred vision, ↑ LFT
	Clonidine	PO, IV, epidural, topical	PO: 0.3–0.4 mg epidural: 30–40 mcg/h	Hypotension, bradycardia, sleepiness, dizziness, dry mouth, decreased bowel motility
TCA's	Amitriptyline	PO	10–25 mg qhs, titrate up to 25–150 mg qhs over several d	Sleepiness, dry mouth, ↑ HR, blurred vision, urinary retention, constipation, confusion
	Nortriptyline	PO	10–25 mg qhs, titrate up to 25–150 mg qhs over several d	Sleepiness, dry mouth, ↑ HR, blurred vision, urinary retention, constipation, confusion

	Duloxetine	PO	30–60 mg/d	Nausea, dry mouth, headache, sleepiness
SNRI	Lorazepam	IV, IM, PO	IV/IM: 0.02–0.08 mg/kg PO: 2–3 mg	Resp depression (if given with opioids)
	Ondansetron	IV	IV: 4 mg Peds IV: 0.05–0.075 mg/kg	Headache, dizziness, sedation, shivers, ↑ LFT
	Benadryl	IV, PO	IV: 10–50 mg q6–8h Peds IV: 5 mg/kg/d in 4 divided doses (max 300 mg)	Tachycardia, dizziness, seizures, urinary retention
	Lidocaine	IV, topical	IV: 0.5–2 mg/kg/h topical patch: 12 h on 12 h off	Tachyphylaxis, systemic toxicity, topical irritation

TCA, tricyclic antidepressant; SNRI, selective serotonin–norepinephrine reuptake inhibitor.

ANALGESIC DELIVERY SYSTEMS

PO
- Not optimal for immediate postop pain (delayed time to peak effect)
- Opioids commonly combined with COX inhibitors

SC/IM
- Less desirable routes (pain on injection & erratic absorption)
- Cyclical period of sedation → analgesia → inadequate analgesia common

IV
- Requires close respiratory monitoring
- Common in PACU, ICU, & specialized units

Patient-Controlled Analgesia (PCA)
- Allows the pt to self-administer opioids with button push
- Physician specifies: Dose/minimum time period between doses (lockout)/basal infusion rate/max delivered dose in 1 h (i.e., morphine 1/10/0/5)

PCA Guidelines: Adult					
Opioid	Demand Dose	Dose Range	Lockout Interval	1-h Limit	Basal Infusion
Morphine	1 mg	0.5–3 mg	5–20 min	10 mg	0–10 mg/h
Fentanyl	15 mcg	10–50 mcg	3–10 min	100 mcg	0–100 mcg/h
Hydromorphone	0.2 mg	0.1–0.5 mg	5–15 min	1.5 mg	0–0.5 mg/h
Meperidine	7.5 mg	4–15 mg	5–15 min	75 mg	0–30 mg/h
Methadone	0.2 mg	0.1–0.4 mg	10–15 min	2 mg	20 mcg/kg

Continuous and PNCA* Guidelines: Pediatric				
Opioid	Initial Bolus	Demand Dose	Lockout	Infusion
Morphine	0.1 mg/kg	0.01–0.02 mg/kg	7–15 min	0.01 mg/kg/h
Fentanyl	1.5 mcg/kg	0.2–1 mcg/kg	7–15 min	0.15 mcg/kg/h
Hydromorphone	15 mcg/kg	2–6 mcg/kg	7–15 min	3 mcg/kg/h

*Children >6 y old can usually manage PCA. Alternatively, and in children <6 y old a basal infusion or parent/nurse-controlled analgesia (PNCA) are options.

Neuraxial Analgesia
- Intrathecal or epidural routes; effective for postop pain after abd, pelvic, thoracic, and orthopedic surgeries of lower extremity
- Local anesthetics (bupivacaine, lidocaine, ropivacaine) +/– opioids
- Clonidine and buprenorphine can also be added

Epidural Opioids
- Site of action = pre- & postsynaptic receptors in dorsal horn substantia gelatinosa
- Opioid drugs enter CSF at rate dependent on physicochemical properties
  - Molecular weight

- pKa
- oil:water solubility
- Lipid-soluble opioids (sufentanil, fentanyl) enter spinal cord faster, faster onset, faster vascular uptake → shorter duration
- Water-soluble opioids (morphine) have slower onset, longer duration of action

Epidural Placement Level	
Thoracotomy	T4–6
Upper abdominal surgery	T8–9
Lower abdominal surgery	T10–12
Lower extremity/pelvis	L2–4

PCEA* General Guidelines (Nonlabor) Using Common Solutions				
Solution	Demand Dose	Lockout	Infusion Rate Range	1-h Limit
Bupivacaine: 0.0625, 0.125, 0.25% + adjuvant	2–4 mL	10–20 min	3–12 mL/h	20 mL
Ropivacaine: 0.2% + adjuvant	2–4 mL	10–20 min	3–12 mL/h	20 mL
Adjuvants: • Fentanyl 2–5 mcg/mL • Hydromorphone 10–20 mcg/mL • Clonidine 0.75–5 mcg/mL—can cause bradycardia at doses >1 mcg/kg/h • Epinephrine 2 mcg/mL				

*PCEA, patient-controlled epidural analgesia.

Troubleshooting Epidural Catheter Infusions

Signs of Inadequate Epidural Analgesia
- Pain at rest and with movement (pain score >5)
- ↑ HR, ↑ RR
- For thoracic & abd cases:
  - Inability to breathe deeply, cough, use incentive spirometer
- Pain beyond the levels expected to be covered by the epidural, or patchy coverage

Testing of Epidurals
- STEP 1: Assess the pt to ensure placement of epidural should cover surgical site
- STEP 2: Test the pt's sensory level using ice
- STEP 3: Inspect the catheter to ensure it has not migrated out of the epidural space
- STEP 4: Prepare either 2% lidocaine with 1:200,000 epi or 0.25% bupivacaine with 1:200,000 epi
- STEP 5: Get baseline vital signs, and ensure pt will tolerate a bolus (anticipate up to 10–20-point drop in SBP)
- STEP 6: Bolus 2–3 mL of local anesthetic via epidural → check BP, motor/sensory block & pain relief
  - May repeat 3 mL after 3–5 min
  - Consider replacing epidural if no pain relief after 8 mL of test dose over 10–15 min
- STEP 7: Monitor pt for 20–30 min, checking BP, pain relief, and signs of toxicity

"Splitting" Epidural with IV PCA
- Technique: Add IV PCA in addition to epidural infusion (*must simultaneously remove opioids from epidural infusion*)
- May be necessary for:
  - Pt with opioid dependence (requires higher dose of opioid)
  - Incomplete incisional coverage from epidural (i.e., referred pain to shoulder from diaphragm irritation)
  - Upper & lower body surgeries (trauma victims)
  - Large surgical incision
  - Lower level epidural catheter placement

Treatment of Side Effects from Epidural Analgesia	
Pruritus	Nalbuphine 5–10 mg IV/IM
	Benadryl 25–50 mg IV
	Naloxone 40–80 mcg IV
Nausea/vomiting	Metoclopramide 10 mg IV
	Nalbuphine 10 mg IV
	Naloxone 40–80 mcg IV
Respiratory depression	Naloxone 40–100 mcg IV, repeat as needed

Intrathecal Opioids
- Can be added to spinal anesthesia
- Act on substantia gelatinosa of the spinal cord
- Side effects mediated by mu receptors (in brain & brainstem)

Intrathecal Opioids				
Opioid	Dose	Duration	Indications	Side Effects
Morphine	0.2–0.4 mg	24 h	Good spread & long duration of action	Nausea, vomiting resp depression, sedation, itching, urinary retention
Fentanyl	12.5–25 mcg	3–4 h	For segmental spread	Nausea, resp depression
Sufentanil	5–10 mcg	2–4 h	Very lipid soluble & has segmental spread	Nausea, resp depression
Meperidine	10 mg	3–6 h	In addition to opioid effect has local anesthetic effect	Hypotension

MANAGING SIDE EFFECTS

Opioid Side Effects	Opioid Receptor	Treatments
Nausea/vomiting	Mu1, Mu2	Switch/wean agent, ondansetron, phenergan, prochlorperazine, haloperidol, metoclopramide
Allergic reaction		Switch agent, diphenhydramine, epinephrine
Respiratory depression	Mu2	Support airway, ↓ dose, consider naloxone
Pruritus	Mu (neuraxial)	Switch agent, naloxone/nalbuphine (antihistamines not very effective)
Delirium, dysphoria	Mu1, kappa	Switch agent, ↓ dose, haloperidol, olanzapine
Constipation	Mu, kappa	Laxatives (senna, lactulose) + stool softeners (Colace)
Sedation	Mu1, kappa	↓ Dose, hold anxiolytics, consider CNS stimulants if persistent
Urinary retention	Mu2	↓ Dose, discontinue agent, place urinary catheter

ACUTE ON CHRONIC PAIN

Opioid Receptor Mixed Agonists/Antagonists
- Less misuse potential because they have a ceiling effect, so commonly used for maintenance of chronic pain
- These drugs will block the effects of pure opioid agonists
- Produce partial agonist effects at κ (kappa) and/or δ (delta) opioid receptors
- Usually these are tapered off before surgery and replaced by pure agonists so that pain can be better managed

Mixed Opioid Agonists/Antagonists			
Drug	Dose	Potency	Side Effects
Naloxone	40–100 mcg IV q3–5min prn		Sweating, nausea, vomiting, nervousness
Nalbuphine	2.5–10 mg IV q4prn	1:1 morphine	Drowsiness, dizziness, nausea, mouth pain

Buprenorphine (Suboxone—buprenorphine/naloxone)	0.4 mg IV q4–6h	25× morphine	Drowsiness, dizziness, nausea, mouth pain
Pentazocine (Talwin—pentazocine/naloxone)	50 mg PO q4–6h	1/3 morphine	Drowsiness, dizziness
Butorphanol	0.5–2 mg IV q4h	5× morphine	Drowsiness, dizziness, nausea

Definitions
- *Opioid rotation*—switching to a different opioid to provide better pain control, in response to organ dz, and to avoid the need for dose escalation; works due to principle of incomplete cross tolerance
- *Incomplete cross tolerance*—different opioids interact with the receptors differently, so when a pt becomes tolerant to one agent, they may not be equally tolerant to another. Thus when switching, it is essential to use lower than equianalgesic doses (typically 25% reduction).

Opioid Rotation (Example)	
1. Calculate total 24-h opioid dose	1. Morphine 30 mg PO q6h = 120 mg in 24 h
2. Find new opioid on equianalgesic table	2. Hydromorphone 7.5 mg = 30 mg morphine
3. Solve equation for new dose	3. 120 mg/30 mg = 4 × 7.5 → 30 mg hydromorphone in 24 h
4. Divide new 24-h dose by # doses/d	4. 30 mg/4 doses = 7.5 mg q6h
5. ↓ Calc dose by 25–50%	5. 33% reduction = 5 mg hydromorphone PO q6h
6. Titrate to clinical effect	

JONATHAN P. WANDERER

HYPOTENSION

Common Causes of Hypotension in the PACU	
• Hypovolemia	• MI/↓ myocardial contractility
• Bleeding	• Cardiac tamponade
• Sepsis/↓ SVR	• Congestive heart failure
• Cardiac arrhythmias	• Anaphylaxis/anaphylactoid reaction
• Drugs/anesthesia (spinal/epidural)	• Pneumothorax
• Error in measurement (inappropriate cuff size, machine malfunction)	• Adrenal insufficiency/severe hypothyroidism
• Pulmonary embolism	

Source: Adapted from Rose DK, Cohen MM, DeBoer DP. Cardiovascular events in postanesthesia care unit: Contribution of risk factors. Anesthesiology 1996;84:772–781.

Initial Diagnosis & Management
1. Examine & stabilize—check **A**irway, **B**reathing, & **C**irculation
2. Fluid resuscitate—obtain adequate venous access
3. Review data—pt Hx, anesthesia record, surgical procedure, estimated blood loss, PACU data
4. Consider laboratory studies
   • ABG—assess oxygenation & acid–base status
   • CBC—assess hemoglobin & platelet level (also consider coagulation studies)
   • ECG—assess for arrhythmias (also consider cardiac enzymes)
   • CXR—rule out pneumothorax/hemothorax/cardiomegaly
   • Blood cultures—esp if sepsis suspected
   • Transthoracic/transesophageal echo—assess cardiac contractility, LV/RV function, LV filling, IVC collapse, valvular abnl
5. Consider invasive/noninvasive monitoring—arterial BP, CVP, pulmonary artery catheter, noninvasive cardiac output monitor
6. Initiate pressor/inotropic support—phenylephrine, norepinephrine, dopamine
7. Obtain consultations as needed—cardiology, ICU, surgery

Management of Specific Conditions
Hypovolemia

Diagnosis	Tachycardia, hypotension, low CVP/PCWP, respiratory variation in arterial waveform, IVC collapse/underfilled LV on echo
Treatment	Fluid resuscitation, assess for causes (ongoing bleeding, diuresis, high NG output)

Bleeding

Diagnosis	Tachycardia, anemia, hypovolemia, sanguineous drain output
Treatment	Fluid resuscitation, blood transfusion, correct coagulopathy & thrombocytopenia, treat hypothermia, consider return to OR

Sepsis

Diagnosis	Fever, leukocytosis, tachycardia, hypovolemia, lactic acidosis
Treatment	Fluid resuscitation, obtain blood/specific cultures, initiate broad-spectrum antibiotics

Myocardial Infarction/Ischemia

Diagnosis	12-lead ECG, TTE/TEE, cardiac enzymes, cardiology consult
Treatment	Cautious fluid resuscitation, aspirin, discuss with cardiologist & surgeon the role of heparinization/cardiac cath/antiplatelet agents; consider inotropic/vasopressor/IABP support; may initiate diuresis/β-blockade once BP stabilized

Arrhythmias

Diagnosis	12-lead ECG, cardiac enzymes, check electrolytes, ABG
Treatment	Treat the cause, follow ACLS protocol • Tachyarrhythmia: Electrical/chemical cardioversion, correct electrolytes, cardiology consultation, maintenance antiarrhythmics • Bradyarrhythmia: Atropine/epinephrine/dopamine, transcutaneous transvenous pacing, cardiology consult

Drugs

Treatment	Stop the drug, administer antagonist agent (e.g., naloxone for morphine)

Pulmonary Embolism

Diagnosis	ECG → sinus tach/$S_1Q_3T_3$; ultrasound (US) of lower ext; D-dimer not helpful TTE/TEE → rule out central pulm embolism/assess RV dysfx scan/CT chest pulm angiogram when stable
Treatment	Cautious fluid resuscitation, invasive monitoring, inotropes/pressors Consider thromboembolectomy/catheter-directed thrombolysis/anticoagulation/IVC filter placement

Congestive Heart Failure

Diagnosis	Bibasilar crackles, frothy sputum on examination Chest x-ray → cephalization of blood vessels, pulmonary edema, ↑ cardiac shadow Invasive hemodynamic monitoring shows ↓ cardiac output, ↑ filling pressures
Treatment	Supplemental O_2, diuresis, digoxin/inotropic support

Anaphylaxis

Diagnosis	Tachycardia, vasodilatory shock (↓ SVR, ↑ cardiac output), rash, wheezing Check serum tryptase & eosinophil count, consult allergy
Treatment	Remove causative agent, fluid resuscitation, diphenhydramine, steroids, epinephrine

Pericardial Tamponade

Causes	Postcardiac surgery bleeding, trauma, dissecting thoracic aneurysm, procedure related (e.g., s/p CVP placement, coronary cath)	
Diagnosis	• Beck triad:	Hypotension, jugular venous distension, muffled heart sounds
	• Pulsus paradoxus:	↓ Of >10 mmHg in systolic BP with inspiration
	• ECG:	Nonspecific ST-segment changes, low-voltage QRS
	• Chest x-ray:	Enlarged cardiac shadow
	• Echo:	Diagnostic & may assist in therapeutic pericardiocentesis
Treatment	Fluid resuscitation, pericardiocentesis, surgical repair of bleeding site	

Pneumothorax

Diagnosis	↓ Breath sounds, ↓ lung markings on chest x-ray
Treatment	Needle decompression/chest tube placement, surgery consult

Errors in Measurement

Diagnosis	Inappropriate BP cuff size, incorrect transducer level, poor arterial waveform (under/overdamped), machine malfunction
Treatment	Place appropriate size BP cuff, manual measurement, check a-line waveform, zero transducer at appropriate level, check equipment

Endocrine Disorders: Adrenal Insufficiency

Diagnosis	ACTH stim test; random cortisol levels nonspecific & unhelpful
Treatment	Fluids, administer hydrocortisone, endocrinology consult

Endocrine Disorders: Severe Hypothyroidism

Diagnosis	Hypothermia, bradycardia, high TSH level, low free T_3 & T_4 levels
Treatment	Fluid resuscitation, levothyroxine administration, endocrinology consult

Bleeding

Common Causes
- Surgical bleeding
- Coagulopathy
- Thrombocytopenia

Diagnosis
- Bleeding may be obvious or occult
- Important to examine surgical drains/surgical site
- Signs of hypovolemia (tachycardia, tachypnea, ↓ urine output) may suggest bleeding

Management
- Consult surgeon, place large-bore IVs, & initiate fluid resuscitation
- Send CBC, PT, PTT, INR, & fibrinogen, & request blood cross-match
- Transfuse: PRBCs based on hemoglobin level, pt's condition, & coexisting dz FFP to correct coagulopathy
- Cryoprecipitate if evidence of hypofibrinogenemia
- Platelets if level <50,000–100,000 or previous exposure to antiplatelet agents
- Consider use of recombinant factor 7 in uncontrolled, diffuse, postop bleeding
- Assess for evidence of DIC (↓ fibrinogen, + FDP/D-dimer, ↑ PT/PTT, ↓ platelets)
  → Occurs in mismatch transfusion, placental abruption, intrauterine fetal demise, underlying malignancy, complex infections
  → Treat with transfusion of FFP, cryoprecipitate, & platelets
- Maintain normothermia & consider calcium administration during massive transfusion
- Alert OR personnel about need for possible take back

HYPERTENSION

Common Causes of Hypertension in the PACU	
• Pain	• Essential hypertension/missed medications
• Anxiety	• Fluid overload
• Respiratory insufficiency (hypoxia, hypercarbia)	• Endocrine dz (thyroid storm, pheochromocytoma)
• Hypothermia/shivering	• Error in measurement (inappropriate cuff size, machine malfunction)
• ↑ Sympathetic activity	
• ↑ ICP	

Diagnosis and Management
- Treat the underlying cause
- Resume home antihypertensives as soon as possible
- For initial management consider:
  Labetalol 5–40 mg IV bolus q10min or
  Hydralazine 2.5–20 mg IV bolus q10–20min or
  Lopressor 2.5–10 mg IV bolus
- For severe hypertension, consider vasodilator infusion
  Sodium nitroprusside (0.25–10 mcg/kg/min) or
  Nitroglycerine (10–100 mcg/min)
  Esmolol, nicardipine, cardizem infusions may also be used

RESPIRATORY AND AIRWAY PROBLEMS

Common Causes of Respiratory Insufficiency in the PACU		
Hypoventilation	**Upper Airway Obstruction**	**Hypoxemia**
• Residual anesthesia	• Airway edema	• Atelectasis
• Residual muscle relaxant	• Trauma	• Asthma/COPD exacerbation
• Postop opioids	• Vocal cord paralysis	• CHF/fluid overload
• Splinting $2°$ to pain	• Arytenoid dislocation	• Pulmonary embolism
• Tight abdominal binder	• Secretions	• ALI/ARDS
	• Foreign body	• Aspiration

• Obstructive sleep apnea/obesity	• Laryngospasm	• Pneumo/hemothorax pleural effusion
• Premature infants/neonates	• Anxiety/Munchausen stridor	• Diaphragmatic injury/paralysis
		• Pneumonia

Source: Adapted from Rose DK, Cohen MM, Wigglesworth DF, et al. Critical respiratory events in the postanesthesia care unit: patient, surgical, and anesthetic factors. *Anesthesiology* 1994;81:410–418.

Respiratory Insufficiency: Diagnosis & Management
1. Assess **A**irway, **B**reathing, **C**irculation
2. ↑ Delivered FiO$_2$, ↑ flow rate, & consider nonrebreather or shovel mask
3. Consider jaw thrust/chin lift, placement of oral/nasal airway
4. Consider positive-pressure ventilation with bag–valve mask
5. Consider intubation vs. noninvasive ventilation (CPAP/BiPAP)
6. Review pt Hx, OR & postop course, fluid status, & medications administered
7. Consider ABG, chest x-ray (rule out pneumothorax/pulmonary edema)

Respiratory Insufficiency: Management of Specific Conditions
Hypoventilation

Diagnosis	Hypoventilation/inadequate ventilation for sufficient gas exchange ↑ PaCO$_2$ & respiratory acidosis

Treatment of Hypoventilation	
Suspected Cause	**Therapy**
Residual inhalational/IV anesthesia	Arouse pt, encourage breathing/coughing
Residual muscle relaxant	Administer reversal (neostigmine or sugammadex)
Postop narcotic administration	Administer naloxone
Splinting 2° to pain	Initiate pain control, consider PCA/regional analgesia
Tight abdominal binder	Release binder, consult surgeon
Obstructive sleep apnea/obesity	Reposition pt, consider BiPAP
Premature infants/neonates	Supplemental O$_2$, consider acetaminophen/regional analgesia instead of narcotics

Fluid Overload/Pulmonary Edema

Diagnosis	Hypoxemia on ABG, high CVP/PCWP Chest x-ray: ↑ Pulmonary vasculature, ↑ interstitial/alveolar fluid, pleural effusion, fluid in fissure
Treatment	Stop IV fluids; administer diuretics (furosemide 20–100 mg IV) Provide supplemental O$_2$; consider noninvasive mechanical ventilation

Atelectasis

Diagnosis	↓ Breath sounds, opacification on chest x-ray
Treatment	Incentive spirometry; inhaled *N*-acetylcysteine to loosen secretions; reposition pt; CPAP/BiPAP; bronchoscopy to remove impacted secretions; chest physiotherapy; positive-pressure ventilation with PEEP

Asthma/COPD Exacerbation

Diagnosis	Wheezing on auscultation
Treatment	Albuterol/atrovent; steroids (methylprednisolone 125 mg IV); cromolyn sodium; CPAP/BiPAP; severe bronchospasm may require intubation Aminophylline (6 mg/kg IV load, followed by infusion 0.5–1 mg/kg/h)

Pulmonary Embolism

Diagnosis	ECG → sinus tach/S$_1$Q$_3$T$_3$; US of lower ext; D-dimer not helpful TTE/TEE → rule out central pulm embolism/assess RV dysfx CT chest/scan/pulm angiogram when stable
Treatment	Cautious fluid resuscitation, invasive monitoring, inotropes/pressors, consider thromboembolectomy/catheter-directed thrombolysis/anticoagulation/IVC filter placement

Acute Lung Injury (ALI)/Acute Respiratory Distress Syndrome (ARDS)

Diagnosis	ARDS = acute respiratory failure without evidence of left heart failure Bilateral infiltrates on chest x-ray, PaO_2/FiO_2 ratio <200 ALI = (ARDS features + PaO_2/FiO_2 ratio <300)
Treatment	Treat the underlying cause & maintain lung protective ventilation (See ARDS section in Chapter 19, Thoracic Surgery)

Aspiration

Diagnosis	Chest x-ray may reveal foreign body, infiltrates, atelectasis or collapse
Treatment	Supportive care for small aspirations (no respiratory compromise) Large aspirations: Rapid sequence intubation, gastric decompression, mechanical ventilation with high PEEP, bronchoscopy to remove large foreign bodies; prophylactic antibiotics & steroids are ineffective; bronchoalveolar lavage & routine suctioning should not be performed Prevent recurrence: Elevate head of bed, avoid sedation, place NG tube

Upper Airway Obstruction/Stridor

Causes	Airway edema/trauma, vocal cord paralysis, arytenoid dislocation, secretions, foreign body
Treatment	Racemic epinephrine, dexamethasone, humidified air, heliox Treat secretions with suctioning & admin of glycopyrrolate (0.2 mg IV) Severe edema/trauma may necessitate reintubation Obtain ENT consult for vocal cord paralysis/arytenoid dislocation/removal of foreign body

Pneumothorax/Hemothorax/Pleural Effusion

Diagnosis	Chest x-ray diagnostic most of the time
Treatment	Needle decompression of chest (2nd intercostal space in midclavicular line), chest tube decompression (also see Chapter 12, Procedures in Anesthesia) Exploratory thoracotomy for large hemothorax/ongoing bleeding

Diaphragmatic Injury/Paralysis

Diagnosis	Elevation of hemidiaphragm on chest x-ray
Treatment	Paralysis 2° to regional blocks are usually temporary Supportive treatment with ↑ FiO_2, reassurance, noninvasive ventilation Large diaphragmatic injury may require surgical repair

Pneumonia

Diagnosis	Fever, cough, leukocytosis, new infiltrate on chest x-ray Obtain respiratory secretions & blood cultures
Treatment	Broad-spectrum antibiotics

Laryngospasm

Diagnosis	Laryngospasm = involuntary contraction & closure of vocal cords Presence of inspiratory stridor, ↑ inspiratory effort, poor air exchange → leading to ↓ SpO_2, pulmonary edema, cardiac arrest Risk factors: Young age, upper respiratory infection, GERD, obesity, ENT surgery, obstructive sleep apnea
Treatment	Cessation of stimulation, positive-pressure ventilation with 100% O_2 if positive-pressure ventilation is ineffective Consider inducing anesthesia with propofol Consider inducing muscle relaxation with succinylcholine, 4% of pts with laryngospasm develop negative pressure pulmonary edema → consider mechanical ventilation with PEEP & diuresis

Anxiety/Munchausen Stridor

Diagnosis	Episodic inspiratory stridor (esp to attract attention), nl flow volume loops refractory to medical management of inspiratory stridor Risk factors include female, type A personality, anxiety d/o, GERD Fiberoptic laryngoscopy reveals posterior diamond-shaped glottis
Treatment	Pt education, speech therapy, benzodiazepines (lorazepam 1–2 mg IV)

NEUROLOGIC PROBLEMS

Common Problems

Delayed awakening, emergence delirium/confusion, anxiety/panic attack, peripheral neuropathy

Delayed Awakening (see Chapter 11, Common Intraoperative Problems)

Definition	Delayed awakening is said to occur when a pt fails to regain appropriate level of consciousness following general anesthesia

Causes of Delayed Awakening in PACU	
Anesthesia-related	Residual anesthetic Residual muscle relaxant, pseudocholinesterase deficiency Excessive narcotics
Metabolic	Hypothermia Hypoxemia Hypercarbia/hyponatremia/hypocalcemia/hypoglycemia Renal/hepatic failure
Intracranial event	Stroke/cerebrovascular accident (CVA) Seizure Intracranial hypertension

Diagnosis	Perform complete neuro assessment (cranial, motor, & sensory nerves)
	Review anesthetic record for drugs/doses
	Check for residual muscle relaxant with train-of-four/tetany
	Send ABG, serum sodium/calcium/glucose levels, check pt temp
	Consider application of bispectral index/EEG
	   → Low bispectral index may be suggestive of residual anesthetic
	   → EEG can assess for seizure activity
	Consider neurologic imaging to assess for stroke (noncontrast CT/MRI brain)
	Consider pseudocholinesterase deficiency (family Hx, pseudocholinesterase level, dibucaine number)

Treatment	Consider narcotic reversal if slow respiratory rate + pinpoint pupils → administer naloxone (0.04 mg IV q2min up to 0.2 mg IV) Consider benzo reversal with flumazenil (0.2 mg IV q2min up to 1 mg IV) Reverse muscle relaxants, correct electrolyte abnl, rewarm pt as indicated

Stroke

Risk factors	Geriatric pts, Hx of TIA/stroke, cardiac surgery (highest risk factor), aortic/carotid surgery, craniotomy, intraoperative hypotension, hypoxia, atrial fibrillation
Treatment	Consult neurology, maintain adequate SpO_2 & cerebral perfusion pressure

Seizure

Causes	Epilepsy d/o Hx, preop cessation of anticonvulsants, stroke, hypoxia, hypoglycemia, hyponatremia, hypocalcemia, hypophosphatemia, trauma, hypotension, EtOH withdrawal, local anesthetic overdose
Treatment	Benzodiazepine (lorazepam 1–5 mg IV) for ongoing seizures Provide supplemental O_2 & secure airway if needed Consult neurology

Intracranial Hypertension

Diagnosis	Place intracranial pressure monitor
Treatment	Hyperventilate pt to lower $PaCO_2$ Maintain CPP Consider administration of mannitol, furosemide, 3% saline Consider deep sedation/muscle relaxation/hypothermia in cases of refractory high ICP

Emergence Delirium/Confusion

Risk factors	High preop anxiety, benzodiazepine/ketamine use, age (toddlers & geriatrics), hypoxia, hypercarbia, hyponatremia, EtOH withdrawal, intubated pts, presence of Foley catheter
Diagnosis	Check ABG, electrolytes, consider CT scan of brain
Treatment	Treat underlying cause Reorient pt & avoid aggravating factors Haloperidol (2.5–10 mg IV)/soft limb restraints for combative pts

Anxiety/Panic Attack

Treatment	Reassurance, de-environmentalization, pain management helpful Consider benzodiazepines (lorazepam 1–2 mg IV or midazolam 1–2 mg IV)

Peripheral Neuropathy (see Chapter 15, Complications of Anesthesia)

Risk factors	Excessive stretch, compression, direct trauma, positioning, diabetes, male, BMI >37 or <24, prolonged hospital stay Ulnar neuropathy is most common
Treatment	Sensory neuropathies: Usually resolve in 1–2 wk Motor neuropathies: Require neurologist consult, EMG, physical therapy

---

POSTOPERATIVE NAUSEA AND VOMITING (PONV)

See Chapter 30, Postoperative Nausea and Vomiting

PACU DISCHARGE CRITERIA

- PACU discharge criteria are usually based on modified Aldrete score *(Anesthesiology 2002;96:742)*
- Assessment parameters include vitals, mental status, respiratory status, activity, surgical site status, pain control, recovery from regional anesthesia, and postop nausea or vomiting
- Clinical judgment should always supersede any score or criterion
- Postanesthesia recovery is divided into 2 phases
  Phase 1: Starts with pt entering PACU from OR till criteria are met for transfer to phase 2 in PACU/hospital room/ICU
  - *Pts are not discharged home from phase 1*
  - Some pts who meet criteria for phase 2 recovery may be fast tracked directly from OR to phase 2 recovery bypassing phase 1, if permitted by the hospital policy
  Phase 2: Starts with completion of phase 1, ends with pt discharge to home
  (J Clin Anesth 1995;7:89)

Guidelines for Discharge from Phase 2
- Redocumentation of vitals, postanesthesia recovery score
- Acceptable surgical site condition
- Adequate pain control (<3 out of 10 or tolerable)
- Ability to ambulate
- Recovery from regional anesthesia (except for peripheral nerve block)
- Discharge to a responsible individual
- Postanesthesia recovery score of ≥9
- Written & verbal instructions provided prior to discharge

Common Discharge Issues
- Passing of urine is **not** a mandatory requirement
- Ability to drink and retain fluids is **not** mandatory prior to discharge
- There is **no** minimum PACU stay period
- Responsible individual to accompany the pt home should be mandatory
(Anesthesiology 2013;118(2):291–307)

COMPLICATIONS OF ANESTHESIA

MICHAEL W. SANFORD • DAVID A. NAKATA

INTRODUCTION

Complications arise from human error, equipment malfunctions, and pt comorbidities.

PERIPHERAL NERVE INJURY

Classification of Peripheral Nerve Lesions

Neurapraxia: No peripheral degeneration → rapid recovery

Axonotmesis: Associated with axonal degeneration without complete destruction → recovery slow but typically complete

Neurotmesis: Separation of related parts of nerve occurs → recovery is poor

Anesthesia-related Causes

Ischemia secondary to

- Nerve stretch: Tension within axon leads to compression of arterial & venous plexus
- Direct nerve compression: Compressive forces > mean capillary pressure (35 mmHg) → resistance to flow & ischemia
- Both stretch & compression can act to simultaneously impact nerves (especially ulnar nerve, brachial plexus, sciatic nerve)

Duration of Ischemia

- Unknown what peripheral nerve ischemic time → permanent damage
- Comorbidities that ↓ vascular supply may ↓ time required before damage
- Vascular tourniquets (e.g., in orthopedic surgery) shown to produce reversible nerve conduction abnormalities
  → Tourniquet times <2 h thought to be well tolerated
  → Compression unlikely cause of postop neuropathy in short cases

Other Factors Impacting Peripheral Nerves

- Coexisting dz: Diabetes mellitus, nerve entrapment syndromes (osteo- & rheumatoid arthritis, previous trauma, tissue edema), metabolic abnormalities (malnutrition, vitamin deficiencies), drug related (chemotherapy), hereditary neuropathies, hypertension, tobacco use
- Coexisting issues may lead to neuropathies 2° to "double-crush syndrome" (two separate causes of nerve injury potentiate severity of injury)

Summary of ASA Practice Advisory: Prevention of Peripheral Neuropathy	
Preop assessment	• Helpful to ascertain that pts can comfortably tolerate anticipated operative position
Upper-extremity positioning	• Limit arm abduction to 90° in supine pts. Prone pts may comfortably tolerate arm abduction >90° • Position arms to ↓ pressure on postcondylar groove of humerus (ulnar groove); when arms tucked at side, neutral forearm position is recommended; when arms abducted on armboards, either supination or neutral forearm position acceptable • Avoid prolonged pressure on radial nerve in spiral groove of humerus • Extension of elbow beyond comfortable range may stretch the median nerve
Lower-extremity positioning	• Lithotomy positions that stretch hamstring muscle group beyond comfortable range may stretch the sciatic nerve • Avoid prolonged pressure on peroneal nerve at fibular head • Avoid extension or flexion of hip to ↓ risk of femoral neuropathy
Protective padding	• Padded armboards may ↓ risk of upper-extremity neuropathy • Chest rolls in laterally positioned pts may ↓ risk of upper-extremity neuropathies • Padding at elbow & fibular head may ↓ risk of upper- & lower-extremity neuropathies, respectively
Equipment	• Properly functioning automated BP cuffs on upper arms do not affect risk of upper-extremity neuropathies • Shoulder braces in steep head-down positions may ↑ risk of brachial plexus neuropathies

Postop assessment	• Simple postop assessment of extremity nerve function may lead to early recognition of peripheral neuropathies
Documentation	• Charting specific positioning actions during care of pts may result in improvements of care by helping practitioners focus attention on relevant aspects of pt positioning & providing information that continuous improvement processes lead to refinement in pt care

Source: Practice advisory for the prevention of perioperative peripheral neuropathies 2018: an updated report by the American Society of Anesthesiologists Task Force on prevention of perioperative peripheral neuropathies. Anesthesiology 2018;128(1):11–26.

AIRWAY/DENTAL COMPLICATIONS

Airway Complications

Incidence
- Unknown owing to varying significance/detection of injuries
- Minor trauma to larynx & pharynx may be as common as 6%
- Damage typically ↑ in relation to duration of intubation (many injuries result from placement of endotracheal tube)
- Many injuries occur during routine, "easy" intubations
- Delayed, chronic complications often present wk to even mo after extubation, particularly with prolonged intubations (>5 d)

Risk Factors for Intubation Trauma
- Difficult, traumatic, multiple attempts at intubation
- Laryngeal abnormalities (past trauma, inflammatory conditions, infection)
- Movement of endotracheal tube (tube manipulation/surgical repositioning, coughing/bucking)
- Impaired clearance of secretions
- Gastroesophageal reflux

Sites of Injury		
Nasal	Nasal alar necrosis	Preventable by careful (ETT) positioning
	Sinusitis	Incidence ↑ with duration of intubation (up to 20% with nasal intubation >5 d)
Oropharyngeal	Contusion/lacerations of lips or pharynx	Usually 2° to trauma from laryngoscope blade or ETT; rarely serious bleeding
	Dental trauma	Common (see discussion later)
Laryngeal & tracheal injury	Vocal cord/mucosal edema	Most significant complication early after extubation; presents with airway obstruction • Acute obstruction esp worrisome in children (smaller airway diameter) • Incidence of symptomatic laryngeal/tracheal edema up to 4% in kids • Tracheal erosion 2° to ETT trauma → tracheoesophageal fistula/tracheomalacia
	Granuloma formation	More common in adults, particularly women
	Vocal cord dysfunction	• May occur 2° to direct trauma, recurrent laryngeal nerve injury, arytenoid dislocation • Presents with partial airway obstruction/dysphonia • Bilateral vocal cord dysfunction presents as complete airway obstruction (requiring emergency airway) • May evaluate mobility with direct laryngoscopy under GA
	Tracheobronchial rupture	• Suspect with subcutaneous emphysema, respiratory distress, pneumomediastinum, & pneumothorax • May lead to mediastinitis & death

Pulmonary	*Aspiration*	• Occurs up to 0.05%, usually during induction • Ranges from benign mild inflammation to severe inflammation, pneumonitis, asphyxiation from airway obstruction, or lethal infectious pneumonia • Risk factors include emergency surgery, unanticipated airway difficulty, GI obstruction • Prevention with nonparticulate antacids, H_2 receptor antagonists, or gastroprokinetic agents
Esophageal	*Esophageal/ pharyngeal perforation*	• Often delayed presentation with mortality 25–50% • Associated with difficult intubation, elderly, female • Risk ↑ by insertion of devices such as TEE probes & esophageal dilators

Prevention
• Use small ETTs with lowest possible cuff pressures (leak <30 cm in pediatric pts)
• Limit use of adjuncts (such as intubating stylets)
• Wean ventilator to minimize duration of intubation
• Treat airway infections aggressively & early
• Minimize aspiration risk (when risk factors present)
• Perform detailed assessment to prevent unanticipated airway difficulty (to ↓ chance of otherwise preventable airway injury)
• Prepare alternative plans if intubation fails
• Discuss risk of airway injury with pts preop (shown to ↓ litigation)

Management
• Acute airway edema/stridor: Nebulized racemic epinephrine; dexamethasone controversial
• Prolonged intubation (>5 d): Consider laryngeal evaluation to evaluate for injury
• Chronic injury from repeated/prolonged intubation: Surgical correction may be required
• Tracheobronchial rupture: Emergent surgical correction

Obtain follow-up if concerned about airway trauma
• Inform pts if airway management was difficult/nonstandard

Dental Injuries
• Dental trauma: Most common permanent airway injury & leading source of malpractice claims (30–40%)
• Injuries: Fractured teeth, displaced restorations, subluxation, & avulsion (upper incisors most commonly affected secondary to use as fulcrum for laryngoscope)
• Deciduous tooth loss → can result in problems with permanent teeth
• Adverse outcomes → related to aspiration of teeth/restorations

Incidence
• Overall incidence: Reports range from 0.02–5% (75% of injuries occur during intubation)
• Injuries can occur during maintenance (poorly positioned airway, bite block, masseter spasm during wakeup)

Risk Factors
• Tracheal intubation; poor dentition/periodontal dz; difficult airway characteristics; past dental restoration/endodontic treatment; elderly pts; brittle enamel; loose deciduous teeth; inexperienced laryngoscopist

Prevention
• Detailed preop Hx & examination:
  → Caries/loose teeth, prostheses, past dental work
  → Assess mouth opening
  → Evaluate dentition, evidence of periodontal dz, tooth hypermobility
  → Document pre-existing conditions (reduces litigation if damage occurs)
• Consider tooth protection
  → Protectors (prefabricated rubber/custom-made by dentist)

Management
• Loosened tooth
  Return to original position promptly; splint with tape/suture

- Displaced fragment of tooth/restoration:
  Locate & recover all pieces; consider radiographs (chest, lateral head, & neck) to exclude passage through glottis
- Avulsed tooth
  Immediately recover tooth and assess if replacement feasible
  Avoid wiping or drying root surface
  Consider temporary splint with tape/suture
  If aspiration concern prevents immediate reimplantation
  → carefully place tooth in suitable medium (saline/milk)

Immediate dental referral, injury documentation, & discussion with pt important
- Most hospitals require filing an incident report
- Reimbursement responsibility depends on hospital policy

Burns
Intraoperative burns are rare; can be devastating/fatal

Surgical Fire
- 600 surgical fires per y in the United States
- Fire requires O_2, flammable materials, & ignition source
  → O_2 commonly administered in OR (endotracheal, nasal cannula)
  → Flammable materials = surgical drapes, alcohol prep solutions, plastic ETTs
  → Ignition sources = laser, electrosurgical units (ESUs), cautery
- Head & neck surgeries represent most cases involving fire in OR
  → Higher risk since nasal cannulas + laser/electrocautery → combustion
  → ETT carrying enriched O_2 can also ignite, leading to a "blowtorch" effect during positive-pressure ventilation

Airway Fire
- Prevention: ↓ FiO_2 during lasering; use heliox; use fire resistant ETTs; wrap ETT in metal tape; fill ETT cuff with saline, not air
- Management: Remove ETT/stop ventilation, discontinue O_2, douse fire with saline/water, mask-ventilate pt; perform bronchoscopy to assess airway damage

Electrocautery/Electrosurgical Unit
- Current path: Electrosurgical pencil → through pt → out grounding pad
- Current density dissipated over large surface area → limits risk of burn (because of low impedance return electrode)
- ESU-associated burns:
  → Improper placement of return electrode (↓ contact surface area)
  → Fluids (blood, irrigation, skin prep) cause improper electrode contact
  → Avoid placement of return electrode over bony prominences
  → ESUs can serve as ignition source (esp if ↑ O_2 conc in use)

Magnetic Resonance Imaging
- Complications usually involve metallic objects flying into magnetic field & burns
- MRI radio frequency can cause heating of current conducting materials:
  → ECG cables & electrodes
  Remove excess cables & avoid cable contact with skin
  Do not loop cables, ensure that ECG electrodes are firmly attached
  → Medicated patches
  Some contain aluminized backing (can heat in MRI)
  Avoid testosterone, nitro, nicotine, scopolamine, clonidine patches

Perioperative Blindness

Summary of ASA Practice Advisory: Perioperative Visual Loss & Spine Surgery
- Prone spine surgery pts who undergo prolonged operations and/or have substantial blood loss are at ↑ risk of perioperative visual loss
- Inform high-risk pts of the small, unpredictable risk of visual loss
- Avoid deliberate hypotension in high risk pts unless essential
- Use colloids along with crystalloids to maintain volume in pts with significant blood loss
- No transfusion threshold known to eliminate risk of visual loss 2° to anemia
- Position high-risk pts head level to or higher than heart; consider staged procedures

Source: Practice advisory for perioperative visual loss associated with spine surgery 2019: an updated report by the American Society of Anesthesiologists Task Force on Perioperative Visual Loss, the North American Neuro-Ophthalmology Society, and the Society for Neuroscience in Anesthesiology and Critical Care. *Anesthesiology* 2019;130:12–30.

ENHANCED RECOVERY AFTER SURGERY (ERAS)

BRIAN F. S. ALLEN • ADAM B. KING • MATTHEW D. McEVOY

3 factors that most commonly affect hospital length of stay: **pain**, **postoperative ileus**, and **immobilization** (Colorectal Dis 2006;8(6):506–13)

Many postoperative complications are related to inflammatory response generated due to surgery and perioperative management. Thus, many postoperative complications are thought to be preventable. ERAS protocols are shown to reduce surgical complications and hospital length of stay by 30% (Br J Surg 2014;101(3):172–88).

ERAS protocols aim to minimize these complications by standardized multimodal pain management with opioid avoidance, goal-directed fluid therapy, early ambulation, early refeeding, reduction of surgical site infection, and ileus and nausea prevention.

Enhanced Recovery After Surgery (ERAS) Pathways

- Pathways seek to improve outcomes, reduce cost, and speed recovery
- Focused interventions in the perioperative period focusing on:
  - Goal-directed fluid and hemodynamic therapy (GDFT/GDHT)
  - Non-Opioid Multimodal Analgesia (NOMA)
  - Prevention of postoperative nausea and vomiting (PONV)
  - Ileus prevention and early oral intake
  - Early ambulation

Components of a Typical Enhanced Recovery Pathway

Preoperative	Intraoperative	Postoperative
Pt education session	Use of regional anesthesia	Multimodal analgesia
Medical optimization	Standardized anesthetic	No or low opioid strategy
Evaluation by anesthesiology	Standardized surgical technique	Early mobilization
Nutritional assessment	Standardized nausea prevention	Early oral intake
Discharge planning	Goal-directed fluid therapy	Goal-directed discharge
Fluid & carbohydrate loading	No routine urinary catheters	Early removal of catheters
Thromboprophylaxis	No routine nasogastric tubes	Thromboprophylaxis
No/selective bowel prep		Audit compliance & outcomes

While initially developed in colorectal surgery, the benefits of ERAS protocols have been extended to other surgical populations including: Cystectomy, bariatric surgery, gastrectomy, liver surgery, pancreaticoduodenectomy, and total joint replacement

Agency for Healthcare Research and Quality

Enhanced Recovery Pathway Publications

Surgical type	Citation
Gynecologic surgery	Reg Anesth Pain Med 2019;44:437–46
Hip fracture	Anesth Analg 2018:1–11
Total knee arthroplasty	Anesth Analg 2019;128:441–53
Total hip arthroplasty	Anesth Analg 2019;128:454–65
Bariatric Surgery	Anesth Analg 2019 [epub ahead of print]

The principles underlying an ERAS Care Pathway are similar across many surgical pt populations, but no single approach has been shown superior to any other. Of note, 5 components have the strongest evidence: (1) Pt education, (2) thoracic epidural for open abdominal procedures, (3) targeted euvolemia/zero fluid balance, (4) no routine nasogastric decompression, (5) early feeding after surgery (JAMA 2019;321:1049–2).

Below are details of one such pathway at our institution, the ERAS Pathway for Colorectal Surgical Patients. Note that application in practice, particularly of multimodal analgesia and GDFT, requires assessment of the individual pt when selecting appropriate doses and medications.

Example of an Enhanced Recovery Pathway for Colorectal Surgical Pts[a]	
Preoperative	• Pt able to drink clear liquids until 2 h prior to surgery • Preoperative multimodal analgesia • Gabapentin (100–600 mg PO depending on age) • Acetaminophen (500–1,000 mg PO depending on weight) • Regional or neuraxial anesthesia performed • Thromboprophylaxis administered • Perioperative antibiotics (completed prior to incision)
Intraoperative	• Standardized surgical technique • Standardized anesthesia technique • Multimodal analgesia • Opioid minimization • Ketamine bolus (0.5 mg/kg) + infusion (5 mcg/kg/min) • Lidocaine bolus (100 mg) + infusion (2 mg/min) • Ketorolac 30 mg IV at discretion of surgeon and anesthesiologist • PONV prophylaxis (based on number of Apfel risk factors) • Targeting euvolumia; GDFT/GDHT with monitor[c] if open/high-risk • IVF: Plasma-lyte, Normosol, or LR; no normal saline • Normothermia (goal: Temp >36°C) • Glycemic control (goal: Glucose <180 mg/dL) • No routine nasogastric tube placement
Postoperative	• Early enteral nutrition: Clear liquids started POD1 • Ambulation by morning of POD1 (encouraged POD0) • Multimodal analgesia • *Scheduled* acetaminophen (500–1,000 mg PO q8h) • *Scheduled* gabapentin (100–600 mg PO q8h) • *Scheduled* ketorolac (15–30 mg IV) q6h ×3 d[b] • Lidocaine infusion (1–2 mg/min) × 24 h postoperatively • Ketamine infusion (2.5 mcg/kg/min) × 48 h • If open, no lidocaine/ketamine infusion and epidural in place until pt has return of bowel function • Oxycodone (5 mg PO q6h) PRN • Aggressive treatment of nausea or emesis • Discontinuation of maintenance IVF once pt tolerates >300 mL of PO fluid in 8 h • Early removal of urinary catheters • Discharge once the following goals are achieved: • Drinking and eating • Analgesia with oral medications • Mobilizing • Urinating without a catheter

[a]Based on Vanderbilt University Medical Center Enhanced Recovery Pathway for Colorectal Surgery Patients.
[b]Dose reduced for CrCl <30 mL/min, Weight <50 kg, or age >65; avoided if contraindications (eg, h/o bleeding ulcer).
POD, postoperative d; PO, by mouth
[c]Monitor = consider monitor that can provide indices of preload (PPV, SVV, ΔSV) and cardiac output.

ERAS 16-2

TRAUMA, BURN, AND CRITICAL CARE MANAGEMENT

JOSEPH R. PAWLOWSKI • DANIEL W. JOHNSON

INTRODUCTION

Also see Frendl G, Urman RD. *Pocket ICU*. 2nd ed. Philadelphia, PA: Lippincott Williams & Wilkins; 2017.

AIRWAY MANAGEMENT FOR TRAUMA

Intubation Indications
• Hypoxia, hypercarbia, trauma to the airway, severe shock, poor mental status (inability to protect airway or cooperate with procedures), severe head injury (GCS <8), inhalational injury

Intubation Considerations
• Higher incidence of difficult airway with trauma
• Facial and airway injuries
• May need emergent surgical airway management (notify surgeon early)
• Intubation often occurs prior to determination of cervical spine stability
• Must assume cervical spine instability during intubation (collar likely in place prior to airway management)
• Mask ventilation: Chin-lift contraindicated, jaw-thrust maneuver acceptable
• In-line stabilization of C-spine: Assistant holds head firmly in neutral/stable position using two-handed manual inline stabilization
• Remove collar immediately following onset of neuromuscular blockade
  • Allows normal mouth opening for laryngoscopy
  • Improves ease of mask ventilation
  • Allows access to the neck (for surgical airway)
• No evidence suggesting superiority of one method of intubation over another
• Perform RSI with careful direct or video laryngoscopy limiting spine movement → Obtain good intubating conditions in short amount of time
• Consider awake/asleep fiberoptic intubation (FOI) only if the pt has isolated neck, facial, or airway injury making FOI the safest method, or use induction with maintenance of spontaneous ventilation during laryngoscopy, use of a lighted stylet, early tracheostomy (especially in pts with facial/laryngeal injury)
• FOI may not be appropriate for pts with significant bleeding at the airway. Instead, surgical airway may be the fastest and safest method.

Induction Considerations
• Goal: Avoid hypotension (damaged tissue will tolerate ischemia poorly)
• All trauma pts considered "full stomach" (consider rapid sequence induction)
• Tailor induction to minimize hypotension
• Pts *in extremis* may require little/no sedation for intubation
• If succinylcholine is contraindicated, consider rocuronium 1.2 mg/kg IV
  • Succinylcholine is contraindicated after the 1st 12 h following major burn, immobilization, or denervation due to upregulation of acetylcholine receptors
  • After 24 h, risk of hyperkalemic cardiac arrest rises further

Acute Spinal Cord Injury (ASCI)
General Considerations
• Most injuries from fracture/dislocation of vertebral column
• Major causes of death in spinal cord–injured pts are aspiration and shock

Anesthesia Considerations
• Movement of pt: C-spine stabilization or log-rolling must be performed carefully to maintain spine alignment
• Pt positioning: If turning prone, ensure endotracheal tube is secure
• Impairment of pulmonary mechanics: In pts with high spinal cord injuries, muscular control of ventilation may be impaired (can lead to atelectasis → ↓ in FRC →V–Q mismatch)
• Often increased vagal tone in cervical spine injuries; pts may have bradycardic events/arrest during suctioning/positioning

Significance of Spinal Cord Injury Site (Most Common Injury Sites: C5–6, T12–L1)
C3	→ Impaired innervation of diaphragm/necessitates ventilatory support
C7	→ Reduced vital capacity/FEV$_1$ (up to 70%)
T1	→ At least incomplete tetraplegia
T4	→ Bradycardia is possible
T7	→ Reduced strength of accessory muscles of breathing
L4	→ At least incomplete paraplegia

Steroid Therapy for Acute Spinal Cord Injury
- High-dose steroid (methylprednisolone) therapy is not recommended to improve motor outcomes after ASCI (Neurosurgery 2013;72(3):93–105), although some surgeons consider it a treatment option
  - If used, must be initiated within 8 h of injury
  - Methylprednisolone loading dose 30 mg/kg IV over 1 h followed by:
    - 5.4 mg/kg/h IV infusion for next 23 h if started within 0–3 h of injury
    - 5.4 mg/kg/h IV infusion for 47 h if started within 3–8 h of injury
- Steroid use is associated with increased mortality in pts with moderate to severe traumatic brain injury, and should be avoided in these cases
- No evidence supports the use of steroids in penetrating ASCI
- Must administer stress ulcer & hyperglycemia prophylaxis during steroid therapy

Neurogenic Shock
- Triad of hypotension, bradycardia, and hypothermia from functional sympathectomy (loss of vascular tone) and/or loss of cardiac inotropy/chronotropy secondary to high spinal cord injury
- More common in mid-thoracic injuries and higher
- In high cord injuries, loss of cardiac accelerator function & unopposed parasympathetic tone contribute to bradycardia (exacerbates impaired cardiac output)
- Consider anticholinergics/β-agonists to ↑ heart rate
- Consider α-agonists to restore peripheral vascular tone & improve venous return

Spinal Shock
- Disruption of all cord function caudal to spinal cord injury
- Causes flaccid weakness/lack of spinal arc reflexes at and below injury

Autonomic Hyperreflexia
- Most common in injuries above T6, occurs wk to mo after the acute injury
- Results from loss of descending inhibitory impulses + sympathetic system overactivity
- Stimulation below injury level (bladder distention, surgical stimulation) causes:
  - Vasoconstriction/hypertension below injury
  - Reflex bradycardia & dysrhythmias
  - Vasodilation above injury
- Symptoms: Headaches, blurred vision, seizures, cerebral hemorrhage, pulmonary edema 2° to left heart failure, loss of consciousness, nasal congestion, cutaneous flushing
- Treatment:
  - Remove stimulus
  - Consider atropine for severe bradycardia
  - Hypertension treated with direct vasodilators (nitroprusside/nitroglycerin), α-blockers (prazosin), ganglionic blockers (trimethaphan)
  - Consider using general anesthesia or spinal; epidural may not be as effective because of sacral sparing effect

Intraoperative Trauma Management

Trauma Room Setup
Anesthesia machine on, fully checked & primed with 100% oxygen
OR table in correct position
Thermostat ↑ (ahead of time) to warm room
Airway equipment (including suction) available & difficult airway cart nearby
Standard monitors; invasive pressure transducers
Anesthetic & vasoactive drugs
Defibrillator available

| Forced-air warming apparatus & blankets |
| IV tubing (must be primed); fluid warmer |
| Inflatable pressure bags and rapid infusion device |
| Supplies for large-bore IV, arterial, central access |

Goal: Optimize pt stability while not delaying surgical control of bleeding. Clear communication must be maintained despite chaotic environment.

Maintenance of Anesthesia
- Overall goal is to avoid and treat the "lethal triad": Acidosis, hypothermia, coagulopathy
- Maintenance options may include a combination of hypnotic, analgesic, and neuromuscular blocking agents
- "Damage control" surgery refers to the standard strategy of focusing initial surgical efforts on stopping bleeding and limiting contamination, delaying definitive repair
- Normal doses of volatile agent may cause hypotension in unstable pts
- Nitrous oxide typically avoided due to potential pneumothorax/other air collections
- Trauma pts are at high risk of intraoperative recall (consider processed EEG monitoring)

Management of Hypotension
- Ensure adequate cardiac preload (volume resuscitation)
  - If pt is rapidly exsanguinating, instruct the surgeon to aggressively pack, apply pressure to the bleeding area, and/or clamp proximal to injury until adequate volume can be administered
- Vasopressors/inotropes as necessary, consider categories of shock:
  - Hypovolemic shock (hemorrhage)
  - Cardiogenic shock (myocardial injury/pre-existing heart dz)
  - Obstructive shock (pericardial tamponade, tension pneumothorax, pulmonary emboli)
  - Distributive shock (SIRS/sepsis, anaphylaxis)
  - Neurogenic shock (cord injury)
- Communicate hemodynamic status to the surgical team
  - Surgeons can often adjust clamp/pack placement, or organ manipulation to help if needed
- Consider concomitant intoxication as a cause of cardiovascular instability and/or altered mental status

Emergence/Transport
Preparation before transporting intubated/sedated pt to the ICU includes:
- Functioning bag valve mask + full oxygen tank
- Equipment for mask ventilation/reintubation
- Emergency drugs (phenylephrine, ephedrine, atropine, epinephrine, succinylcholine)
- Transport monitor (SpO$_2$, ECG, blood pressure; consider capnography)
- Assistance to move the bed & secure elevators
Considerations during emergence:
- Severe hypertension may disrupt clots
- Airway may be edematous after volume resuscitation
  - An "easy airway" at induction might be difficult after massive fluid administration
  - Ensure help and equipment for rapid reintubation available

Fluid Resuscitation
Overall goal: Maintain perfusion to vital organs while surgeon controls hemorrhage

Goals for Early Resuscitation of the Trauma Patient in Hemorrhagic Shock
Maintain SBP 90–110 or MAP 60–70 (goal may be higher if pt has neurologic injury)
Maintain Hgb 7–9
Maintain INR <1.8
Maintain platelets >50,000
Maintain normal serum ionized Ca^{2+}
Maintain core temperature >35°C
Prevent acidosis from worsening

Obtain Adequate Vascular Access
- Peripheral IVs (14G catheters—can deliver up to 500 mL/min)
- Peripheral rapid infusion catheter (can deliver 850 mL/min)
- 9-Fr central venous "introducer" catheter (can deliver 1,000 mL/min) (Note: PICCs and triple-lumen catheters deliver at far slower rates than large-bore IVs)
- Consider rapid infusion devices and/or pressure bags (must take care to avoid administration of IV air when giving fluids under pressure)

Fluid Resuscitation
- Choice of fluid is debated; most experts agree that warmed lactated Ringer's or other balanced crystalloids are the initial fluid of choice, while blood is obtained
- Colloids are more expensive and their superiority over crystalloids is not supported by evidence. Colloids are contraindicated in head trauma.
- Avoid excessive administration of fluids (causes dilution of platelets/coagulation factors, reversal of compensatory vasoconstriction, breakage of clots due to rapid volume expansion)

Transfusion Therapy (see Chapter 10, Fluids, Electrolytes, & Transfusion Therapy)
- *Packed red blood cells (PRBCs)*
- Uncross-matched blood (type O)—use if pt has unstable hemorrhagic shock
- Type-specific blood—substitute for type O as soon as possible
- Transfusion rate depends on bleeding rate
- Goal is to maintain Hb above 7–9 (recheck frequently)
- *Fresh frozen plasma (FFP) and platelets*
  - For massive hemorrhage/transfusion, evidence supports the use of a 1:1:1 strategy:
    - For every unit of PRBCs transfused, give 1 unit of FFP
    - For every 6 units of FFP and PRBCs, give 1 **dose** of platelets (a "6-pack" of platelets from conventional donation, or 1 unit of apheresis platelets)
  - ABO compatibility required for FFP; Rh compatibility not required
  - INR <1.8 and platelet count >50,000 are generally desirable
- *Adverse effects of massive transfusion*
  - Calcium depletion $2°$ to citrate chelation
  - Transfusion reaction (given cumulative risk of clerical errors)
  - Hyperkalemia (secondary to hemolysis in stored blood)
  - Transfusion-related acute lung injury (TRALI)
  - Volume overload/congestive heart failure (CHF)

Monitoring during Fluid Resuscitation in OR
- Pulse pressure variation and systolic pressure variation
- Transesophageal echocardiography
- Urine output
- Serum markers of global tissue perfusion (degree of acidosis, base deficit, lactate, central/mixed venous O_2 saturation)

Rhabdomyolysis	
Definition	Acute disintegration of striated muscle
Causes	Trauma, crush injury, electrical shock, CPR, ischemia, arterial occlusion (including cross-clamp and REBOA), compartment syndrome, DIC, burn injury, hypothermia, medications, & illicit drugs
Signs/ symptoms	Acute myalgias/pigmenturia
	↑ Serum CK, myoglobin, potassium, urea, & phosphorus
	Arrhythmias (caused by excess potassium + hypocalcemia)
Consequence	Free myoglobin toxic to renal tubules → acute kidney injury
Course	CK levels typically peak 2–5 d after initial insult
	Levels >16,000 U/L more likely to cause kidney injury
	Hypocalcemia (from influx/deposition of Ca^{2+} in damaged muscle) may occur
Therapy	Restore blood flow to ischemic areas
	IV fluids (maintain urine output 200 mL/h until CK levels ↓)
	Mannitol and sodium bicarbonate are **not** supported by evidence
	Treat hypocalcemia if tetany/severe hyperkalemia develops
	Treat compartment syndrome if it develops
	Dialysis if fluid resuscitation fails to correct intractable hyperkalemia and/ or acidosis

Necrotizing Fasciitis/Myonecrosis	
Definitions	Deep infection that involves fascia & subcutaneous tissue; myonecrosis indicates muscle involvement
Signs/symptoms	Cellulitis, ↑ temp, lethargy, subcutaneous tissue has hard, "wooden" feel, pain out of proportion to examination; gas gangrene = severe fulminant clostridial myonecrosis (may also see crepitus)
Pathology	Typically Group A streptococcal species, *Staph aureus*, anaerobic streptococcal species & bowel flora
Course	Infections can spread rapidly/cause systemic toxicity; mortality is high
Treatment	Early surgical debridement & broad-spectrum antibiotics

Nutrition
Enteral feeding—preferred over parenteral nutrition (promotes maintenance of intestinal tissue)

Total Parenteral Nutrition (TPN)
- Use only when adequate enteral feeding not possible
- Must be given centrally (due to ↑ osmolarity)
- Typical TPN formula: Carbohydrates 50–60%, proteins 15–25%, lipids 20–30% Insulin therapy/frequent glucose monitoring required to avoid hyperglycemia → insulin can be added to TPN solution
- Monitor labs at least weekly: Electrolytes, aminotransferases, alkaline phosphatase, bilirubin, triglycerides, cholesterol, prealbumin, and transferrin
- Complications
  → Infection/sepsis, excessive CO_2 production, hepatic steatosis, hyperglycemia, hyperlipidemia, impaired immune function, electrolyte derangements, muscle weakness
- Intraoperative management
  → Avoid abrupt cessation of TPN without replacing carbohydrate source (risk of hypoglycemia)

Glycemic Control in ICU Patients
- Conventional glucose maintenance (<180) is superior to aggressive glucose maintenance (80–110)
  → Increased risks of aggressive glycemic control = hypoglycemia, death

---

BURN MANAGEMENT

Pathophysiology
- Skin destruction → impairs heat regulation, fluid/electrolyte maintenance, microbial barrier
- Circulating mediators trigger systemic inflammatory response
  → Hypermetabolism, immunosuppression, & alteration in cell membrane permeability
  → Massive fluid shifts from vascular compartment to burned tissue
  → Edema occurs in burned tissue as well as in unaffected tissues
  → Fluid loss from intravascular space can cause hypovolemic shock

Initial Evaluation and Management
Depth of burn injury: 1st, 2nd, & 3rd degree classification system replaced by:
- Superficial → involves only the epidermis, painful, dry, red
- Partial-thickness
  - Superficial partial-thickness → involves the epidermis & dermis, blisters and blanches with pressure
  - Deep partial-thickness → extends into deeper dermis, involves hair follicles and glands, does not blanch
- Full thickness → destroys all layers of dermis and may extend to subcutaneous tissue
- Extension to deep tissues (4th degree) → extends through skin into underlying soft tissue, muscle, and/or bone
Total body surface area (TBSA; Fig. 17-1)
- "Rule of nines" estimates surface area burned in adult pts (Fig. 17-1)
  → Head & each upper extremity represent = 9% TBSA
  → Anterior trunk, posterior trunk, & each lower extremity = 18% TBSA
  → Less accurate in children, due to different bodily proportions (Fig. 17-1)
Referral to a designated burn center

Figure 17-1 Rule of nines.

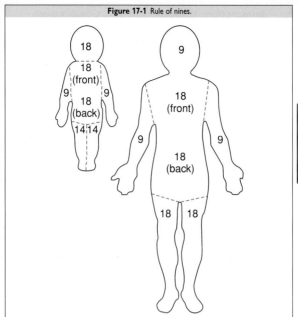

(Courtesy of J. Ehrenfeld, MD.)

- Transfer pt once stabilized if: Any 3rd-degree burn; burn is >10% TBSA; burn involves hands, feet, face, perineum, or major joints; electrical or chemical burns; inhalation injury; complex co-morbidity; burned children

Baux score – mortality risk
- Age + TBSA + 17 (if inhalation injury present).
- Score of 110 = 50% mortality (*J Trauma Acute Care Surg* 2012;72(1):251–256)

Airway and Respiratory Management
- Deliver maximal FiO$_2$ during initial resuscitation of major burn victims
- Inspiration of hot gases
  → Can cause direct airway damage/obstruction from edema
- Tracheal intubation usually indicated in large burns → perform before airway edema renders this impossible
- Suspect possible inhalation injury when head/neck involved (singed nasal hairs, swelling of nose, mouth, lips, throat; cough productive of soot)
- Chest wall expansion may be ↓ in major chest burns → consider emergency escharotomies
  → All inhalational injuries = potential "difficult airway" (due to cord edema); prep for surgical airway

Cardiovascular and Fluid Management
- Parkland formula: 4 mL of lactated Ringer's per kg per % TBSA burn in initial 24 h
  - Half of calculated fluid given during 1st 8-h postburn, remainder over next 16 h (e.g., 70 kg man with 60% TBSA burn needs 4 × 70 × 60 = 16,800 mL; give 8,400 mL of LR during 0–8 h after burn, 8,400 mL during 8–24 h)
  - Pt's daily maintenance fluid should be given concurrently
- Cardiac output reduced immediately postburn (↓ circulating vol + direct myocardial depression)
- 3–5 d postburn, hypermetabolic state → ↑ cardiac output (2–3 × normal), ↓ SVR

INTRAOPERATIVE MANAGEMENT: GENERAL CONSIDERATIONS

Airway management:	Often challenging → from edema/deformity of normal anatomy. NG tube should be placed early (pts often develop ileus after burn)
Monitors:	ASA standards, must have temp monitoring, consider CVP line
Resuscitation:	Correct acidosis/electrolyte abnl, address coagulopathies; expect large volume blood loss during excision & grafting (order adequate colloid/blood products in advance) (obtain IV access for large volume resuscitation)
Warming modalities:	Cover pt, ↑ OR temp, warm all fluids, use warming blankets; heat often lost during pt transport to & from OR

Anesthesia for Burn Surgery

Relaxants:	Depolarizing agent succinylcholine is dangerous after initial 12 h (potential for profound hyperkalemia & subsequent cardiac arrest)
	Burn pts exhibit ↓ response nondepolarizing agents, often need ↑ dose
Induction:	Consider ketamine in pts with uncertain CV/volume status
Maintenance:	After early course (during which high FiO₂ desirable), nitrous oxide may be added
Analgesia:	↑ Opioid requirements due to tolerance & ↑ in volume of distribution

SEPSIS AND SEPTIC SHOCK

Definitions:
- **Sepsis** is life-threatening organ dysfunction caused by a dysregulated host response to infection (*JAMA* 2016;315(8):801–810)
  - Organ dysfunction is an ↑ of two or more points in the SOFA score
- **Septic shock** is a subset of sepsis in which particularly profound circulatory, cellular, and metabolic abnormalities are associated with a greater risk of mortality than with sepsis alone

SOFA Score		
Lung: Respiration	PaO_2/FiO_2 >400	0 points
	PaO_2/FiO_2 301–400	1 point
	PaO_2/FiO_2 <301	2 points
	PaO_2/FiO_2 101–200 with ventilatory support	3 points
	PaO_2/FiO_2 <101 with ventilatory support	4 points
Coagulation: Platelets	>150 ×10³/mm³	0 points
	101–150 ×10³/mm³	1 point
	51–100 ×10³/mm³	2 points
	21–50 ×10³/mm³	3 points
	<21 ×10³/mm³	4 points
Liver: Bilirubin	<1.2 mg/dL	0 points
	1.2–1.9 mg/dL	1 point
	2–5.9 mg/dL	2 points
	6–11.9 mg/dL	3 points
	>12 mg/dL	4 points
Cardiovascular: Blood pressure	Hypotension absent	0 points
	Mean arterial pressure <70 mmHg	1 point
	On dopamine ≤5 mcg/kg/min or any dobutamine	2 points
	On dopamine >5 mcg/kg/min, epinephrine ≤0.1 mcg/kg/min, or norepinephrine ≤0.1 mcg/kg/min	3 points
	On dopamine >15 mcg/kg/min, epinephrine >0.1 mcg/kg/min, or norepinephrine >0.1 mcg/kg/min	4 points
Brain: Glasgow coma score (GCS)	15	0 points
	13–14	1 point
	10–12	2 points
	6–9	3 points
	<6	4 points

Kidney: Renal function	Creatinine <1.2 mg/dL	0 points
	Creatinine 1.2–1.9 mg/dL	1 point
	Creatinine 2–3.4 mg/dL	2 points
	Creatinine 3.5–4.9 mg/dL or urine output 200–500 mL/d	3 points
	Creatinine >5 mg/dL or urine output <200 mL/d	4 points

Screening for Early Sepsis
- Quick SOFA (qSOFA) score useful in pts with suspected infection outside of the ICU. Greater predictive validity for in-hospital mortality than SOFA and SIRS (*JAMA 2016;315(8):801–810*)

qSOFA Score		
Altered mental status	GCS < 15	1 point
Fast respiratory rate	Rate ≥22 breaths/min	1 point
Low blood pressure	Systolic blood pressure ≤100 mmHg	1 point
A score of 2 or 3 predicts greater chance of mortality		

Acute Physiology and Chronic Health Evaluation (APACHE) II Score
- Most commonly used ICU illness scoring system: ↑ Score = ↑ dz severity/risk of death
- Useful in initial evaluation of pts with sepsis
- Calculated based on temp, MAP, heart rate, respiratory rate, $P(A-a)O_2$ or PaO_2 (depending on FiO_2), arterial pH, sodium, potassium, creatinine, hematocrit, WBC count, GCS score, HCO_3, age, and chronic health status
- Several web-based calculators available (http://www.sfar.org/scores2/apache22.html)

Associated Problems in Sepsis
- Shock (from vasodilation, intravascular depletion +/– myocardial depression)
- Respiratory failure (from endothelial injury → alveolar capillary leak → impaired oxygenation)
- Acute respiratory distress syndrome (ARDS)
- Renal failure/metabolic acidosis
- Disseminated intravascular coagulopathy (DIC)
- Multiple organ dysfunction syndrome

Early Quantitative Fluid Resuscitation
- Overall goal: Maintain perfusion to organs while infection is treated
  - Most important factor for survival: EARLY administration of antibiotics
- Specific goals for fluid administration include:
  - CVP 8–12 mmHg
  - MAP >65 mmHg
  - Urine output >0.5 mL/kg/h

Markers of Resuscitation in Sepsis
- Trend of lactic acid level or base deficit
- Continuous or intermittent central or mixed venous oxygen saturation monitoring: Inadequate tissue perfusion → rise in oxygen extraction → low SvO_2 or $ScvO_2$

MANAGEMENT OF SEPSIS

Summary of Recommendations from the Surviving Sepsis Guidelines 2016 (*Crit Care Med 2017;45(3):486–552*)

The following evidence-based classification is used to grade the quality of evidence and the strength of recommendations:

Quality of evidence: High, Moderate, Low, Very Low

Strength of recommendation: Strong, Weak

Ungraded strong recommendation: Best Practice Statement (BPS)

- **Screening for sepsis and performance improvement**
  Hospitals should have a performance improvement program for sepsis, including sepsis screening for acutely ill, high-risk pts (BPS)
- **Initial resuscitation**
  - Treatment and resuscitation for sepsis should begin immediately (BPS)
  - To resuscitate hypoperfusion, at least 30 mL/kg of IV crystalloid fluid should be given within the 1st 3 h (strong recommendation, low quality evidence), and additional fluids guided by frequent reassessment of hemodynamics (BPS)

- Further hemodynamic assessment (such as assessing cardiac function) should occur to determine the type of shock (BPS)
- Dynamic over static variables should be used to predict fluid responsiveness, where available (weak recommendation, low quality evidence)
- Initial target mean arterial pressure (MAP) of 65 mmHg should be the goal in pts with septic shock requiring vasopressors (strong recommendation, moderate evidence)
- Resuscitation should be guided by normalizing lactate in pts with elevated lactate levels (weak recommendation, low quality evidence)
- **Diagnosis**
  - Appropriate routine microbiologic cultures should be obtained before starting antimicrobial therapy in pts with suspected sepsis or septic shock, if doing so results in no substantial delay in starting antimicrobials (BPS)
  - Appropriate cultures always include at least two sets of blood cultures (aerobic and anaerobic)
- **Antimicrobial therapy**
  - IV antimicrobials should be initiated as soon as possible after recognition and within 1 h (strong recommendation, moderate quality evidence)
  - Empiric therapy should have activity against all likely pathogens (strong recommendation, moderate quality evidence)
  - Narrow empiric therapy once pathogen sensitivities are established and/or clinical improvement is noted (BPS)
  - Antimicrobial prophylaxis is not recommended in pts with severe inflammatory states that are not infectious (BPS)
  - Empiric therapy should be aimed at the most likely bacterial pathogen (weak recommendation, low quality evidence)
  - Combination therapy should not routinely be used for ongoing treatment of most other serious infections (weak recommendation, low quality evidence)
  - Combination therapy should not be used for routine treatment of neutropenic sepsis/bacteremia (strong recommendation, moderate quality evidence)
  - Combination therapy should be de-escalated within the 1st few d in response to clinical improvement (BPS)
  - Antimicrobial therapy lasting 7–10 d is adequate for most infections (weak recommendation, low quality evidence)
  - Longer courses of antibiotics are appropriate for pts who have slow clinical response, undrainable foci of infection, S. aureus infection, some fungal and viral infections, or immunologic deficiencies (weak recommendation, low quality evidence)
  - Shorter courses of antibiotics are appropriate for pts who quickly improve following effective source control of intra-abdominal or urinary sepsis and those with anatomically uncomplicated pyelonephritis (weak recommendation, low quality evidence)
  - Daily assessment for de-escalation of antibiotics should occur (BPS)
  - Procalcitonin levels can be used to support shortening the duration of antimicrobial therapy (weak recommendation, low quality evidence)
  - Procalcitonin levels can be used to support discontinuing empiric antibiotics in pts who subsequently have limited evidence of infection (weak recommendation, low quality evidence)
- **Source control**
  - A specific anatomic source of infection requiring emergent source control should be identified as rapidly as possible, and any required source control intervention be implemented as soon as possible (BPS)
  - Intravascular access devices that are a possible source should be removed as promptly as possible after other vascular access is established (BPS)
- **Fluid therapy**
  - A fluid challenge technique should be applied when giving fluids as long as hemodynamic factors continue to improve (BPS)
  - Crystalloids are the fluid of choice for initial resuscitation and subsequent volume replacement (strong recommendation, moderate quality evidence)
  - Balanced crystalloids or saline should be used for fluids (weak recommendation, low quality evidence)
  - Albumin can be added to crystalloids when pts require a substantial amount of crystalloid for resuscitation (weak recommendation, low quality evidence)
  - Recommend against hydroxyethyl starches (HESs) (strong recommendation, high quality evidence)
  - Use crystalloids over gelatins when resuscitating pts (weak recommendation, low quality evidence)

- **Vasopressor therapy**
  - Norepinephrine should be the 1st-line pressor used (strong recommendation, moderate quality evidence)
  - Add either vasopressin (up to 0.03 U/min) (weak recommendation, moderate quality evidence) or epinephrine (weak recommendation, low quality evidence) to norepinephrine with the intent of raising MAP to target, or adding vasopressin to ↓ norepinephrine dosage (weak recommendation, moderate quality evidence)
  - Use dopamine only in select pts (e.g., pts with bradycardia and low risk of tachyarrhythmias) (weak recommendation, low quality evidence)
  - Low-dose dopamine for renal protection is not recommended (strong recommendation, high quality evidence)
  - Use dobutamine in pts who show evidence of persistent hypoperfusion despite adequate fluid loading and use of vasopressors (weak recommendation, low quality evidence)
  - All pts requiring vasopressors should have an arterial line placed as soon as practical (weak recommendation, very low quality evidence)
- **Corticosteroids**
  - IV hydrocortisone is not recommended unless fluid resuscitation and vasopressor therapy are unable to restore hemodynamic stability (weak recommendation, low quality evidence)
- **Blood products**
  - Transfuse RBCs only when hemoglobin concentration decreases to <7 g/dL unless there is myocardial ischemia, severe hypoxemia, or acute hemorrhage (strong recommendation, high quality evidence)
  - Erythropoietin to treat anemia associated with sepsis is not recommended (strong recommendation, moderate quality evidence)
  - Fresh frozen plasma should not be used to correct clotting abnormalities unless there is bleeding or a planned invasive procedure (weak recommendation, very low quality evidence)
  - Transfuse platelets when counts are <10,000/mm^3 in the absence of bleeding and when counts are <20,000/mm^3 if the pt has a significant risk of bleeding. Higher platelet counts (>50,000/mm^3) for active bleeding or procedures (weak recommendation, very low quality evidence)
- **Immunoglobulins**
  - The use of IV immunoglobulins is not recommended (weak recommendation, low quality evidence)
- **Blood purification**
  - No recommendation is made (e.g., plasma exchange, plasma filtration)
- **Anticoagulants**
  - Antithrombin is not recommended (strong recommendation, moderate quality evidence)
  - No recommendation is made regarding thrombomodulin or heparin
- **Mechanical ventilation**
  - Target tidal volume of 6 mL/kg predicted body weight should be used in adults with sepsis-induced ARDS (strong recommendation, high quality evidence)
  - Plateau pressures should have an upper limit goal of 30 cm H_2O in pts with severe ARDS (strong recommendation, moderate quality evidence)
  - Higher PEEP over lower PEEP should be used in moderate to severe ARDS (weak recommendation, moderate quality evidence)
  - Prone over supine positioning should be used in adults with ARDS and a PaO$_2$/FIO$_2$ ratio <150 (strong recommendation, moderate quality evidence)
  - Neuromuscular blockade should be used for <48 h (weak recommendation, moderate quality evidence)
  - β-2 agonists are not recommended to treat ARDS without bronchospasm (strong recommendation, moderate quality evidence)
  - Routine use of the PA catheter is not recommended (strong recommendation, high quality evidence)
  - Mechanically ventilated pts should have the head of the bed elevated between 30° and 45° to limit aspiration risk (strong recommendation, low quality evidence)
  - Spontaneous breathing trials should be used in pts who are ready for weaning (strong recommendation, high quality evidence)
- **Sedation and analgesia**
  - Continuous or intermittent sedation should be minimized, targeting specific titration end points (BPS)

- **Glucose control**
  - A protocolized approach should commence when 2 consecutive blood glucoses are >180 mg/dL, and target an upper glucose level of ≤180 mg/dL (strong recommendation, high quality evidence)
  - Blood glucose should be monitored every 1–2 h until values and insulin rates are stable, and every 4 h thereafter in pts on insulin infusion (BPS)
  - Arterial blood rather than capillary blood should be used for point-of-care testing if pts have arterial catheters (weak recommendation, low quality evidence)
- **Renal replacement therapy**
  - Either continuous or intermittent RRT should be used in pts with sepsis and acute kidney injury (weak recommendation, moderate quality evidence)
  - CRRT should be used to facilitate fluid balance management in hemodynamically unstable pts (weak recommendation, very low quality evidence)
  - RRT should not be used in pts with acute kidney injury for creatinine ↑ or oliguria without other definitive indications for dialysis (weak recommendation, low quality evidence)
- **Bicarbonate therapy**
  - Sodium bicarbonate should not be used in pts with hypoperfusion-induced lactic acidemia unless pH <7.15 (weak recommendation, moderate quality evidence)
- **Venous thromboembolism (VTE) prophylaxis**
  - Prophylaxis with unfractionated heparin (UFH) or low–molecular-weight heparin (LMWH) should be used unless contraindicated (strong recommendation, moderate quality evidence)
  - LMWH rather than UFH should be used unless LMWH is contraindicated (strong recommendation, moderate quality evidence)
  - Combination pharmacologic VTE prophylaxis and mechanical prophylaxis should be used if possible (weak recommendation, low quality evidence)
- **Stress ulcer prophylaxis**
  - Either proton pump inhibitors or histamine-2 receptor antagonists should be used in pts who have risk factors for gastrointestinal bleeding (weak recommendation, low quality evidence)
- **Nutrition**
  - Start enteral nutrition early. Early parenteral nutrition alone or in combination with enteral feedings is not recommended (strong recommendation, moderate quality evidence)
  - Use IV glucose and advance feeds as tolerated over the 1st 7 d rather than initiate parenteral nutrition (strong recommendation, moderate quality evidence)
  - Feeding tubes should be placed postpyloric in pts with feeding intolerance or who are considered to be at high risk of aspiration (weak recommendation, low quality evidence)
- **Goals of care, communication of prognosis**
  - Discuss with pts and families (BPS)
  - Integrate goals of care into 1 treatment plan, including palliative care plans and end-of-life planning (strong recommendation, moderate quality evidence)
  - Goals of care should be addressed as early as possible but no later than 72 h after ICU admission (weak recommendation, low quality evidence)

An Approach to Sedation of ICU Patients
- Evaluate and treat pain (uncontrolled pain = risk factor for delirium)
- Evaluate and address delirium
- Evaluate Richmond Agitation Sedation Scale (RASS) for level of sedation
  If oversedated, hold analgesics and/or sedatives until RASS is at goal, then reduce the amount of analgesics/sedatives from prior regimen
  If undersedated and receiving mechanical ventilation, titrate propofol until goal RASS is achieved
  If undersedated and NOT receiving mechanical ventilation, consider adding the following agents:
  - Dexmedetomidine 0.2–1 mcg/kg/h. Avoid using a loading dose to reduce the risk of bradycardia and hypotension.
  - Typical (haloperidol) and atypical (quetiapine) antipsychotics
  - Centrally acting cardiovascular medications (e.g., clonidine, propranolol) which have mild sedating effects
  - Minimize the use of benzodiazepines (particularly in elderly or delirious pts)

Transfusion of Red Blood Cells (RBCs) in the Critically-Ill Patient

In 2009, the Society of Critical Care Medicine published the results of an exhaustive analysis of trials

Key recommendations:

- RBCs should be transfused when a critically ill pt is suffering from hemorrhagic shock
- For hemodynamically stable pts transfusion of RBCs to maintain a hemoglobin ≥7 g/dL is as effective as transfusion to maintain a hemoglobin of ≥10 g/dL. A possible exception to this is *acute* myocardial ischemia. In the setting of stable cardiac dz, there is no clear benefit to maintaining hemoglobin ≥10 g/dL
- In the absence of ongoing hemorrhage, RBCs should be transfused as single units
- Transfusion should be avoided in ALI/ARDS pts unless absolutely necessary
- Transfusion decisions must be tailored to individual pts' situations. Rigid protocols should be avoided

Bioterrorism and Chemical Warfare Agents			
Potential Agent	Effect	Treatment	Staff Protection
Botulinum	Paralysis (symmetric descending weakness)	Trivalent botulism antitoxin or botulism immune globulin	Universal precautions
Nerve agents (Sarin, VX)	Cholinergic crisis	Atropine repeated q5–10min and pralidoxime followed by infusion	Level C chemical protection suits & filtration breathing apparatus
Cyanide	Inhibits aerobic respiration → lethal metabolic acidosis	Na thiosulfate, Na nitrite, hydroxocobalamin	Level C chemical protection suits & filtration breathing apparatus
Bacillus anthracis (Anthrax)	Mediastinitis, meningitis, multiorgan failure	Ciprofloxacin, doxycycline, penicillin, and streptomycin	Isolation, vaccination
Variola virus (smallpox)	Rash, pneumonia	Cidofovir	Isolation, vaccination with vaccinia immunoglobulin

ICU Medications			
		Dose	
Drug	Class	per kg	average
Pressors, Inotropes, and Chronotropes			
Phenylephrine	α_1	10–300 mcg/min	
Norepinephrine	$\alpha_1 > \beta_1$	1–40 mcg/min	
Vasopressin	V_1	0.01–0.1 U/min (usually <0.04)	
Epinephrine	$\alpha_1, \alpha_2, \beta_1, \beta_2$	2–20 mcg/min	
Isoproterenol	β_1, β_2	0.1–10 mcg/min	
Dopamine	D	0.5–2 mcg/kg/min	50–200 mcg/min
	β, D	2–10 mcg/kg/min	200–500 mcg/min
	α, β, D	>10 mcg/kg/min	500–1,000 mcg/min
Dobutamine	$\beta_1 > \beta_2$	2–20 mcg/kg/min	50–1,000 mcg/min
Milrinone	PDE	±50 mcg/kg over 10 min then 0.25–0.75 mcg/kg/min (consider avoiding the loading dose)	3–4 mg over 10 min then 20–50 mcg/min
Vasodilators			
Nitroglycerin	NO	5–500 mcg/min	
Nitroprusside	NO	0.25–10 mcg/kg/min	10–800 mcg/min
Nicardipine	CCB	2.5–15 mg/h (titrate by 2.5)	
Labetalol	α_1, β_1, and β_2 blocker	5–80 mg q10min or 10–120 mg/h	
Fenoldopam	D	0.1–1.6 mcg/kg/min	10–120 mcg/min
Clevidipine	CCB	1–32 mg/h	
Epoprostenol	vasodilator	2–20 ng/kg/min	

Antiarrhythmics

Drug	Class		
Amiodarone	K et al. (Class III)	150 mg over 10 min, then 1 mg/min × 6 h, then 0.5 mg/min × 18 h	
Lidocaine	Na channel (Class IB)	1–1.5 mg/kg then 1–4 mg/min	100 mg then 1–4 mg/min
Procainamide	Na channel (Class IA)	17 mg/kg over 60 min then 1–4 mg/min	1 g over 60 min then 1–4 mg/min
Ibutilide	K channel (Class III)	1 mg over 10 min, may repeat × 1	
Propranolol	β blocker	0.5–1 mg q5min then 1–10 mg/h	
Esmolol	$\beta_1 > \beta_2$ blocker	500–1,000 mcg/kg then 50–200 mcg/kg/min	20–40 mg over 1 min then 2–20 mg/min
Verapamil	CCB	2.5–5 mg over 1–2′, repeat 5–10 mg in 15–30′ prn 5–20 mg/h	
Diltiazem	CCB	0.25 mg/kg over 2 min reload 0.35 mg/kg × 1 prn then 5–15 mg/h	20 mg over 2 min reload 25 mg × 1 prn then 5–15 mg/h
Adenosine	purinergic	6 mg rapid push; if no response: 12 mg → 12–18 mg	

Sedation

Drug	Class		
Morphine	opioid	1–30 mg/h	
Fentanyl	opioid	50–100 mcg then 50–800 mcg/h	
Hydromorphone	opioid	0.5–2 mg, then 0.5–3 mg/h	
Remifentanil	opioid		
Propofol	anesthetic	1–3 mg/kg then 10–150 mcg/kg/min	50–200 mg then 20–400 mg/h
Dexmedetomidine	α_2 agonist	0.2–1.5 mcg/kg/h	
Diazepam	BDZ	1–5 mg q1–2h then q6h prn	
Midazolam	BDZ	0.5–2 mg q5min prn; 0.02–0.1 mg/kg/h or 1–10 mg/h	
Lorazepam	BDZ	0.01–0.1 mg/kg/h	
Naloxone	opioid antag.	0.4–2 mg q2–3min to total of 10 mg	
Flumazenil	BDZ antag.	0.2 mg over 30 s, then 0.3 mg over 30 s prn may repeat 0.5 mg over 30 s to total of 3 mg	

Miscellaneous

Drug	Class		
Aminophylline	PDE	5.5 mg/kg over 20 min then 0.5–1 mg/kg/h	250–500 mg then 10–80 mg/h
Octreotide	somatostatin analog	50 mcg then 50 mcg/h	
Glucagon	hormone	3–10 mg IV slowly over 3–5 min then 3–5 mg/h	
Mannitol	osmole	1.5–2 g/kg over 30–60 min repeat q6–12h to keep osm 310–320	

Partially adapted from Sabatine MS. *Pocket Medicine*. 7th ed. Philadelphia, PA: Wolters Kluwer; 2020.

MUOI A. TRINH • LINDA SHORE-LESSERSON • AMANDA J. RHEE

NORMAL CARDIOVASCULAR PHYSIOLOGY

Coronary Artery Anatomy			
Major Vessel	**Branch 1**	**Branch 2**	**Supply**
Left main coronary artery	Left anterior descending (LAD) coronary artery	Septal branches	Anterior 2/3 of interventricular septum, apical anterior papillary muscle
	Circumflex artery	Diagonal branches	Anterior surface of left ventricle
		Obtuse marginal branches	Lateral & posterior wall of left ventricle, anterolateral papillary muscle; *left dominant:* Gives rise to posterior descending artery (PDA) which supplies inferior & posterior ventricles, posterior 1/3 of interventricular septum
Right main coronary artery	Acute marginal branches		Right ventricle
	AV nodal artery		AV node
	Usually SA nodal artery		SA node
	Posterior descending artery (*right dominant 85%*)		Inferior & posterior ventricles, posterior 1/3 of interventricular septum, posteromedial papillary muscle

Cardiac Cycle: Definitions & Equations
- **Systole** = isovolumic ventricular contraction & ejection
- **Diastole** = isovolumic ventricular relaxation & filling
- **Cardiac output (CO)** = stroke volume × heart rate → volume of blood pumped by each ventricle per min
- **Stroke volume (SV)** = amount of blood pumped out of each ventricle during systole
- **Cardiac reserve** = difference between cardiac output at rest & the max volume of blood the heart is capable of pumping per min
- **Preload** = volume of blood in ventricle before systole, used to estimate left ventricular end diastolic volume (LVEDV)
- **Starling law** = contractility depends on muscle fiber length (Fig. 18-1)
- **Afterload** = resistance to ejection of blood by each ventricle
- **Coronary perfusion pressure (CPP)** = aortic diastolic BP – LVEDP
- **Left ventricular wall tension** → Law of Laplace: $T = p \times r/(2 \times t)$ where T = wall tension, p = pressure, r = radius, t = wall thickness
- **Fick equation:**

Cardiac output = O_2 consumption/([arterial O_2 content] − [venous O_2 content])

To Calculate Variables of Cardiovascular Function		
Variable	**Formula**	**Normal Value with Units**
Cardiac index	CO/BSA	2.8–4.2 L/min/m²
SVR (TPR)	[(MAP – CVP) × 80]/CO	1,200–1,500 dyn·s/cm⁵
PVR	[(MPAP – PCWP) × 80]/CO	100–300 dyn·s/cm⁵
SV	(CO × 1,000)/HR	60–90 mL/beat
SI	SV/BSA	20–65 mL/beat/m²
LV stroke work index	0.0136 (MAP – PCWP) × SI	46–60 g × m/beat/m²
RV stroke work index	0.0136 (MPAP – CVP) × SI	30–65 g × m/beat/m²
MAP	DBP + (SBP – DBP)/3	50–70 mmHg

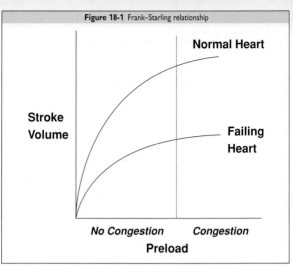

Figure 18-1 Frank–Starling relationship

Stroke Volume

Normal Heart

Failing Heart

No Congestion | Congestion

Preload

(Image courtesy of J. Ehrenfeld.)

COMMON DISEASE STATES AFFECTING THE HEART

Coronary Artery Disease & Acute Coronary Syndromes	
Coronary artery dz	Atherosclerotic narrowing of one or more coronary arteries
Ischemic heart dz	Coronary blood flow does not meet requirements of myocardial O₂ demand
Acute coronary syndrome	Life-threatening conditions that result from CAD or coronary spasm (unstable angina, acute myocardial infarction, coronary emboli)
Risk factors:	Age, cigarette smoking, hypercholesterolemia, HTN, diabetes, obesity, family Hx
Angina pectoris	Chest discomfort resulting from myocardial ischemia
Stable angina	Chronic angina pectoris brought on by exertion & relieved by rest (can get temporary ST seg changes without myocardial damage)
Unstable angina	↑ Duration & frequency of angina pectoris produced by less exertion or at rest (myocardial infarction likely to result if left untreated)
Variant angina	Anginal discomfort at rest; results from coronary artery vasospasm (ST changes can occur, usually elevation)
Non–ST-segment elevation MI (NSTEMI)	Partially occlusive thrombus without myocardial necrosis
ST-segment elevation MI (STEMI)	Coronary thrombus completely obstructs coronary artery, causing transmural necrosis

Determinants of Myocardial Perfusion
Supply: CPP, HR, PaO_2, coronary artery diameter
Demand: Myocardial O_2 consumption, HR, LV wall tension, contractility, conduction, relaxation

Treatment of Coronary Artery Disease & Acute Coronary Syndromes

Stable angina	Sublingual nitroglycerin
Unstable angina/ NSTEMI	**MONA—m**orphine, **O₂**, **n**itroglycerine, **A**SA
	Medical therapy—nitroglycerine, β-blockade, P2Y12 inhibitor (clopidogrel, ticagrelor), heparin (UFH or LMWH), glycoprotein IIb/IIIa inhibitor (abciximab, eptifibatide, tirofiban), direct thrombin inhibitor (bivalirudin), fondaparinux
	Adjunctive therapy—ACE inhibitors, ARBs, HMG-CoA reductase inhibitors (statins)
	Percutaneous coronary intervention (PCI) within 48 h for shock
STEMI	**MONA—m**orphine, **O₂**, **n**itroglycerine, **A**SA
	Medical therapy—P2Y12 inhibitor (clopidogrel, prasugrel, ticagrelor), glycoprotein IIb/IIIa inhibitor (abciximab, eptifibatide, tirofiban), heparin (UFH or LMWH), β-adrenergic receptor blockers, fondaparinux (should not be used alone), angiotensin-converting enzyme inhibitor, statin therapy
	Adjunctive therapy: ACE inhibitors, ARBs, HMG-CoA reductase inhibitors (statins)
	If symptom onset within prior 12–24 h and candidate for reperfusion: **PCI-capable hosp FMC to device time <90 min. Non-PCI capable hosp:** Immediate transfer to primary PCI hosp: FMC-device ≤120 min/if expected to be >120 min, give fibrinolytic within 30 min and transfer when can
	If STEMI with out of hospital cardiac arrest—therapeutic hypothermia and PCI

Description of Coronary Artery Disease Treatments

PCIs	Persistent anginal episodes; significant stenosis of 1–2 coronary arteries, favorable anatomy, STEMI, acute MI with cardiogenic shock
CABG	>50% stenosis of left main coronary artery; ≥70% stenosis in 3 major arteries, 1 VD with angina, 2–3 vessel dz with reduced LV contractile fx or diabetes; STEMI with coronary anatomy not amendable to PCI with ongoing ischemia, cardiogenic shock, severe HF; life-threatening arrhythmias with LM dz >50% or 3 VD

Hypertension (HTN)

Stage 1 HTN: SBP >130–139 or DBP >80–89 in cardiovascular dz, diabetes, or chronic kidney dz
Stage 2 HTN: SBP ≥140 or DBP ≥90

- Essential HTN (1° HTN)—no definable cause (95% of pts)
- 2° HTN: Iatrogenic (meds), renal, aortic coarctation, pheochromocytoma, adrenocortical hormone excess, thyroid hormone abnormal, estrogen therapy, Cushing dz
- Consequences of HTN
  - Organ damage: Ventricular hypertrophy, systolic dysfunction, CAD, stroke, abd aortic aneurysm, aortic dissection
  - Hypertensive urgency: BP >180 or DBP >120 without end-organ damage
    Hypertensive emergency: When this level of hypertension is associated with end-organ damage, including encephalopathy—headache, blurred vision, confusion, somnolence, coma
- Treatment: Diuretics, sympatholytic agents (β-blockers/α-2 agonists/α-1 antagonists), vasodilators (Ca-channel blockers, ACE inhibitors, ARBs), nitrates
- Anesthetic considerations
  - Monitoring: BP cuff vs. arterial line as indicated
  - Goal: Keep BP within 20% of baseline

Valvular Disease

Mitral Stenosis

Causes: Rheumatic fever, congenital stenosis, degenerative calcification, endocarditis

Pathophysiology

- ↑ LA pressure → pulmonary edema, LV hypertrophy
- Atrial fibrillation may result from LA dilation, LA thrombus from stasis of flow
- Develop pulmonary HTN
- Stroke volume is fixed

Clinical Feature

- High-pitched "opening snap" followed by low-frequency diastolic rumble

Classification

- Mild: MVA 1.5–2 cm², moderate: MVA 1–1.5 cm², severe: MVA ≤1 cm²

Treatment
- Medical therapy; balloon mitral valvuloplasty; open mitral commissurotomy; mitral valve repair/replacement

Anesthetic Management
- Maintain sinus rhythm (atrial kick provides 40% vent filling)
- Maintain preload & SV to avoid drop in SVR
- Maintain normal HR (to allow time for filling)
- Prevent ↑ in PVR (avoid hypoxia, hypercarbia, acidosis, pain)

Mitral Regurgitation
Causes: Myxomatous dz (mitral valve prolapse [MVP]), ischemic heart dz, heart failure, annular dilation, endocarditis, rheumatic heart dz, hypertrophic cardiomyopathy (SAM), myocardial infarction (necrotic papillary muscle, ruptured chordae)

Pathophysiology
- Severity determined by
  - Systolic pressure gradient between LV and LA
  - Systemic vascular resistance opposing forward LV blood flow
  - Left atrial compliance
  - Duration of regurgitation with each systole
- **Regurgitant fraction** = volume of MR/total LV stroke volume (>0.6 = severe)
- **Acute MR:** ↑ Pulmonary pressure & pulmonary congestion
- **Chronic MR:** ↑ LA size & compliance

Clinical Features
- Apical holosystolic murmur radiating to axilla

Treatment
- Medical therapy; mitral valve repair/replacement, Mitraclip

Anesthetic Management
- Maintain HR normal or high (decrease regurgitant fraction)
- Avoid myocardial depression
- Avoid ↑ SVR (can worsen regurgitation)
- Initiate prophylaxis against endocarditis
- PA catheter v waves increase as regurgitant fraction increases

Aortic Stenosis
Causes: Bicuspid AV, senile degenerative dz, rheumatic fever
Risk factors: Male gender, hypercholesterolemia, smoking

Pathophysiology
- Blood flow across valve is obstructed during systole
- Concentric LV hypertrophy
- Dependence on atrial kick to fill stiff ventricle
- Stroke volume is fixed
- Compression of subendocardial vessels → ischemia

Symptoms & Severity
- Angina—median survival 5 y
- Syncope—median survival 3 y
- Congestive heart failure—median survival 2 y

Clinical Features
- Harsh, holosystolic, crescendo–decrescendo murmur

Classification
- Mild = valve area <2.5 cm^2, moderate </ = 1–2.5 cm^2, severe <1 cm^2

Treatment
- Percutaneous balloon valvuloplasty, percutaneous transcatheter aortic valve replacement (TAVR), surgical AVR

Anesthetic Management
- Maintain sinus rhythm (atrial kick provides up to 40% of preload)
- Maintain slow to normal HR to allow time for ventricular filling
- Avoid ↓ SVR (will ↓ CO because of fixed SV) → because of this, spinal anesthesia is relatively contraindicated in the setting of severe AS
- Initiate prophylaxis against endocarditis
- Avoid myocardial depression as stroke volume is fixed
- Consider arterial line placement for severe AS
- Consider percutaneous pacing capability in case of cardiac arrest (chest compressions usually ineffective)

Aortic Regurgitation (AR)
Causes: Leaflet abnormalities (rheumatic heart dz, endocarditis, bicuspid valve), dilation of aortic root (aortic aneurysm/dissection, Marfan syndrome, syphilis, cystic medial necrosis)

Pathophysiology
- Acute = surgical emergency—systemic hypotension, pulm HTN, and pulm edema (sudden ↑ LV diastolic pressure backs up to pulm circulation)
- Chronic—LV compensates with dilation & hypertrophy → heart failure

Clinical Features
- Bounding pulses from widening pulse pressure
- Austin Flint murmur—turbulent flow across mitral valve during diastole due to AR jet

Treatment
- Asymptomatic—nifedipine, ACE inhibitor, diuretics
- Symptomatic—aortic valve replacement

Anesthetic Management
- Maintain sinus rhythm
- Maintain normal to high normal heart rate
- Avoid ↑ SVR (will worsen regurgitant fraction)
- Avoid myocardial depression
- Initiate prophylaxis against endocarditis
- Consider vasodilators (nitroprusside) to ↓ afterload

Pulmonic Stenosis
Causes: Congenital deformity, carcinoid heart dz

Classification
- Mild: Pressure gradient <40 mmHg, moderate 40–80 mmHg, severe >80 mmHg
- Treatment
- Balloon valvuloplasty; valve replacement

Pulmonic Regurgitation
Causes: Annular dilation 2° enlarged pulm artery in pulm HTN, congenital/carcinoid heart dz

Tricuspid Stenosis
Causes: Congenital, rheumatic heart dz, right atrial tumor, endocarditis

Tricuspid Regurgitation
Causes: Congenital, endocarditis, carcinoid heart dz, secondary event from mitral valve or left-sided heart dz

Hypertrophic Cardiomyopathy (HCM)
Causes: Genetic, mixed, acquired (AS, chronic hypertension)

Pathophysiology
- LV outflow obstruction (asymmetrical hypertrophic septum, turbulent LV ejection)
- LVH & RA enlargement, ↑ myocardial O_2 consumption → subendocardial ischemia

Clinical Features
- Mitral regurgitation from SAM (systolic anterior motion of anterior mitral leaflet) ↑ risk of sudden death

Anesthetic Management
- Maintain slow HR (to allow for ventricular filling)
- Maintain sinus rhythm
- Maintain low to normal contractility
- Maintain preload & afterload
- Treatments include β-blockers, verapamil, pacing, ICD, surgical myectomy

Anesthetic Goals in Valvular Disease					
	Preload	Afterload	HR	SVR	Contractility
Tricuspid stenosis	High normal	High	Low	High	Maintain
Tricuspid regurg	High normal	Low	High normal	Low	Maintain
Pulm stenosis	High	High	Low	High	Maintain
Pulm insuff	High normal	Low	High normal	Low	Maintain
Mitral stenosis	High normal	High	Low	High	Maintain
Mitral regurg	High normal	Low	High normal	Low	Maintain
Aortic stenosis	High	High	Low	High	Maintain

Aortic insuff	High	Low	High normal	Low	High
CAD	Normal	Low normal	Low	High	Normal
HCM	High	High	Low	High	Low normal
ICM	High	Low	High normal	High	High
Tamponade	High	Low	High	High	High

HEART BLOCKS/ARRHYTHMIAS (SEE CHAPTER 35, ELECTROCARDIOGRAM [ECG] INTERPRETATION)

Bradyarrhythmias—HR <60 bpm
Sick sinus syndrome—intrinsic SA node dysfx → inappropriate bradycardia
Treatment: Anticholinergics, β-adrenergic agents (isoproterenol), pacing
Rhythms that emerge from more distal latent intrinsic pacemakers of the heart with SA node dysfunction:

  Junctional escape rhythm—narrow complex (40–60 bpm)
  Ventricular escape rhythm—wide complex (30–40 bpm)
• Conduction defects below AV node within His–Purkinje system:
  → *Left bundle branch block (LBBB)*
  → *Right bundle branch block (RBBB)*
  → *Interventricular conduction delay*

Atrioventricular Conduction System
1° AV block—PR interval increased to >0.2 s
2° AV block
  → **Mobitz type I** (Wenckebach)—AV delay (PR interval) gradually ↑ with each beat until QRS is dropped after P wave. *Treatment*—only if symptomatic: Atropine, isoproterenol, permanent pacemaker for persistent block
  → **Mobitz type II**—sudden unpredictable dropped QRS which is not associated with progressive PR interval prolongation. *Treatment: Permanent pacemaker—as this may progress to 3° AV block*
3° AV block—"complete heart block" or "atrioventricular dissociation"
  → no relationship between P wave & QRS. *Treatment: Permanent pacemaker*

Perioperative Considerations
• Indications for temporary perioperative pacemaker insertion are same as indications outside the setting of surgery

Tachyarrhythmias—HR >100 bpm
Supraventricular Arrhythmias
Sinus Tachycardia
Premature Atrial Beats
  Treatment—only if symptomatic: β-blockers
Atrial Flutter—atria @ 180–350 bpm, ventricular rate 150 (2:1 AV block)
  Treatment: Unstable—electrical DC cardioversion; stable—β- & Ca-channel blockers, burst pacing
Atrial fibrillation—atria @ 350–600 bpm, ventricular rate variable
  Treatment: Unstable—cardioversion (if <48 h) & DC cardioversion with anticoagulation (heparin, apixaban) (if >48 h or unknown duration); stable—anticoagulation 3 wk or echocardiogram to rule out clot, then DC cardioversion; β- & Ca-channel blockers, IC and III antiarrhythmic drugs
Paroxysmal SVT—ventricular rate 140–250, narrow complex, hidden P's
Treatment: Vagal maneuvers, β- & Ca-channel blockers, RFA

AV Reentrant Tachycardia
Wolff–Parkinson–White: PR interval shortened, β-wave, wide QRS
  Treatment: RFA, β- & Ca-channel blockers, avoid procainamide

Ventricular Arrhythmias
Premature ventricular contractions—widened QRS
  Couplet—2 in a row, bigeminy—every other beat is PVC
Ventricular Tachycardia—3 or more PVC in a row, 100–200 bpm
Sustained VT—persists for 30 s or more
Nonsustained VT—persists for <30 s
  Treatment: Symptomatic but stable → electrical cardioversion (200 J monophasic, 100 J biphasic); asymptomatic nonsustained VT → β-blockers; unstable—see ACLS protocol (CPR, cardioversion, epinephrine, vasopressin, amiodarone, lidocaine)

Torsades de Pointes—polymorphic VT with QRS twisting about baseline
  Treatment—MgSO$_4$ 1–2 g IV
Ventricular fibrillation—irregular ECG without discrete QRSs
  Treatment—see ACLS protocol, CPR, cardioversion, epinephrine, vasopressin, amiodarone, lidocaine
Asystole—no electrical activity
  Treatment—see ACLS protocol, CPR, epinephrine

Intra-aortic Balloon Pump

Balloon placed in descending aorta (distal to L subclavian artery proximal to SMA) & synchronized with ECG. Balloon *inflates* at onset of diastole, *deflates* during systole (triggered by R wave, arterial line, or pacer).

Blood displacement	Proximal displacement—improves coronary artery perfusion; distal displacement—improves systemic perfusion

Goals: ↓ Afterload, ↓ wall tension, LVEDP & LVEDV (↓ in myocardial O$_2$ consumption); ↑ arterial & aortic diastolic pressures improved coronary artery perfusion

Indications & Contraindications for Intra-aortic Balloon Pump	
Indications	**Contraindications**
Complications of myocardial ischemia • Hemodynamic: Cardiogenic shock • Mechanical: MR, VSD • Intractable dysrhythmias • Postinfarct angina	• Severe aortic insufficiency • Inability to insert • Irreversible cardiac dz (not transplant candidate) • Irreversible brain damage
Acute cardiac instability • Angina: Unstable, preinfarction • Cath lab mishap: Failed PTCA • Bridge to transplantation • Cardiac contusion • Septic shock	

Source: Adapted from Barash PG. *Clinical Anesthesia.* 5th ed. Philadelphia, PA: Lippincott Williams & Wilkins; 2006.

Cardiovascular Implantable Electronic Device (CIED)

Pacemaker indications: Sick sinus syndrome, tachy-brady syndrome, severe heart block
Asynchronous vs. synchronous:
• **Synchronous (demand) mode**—pacer senses P wave, R wave or both; pacer is either **triggered** or **inhibited** by sensed signal
• **Asynchronous mode**—pacer fires regardless of pt's intrinsic rhythm
  → Only used in perioperative situations or if ablation/surgery has removed conduction
Biventricular pacing for congestive heart failure
• ↑ Depolarization of LV; synchronizes contraction of ventricles; increase cardiac output

Generic Pacemaker Codes				
Pacing Chamber	**Sensing Chamber**	**Response to Sensing**	**Programmability**	**Anti-tachyarrhythmia Function (s)**
O = none	O = none	O = none	O = none	O = none
A = atrium	A = atrium	I = inhibited	R = rate modulation	P = Pacing (antitachyarrhythmia)
V = ventricle	V = ventricle	T = triggered	P = simple programmable	S = Shock
D = dual (A + V)	D = dual (A + V)	D = dual (T + I)	M = Multiprogrammable	D = Dual (P + S)
			C = communicating	

Commonly Used Pacing Mode			
Mode	**Description**	**Function**	**Indication**
AOO	Atrial asynchronous	A pacing	Bradydysrhythmias
VOO	Vent asynchronous	V pacing	Bradydysrhythmias
DOO	Atrial & vent. asynchronous	AV pacing	Bradydysrhythmias

VAT	Atrial sensed & vent triggered	V paced, A sensed, sensed A beat triggers V output	Complete heart block with normal SA node
VVI	Vent noncompetitive	V pacing on demand, sensed V beat inhibits paced V beat	Sinus node dysfx, chronic Afib, complete block
DDD	Universal	A paced, V paced, AV sensed, sensed A inhibits A output, sensed A triggers V output, sensed V inhibits V output	Sinus brady, sinus tachy, complete block, 2° AV block

Anesthetic Considerations for Pacemakers
- Careful Hx, medical records, device information cards, and chest radiograph can help identify device vendor
- Device should have been checked in last 6 mo to determine pacing burden, >40% is considered pacing
- Electromagnetic interference (EMI), evoked potential monitors, nerve stimulators, radiofrequency ablation, and lithotripsy can inhibit demand pacing
  → Bipolar electrocautery is preferred, low monopolar electrocautery can be used in short, frequent bursts
- Consider conversion to an asynchronous mode (VOO) with **magnet** or programming if significant EMI is planned superior to the umbilicus
- MRI can convert pacer to asynchronous mode
- Defibrillator pads should be applied when asynchronous mode is activated in case "R on T" event is triggered resulting in ventricular tachycardia
- EMI dispersal pads should be placed far from pulse generator
- Hyper/hypokalemia can alter pacing thresholds
- Place pacing or defibrillation pads at least 1 in away from pulse generator
- Consider interrogating pacemaker at the end of the case to ensure proper functioning

Implantable Cardiac Defibrillator (ICD)
Indications: Survival of sudden cardiac death episode, sustained VT, cardiac resynchronization therapy (EF <35%), syncope from VT low EF/HCM
Anesthetic management
- Deactivate with magnet (vendor-specific) or programming (preferred)
  → Electrocautery can trigger defib or interfere with proper function
- Lithotripsy should be avoided
- Magnetic field can cause ICD leads to damage heart. Recent ICD are "MRI conditional"; Both lead and pulse generator need to be interrogated or identified and determined MRI compatibility
- External defibrillator should be available in the OR

CARDIOPULMONARY BYPASS MACHINE

- **Basic circuit:** Blood goes from pt → venous cannula → venous reservoir → oxygenator → heat exchanger → main pump → arterial filter → arterial cannula → pt
- Other components
  Cardiotomy suction—removes blood from field for salvage
  LV vent—prevent LV dilation from filling by Thebesian veins & bronchial arteries
  Cardioplegia pump—administers cardioplegic solution
  Ultrafilter—hemoconcentrates blood by removing water & electrolytes
- Cardioplegic solution—high in potassium (K^+)
  Anterograde cardioplegia—catheter in aortic root or coronary artery ostia; flow into coronary arteries
  Retrograde cardioplegia—catheter in right atrium to coronary sinus; flow into coronary veins
- Main pump:
Roller head—generates nonpulsatile flow
Centrifugal pump—flow is pressure dependent, less traumatic to RBC
Oxygenator—membrane oxygenator less traumatic than bubble

Cardiopulmonary Bypass Preanesthetic Management
Monitoring/Access
- Arterial line: Bypass pumps usually nonpulsatile (NIBP usually will not work)
- CVP/PA: Place before or after induction depending on vascular access; consider PA line for complex cases, or significant myocardial dz
- TEE: Place probe after induction, evaluate pathology and manage hemodynamics
- Establish large-bore IV access (18G or larger)

Premedication
- Pts may develop myocardial ischemia with stress/anxiety → consider lorazepam 2–3 mg/midazolam 1–2 mg preoperatively
- Supplement O_2 as needed

Induction
- Consider high-dose narcotic induction (can minimize myocardial depression)
- Fentanyl (7–15 mcg/kg), sufentanil (0.25–20 mcg/kg) or remifentanil (1 mcg/kg, then 0.2–1 mcg/kg/min)
  → May give small amount of paralytic prior to induction (avoid chest wall rigidity)
- Consider etomidate for pts with impaired myocardial fx; otherwise
  → Propofol
- Sevoflurane/isoflurane acceptable provided that hemodynamics (esp BP) is well controlled
- Ketamine may increase risk of myocardial ischemia
- Nitrous oxide generally avoided → risk of expansion of gaseous emboli in open heart procedures
- Paralytics: Vecuronium, rocuronium, cisatracurium, pancuronium (may cause tachycardia)

Fast-tracking in Cardiac Surgery
- Early extubation (within 6-h postop)
  Advantages: Reduced ICU stay, lower costs
- Used for low-risk cases/pts, in OPCAB, short bypass runs
- Must be planned in advance: Limit IV fluids, narcotics, keep pt warm

Cardiopulmonary Bypass Anesthetic Considerations
Prebypass
- Lungs down while sawing through sternum if oscillating saw not used
- Consider use of antifibrinolytic agent to reduce bleeding *(see table "Antifibrinolytics")*
  Aminocaproic acid or tranexamic acid ↓ bleeding by plasmin inhibition
  Aprotinin (not universally available; see table "Antifibrinolytics")
  - Potential ↓ bleeding, transfusions, reoperation for bleeding
  - May be assoc with postop renal failure, ↑ mortality
- Aortic cannulation
  Lower SBP to 90–120 mmHg before cannulation
  Complications: Aortic dissection, emboli, bleeding, hypotension
- Heparinization—prior to initiation of bypass

Heparin
- Mechanism: Binds to antithrombin III → potentiates inhibition of factor X and thrombin
- CPB dose: 300–400 units/kg → check ACT (goal >400 s)
- Heparin resistance: Antithrombin III deficiency, prior heparin therapy, oral contraceptive use, ↑ age
- Management of heparin resistance: Give additional dose of heparin; antithrombin III concentrate, FFP to raise antithrombin levels if antithrombin III not available (↑ antithrombin levels)
- Complications: Bleeding, thrombocytopenia (HIT) → heparin alternatives: Bivalirudin, Danaparoid sodium, r-hirudin, epoprostenol sodium

Protamine
- Mechanism: Base that ionically binds heparin (acid) by forming a stable/inactive complex
- CPB dose: 1 mg for 100 units of heparin; give small test dose 1st to check for allergic response (signs: Hypotension, anaphylaxis, anaphylactoid reaction, bronchospasm, pulm HTN)
- Goal ACT postbypass: <120–130
- Increased risk of protamine reaction: Prior exposure, NPH/PZI insulin, rapid infusion, seafood allergy
- **Note: Never give protamine while still on bypass!**

Sternotomy
- Short but painful stimulus → ensure pt is adequately anesthetized, disconnect pt from ventilator to avoid pericardial/lung injury

During Bypass
- Ventilator turned off (do not forget to turn back on later)
- Volatile agent can be provided by perfusionist through pump
- Consider administer narcotic (fentanyl) plus a benzodiazepine (midazolam) by either bolus dosing or infusion
- Consider insulin infusion for diabetic pts, maintain glucose <180 mg/dL

Potential Catastrophes During Bypass
- Aortic dissection
  - Stop CPB, choose alternate cannulation site, replace/repair dissected artery
- Inadvertent carotid/innominate artery cannulation
  - Treat ensuing cerebral edema, reposition aortic cannula
- Reversed cannulation
  - Stop CPB, evacuate air, reposition cannulas, restart CPB
- Obstruction to venous return
  - Reduce pump flow, treat cause (air lock evacuation, unkink tubing)
- Massive air embolism
  - Stop CPB, place pt in Trendelenburg, remove air
- Protamine administration during CPB will result in catastrophic clotting

During Rewarming
- When primary anesthetic is narcotic, recall occurs most often during rewarming
- Consider using small doses of scopolamine/benzodiazepines

Weaning Off Bypass
- Core temperature should be at least 36°C
- Check K^+, glucose, Hct before weaning
- Positive-pressure ventilation to evacuate air from heart, great vessels, & grafts
- Reversal of heparin anticoagulation is with 1 mg of protamine for every 100 units heparin given slowly, administration before cessation of CPB or while coronary suckers are being used can cause a clotting of bypass pumps
- Check rate and rhythm → may need temporary pacing
- Consider preop and current ventricular function
- Support SVR → goal 1,000–1,200 dyn s/cm⁵. Maintain cardiac output with vasodilators (nitroglycerine, nitroprusside, nicardipine) and inotropes (norepinephrine, dopamine, dobutamine, epinephrine, milrinone). Support blood pressure with vasopressors (phenylephrine, norepinephrine, fondaparinux) as needed

Failure to Wean from CPB
- LV/RV/respiratory failure
  Ventilatory—"pump lung" ARDS, bronchospasm, secretions, pneumothorax, hemothorax
  Preload problems
  Ischemia: Graft failure, inadequate coronary blood flow, prior MI reperfusion injury after cardioplegia aortic dissection
- Valve failure
  Pulmonary hypertension (RV failure)
  Others: Inhalational agents, β- & Ca-channel blockers acidosis, electrolyte abnl, hypocalcemia, hyper/hypokalemia, hypothermia
- Low SVR
  Medications: Vasodilators, inhalational agents, protamine
  Hemodilution, anemia, hyperthermia, sepsis, anaphylaxis/anaphylactoid rxn

Alpha Stat Vs. pH Stat
Alpha stat arterial blood gases are **not** temperature-corrected
- During hypothermic CPB, hypothermic alkaline drift occurs
- Prioritizes maintenance of $[OH^-]$ to $[H^+]$ ratio both inside & outside cell
- Benefit: Appears to have improved neurologic outcome
- Con: Allows leftward shift of oxyhemoglobin dissociation curve, slow cooling

pH stat arterial blood gases are **temperature-corrected**
- CO_2 added to oxygenator, which counteracts alkaline drift at lower temperature resulting in a sample which is then heated to 37°C
- Prioritizes maintenance of extracellular pH
- Benefit: Cerebral vasodilation, faster cooling, counteracts leftward shift of oxyhemoglobin dissociation curve
- Con: ↑ Flow may carry ↑ embolic load to brain

Which to use? pH stat may offer protection in neonatal & infant cardiac surgery, alpha stat most commonly used today in adults

Postop Complications
- Common reasons for pt return to the OR
  - Persistent bleeding, excessive blood loss, cardiac tamponade, unexplained poor cardiac performance

- Postoperative bleeding
  - Inadequate surgical hemostasis → return to OR coagulopathy—due to ↓ platelet count or fx, hemodilution or depletion of coagulation factors, fibrinolysis, insufficient protamine reversal, "heparin rebound"
- Pericardial tamponade
  - Suspect in postop cardiac pts with hemodynamic deterioration
  - Postop bleeding into pericardial sac → ↑ intrapericardial pressure & ↓ venous return
  - TEE findings: See systolic R atrial & diastolic R ventricular collapse
  - Stroke volume is ↓ & CO becomes dependent on HR
    - Compensatory tachycardia, peripheral vasoconstriction are seen
  - Management: Keep pt "full, fast, tight"
    Goal = maintain preload, contractility, CO; normal to high HR
    Ventilate with ↑ rate, ↓ tidal volume, ↓ PIP, avoid PEEP
    Treatment: Surgical exploration, pericardiocentesis

TRANSESOPHAGEAL ECHOCARDIOGRAPHY (TEE)

- 2013 ASE Guidelines for perioperative TEE assessment

Indications:

Evaluation of cardiac and aortic structures where the findings will alter management and TTE is nondiagnostic or TTE is deferred

Intraoperative TEE

Guidance of management of catheter-based intracardiac procedures (occluder devices, percutaneous valvular procedures)

Critically ill pts

Noncardiac surgery—use when the nature of the planned surgery or pt's known or suspected cardiovascular pathology could result in severe hemodynamic, pulmonary, or neurologic compromise, or when unexplained life-threatening circulatory instability persists despite corrective therapy

Critical care—use when diagnostic information required for management cannot be obtained by transthoracic echocardiography or other tests in a timely manner

Contraindications:

Absolute—esophageal stricture/tumor/perforation/laceration/diverticulum, perforated viscus, active upper GI bleed

Relative—Barrett esophagus, symptomatic hiatal hernia, Hx of radiation to neck/mediastinum, GI surgery, recent upper GI bleed, dysphagia, restriction to neck mobility, esophageal varices, coagulopathy, active esophagitis, active peptic ulcer dz

TEE strategies for pt with above contraindications—consider other imaging modalities (epicardial echocardiography), using a smaller probe, limiting the examination and avoiding unnecessary probe manipulation, using the most experienced echocardiographer

- Intraoperative TEE complications: Overall: 0.2%, major morbidity 0–1/2%, esophageal perforation 0–0.3%, odynophagia 0.1%
- ASE/SCA 28 views when performing a comprehensive TEE exam (Fig. 18-2)

CARDIAC PHARMACOLOGY (SEE CHAPTER 2F, VASOACTIVE, AUTONOMIC, AND CARDIOVASCULAR DRUGS)

Heart Failure Drugs			
Name	Mechanism of Action	Dosing	Comment
Milrinone	Phosphodiesterase inhibitor	50 mg/kg over 10 min loading dose followed by 0.375–0.75 mg/kg/min. Max 1.13 mg/kg/d	Increased inotropy and vasodilation
Levosimendan (not available in the US)	Calcium-sensitizing drug that stabilizes the troponin molecule in cardiac muscle	12–24 mcg/kg loading dose followed by 0.1–0.2 mcg/kg/min for 24 h	Increased inotropy and vasodilation. May be associated with hepatic dysfunction
Natrecor (nesiritide)	Recombinant form of human brain natriuretic peptide	2 mcg/kg loading dose followed by 0.01 mcg/kg/min for 24–48 h	Venous and arterial vasodilation. Diuresis. It does not affect cardiac contractility

Figure 18-2 SE/SCA 28 views when performing a comprehensive TEE exam

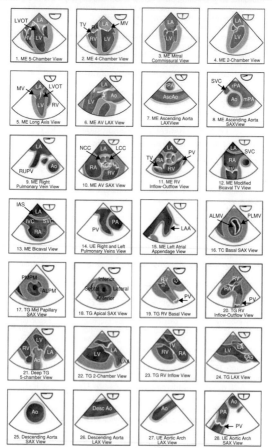

(Reproduced with modification and permission from Hahn RT, Abraham T, Adams MS, et al. Guidelines and standard for performing a comprehensive transesophageal echocardiographic examination: Recommendations from the American Society of Echocardiography and the Society of Cardiovascular Anesthesiologists. *J am Soc Echocardiogr* 2013;26:921–964.)

		Antifibrinolytics[a]		
Drug & Class	Mechanism	Advantages	Disadvantages	Dose
e-Aminocaproic acid: Lysine analog	Binds to lysine binding sites on plasminogen and fibrinogen, thereby inhibiting plasminogen activation and preventing plasmin release	• ↓ Mediastinal bleeding • May ↓ transfusion requirements	• No effect on reop rate • End-organ safety not well established • May cause thrombosis	• Load 100–150 mg/kg followed by infusion of 10–15 mg/kg/h • Load 10 g × 3: Baseline, CPB, and postprotamine
Tranexamic acid: Lysine analog	Same as above	10 times the potency of e-aminocaproic acid	• Dosing rate not well standardized in the literature • May cause thrombosis • Question of neurologic toxicity at high dose	• Low dose: Load 10–15 mg/kg followed by infusion of 1–1.5 mg/kg/h • High dose: Load 100–150 mg/kg followed by infusion rate 10 mg/kg/h
Aprotinin[b]: Nonspecific protease inhibitor (Note: This drug has been removed from the market in many countries)	Inhibits proteases kallikrein, plasmin, and others leading to inhibition of intrinsic coagulation cascade, complement activation, fibrinolysis, and bradykinin formation	• Most evidence for decreased postoperative bleeding and transfusion requirements • Reduces reoperation for bleeding • May reduce stroke rate	• May be associated with renal dysfunction and transient elevated creatinine • Allergy potential: IgG formation because it is derived from compound extracted from beef lung • Association with mortality not well defined • High cost	• 1 mL test dose, wait 10 min, to assess for possible anaphylactic response "high-dose regimen" • 2 × 106 KIU (280 mg) over 20 min followed by an infusion of 5 × 105 KIU (70 mg) per h • Half-dose regime is half of the high dose above

[a]Administration of antifibrinolytics is contraindicated in disseminated intravascular anticoagulation (except in the context of CPB) and upper urinary tract bleeding owing to the risk of thrombosis.
[b]Aprotinin caused a higher mortality rate and a higher Cr level than aminocaproic acid or no antifibrinolytic agent.
From Shaw AD, Stafford-Smith M, White WD, et al. The effect of aprotinin outcome after coronary artery bypass grafting. N Engl J Med 2008;21;358(8):784–793.

TRANSCATHETER AORTIC VALVE IMPLANTATION (TAVI)/ REPLACEMENT (TAVR)

Replacement of native stenotic AV using a catheter delivery prosthesis
- Advantages: No sternotomy, no CPB, less anticoagulation
- Indication: Severe AS
- Contraindication: Life expectancy <1 y, procedure will not improve quality of life, co-existing heart valve/coronary dz requiring surgical intervention, active endocarditis, recent thrombus, noncalcific AV
- Approach: Retrograde-femoral artery, subclavian artery, axillary artery, ascending aorta (mini-sternotomy); anterograde-transapical mini-thoracotomy

Anesthetic Management:
- May be performed under GA or MAC. Consider pt factors
- Maintain sinus rhythm
- Maintain CPP and SVR
- A-line monitoring needed for hemodynamics during rapid ventricular pacing
- Transvenous pacing wire placement may be needed if patient is at higher risk for developing heart block
- Consider central line for vasoactive and inotropes
- TEE/TTE used to confirm diagnosis, evaluate seating of prosthesis, assess LV/RV function, monitor for complications. Consider GA if TEE used, MAC if TTE used
- Anticoagulation with heparin to ACT >250 s
- Prior to deployment rapid ventricular pacing decreases cardiac ejection
- Decrease in MAP during pacing should be treated with alpha agent or vasopressor (phenylephrine, vasopressin, norepinephrine). Avoid inotropes as increased contractility can dislodge valve

Risk Stratification			
Prohibitive	**High**	**Intermediate**	**Low**
STS-PROM >50%	STS PROM ≥8%	STS PROM ≥4–8%	STS PROM <4%
Dz affecting ≥3 major organ systems	Dz affecting ≥2 major organ systems	Dz affecting 1 major organ system	No major organ dysfunction
Anatomic factors prohibiting surgery (chest radiation, severe calcification of aorta)	Significant frailty	Mild frailty	No frailty

STS-PROM—Society of Thoracic Surgeons Predicted Risk of Mortality (30 d).

TAVR Systems	
Edwards Life Science (Sapien 3™, Sapien XT™, Sapien 3 Ultra™)	**Medtronic (CoreValve™, Evolut™ R, and Evolut™ PRO)**
Balloon expandable, bovine pericardium	Self-expanding, retractable valve
Rapid ventricular pacing 180 bpm for deployment	Pacing may be used in difficult cases
Incidence of heart block 5–9%	Incidence of heart block 16–20%

KARA K. SIEGRIST • RYAN J. LEFEVRE • FREDERIC T. BILLINGS, IV

PREOPERATIVE EVALUATION FOR THORACIC SURGERY

- Hx of shortness of breath, asthma, exercise tolerance, cough
  - Medication use for obstructive or restrictive dz, with particular attention to frequency of use and need for bronchodilators and steroids
  - Smoking Hx
  - Exercise tolerance (<2 flights of stairs = poor prognostic indicator)
  - If malignancy present, risk of mass effect should be assessed using CXR or CT/MRI as well as screening for paraneoplastic metabolic derangements
- Assessment of respiratory function ("3-legged stool") to predict complications

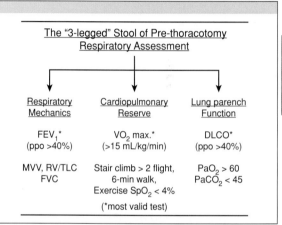

The "3-legged" Stool of Pre-thoracotomy Respiratory Assessment

Respiratory Mechanics	Cardiopulmonary Reserve	Lung parenchyma Function
FEV_1* (ppo >40%)	VO_2 max.* (>15 mL/kg/min)	DLCO* (ppo >40%)
MVV, RV/TLC FVC	Stair climb > 2 flight, 6-min walk, Exercise SpO_2 < 4%	PaO_2 > 60 $PaCO_2$ < 45

(*most valid test)

- Respiratory mechanics are assessed by spirometry (Table—Pulmonary Function Tests)
  - A low-predicted postoperative FEV_1 (ppoFEV_1) is the best predictor of postthoracotomy respiratory complications
  - ppoFEV_1 = preopFEV_1 × (1 – % functional lung tissue removed/100%)
    - >40% = low risk for postop pulmonary complications
    - <30% = high risk for postop pulmonary complications
- Cardiopulmonary reserve is assessed by oxygen delivery
  - VO_2 max
    - >20 cc/kg/min = low risk
    - <15 cc/kg/min = high risk
- Lung parenchymal function is assessed by gas exchange
  - DLCO
    - ppo >40% = low risk
  - Room air arterial blood gas
    - PaO_2 <60 mmHg or $PaCO_2$ >45 mmHg worse prognosis
- Chest x-ray is used to evaluate major anatomical abnormalities, major vascular pathology, lung parenchyma, and effusions

Pulmonary Function Tests		
	Obstructive (COPD/asthma)	Restrictive
Vital capacity	NC or ↓	↓
Total lung capacity	NC or ↑	↓
Residual volume	↑	↓
FEV_1/FVC	↓	NC or ↑
Forced max exp flow (FEF$_{25-75\%}$)	↓	NC

Common causes of abnormal PFTs:
- Pregnancy: ↓ FRC, ↓ RV, ↓ ERV
- Elderly: ↑ FRC, ↑ RV, ↑ lung compliance, ↓ FEV$_1$
- Obesity: ↓ FRC, ↓ VC, ↓ ERV, ↓ IRV
- General anesthesia: ↓ FRC

COMMON DISEASE STATES OF THE LUNG

COPD
- Typically slowly progressive, associated with obstruction of small airways and emphysema; highly associated with cigarette smoking
- May be associated with chronic bronchitis
- Spirometry:
  - Severe: FEV$_1$ <35% predicted
- Incidence ≈7–8% of US adults
- Treatment focused on relieving expiratory obstruction
  - Inhaled β$_2$-agonists: Albuterol/metaproterenol/salmeterol
  - Inhaled anticholinergics: Ipratropium/glycopyrrolate/atropine/tiotropium
  - Inhaled or systemic steroids
    - Consider stress-dose steroids perioperatively if on chronic systemic therapy
  - Antibiotics for bronchitis/other infections
- Anesthetic management
  - Preoperative treatment of atelectasis, bronchospasm, infections, and pulmonary edema, in particular with inhaled bronchodilator therapy
- Continue baseline medications
- Pts may have erythrocytosis, pulm HTN, cor pulmonale, RV failure
  - Pts with ppoFEV$_1$ <40% should have TTE to assess RV function
- Smoking cessation (several wk if possible)
  - Nicotine ↑ HR, BP, and wound infections
  - Carbon monoxide decreases O$_2$ delivery
- Maintain adequate anesthetic depth to limit bronchospasm
  - Lidocaine may ↓ airway reactivity at intubation
  - Volatile anesthetics ↑ bronchodilation
  - Avoid nitrous oxide if emphysematous bullae present as can ↑ risk of rupture and subsequent pneumothorax
  - Limit tidal volume (6 mL/kg) to minimize P$_{aw}$ & limit PEEP (risk of bullae rupture/pneumothorax)
  - Adequate expiratory time to avoid air trapping/auto-PEEP (↓I:E ratio). Increased airway pressures during volume control ventilation or decreased tidal volume during pressure control ventilation are signs of air trapping.
  - Consider deep extubation if no GERD & mask airway adequate to limit bronchospasm during stage II anesthesia and emergence
  - COPD pts have ↑ risk of postop respiratory failure
    - Supplemental oxygen may suppress respiratory drive and ↑ dead space
    - Avoidance of narcotic therapy postoperatively to maintain respiratory drive; consider multimodal non-narcotic analgesia and/or regional anesthesia

Asthma
- Episodic lower airway obstruction due to bronchospasm & inflammation
- Normal spirometry between exacerbations (may develop chronic obstruction in severe, chronic dz)
- Inciting factors: Cold, pollen, dust, exercise, aspirin/NSAIDs, infections
- Incidence ≈5% of US adults
- Treatment focused on increasing bronchial diameter
  - Inhaled short-acting β$_2$-agonists for acute treatment: Albuterol/metaproterenol
  - Inhaled long-acting β$_2$-agonists for chronic treatment: Salmeterol/formoterol
  - Inhaled anticholinergics: Ipratropium
  - PO antileukotrienes (not useful for acute attacks) → montelukast/zileuton/zafirlukast
  - Theophylline
  - Inhaled Cromolyn (not useful for acute attacks)
  - Inhaled or systemic steroids
  - Supplemental oxygen (severe dz)
- Anesthetic management
  - Hx
  - Precipitating factors

- Recent ER visits or hospitalizations
- Current status vs. baseline
- Exercise tolerance
- Climbing 2+ flights of stairs = lower risk
- Continue preop pulmonary medications in particular inhaled bronchodilator therapy
- Consider stress-dose steroid if chronic steroid treatment
- Maintain adequate anesthetic depth to limit bronchospasm
- Volatile anesthetics and ketamine ↑ bronchodilation

Intraoperative Wheezing Patient Management

Differential diagnosis
- Bronchospasm, mechanical obstruction (tube kinking), secretions, pneumothorax, pulmonary edema

Management
- Ensure adequate depth of anesthesia, inhaled short-acting β-agonist (albuterol), consider IV lidocaine, consider IV epinephrine if refractory or no air movement, consider magnesium, ketamine, anticholinergics (ipratropium, atropine)
- Consider deep extubation IF no GE reflux & mask airway adequate

---

Pulmonary Edema

- Etiologies
  - Cardiac
    - Myocardial dysfunction (most common), rhythm disturbances, valvular decompensation
  - Noncardiac (capillary leak)
    - Sepsis/sepsis syndrome, inhalation injury, hypertension (severe), neurogenic, negative pressure (e.g., postlaryngospasm), transfusion-related acute lung injury (TRALI), transfusion-related circulatory overload (TACO)
- Diagnosis
  - Hypoxemia (relative or absolute); rales on auscultation; airway secretions ("pink froth")
- Treatment focused on relieving venous congestion, increasing alveolar pressure and cardiac output
  - Mechanical ventilation (± PEEP)
  - Venodilatation—nitroglycerin (if ischemia suspected)
  - Diuresis—furosemide
  - Inotrope (if low cardiac output)—dobutamine/milrinone/epinephrine
  - Cardioversion for dysrhythmias
  - Consider intra-aortic balloon pump (for ischemia/infarction)
  - Consider veno-venous (VV) ECMO if refractory hypoxia or hypercarbia
- Anesthetic management
  - Invasive monitoring
    - Arterial line
    - Consider CVP or PA catheter, particularly for cardiac causes (heart failure or mitral regurgitation)
    - Consider transesophageal echo if available
  - Minimize myocardial depression
    - Consider etomidate for induction, opioids for maintenance
  - Avoid hypervolemia
  - Consider inotropic support

ARDS (see also Chapter 17, Trauma, Burn, and Critical Care Management)

- Diffuse, patchy pulmonary injury without cardiac failure
- Etiologies: Sepsis, aspiration, pancreatitis, pneumonia, inhalation injury, near drowning
- Leads to atelectasis, ↓ FVC, VQ mismatch
- Treatment focused on minimizing lung injury
  - Treat underlying cause (e.g., infection)
  - Avoid hypervolemia
  - Mechanical ventilation to avoid volutrauma and barotrauma (N Engl J Med 2000;342:1301)
    - Limit P_{aw} ≤30 cm H_2O
    - Tidal volume ≤6 mL/kg
    - PEEP
    - Permissive hypercapnia to pH 7.25–7.3
- Anesthetic management
  - Mechanical ventilation per ARDSnet (see above)
  - Volatile anesthetic for bronchodilation
  - Opioid: Can improve comfort during mechanical ventilation

Restrictive Lung Disease
- ↓ FRC leads to rapid hypoxemia upon brief apnea
- Ventilation management
  - Use lower tidal volume since P_{aw} ↑ rapidly with large tidal volume
  - ↑ Ventilation rate to maintain minute ventilation
  - Institute PEEP
- Anesthetic management
  - Consider feasibility of regional technique
  - General anesthesia
  - Anticipate hypoxemia on apnea at induction. Preoxygenation important
    - Avoid large TV
    - Minimize residual respiratory depressants
    - Bleomycin-related pulm fibrosis: Use FiO_2 ≤40% & ↓ fluids

Pulmonary Hypertension Management
- Nonpharmacologic
  - Avoid factors which ↑ pulmonary vascular resistance (PVR): Hypoxemia/atelectasis/acidosis/hypercarbia/hypothermia/sympathetic stimulation
- Treatment focused on reducing PVR and increasing RV contractility
  - Prostanoids (epoprostenol, iloprost, treprostinil)
  - Phosphodiesterase inhibitors (sildenafil, tadalafil, milrinone)
  - Endothelin antagonists (bosentan, ambrisentan)
  - Inhaled nitric oxide (NO)
  - sGC stimulators (riociguat) may be associated with ↓ BP due to vasoplegia
  - Dobutamine, Epinephrine infusion for right ventricular support
  - Consider preoperative ECMO/Cardiac anesthesia consult if severe

LUNG ISOLATION AND ONE-LUNG VENTILATION (OLV)

Absolute Indications for OLV	Relative Indications for OLV
• Isolation of healthy lung from contamination (infection, hemorrhage) • Control of ventilation distribution (bronchopleural fistula, bronchopleural cutaneous fistula, cyst, bullae, trauma/bronchial injury) • Unilateral lung lavage • Video-assisted thoracoscopic surgery (VATS)	• High-priority surgical exposure (thoracic aortic aneurysm, pneumonectomy, upper lobectomy) • Low-priority surgical exposure (esophageal surgery, middle/lower lobectomy, thoracoscopy)

Double-Lumen Tubes (DLTs)
- Left-sided DLTs are much more frequently used since a right-sided DLT may obstruct right upper lobe bronchus
- Right-sided DLTs have an orifice in the bronchial lumen that must be aligned with right upper lobe (often times difficult due to inconsistent anatomy and tube sizing)
- Tube size selection is based on the pt height:
  Men: <170 cm use 39Fr, >170 cm use 41Fr
  Women: <160 cm use 35Fr, >160 cm use 37Fr
- Typical tube depth at upper incisors (adults)
  Males 29–31 cm, females 27–29 cm

Technique for Double-Lumen Tube Placement

• Perform laryngoscopy to optimize view of the glottis
• Insert bronchial cuff just below cords with tube bend pointed anteriorly (aids initial insertion)
• Remove stylet
• Advance DLT while rotating tube to midline (90° left for left DLT) until well seated
• Inflate tracheal cuff, connect adaptor and circuit, & confirm tracheal placement
  • Breath sounds should be equal on both sides
• Inflate bronchial cuff gently (rarely >2 mL air)
• Recheck breath sounds listening in axilla
• Selectively clamp & recheck R/L breath sounds
  • Changes may be difficult to detect if soft baseline breath sounds (e.g., COPD)
• Verify position with bronchoscope since malposition often missed by auscultation alone
  • Verify bronchial cuff down proper mainstem bronchus
    • Airway rings visualized anteriorly, longitudinal muscular fibers posterior

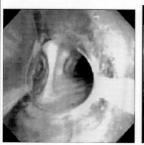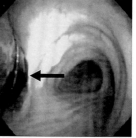

(From Eisenkraft JB, Cohen E, Neustein SM. Anesthesia for Thoracic Surgery. In: Barash PG, Callan MK, Cullen BF, Stock MC, Stoelting RK, Ortega R, Sharar SR, Holt N, eds. *Clinical Anesthesia*. 8th ed. Philadelphia, PA: Wolters Kluwer; 2018:1045.)

- Identify right-upper-lobe bronchus open
- Ensure no bronchial cuff herniation over carina upon inflation
- DLT often migrates with pt lateral repositioning
- Recheck DLT position after final pt positioning
  - Picture on the left demonstrates appropriately positioned L DLT. Picture on the right demonstrates incorrectly positioned L DLT since bronchial cuff is above carina

Troubleshooting Double-Lumen Tube Malposition

- Recheck adequate balloon inflation if air leak
- Consider returning to 2-lung ventilation (if hypoxemic/inadequate ventilation)
- Recheck position with bronchoscope
- If large ↑ P_{aw} or no TV with 1 lung ventilation, hypoventilation, hypoxia, barotrauma, or pneumothorax may develop
  - Consider tube too shallow or too deep if ventilating tracheal lumen. Bronchial cuff may be in trachea occluding ventilation via tracheal lumen or tube may be deep in mainstem bronchus and tracheal lumen orifice pushed up against airway wall
- If right lung will not fully deflate, recheck patency of R upper lobe bronchus with fiberscope
- If tube is on wrong side or unsure, to reposition:
  - Insert bronchoscope through bronchial lumen into airway
  - Deflate both cuffs & pull tube back so bronchial cuff is below cords but above carina (~21 cm at teeth in an adult [i.e., standard single-lumen ET tube depth])
  - Advance bronchoscope down desired mainstem bronchus (left for left-sided tube)
  - Advance tube over bronchoscope
  - Remove bronchoscope from bronchial lumen
  - Advance bronchoscope into tracheal lumen to confirm appropriate tube position (see figure above)

Troubleshooting Double-Lumen Tubes: Both Cuffs Inflated & 1 Lumen Clamped

	Tracheal Side Ventilated	Bronchial Side Ventilated	Problem
Breath sounds	Clear or absent ventilation	Clear on bronchial side, but ↑ airway pressures	DLT too deep
	Absent ventilation	Both sides ventilated	DLT too shallow
	Absent or on wrong side	Wrong side only	DLT on wrong side

Adapted from Dunn P. *Clinical Anesthesia Procedures of the MGH*. 7th ed. Philadelphia, PA: Lippincott William & Wilkins.

Bronchial Blockers

- Pros: Only requires single-lumen ETT placement which can be easier if difficult airway or abnormal anatomy; no cuff damage risk during intubation; no need for ETT exchange at the end of case; easy recognition of anatomy since carina is at the tip of a single-lumen ETT

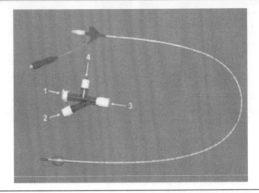

The wire-guided endobronchial blocker (Arndt blocker) and the multiport connector; 1, fiberoptic bronchoscope; 2, blocker port; 3, endotracheal tube connector port; 4, ventilation port.

From Campos JH. An update on bronchial blockers during lung separation techniques in adults. *Anesth Analg* 2003;97(5):1266–74.

- Cons: Can be more labor intensive (both initial positioning and repositioning during case since more prone to dislodgement), smaller suctioning channel; more difficult intraop conversion from 1- to 2-lung ventilation
- Insertion:
  - Ensure adequate time for deflation of lung since there limited suction port
  - Insert bronchoscope and bronchial blocker through multipronged connector
  - Snare bronchial blocker around bronchoscope and advance while holding snare tightly closed into desired bronchial lumen
  - Inflate bronchial blocker balloon in desired bronchus
  - Snare can be removed to provide a suction channel, but snare cannot be replaced once removed, thereby limiting the ability to reposition blocker
  - Some brands of blockers use a steerable wheel instead of a snare for guidance

Physiology of 1-Lung Ventilation
- 1-lung ventilation of the dependent (bottom) lung in lateral position
  - Gravity causes ↑ blood flow to dependent lung decreasing pulmonary shunt since decreased blood flow to nondependent lung which is not being ventilated
  - Positive-pressure ventilation, however, increases shunt since nondependent nonventilated lung is isolated from the positive pressure
- Lateral positioning with open chest
  - ↑ Blood flow to dependent lung
  - ↓ Effective compliance in dependent lung
  - ↓ FRC
  - Shunt from blood flow through nondependent nonventilated lung results in hypoxia
  - Impaired ventilation of dependent ventilated lung results in hypercapnia, acidosis
- Hypoxic pulmonary vasoconstriction (HPV)
  - Vasoconstriction of pulmonary arteries in presence of alveolar hypoxia secondary to nonventilation redirects blood to alveoli with higher O_2 tension (i.e., the ventilated lung)
  - HPV is inhibited by vasodilators (e.g., nitroprusside, nitroglycerine), alkalemia, hypocarbia, and volatile anesthetics

Anesthesia for 1-Lung Ventilation
- Invasive monitoring
  - Arterial line indications: Surgery near hilum (lobectomy, large wedge resection), compromised respiratory system (COPD, pulm HTN), or compromised cardiac Hx (myocardial ischemia, arrhythmia)
  - Pulmonary artery catheterization indications: Severe cardiac dz or severe pulmonary hypertension
    - Monitor PA, P_{cw} for left heart filling pressures
    - PA catheter usually floats to the R lung

- Risks: Dysrhythmias, PA rupture
- No proven improvement in outcomes with routine use
- Low tidal volume 4–5 mL/kg; plateau pressure <25 cm H_2O; peak pressure <35 cm H_2O
  - Smaller TV ↑ risk atelectasis
  - Larger TV ↑ shunting to nonventilated lung, ↑ risk barotraumas to ventilated lung; ↑ mediastinal movement causing difficult surgical visualization and dissection
- Permissive hypercapnia
- Minimize FiO_2 to maintain SaO_2 >92%, but FiO_2 <1.0 often not tolerated due to shunt
- Limit time on 1-lung ventilation
- ↑ Incidence of hypoxemia with:
  - Right lung deflation (R lung is 10% larger than L lung, therefore increased shunt) Supine position
- Judicious IV fluid administration
  - Excessive IV fluid administration can lead to pulmonary edema in dependent lung and worsen shunt
  - Atrial distention can lead to ↑ risk of postoperative atrial arrhythmias
- Management of inadequate ventilation during OLV
  - Maximize minute ventilation while limiting volutrauma and barotrauma
  - Pressure control ventilation to provide greater tidal volume for same pressure
  - Reduce I:E ratio provide more inspiratory time and therefore more tidal volume for same pressure, but beware of air trapping
  - ↑ Respiratory rate, but beware of air trapping
  - Note: Increased dead space ventilation:alveolar ventilation with DLT due to smaller tidal volumes, bigger ET tube will significantly ↑ the alveolar dead space: ↑ $EtCO_2$:$PaCO_2$ gradient (from a gradient of 5–10 to 15–30 mmHg).
- Signs of alveolar air trapping
  - Decreased compliance from air trapping will result in higher airway pressures for same tidal volume (VC ventilation) or smaller tidal volume for same airway pressure (PC ventilation)
  - Decreased cardiac output secondary to reduced cardiac filling will result in hypotension
- Treatment of alveolar air trapping
  - Disconnect circuit and reinstitute ventilation with longer expiratory time +/– PEEP

Anesthetic Techniques—Specific Surgical Procedures
Video-Assisted Thoracic Surgery (VATS)
- Preop evaluation
  - Discuss potential for open thoracotomy and postoperative mechanical ventilation
- Complications
  - Bleeding, lung injury (air leak)
- Anesthetic management
  - General anesthesia most common
  - 2 large-bore IVs
  - Arterial line indications: Surgery near hilum (lobectomy, large wedge resection), compromised respiratory system (COPD, pulm HTN), or compromised cardiac Hx (myocardial ischemia, arrhythmia)
  - Double-lumen endotracheal tube or alternative lung isolation technique (see "Lung Isolation" section above)
- Consider slightly lower TV (e.g., 4–5 mL/kg) to ↓ mediastinal shift and improve operating conditions
  - Muscle relaxation (see "Mediastinoscopy" below)
  - Consider a neuraxial anesthetic (epidural) or other regional technique (intercostal blocks, paravertebral, etc.) if ↑ likelihood of conversion to open thoracotomy
- Postop chest x-ray

Pneumonectomy
- Preop evaluation
  - See "PFTs/Evaluation of Lung Resectability" above
  - ↑ Risk of morbidity with right vs. left pneumonectomy, trauma, massive hemoptysis, Hx of cardiac dz, >10% preop weight loss
  - Optimize treatment of existing pulmonary/cardiac dz
  - Encourage smoking cessation
- Complications
  - Bleeding, airway (stump) leak, cardiac dysrhythmias (consider role of β-blocker), cardiac herniation through pericardial defect, pulmonary edema, myocardial infarction, intracardiac shunt (can get ↑ R heart pressure, shunting via PFO)

- Anesthetic management
  - Arterial catheter
  - 2 large-bore IVs or central line
- Airway
  - DLT to nonoperative side or bronchial blocker
    - May consider L sided DLT if L pneumonectomy and pull tube above the carina prior to bronchial resection
  - Risk of intraop dislodgement with either technique
  - Risk of bronchial stump damage with manipulations
- Muscle relaxation
- Limit intraop fluids

Mediastinoscopy
- Preop evaluation
  - Airway: Mass effects on trachea and bronchi, great vessels
  - Hx: CV problems, stroke, SVC syndrome, Lambert–Eaton syndrome
- Complications
  - Hemorrhage (can be severe if great vessel injury), pneumothorax, chylothorax, recurrent laryngeal nerve injury, air embolization
- Anesthetic management
  - General anesthesia
  - Anterior mediastinal mass compression of airway can result in complete obstruction upon induction of general anesthesia
  - Inhalational or IV induction with maintenance of spontaneous ventilation
  - Consider awake intubation if significant symptoms
  - If airway collapse does occur, consider repositioning ET tube, advancing ET tube past mass, or rigid bronchoscopy
  - Consider preinduction cardiopulmonary bypass or VA ECMO cannulation in extreme risk pts
- Vascular access
  - 2 large-bore IVs
  - Arterial line in right radial (monitors brachiocephalic artery compression by mediastinoscope—especially important in pts with poor cerebral collateral circulation)
- Avoid nitrous oxide
- Muscle relaxation
  - Movement ↑ risk of surgical trauma
  - Cough/strain ↑ thoracic venous engorgement
  - Spontaneous ventilation may ↑ risk air embolism
- Postop chest x-ray

Mediastinal Mass Considerations
- Preop evaluation
  - ↑ Risk of tracheobronchial obstruction with:
    - Orthopnea
    - Large airway compression on imaging
    - Flattened expiratory limb of flow-volume loop on PFTs
- Evaluate for evidence of superior vena cava syndrome
  - Upper-extremity/facial edema (may indicate airway edema)
  - Dilated upper-extremity veins
  - Headache, CNS changes
  - Consider preop steroid, diuretic, elevation of head of bed
- Hx syncope with position or Valsalva suggests
  - Cardiac/PA compression with hypotension
  - Critical tracheobronchial obstruction
  - Consider preop echo to evaluation for compression
- Consider preop biopsy/treatment to shrink mass (if severe airway/cardiovascular compression)
- Complications
  - Acute tracheobronchial compression intraop
    - Highest risk is on transition to positive-pressure ventilation
  - Acute cardiac/PA compression with severe hypotension
  - Bleeding (esp with SVC syndrome due to venous engorgement)
  - Smooth emergence & extubation since cough/straining may worsen airway collapse

- Anesthetic management of anterior mediastinal masses:
  - Arterial access preinduction
  - Large-bore/central venous access
  - Consider standby cardiopulmonary bypass or ECMO (femoral cannulation) if airway or cardiovascular compression by mass
  - Rigid bronchoscope available
  - If SVC syndrome:
    - Consider lower-extremity vascular access (more reliable drug/fluid delivery)
    - Avoid jugular or subclavian lines
- Consider spontaneously breathing bronchoscopic exam/intubation if significant airway compression
- Initiate slow, controlled induction
  - Controlled transition from spontaneous ventilation to positive pressure
  - Short-duration relaxant desirable to facilitate tracheal intubation
  - If airway obstruction occurs:
    - Attempt lateral positioning to move mass
    - Resume spontaneous ventilation if possible
    - Attempt to pass tracheal tube beyond obstruction carefully (risk hemorrhage)
    - Attempt rigid bronchoscopy to open airway
    - Consider cardiopulmonary bypass/ECMO (femoral cannulation)

Esophagectomy
- Preop eval
  - Dysphagia (reflux, risk of chronic aspiration)
  - Prior chemo/radiation therapy
  - Risk for cardiac dysrhythmias, esp supraventricular
  - Consider epidural placement for postoperative analgesia given strict NPO status
- Complications
  - Gastroesophageal reflux, esophageal leak, respiratory failure, hypotension, cardiac dysrhythmias
- Anesthetic management
- Rapid sequence induction if aspiration risk
  - Consider cricoid pressure at induction
    - May ↓ lower esophageal sphincter tone
  - Arterial line since surgery in mediastinum with either transhiatal or Ivor Lewis technique
  - Lung isolation for thoracotomy approaches
  - Avoid nitrous oxide (expands bowel gas, need high FiO_2 with 1-LV)
  - Avoid vasopressors (↑ risk anastomotic necrosis and subsequent leak)
    - Intraop use or hypotension associated with ↑ incidence GI anastomotic leak
  - Consider ↓ drug dosages if pt has ↓ serum albumin from malnutrition
  - Monitor glucose closely (especially if pt receiving TPN)
  - Communicate with surgeon regarding esophageal manipulations (e.g., NG tube, esophageal bougie)
  - Intraop hypotension: May be from hypovolemia, surgical compression of heart or great vessels, bleeding
  - If postop mechanical ventilation planned change to standard endotracheal tube at completion of surgery via long exchange catheter or extubation and reintubation based on risk of airway loss from difficult intubation or glottis edema
  - Caution taken in subsequent surgeries for pts postesophagectomy for GI prophylaxis and risk of aspiration; keep head of bed elevated at all times; Rapid sequence induction

Bronchoscopy
- Preop evaluation
  - See above (VATS)
  - Careful attention to paraneoplastic syndromes if malignancy is present and compressing mediastinal masses
- Complications
  - Respiratory acidosis secondary to intermittent ventilation can lead to cardiac dysrhythmias
  - Pneumothorax can occur especially in the setting of endobronchial biopsies. Careful postop evaluation required. Low threshold for postop x-ray.
  - If laser destruction of tumor planned, minimize FiO_2 for risk of spontaneous combustion
  - Mechanical trauma including: Teeth damage, hemorrhage, bronchospasm, perforation of trachea or bronchial tree, edema

- Anesthetic management
  - Consider pretreatment with drying agent (e.g., glycopyrrolate, scopolamine)
  - Topical anesthesia of naso/oropharynx and trachea
  - Inhaled 10 cc nebulized 4% lidocaine and/or viscous 2% lidocaine
  - 1 cc 1% aliquots with bronchoscope onto epiglottis and cords
  - Alternatively, can consider nerve blocks of glossopharyngeal and superior laryngeal nerves with transtracheal block
  - Max dose lidocaine 5 mg/kg
  - If inadequate topicalization, increased likelihood of laryngospasm
- General anesthesia often utilized in combination with topical anesthesia
  - LMA placement unless contraindication (GERD, etc.)
  - Consider TIVA as significant anesthetic gas leak can occur around bronchoscope
  - Controlled ventilation recommended unless contraindication present (obstructing mass, etc.)
  - Neuromuscular blockade can be utilized with careful titration

Enhanced Recovery (ERAS) for Thoracic Surgery
- Mutlifaceted approach focused on reducing length of stay and postoperative complications
- Comprised of pt education, nutritional support, minimizing IV fluids, multimodal analgesia, minimizing opioids, and early ambulation
- Supported by evidence for invasive thoracic surgery (thoracotomy)
- No evidence for improved outcomes in minimally invasive thoracic surgery (VATS)
- Example ERAS protocol for thoracic surgery
  - **Pt education:** Starts in preop visits and includes expectations for surgery, instructions for incentive spirometer, education about PO intake perioperatively
  - **Nutritional support:** Preoperative clear liquid carbohydrate rich drink 2 h prior to surgery. *Caution with esophagectomy pts.* PO intake as soon as tolerated postoperatively
  - **Minimizing IV Fluids:** Goal-directed therapy intraop. D/C maintenance fluids when tolerating PO intake
  - **Multimodal analgesia:** Targeted at reducing opioid and volatile anesthetic requirements.
    - Preop: Acetaminophen, gabapentin
    - Intraop: Ketamine, ketorolac
    - Postop: Acetaminophen, gabapentin, ketorolac
  - **Regional anesthesia:** Targeting further reducing opioid consumption and improving respiratory effort. Paravertebral blocks or intercostal blocks with liposomal bupivacaine may allow for early mobility and ambulation relative to a thoracic epidural
  - **Early ambulation:** Pain control as above, remove lines (Foley, chest tubes, etc.) as quickly as possible

JESSE M. EHRENFELD • RICHARD D. URMAN

INTRODUCTION

Systemic Manifestations of Liver Disease	
Cardiovascular	Cardiomyopathy, ↑ CO, ↓ SVR, pulmonary HTN, ↑ PVR, ↑ total body water, ↓ effective plasma volume, ↓ plasma oncotic pressure
Respiratory	Hypoxemia from intrapulmonary shunts, ↓ FRC, concurrent COPD/pneumonia, pleural effusions, resp alkalosis
Gastrointestinal	↑ Portal hydrostatic pressure → portal HTN → ascites; GI bleeding due to esophageal varices, ↓ gastric emptying
Renal	Acute and chronic kidney injury, hepatorenal syndrome
Hematologic	Anemia, coagulopathy, thrombocytopenia, coagulation imbalance
Neurologic	Encephalopathy, neuropathy, ↑ ICP in acute liver failure
Metabolic	Hypoglycemia, ↓ K, ↓ Na, ↓ albumin

Child–Pugh Classification of Severity of Liver Disease			
	Points Assigned		
Parameter	1	2	3
Ascites	Absent	Slight	Moderate
Bilirubin mg/dL	<2	2–3	>3
Albumin g/dL	>3.5	2.8–3.5	<2.8
Prothrombin time (s over control)	<4	4–6	>6
INR	<1.7	1.7–2.3	>2.3
Encephalopathy	None	Grades 1–2	Grades 3–4
Grade A: Total score = 5–6	→ 1- & 2-y survival = 100% & 85%		
Grade B: Total score = 7–9	→ 1- & 2-y survival = 80% & 60%		
Grade C: Total score = 10–15	→ 1- & 2-y survival = 80% & 60%		

See also Chapter 33, Organ Transplantation

ANESTHETIC CONSIDERATIONS IN ABDOMINAL SURGERY

Preoperative Evaluation
• Fluid status: Pts often hypovolemic
• Inadequate fluid intake (fasting, anorexia)
• Fluid loss (emesis, bowel preps, GI bleeding, fevers = insensible loss)
• Sequestration of fluid from intravascular space (3rd spacing)

Physical Signs of Hypovolemia			
	Fluid Loss (% of Body Weight)		
Sign	5%	10%	15%
Sensorium	Normal	Lethargic	Obtunded
Heart rate	Normal or ↑	↑ >100 bpm	Markedly ↑ >120 bpm
Blood pressure	Normal	Mildly ↓ with resp variation	↓
Orthostatic changes in HR & BP	Absent	Present	Marked
Mucous membranes	Dry	Very dry	Parched
Urine output	Mildly ↓	Moderately ↓	Markedly ↓

Anesthetic Management
Technique
• Abdominal procedures usually require muscle relaxation
  • Epidural analgesia may be beneficial (↓ anesthetic requirements, blunt surgical stress response, ↑ postop pain relief, ↓ postop atelectasis, ↑ postop mobility)

Level of Epidural Catheter Insertion in Relation to Type of Surgery	
Surgical Location	
Pancreas, spleen, esophagus, stomach, liver, gallbladder, ileal loop	T7–T10
Adrenals, small intestine, colon, kidney, ureters, uterus, ovaries, & testes	T8–L1
Prostate, urethra, & rectum	L3–L4

Fluid Management (See Chapter 10, Fluids, Electrolytes, & Transfusion Therapy)
- General strategies
  - Body wt–based formulas: Rough guidelines for fluid replacement
  - Goal-directed strategies: Aimed at optimizing stroke volume, cardiac output, & tissue perfusion. Use mechanical ventilation or fluid bolus–induced variations in pulse pressure (dPP), stroke volume (SV), or cardiac output (CO) to assess fluid responsiveness
- Blood products—should be given based on clinical eval of blood loss (surgical suction canister, sponges) & point-of-care testing (hematocrit, INR, TEG)

Muscle Relaxation
- Usually required for intra-abdominal procedures & abdominal closure
  - Secondary to intraop bowel edema & abdominal distention
- Inhalational agents may potentiate effects of muscle relaxants

Use of Nitrous Oxide (N_2O)
- N_2O diffuses into bowel lumen faster than nitrogen can diffuse out
  - Degree of bowel distention is a function of:
    - N_2O conc, blood flow to the bowel, duration of admin
- Avoid N_2O (relative contraindication) in bowel obstruction
  - May have large initial volume of bowel gas and/or difficult surgical closure
- Causes an obligatory reduction in FiO_2
  - However, ↑ FiO_2 may reduce incidence of surgical wound infection
- May ↑ pulmonary artery pressure (esp in pts with pulmonary HTN)
- Possible ↑ incidence of PONV

Common Intraop Problems
- ↓ FRC, atelectasis, & hypoxemia because of
  - Surgical retraction of abd viscera to improve exposure
  - Insufflation of gas during laparoscopy
  - Trendelenburg position
  - *(Application of PEEP and sigh breaths may reverse those effects)*
- Hypothermia 2° to heat loss: Radiation > convection > conduction > evaporation
  - Most heat loss occurs during 1st h of anesthesia (1–1½°C) *(treat by ↑ OR temp, apply convective warming blankets, warm IV fluids)*
- Hypotension, tachycardia, & facial flushing during bowel manipulation
  - 2° to mediator release (prostaglandin F1-α, a prostanoid)
- Oliguria due to ↑ intra-abd press, retraction of ureters, hypotension or hypovolemia
- Opioid-induced biliary tract spasm
- May interfere with interpretation of intraop cholangiograms *(Reversed by naloxone, nitroglycerin, & glucagon)*
- Hiccups are episodic diaphragmatic spasms relieved by ↑ anesthetic depth, ↑ neuromuscular blockade, drainage of stomach to relieve gastric distention

ALCOHOL ABUSE

Preop Evaluation
- Alcoholic cirrhosis characterized by AST/ALT ratio >2

Anesthetic Considerations
- Acute intoxication: ↓ Anesthetic requirements (2° to EtOH depressant effects)
- Chronic intoxication: ↑ Anesthetic requirements (2° to tolerance)
- Head & cervical spine injury must be considered in intoxicated pts

Postop Considerations
- Unrecognized alcohol abuse may present with delirium tremens
- Often occurs 72 h after last drink (postop d 3)
- Signs: Autonomic hyperactivity, tremors, hallucinations, seizures
- Treatment: Benzodiazepines

Multisystem Involvement in Alcoholic Abuse	
Cardiovascular	Dilated cardiomyopathy, hypertension
Respiratory	COPD (20% of alcohol abuse pts)
Neurologic	Cerebellar degeneration, polyneuropathy
	Nutritional d/o (Wernicke–Korsakoff syndrome)
	Delirium tremens (alcohol withdrawal)
Gastrointestinal	Esophagitis, gastritis, pancreatitis, hepatic cirrhosis
Hematologic	Anemia, thrombocytopenia
Endocrine	↓ Gluconeogenesis (hypoglycemia), hypomagnesemia

ANESTHETIC MANAGEMENT: LIVER SURGERY

General Considerations
- Liver resections often done for metastasis to liver or 1° hepatocellular carcinoma
- Laparoscopic ablation of liver lesions as a palliative option in high-risk pts
- Hypoxemia → 2° hepatopulmonary shunting, atelectasis, ↓ FRC from ascites
- Prior portosystemic shunt ↑ surgical complexity & risk of surgical bleeding

Management of Portal Hypertension
- Pharmacologic: β-Blockers
- Endoscopic: Sclerotherapy & esophageal banding for bleeding varices
- Transjugular intrahepatic portosystemic shunt (TIPS) have replaced surgical shunts, done percutaneously under fluoroscopy
- Surgery: ↑ Risk of encephalopathy, no evidence of better outcome

Monitoring
- A-line & CVP

Anesthetic Technique
- General endotracheal anesthesia
- Thoracic epidural for postop pain control (provided no coagulopathy)
- Aspiration precautions (nonparticulate antacids, rapid-sequence induction)
- Avoid N_2O (risk of bowel expansion & potential ↑ pulm artery pressure)
- Avoid histamine-releasing muscle relaxants (atracurium, mivacurium) to avoid further ↓ blood pressure
- Hyperdynamic circulation in pts with end-stage liver dz may require vasopressor therapy to ↑ systemic afterload
- Concomitant pulmonary HTN in pts with ESLD → avoid hypoxemia, hypercarbia, & metabolic acidosis (worsen pulmonary HTN)
- Careful NG tube placement (concern for coagulopathy + esophageal varices)
- Fluid replacement with isotonic fluids & colloids (pts have ↓ intravascular oncotic pressure)
- Prolonged hepatic "inflow" occlusion (Pringle maneuver: Occlusion of portal vein & hepatic artery) → may lead to coagulopathy & metabolic acidosis

Postop Care
- Bleeding: Surgical vs. coagulopathy
- *Small for size syndrome* in extensive hepatic resections (remaining liver unable to support metabolic functions → ↑ lactate, ↑ liver enzymes, worsening metabolic acidosis)

ANESTHETIC MANAGEMENT: LAPAROSCOPIC SURGERY

General Considerations
- Advantages include smaller incision, ↓ surgical trauma, ↓ postop pain, ↓ pulmonary dysfx, ↓ postop ileus, faster recovery, & ↓ hospital stay
- 3 ports typically inserted into abdomen: (Subumbilical port used for CO_2 insufflation to 12–15 mmHg)

Physiologic Changes During Laparoscopy	
Physiologic Change	**Mechanism**
Respiratory	
↓ Lung compliance	Trendelenburg position, ↑ intra-abd pressure
↑ Ventilation/perfusion mismatch	↓ FRC
↑ Inspiratory pressures	Trendelenburg position, pneumoperitoneum
↑ $PaCO_2$ and ↓ pH	↓ Pulm perfusion, ↓ alveolar ventilation

Cardiovascular	
↑ Systemic vascular resistance, ↑ pulm vascular resistance, ↑ mean arterial pressure	Hypercapnia, ↑ intra-abd pressure, ↑ catecholamine release
↓ Venous return	Vena cava compression
↓ Cardiac output	↓ Preload, ↑ afterload
Neurologic	
↑ Intracranial pressure	Trendelenburg position, ↑ cerebral blood flow due to hypercapnia
Renal	
↓ Urine output	↓ Renal blood flow; ↑ ADH secretion, ↑ IAP

Anesthetic Technique: Laparoscopic Surgery
- General anesthesia with endotracheal intubation and controlled ventilation
- Muscle relaxation to avoid further ↑ in intrathoracic pressure
- Rapid-sequence induction for antireflux procedures and pts with full stomach
- Persistent ↑ ETCO$_2$ despite adequate minute volume may signal subcutaneous emphysema
- Attenuation of hemodynamic changes to peritoneal insufflation:
  - Bradycardia → glycopyrrolate or atropine
  - Decreased CO & hypertension → use volume loading and/or vasopressor
  - Hypertension → use vasodilators

Causes of Hypotension During Laparoscopy	
• Reverse Trendelenburg position	• Venous gas embolism
• Bleeding & hypovolemia	• Tension pneumothorax
• High insufflation pressures	• Tension pneumoperitoneum
• Arrhythmias	• Pericardial tamponade
• Myocardial ischemia	

Monitoring
- Large-bore peripheral IV access (limited access to tucked arms during case)
- Orogastric tube to aspirate gas from stomach prior to trocar placement
- Acute ↑ in peak airway pressure may signal:
  - Endobronchial migration of tube (esp with bed change to Trendelenburg)
  - Pneumothorax (usually accompanied by ↓ SpO$_2$)
- Avoid ↑ peak airway pressure: Use pressure-control ventilation and ↓ exp time (e.g., I/E ratio 1:1.5)
  - Minute volume usually must be ↑ by 20% to maintain normocarbia
- Bradycardia following CO$_2$ insufflation likely vagally mediated
  - May also be 2° to hypercarbia & respiratory acidosis
- Avoid ↑ in insufflation pressure that can compromise venous return (max 12–15 mmHg)

Postop Care
- Shoulder pain (suprascapular nerve irritation)—*treat with NSAIDs*
- Unrecognized intra-abdominal visceral/vascular injury → progressive hypotension, ↑ abdominal girth, ↓ hematocrit
- ↑ Incidence of PONV
- Extensive subcutaneous emphysema may require mechanical ventilation

---

LARGE INTESTINAL SURGERY

Indications
- Colon cancer, diverticulitis, ulcerative colitis, Crohn dz, ischemic colitis, reversal of colostomy

Preop Evaluation
- Preop fasting + bowel prep = large fluid deficit
- Bowel obstruction can ↑ risk for gastric aspiration during induction
- Thoracic epidural analgesia (T8–12) ↓ atelectasis, ↑ early ambulation *(may contribute to hypotension in presence of hypovolemia)*
- *Bilateral TAP catheters to reduce incision pain as part of multimodal analgesia if epidural analgesia contraindicated or undesirable by surgeon or pt (see Chapter 6, Regional Anesthesia)*

Anesthetic Management: Large Intestinal Surgery
- Consider aspiration precautions if pt is obstructed
- Consider stress dose steroids if pt is on preop steroids

- Fluid replacement must account for evaporative losses of exposed viscera
- Mesenteric traction syndrome: Hypotension during bowel surgery from bowel-associated mediator release (vasoactive intestinal peptide)
  - Hypovolemia, surgical bleeding, sepsis 2° to peritoneal fecal spillage

Postop Complications
- Prokinetic agents (metoclopramide) can cause anastomotic dehiscence after colonic surgery
- Postop ileus caused by bowel manipulation, opioids, immobility, lack of enteral feeding, & bowel edema from fluid overload (epidural analgesia may ↓ incidence of ileus)
- Prolonged NG tube placement can lead to ischemic necrosis of nasal septum

SMALL INTESTINAL SURGERY

Indications
- Small bowel obstruction, neoplasms, intussusception, intestinal bleed, resection of carcinoid tumor, Crohn dz

Carcinoid Tumors/Carcinoid Syndrome
- Carcinoid tumors typically asymptomatic
  - May present with abd pain, diarrhea, & intermittent obstruction
- Metastatic carcinoid tumors (hepatic, pulm metastases) systemic symptoms
  → Carcinoid syndrome: Cutaneous flushing, bronchoconstriction, hypotension, diarrhea, & rt-sided valvular lesions
  ↑ 5-hydroxy-indole-acetic acid (>30 mg in 24-h urine)
- Epidural analgesia may exacerbate intraop hypotension (consider use of dilute local anesthetics/narcotics + volume loading)

Monitoring
- Consider TEE for carcinoid (eval rt-sided heart lesions & guide fluid therapy)

Anesthetic Management
- Consider aspiration precautions/rapid-sequence induction for obstruction
- Carcinoid tumors
  - Avoid agents that release histamine (thiopental, succinylcholine, atracurium, morphine)
  - Octreotide (synthetic somatostatin) effective in relieving hypotension (subcutaneous dose 50–500 mcg—half-life of 2.5 h)

Postop Care
- 50% of carcinoid deaths result from cardiac involvement
- Similar considerations as in large intestine surgery

PANCREATIC SURGERY

Indications
- Pancreatic adenocarcinoma resection (Whipple: Pancreatojejunostomy with gastrojejunostomy & choledochojejunostomy)
- Treatment of complications of pancreatitis: Infected pancreatic necrosis, hemorrhagic pancreatitis, drainage of pancreatic pseudocyst

Monitoring
- Pancreatic surgery can be assoc with significant blood loss & fluid shifts (consider A-line, CVP depending on pt comorbidities)

Anesthetic Management
- Consider thoracic epidural analgesia (T6–T10) for postop pain control
- Often feeding tube tip will be adjusted by surgeon during procedure
- Pancreatic surgery for infection may be complicated by sepsis & ARDS requires aggressive fluid resuscitation, vasopressor support (α-agonist, e.g., norepinephrine) & postop mechanical ventilation

Postop Care
- Significant pancreatic resection → insulin insufficiency & new-onset diabetes

SPLENIC SURGERY

Indications
- Splenic injury (blunt or penetrating trauma)
- Idiopathic thrombocytopenic purpura with splenic sequestration of platelets

Preop Preparation
- Periop platelet transfusion *not* warranted (unless platelet count is *<50,000/μL or clinical evidence of coagulopathy*)

Anesthetic Management
- Avoid drugs that interfere with platelet function (NSAIDs)

Postop Care
- Pts should receive pneumococcal, *Haemophilus influenzae*, & meningococcal vaccines

---

HEMORRHOIDECTOMY & DRAINAGE OF PERIRECTAL ABSCESS

Anesthetic Management
- Procedures usually short, often in lithotomy/prone position
- Usually general anesthesia (consider LMA for lithotomy cases)
- Spinals may be used (hypobaric solution for prone case, hyperbaric for lithotomy)
- Deep plane of anesthesia provides sphincter relaxation

Postop Care
- Postop pain can be severe → consider use of local anesthetic infiltration, narcotics, & NSAIDs

---

INGUINAL HERNIORRHAPHY

Anesthetic Management
- Commonly done as an outpt procedure
- Spermatic cord traction may initiate a vagally mediated bradycardia
  - MAC + local anesthesia most common approach
  - Paravertebral block (T10–L2) increasingly used
  - Spinal or general anesthesia may also be used

VENTRAL HERNIORRHAPHY

Preop Considerations
- Staged ventral hernia repair may ↓ incidence of postop respiratory failure (*closure of large abd defects → pulm restriction*)

Monitoring
- Obtain large-bore IV access to replace evaporative fluid losses in large cases

Anesthetic Management
- Consider epidural analgesia (T10–T12) or transversus abdominis plane block (bilateral for midline incisions, unilateral for one-sided hernias)
- Usually done with general endotracheal anesthesia + muscle relaxation
- Smooth emergence impt (no coughing/bucking) to avoid disruption of repair

---

APPENDECTOMY

Preop Evaluation
- Consider preop IV hydration to replace fluid deficits (vomiting, poor intake)

Anesthetic Management
- Performed via open or laparoscopic approach
- General anesthesia with endotracheal tube
- Consider taking aspiration precautions (rapid-sequence induction)

Postop Care
- IV opioids usually sufficient for postop pain management

CHOLECYSTECTOMY

Anesthetic Management
- Performed via open or laparoscopic approach with general endotracheal anesthesia
- Opioid-induced biliary tract spasm
  - May interfere with interpretation of intraop cholangiograms
  - Can be reversed by naloxone, nitroglycerin, & glucagon
- Minimal blood loss unless abdominal vessel injury occurs

Postop Care
- Lap cholecystectomy → less postop pain & earlier discharge (usually same d)

Anesthesia for Aesthetic Surgery

Liposuction
- Most commonly performed plastic surgery procedure
- Performed by inserting hollow rods into skin & suctioning subcutaneous fat
- Tumescent liposuction (pre-aspiration injection of lidocaine and epinephrine-containing wetting solution) is the most common form of liposuction

Anesthetic Techniques
- Pain can be controlled with locally infiltrated lidocaine + IV/oral opioids
- Low-volume procedures → sedation or MAC vs. GA (if pt/provider request)
- Large-volume procedures → consider deep sedation/GA/regional
- Limit IV fluids if large volume of solution is being infused, may require diuresis

Complications
- Lidocaine toxicity (can occur postprocedure 2° to slow systemic absorption)
- Volume overload/CHF
- Hypovolemia, bleeding, PE, fat embolism, hypothermia, body cavity perforation

Mammoplasty
- *Augmentation*—Technique: Usually GA (separation of pectoralis muscle may require paralysis); consider antiemetic prophylaxis
- *Reduction*—Technique: Usually GA; paravertebral blocks/epidural may be used

Blepharoplasty (Lidlift)
- Technique: Local anesthetic infiltration + MAC (so pt can open & close eyes intraop)
- Avoid bucking/coughing during emergence and PONV (may ↑ risk of hematoma)
- Consider propofol/remifentanil infusion for wakeup, PONV prophylaxis
- Complications: Oculocardiac reflex (OCR), retrobulbar hematoma, LA toxicity

Rhytidectomy (Facelift)
- Technique: Usually GA or MAC
- Beware of airway fire with MAC + supplemental O_2 (proximity of cautery & O_2)
- Same emergence and PONV precautions as blepharoplasty

Practice Advisory on Liposuction

Anesthetic Infiltration Solutions

• For small-volume liposuction, wetting solutions with local anesthetics may provide sufficient pain relief without additional anesthesia; pts or providers, however, may prefer sedation/general anesthesia even with small-volume liposuction
• Avoid bupivacaine (Marcaine) as additive to infiltrate solution (severe side effects, slow elimination, & lack of toxicity reversal)
• Lidocaine given in large volumes may cause systemic toxicity. Preventive measures:
  • Limit lidocaine dose to 35–55 mg/kg (this level may not be safe in pts with low protein levels/conditions where lidocaine byproducts accumulate). Levels may peak 8–12 h after infusion
  • Calculate dose for total body weight & ↓ lidocaine concentration if necessary
  • Utilize superwet rather than tumescent technique
  • Avoid lidocaine when utilizing general/regional anesthesia
• Avoid epinephrine in pts with pheochromocytoma, hyperthyroidism, severe HTN, cardiac dz (CAD or arrhythmia), or peripheral vascular dz
• Consider staged infiltration of various sites to ↓ effects of excess epinephrine

Source: Adapted from Iverson RE. Practice advisory on liposuction. *Plast Reconstr Surg* 2004;113(5):1478–1490.

MELISSA L. BELLOMY • BRIAN F. S. ALLEN • MATTHEW D. McEVOY

ANESTHETIC MANAGEMENT: BARIATRIC SURGERY

Types of Bariatric Surgery
- **Vertical band gastroplasty**—creation of small gastric pouch, usually laparoscopic
- **Roux-en-Y gastric bypass**—small gastric pouch anastomosed to proximal jejunum
  - Pts at risk for Iron and B_{12} deficiency, dumping syndrome

Preanesthetic Considerations
- **Obesity-associated comorbidities**
  - HTN, hyperlipidemia, obstructive sleep apnea (OSA), GERD, Type II DM, NASH
  - ↑ Circulating blood volume, ↑ cardiac output → ↑ in O_2 consumption
  - ↓ Lung compliance, ↑V/Q mismatch, ↓ FRC, & shunt→ hypoxemia
  - Long-standing hypoxemia, hypercarbia → pulmonary HTN & right heart failure

WHO Classification of Obesity based on BMI

Underweight	<18.5
Normal range	18.5–24.9
Overweight	25–29.9
Obese	≥30
Obese class I	30–34.9
Obese class II	35–39.9
Obese class III	≥40

BMI = body weight in kg/(height in meters)^2
- Overweight = BMI >25; obesity = BMI >30; morbid obesity = BMI >35

Anesthetic Technique
- General endotracheal anesthesia
- Truncal blocks for laparoscopic procedures, epidural analgesia for open procedures
  - Reduces need for systemic opioids & oversedation in pts with OSA
- Opioid-sparing anesthetic: Preop APAP, gabapentin; intraop lidocaine, ketamine, consider COX II inhibitors or other NSAIDs
- Lung-protective ventilation: TV 6–8 mL/kg IBW + moderate PEEP + IRM breaths
- Goal-directed fluid therapy: Goal is euvolemia with Plasmalyte or LR; no 0.9% saline, use pressors to maintain BP in reverse T-burg instead of high IVF load
- PONV prophylaxis: Multimodal antiemetic regimen based on risk factors

Airway Management
- Specific considerations
  - Key predictors of difficult intubation: Neck circumference >42 cm, Mallampati scores III & IV
  - Risk factors for difficult mask ventilation: Obesity, OSA, ↑ pharyngeal soft tissue
  - Rapid desaturation following induction 2° to ↓ FRC (limited O_2 reserve), ↑ O_2 consumption, & ↑ incidence of airway obstruction
- Management strategies
  - Avoid or ↓ dose of sedative premedication if possible (↓ respiratory depression)
  - Thorough preoxygenation in a 25° head-up position or reverse Trendelenburg
  - Ramped position (align auditory meatus & sternal notch) to improve laryngeal view
  - Consider awake fiberoptic intubation if airway exam concerning
  - Consider using less soluble inhalational agents (i.e., avoid isoflurane)
  - Aspiration precautions with antacids + rapid-sequence induction (↑ risk w/GERD)

Monitoring
- Consider arterial line if: Hypoxemia at rest, LVEF <30–40%; mod–severe pulm HTN; severe AS, AR, or MR; mod–severe MS; or unable to measure BP noninvasively

Drug-Dose Adjustment in Obesity	
Typically, lipophilic drugs dosed by TBW for loading and adjusted by IBW for maintenance.	
Dosage by Total Body Weight (TBW)	**Dosage by Ideal Body Weight (IBW)**
• Benzodiazepine (loading dose) • Propofol • Opioids (loading dose) • Succinylcholine	• Benzodiazepine (maintenance dose) • Nondepolarizing muscle relaxants • Opioids (maintenance dose) *IBW calculation:* *Men = 50 kg + 2.3 kg × (height [in.] − 60)* *Women = 45.5 kg + 2.3 kg × (height [in.] − 60)*
Obese pts typically have ↑ cardiac output, ↑ volume of distribution	

Postop Complications
- ↑ Atelectasis & hypoxemia *(consider semirecumbent position, CPAP, or BiPAP)*
- ↑ Postop hypercarbia, especially in pts w/baseline retention
  - Minimize this risk with opioid-sparing analgesia in intraop and postop periods
- Accidental stapling of NG tube to stomach *(prevent by communication w/surgeons)*
- DVT prophylaxis & early ambulation ↓ risk of thromboembolism

MEREDITH A. KINGETER • AMY C. ROBERTSON

OPEN VASCULAR PROCEDURES

Abdominal Aortic Aneurysm (AAA) Repair

- Indications: Symptomatic aneurysm, asymptomatic (if >5 cm or growing >0.5 cm/ 6 mo), ruptured aneurysm, dissection, trauma, occlusive dz
- Morbidity: **5% periop MI risk** (risks of acute kidney injury, ischemic colitis, spinal ischemia, and death all ↑ if aneurysm ruptured)
- Mortality for ruptured AAA: **50% periop mortality**; 100% mortality without emergent surgical intervention
- Approach: Supraceliac, suprarenal, infrarenal (depends on aneurysm extension)
- Preoperative evaluation
  - Anatomy/location of AAA: Supraceliac vs. infraceliac
  - Coexisting dz: ↑ Prevalence of CAD in TAAA/AAA pts
  - Lab testing: Electrolytes, BUN/Cr, Coags, CBC, type, and screen
- Lines and monitors
  - 2 large-bore peripheral IVs
  - a-Line: Right radial for descending aortic surgery (see below), consider preinduction a-line if pt unstable
  - Central line (recommend 8.5-Fr introducer) for volume infusion and CVP measurement, use goal-directed fluid therapy
  - Consider pulmonary artery catheterization if suprarenal aneurysm or other significant cardiac Hx
  - Consider thoracic (T8–10) epidural for postoperative pain control
  - TEE may be helpful for early detection of myocardial ischemia (especially for higher aneurysms/cross-clamping)
  - Upper and lower body-warming blankets in place (lower should remain **OFF** until after reperfusion & stabilization)
  - Foley catheter: Goal urine output >0.5 mL/kg/h
  - Cell saver, PRBC in the OR; may also need FFP
- Hemodynamic derangements with aortic cross-clamping
  - ↑ In afterload (↑ LVEDP, LVEDV) and PCWP
  - ↑ Catecholamines
  - ↓ Venous capacity → shift of blood volume proximal to clamp
  - ↑ In MAP, CVP → HTN above the cross-clamp
  - ↑ In PVR → increased membrane permeability
  - **10–55% ↓ in CO** (infrarenal lowest, supraceliac highest reduction)
  - **LV dilatation and ↑ LVEDP** → subendocardial ischemia, LV failure, CHF, arrhythmias

Effects of Decreased Perfusion from Aortic Cross-Clamping	
Organ System	**Potential Effects/Complications**
Abdominal viscera	Bowel ischemia
Renal	Acute kidney injury, potential long-term renal dysfunction • ↑ Risk with suprarenal clamp and cross-clamp time >30 min
Extremities	Distal ischemia
Spinal cord	Spinal cord ischemia and paraplegia • Artery of Adamkiewicz arises from aorta: 15% originates between T5 and T8, 60% between T9 and T12, 25% between L1 and L2 • Anterior spinal artery syndrome: 0.2% incidence with elective infrarenal AAA; 8% with elective TAAA or TEVAR; 40% in setting of thoracic dissection or rupture

- Derangements with release of aortic cross-clamp
  - **↓ Afterload and hypotension** (due to ↓ SVR and hypovolemia)
  - Return of cool, acidotic blood to central circulation
  - **Vasodilatory mediators and ischemic factors** from distal tissues
  - Metabolic acidosis, ↑ EtCO$_2$, ↓ SvO$_2$
  - ↑ CVP from return of pooled venous blood
  - **↓ In spinal cord perfusion pressure (SCPP)** 2° to (1) hypercarbia → ↑ cerebral spinal fluid pressure (CSFP), (2) hypotension, (3) metabolic acidosis → ↑ cerebral blood flow → ↑ ICP and CSFP

- Management before cross-clamping
  - Induction of GA: **Maintain BPs near baseline** as HTN can rupture aneurysm, hypotension can cause myocardial ischemia
  - **Control HR** (usually with esmolol)
  - **Maintain relative hypovolemia** during preclamp phase to prevent HTN from increased afterload and ↓ risk of MI during cross-clamp (*do not overhydrate, use vasodilators*)
  - **Avoid HTN response** to cross-clamp: Deepen anesthesia, nitroprusside (causes arteriolar dilation and MAP reduction), nitroglycerin (may prevent myocardial ischemia and ↓ preload)
- Preparation for clamp release
  - Gradually ↑ **preload** with volume
  - **Wean vasodilators** and have vasopressors ready
  - Lighten anesthesia
- Postclamp management
  - Give **fluid bolus or blood products** (if warranted)
  - Gradual release of clamp can ↓ hemodynamic changes
  - If severe hypotension results, ask surgeon to reclamp and reassess
  - **Vasopressors** may be needed
  - ↑ Minute ventilation to normalize EtCO$_2$
  - **ABG** before and after cross-clamp removal (guide fluid and electrolyte management)
  - Monitor HCT and correct coagulopathies
  - Use standard extubation criteria (pts often stay intubated 2° large volume shifts)
- Preventing acute kidney injury
  - Risk: Supraceliac > suprarenal > infrarenal
  - **Maintain renal perfusion pressure** with highest possible MAP that myocardium will tolerate
  - Maintain intravascular volume
  - Consider mannitol (0.5 g/kg before x-clamping), furosemide, Ca^{2+} blockers, dopamine, fenoldopam (*not proven effective*)
- Preventing spinal cord ischemia
  - SCPP = MAP$_d$ (distal mean aortic pressure) − [CSFP or CVP]*
    *whichever is greater
  - Risk factors for paraplegia: Emergent procedure, prolonged cross-clamp time, more extensive aneurysm, advanced age, severe atherosclerotic dz, ligation of spinal collateral arteries
  - **Maintain highest MAP** (distal aortic perfusion pressures) that myocardium can tolerate
  - SSEP monitoring—not useful (2/3 of cord is supplied by anterior spinal artery → motor)
  - Consider partial bypass or shunt to maintain distal perfusion during x-clamp
  - Consider administering steroids and/or barbiturates
  - Consider epidural cooling
  - **CSF drain:** If monitoring distal pressures, aim for SCPP >30 mmHg; can drain CSF via lumbar drain, up to ~15 mL/15 min (*risk of brainstem herniation with rapid or excessive CSF drainage → limit to ~75 mL*)
  - Avoid excessive vasodilators (hypotension → ↓ perfusion, cerebral vasodilation → ↑ ICP transmitted to CSF)
  - Avoid hyperglycemia (consider insulin infusion for glucose >200 mg/dL)
  - Consider mild hypothermia (passive cooling to about 34°C)

Thoracoabdominal Aortic Aneurysm (TAAA) Repair
- Management similar to AAA (see above) with following key points
- Surgical treatment for proximal dissections; distal dissections may be treated medically
- Pharmacologic measures to reduce blood pressure and aortic wall stress; vasodilators (nicardipine or nitroprusside) and β-blockade (esmolol)

Crawford Classification of TAAA (I–IV)
- I: Descending thoracic aortic aneurysm distal to subclavian artery
- II: Aneurysm originating at subclavian artery to distal abdominal aorta
- III: Aneurysm from mid-descending thoracic aorta to distal abdominal aorta
- IV: Abdominal aortic aneurysm (below the diaphragm)

Stanford Classification of TAAA (A–B)
- Type A: Intimal tear (acute) in aorta from ascending aorta to descending aorta
- Type B: Intimal tear (acute or chronic) in aorta from descending aorta down

Possible Associated Findings with TAAA
- Tracheal or bronchial deviation/compression
- Hemoptysis
- Hoarseness and vocal cord paralysis if compression of left recurrent laryngeal nerve
- Superior vena cava syndrome
- Esophageal deviation/compression
- Hemothorax and mediastinal shift if rupture into pleura
- Cardiac tamponade if rupture into pericardium
- Dissection: Incompetence of the aortic valve if extends to aortic root, cardiac tamponade, coronary ischemia
- Reduced distal perfusion

(Adapted from: Dunn P. *Clinical Procedures of the MGH*. Philadelphia, PA: Lippincott Williams & Wilkins.)

Anesthetic Considerations

Surgery on Ascending Aorta	Surgery Involving Aortic Arch	Surgery on Descending Thoracic Aorta
• Median sternotomy and cardiopulmonary bypass (CPB) • Aortic valve replacement and coronary reimplantation often necessary • Anesthesia similar to other cardiac procedures • Radial a-line site determined by the possible need to clamp subclavian or innominate arteries • Nicardipine or nitroprusside for BP control • β-Blockade (esmolol) if dissection; bradycardia can worsen aortic insufficiency (AI) • TEE to detect intimal tear, coronary ostia, AI, assess embolic risk	• Median sternotomy and CPB • Deep hypothermic circulatory arrest (pack head with ice) • Additional cerebral protection measures: Hypothermia to 15°C, steroids, propofol or barbiturate infusion to achieve flat EEG (BIS) • Longer rewarming contributes to coagulopathy and blood loss	• Left thoracotomy without CPB • One-lung ventilation often employed • "Clamp and run" technique • Right atrium to femoral artery partial bypass may be used • Right radial a-line as clamping of the left subclavian artery may be necessary • Spinal cord protection measures • Cross-clamp → sudden ↑ in afterload may precipitate LV failure and myocardial ischemia • Cell saver for autotransfusion • Pulmonary artery catheterization and/or TEE to assist with hemodynamic management

BP Control During TAAA
- If no bypass: Maintain SBP at baseline SBP ¹/₂ of peak aortic cross-clamp SBP
- If bypass: Maintain SBP at baseline SBP
- Vasodilators should be used sparingly (or not at all) during aortic clamp (risk of ↓ spinal cord and renal perfusion)
- ↓ Conc of volatile agent and turn off vasodilators before aortic unclamp
- Volume repletion with colloid, crystalloid, blood products before/after aortic unclamp

Carotid Endarterectomy
- Indication: Hx of stroke, TIA, or significant arterial occlusion on angiography. According to a systematic review published in 2017, endarterectomy was of some benefit for pts with 50–69% symptomatic stenosis and highly beneficial for those with 70–99% stenosis. There was no benefit in pts with near-occlusion carotid dz (*Cochrane Database Syst Rev* 2017;6:CD001081)
- Morbidity 4–10% (primarily neurologic); incidence of concomitant CAD ≈50%; unstable CAD or left main dz are only pts who benefit from coronary revascularization before vascular surgery (*N Engl J Med* 2004;351(27):2795–2804)
- Periop mortality 1–4%

Anesthetic Techniques

	Advantages	Disadvantages
Regional Anesthesia Superficial and deep cervical blocks	Able to monitor for neurologic deficits; pt can verbalize neurologic symptoms Less hemodynamic alterations	"A good general is always better than a bad regional" → if regional not working, pt may be uncomfortable, move, become tachycardic, and necessitate unplanned conversion to general

	Avoidance of pulmonary complications associated with intubation and coughing/bucking at case end Possible reduced length of hospital stay Decreased risk of 30-d postoperative MI when compared to CEA under general anesthesia (Vascular 2015;23(2):113–119)	Some providers give "deep sedation" plus regional anesthesia → *eliminates benefit of awake detection of neurologic deficits* Risk of local anesthesia systemic toxicity ~5% (Lancet 2008;372:2132–2142)
General Anesthesia	Secure airway Potential benefit of ischemic preconditioning Neuroprotection with use of volatile and intravenous anesthetics	Necessitates careful planning and drug management during induction, emergence, and extubation to avoid HTN and coughing Hypotension (minimal surgical stimulation but must keep pt still) No proven difference in postop stroke or mortality with either technique (GA vs. regional) (Vascular 2015;23(2):113–119)

- **Deep cervical block technique**
  - Inject anesthetic at C2, C3, C4 in line drawn between mastoid process and C6 transverse process; needle should have slight caudal and posterior angulation, contact transverse process, withdraw 2 mm and inject; can be done under ultrasound guidance
  - Potential complications: Intra-arterial injection (vertebral artery), Horner syndrome (sympathetic chain), hoarseness (recurrent laryngeal nerve)
- **Superficial cervical block technique**
  - Technique: Inject anesthetic just posterior to sternocleidomastoid (goal to spread anesthetic subcutaneously and behind SCM) at C6 level and fanned 2–3 cm superior and inferior
  - Easy technique, minimal risk, superficial block can be used alone with supplemental wound infiltration and sedation
- Intraoperative shunting
  - Provides **blood flow from common carotid artery to internal carotid artery** (distal/superior to site of cross-clamp)
  - Indicated in pts with significant contralateral dz
  - Stump pressure: Measurement of pressure distal to site of cross-clamp, need to provide well-flushed a-line tubing over drape; *stump pressure <50 mmHg = indication for shunting*
  - Risk of plaque dislodgement, intimal injury, and air embolus
- Hemodynamic management
  - Avoid tachycardia (↑ myocardial O_2 demand) and hypotension (↓ coronary flow)
  - **Maintain MAP slightly above baseline to optimize collateral blood flow**
  - *Phenylephrine infusion → ideal to maintain MAP without raising heart rate*
  - Consider nitroglycerin for reduction of BP at induction/emergence
  - Consider esmolol/metoprolol to prevent tachycardia, *especially during intubation, reversal of neuromuscular blockade, extubation*
  - Consider a-line placement prior to induction in pts with known CAD
- Intraoperative brain monitoring has *not* been shown to improve outcomes
  - Awake: ↓ Cardiac morbidity and HTN
  - Cerebral oximetry: Correlation between arterial blood pressure and cerebral oximetry as a surrogate for cerebral oxygenation is unproven
  - EEG: May correlate with neurologic changes, reflects cortical function only and not deeper structures, cannot identify emboli
  - SSEPs: GA can alter signal, similar sensitivity and specificity as EEG, cannot identify emboli
  - Stump pressure: Poor sensitivity/specificity
  - Transcranial Doppler: Can confirm adequate flow through shunt, identify acute postoperative thrombosis
    - Near-infrared spectroscopy (NIRS): Measures oxygenation in the frontal cortex, interference can occur from noncerebral blood flow and light, cannot identify emboli

- Other intraoperative considerations
  - Ketamine should be used with caution due to an ↑ in cerebral metabolism, adrenergic stimulation, and potential interaction with neurologic monitoring
  - Avoid large doses of opioids as it may lead to delayed emergence and impair neurologic assessment
  - TIVA may be preferred when EP monitoring is utilized
  - Administration of systemic heparin typically occurs prior to carotid artery cross-clamping. Consider protamine administration for reversal of heparin at the completion of the procedure
- Perioperative complications
  - **Cerebral hypoperfusion** (avoid hyperglycemia and hypocapnia)
  - **Intracerebral steal** due to hypercapnia
  - Carotid body manipulation can cause **bradycardia**; *treat with lidocaine infiltration by surgeon or IV atropine*
  - **Intraoperative stroke** (Most intraoperative strokes are the result of thromboembolism and not hypoperfusion. Consider if delayed emergence/mental status change)
  - **Wound hematoma**
    - Diagnosis: Progressive stridor and dyspnea; often difficult to see hematoma (dressings/pt size)
    - **Evacuate hematoma 1st, manipulate airway 2nd**
    - Treatment: **Return to OR stat**—if rapidly deteriorating respiratory status, open wound *prior to airway manipulation;* attempts at intubation can be impossible (may result in airway swelling/bleeding, making situation worse)

Complications of Carotid Endarterectomy
• HTN: Damage to (or local anesthetic at) carotid sinus; ↑ risk for neuro deficits compared to pts with normal BP (due to hyperperfusion); more likely with GA (vs. regional)
• Hypotension: Removal of plaque → ↑ stimulation of baroreceptors; more likely with regional
• MI: Most frequent cause of morbidity/mortality
• Stroke: Usually embolic
• Bleeding: Can lead to airway obstruction from hematoma or edema
• CNS injury: 10% pts; most common nerves—hypoglossal, vagus, recurrent laryngeal, accessory
• Carotid body damage: ↓ Ventilatory response to hypoxemia/hypercapnia; esp impt if 2nd side CEA

VASCULAR   22-5

ENDOVASCULAR PROCEDURES

Endovascular AAA Repair (EVAR)
- Monitoring for most limited to a-line (plus large-bore IV access)
- Pressors/vasodilators usually not needed
- Conversion to open procedure rate <5% (should always anticipate this possibility)
  - Safely performed under general, epidural, or local anesthesia
- General anesthesia
  - Associated with longer hospital stay and increased pulmonary morbidity compared to local and regional anesthesia (*J Vasc Surg* 2011;54:1273–1282)
  - Complex cases or pt refuses regional/MAC
  - Always considered as backup for conversion to open procedure
- Regional anesthesia
  - Spinal: Duration of procedure usually precludes this
  - Epidural: Allows for ideal anesthesia of incision sites (bilateral femoral vascular access); must be prepared to delay case if achieve bloody/traumatic tap or intravascular catheter
  - Regional techniques may ↓ incidence of hypercoagulability and perioperative vessel clot formation (esp for lower-extremity procedures)
- Monitored anesthesia care (sedation) with local anesthesia
  - Pt must remain flat and still for hours on uncomfortable fluoroscopy bed
  - Advantages: Spontaneous ventilation preserving venous return, fewer pulmonary complications, improved immediate postoperative analgesia
- Contrast-induced nephropathy a concern 2° to extensive angiography; consider pre- and postprocedure hydration with normal saline or 5% dextrose/sodium bicarbonate for pts at increased risk

- Special considerations with thoracoabdominal endovascular aneurysm repair (TEVAR)
  - Proper positioning of graft may require temporary apnea and/or hypotension; consider bolus of propofol, nitroglycerine, or esmolol
  - Rarely adenosine is used to induce brief asystole

Carotid Stent Placement
- Commonly done under MAC and local anesthesia
- Requires immobility (minimal head/neck movement) and ability to tolerate fluoroscopy table
- Consider opioid/α-2 agonist technique (may avoid sedation-associated confusion)

Distal Angioplasty/Thrombectomy
- Pts with operative lower limb vascular dz have >50% incidence of concomitant CAD
- Procedure times often long (on uncomfortable fluoroscopy bed); usually best to avoid large dose of sedative and opiate or medications with long duration of action (*problem of confusion or disorientation*)
- Always be prepared for conversion to open procedure
- Regional techniques may ↓ incidence of hypercoagulability and perioperative vessel clot formation (esp for lower-extremity procedures)

PERIPHERAL VASCULAR SURGERY
- Preop risk: Pts often have significant comorbidities (↑ risk of associated CAD)
- Procedures: Bypass grafts (fem-pop, ilio-fem, etc.), embolectomy, pseudoaneurysm repair
- Monitoring: Invasive monitors per pt condition (hemodynamics often labile) (*place a-line in side opposite surgery*)
- Anesthetic
  - General anesthesia/regional/MAC
    - Regional and GA → associated with comparable rates of cardiac morbidity
  - Continuous epidural/spinal
    - Continuous lumbar epidural catheter commonly used
    - Awake pts can notify personnel of acute MI symptoms (chest pain)
  - Helpful for postop pain control
  - Intraop heparin after epidural placement does not ↑ risk of epidural hematoma
  - ↓ Incidence of postop pneumonia with neuraxial anesthesia compared with GA
    (Cochrane Database Syst Rev 2013;7:CD007083)

JOSHUA H. ATKINS

BASIC PRINCIPLES OF NEUROPHYSIOLOGY

Cerebral Metabolic Rate (CMR), Cerebral Blood Flow (CBF), and Autoregulation (Fig. 23-1)

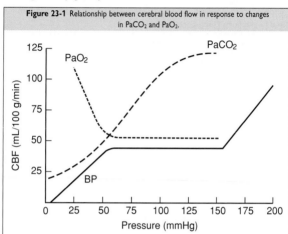

Figure 23-1 Relationship between cerebral blood flow in response to changes in $PaCO_2$ and PaO_2.

(From Dunn P. *Clinical Anesthesia Procedures of the Massachusetts General Hospital.* 7th ed. Philadelphia, PA: Lippincott Williams & Wilkins; 2006.)

- Cerebral perfusion pressure (CPP) = MAP − ICP (or CVP if CVP > ICP)
  - Lack of strong evidence base to guide CPP, likely considerable variation based on factors including injured brain, anesthesia, autoregulatory mechanisms
  - In the absence of other data to guide, Goal of CPP >60 mmHg;
  - Higher pressures needed to achieve adequate tissue O_2 delivery in pts with existing brain pathology/elevated ICP (likely >70 mmHg)
  - Arterial catheter: MAP measured with transducer at tragus to reflect CPP
  - Neurologic exam, EEG/processed, NIRS, TCD, or other CBF monitor can be used to guide CPP, MAP
- Cerebral blood flow in healthy pts is autoregulated (MAP 50–150 mmHg)
  - Global cerebral blood flow ~50 mL/100 g brain/min (~75% to gray matter)
  - In chronic HTN → autoregulation curve shifts to right
  - Modest hypotension may result in hypoperfusion & ischemia
- Extreme hypertension → large increases in CBF & ICP
  - Brain edema, hyperemia, & tissue injury from disruption of BBB
- Blood flow changes with cerebral metabolic rate
  - Brain O_2 delivery closely approximates demand (~50% of O_2 extracted at 1st pass)
  - Blood flow <15 mL/100 g/min → ischemia detectable by EEG
  - Anesthetics, temp, arterial Po_2 & Pco_2, and pathophysiologic states influence relationship between autoregulation of CBF (see Table—Cerebral Blood Flow—Metabolic Rate Coupling (CBF & CMR))
  - Displacement of brain tissue by surgical instruments impairs local perfusion
  - Global brain physiology different than regional/cellular level (e.g., mitochondria)

Cerebral Blood Flow—Metabolic Rate Coupling (CBF & CMR)

- $PaCO_2$ (normal = 20–80 mmHg):
- Hypercarbia: **CBF** ↑, **CMR** ↔ Hypocarbia: **CBF** ↓, **CMR** ↔
  CO_2 response impaired by inhaled potent agents, preserved by IV agents
  CO_2 response curve flattened in presence of chronic hypercapnia
- Profound hypoxia (PaO_2 <50 mmHg): **CBF** ↑, **CMR** ↔
- Temp: **CMR** ↓ **(5–7%/°C), CBF** ↓
- Potent inhalational agents: **CMR** ↓, **CBF** ↑ ("uncouple" metabolic link to CBF)
  Effects may be potentiated by ↓ $PaCO_2$ or IV agents
  Agents also impair blood flow autoregulation
- Nitrous oxide: **CBF** ↑, **CMR** ↑ **(regional, not global)**
  Effect on CMR may be attenuated by combination with other agents
- IV agents (barbiturates/propofol/etomidate/benzodiazepines)
  CMR ↓, **CBF** ↓ (changes small with benzos & narcotics)
  Generally preserve autoregulation and CO_2 responsiveness
  Ketamine = unusual exception: **CBF** ↑, **CMR** ↔ **(may ↑ if used alone)**
- Narcotics: Generally minimal effect on CBF and CMR
- Traumatic brain injury: Heterogeneous response, **CMR** ↓, **CBF** ↑ **(luxury perfusion)**
  Luxury perfusion: CBF exceeds metabolic demand, usually after infarct
- Basal metabolic rate: 3.5 mL O_2/100 g/min
- Avg brain: 1,400 g; avg CaO_2 = 20 mL O_2/100 mL blood
- Global blood flow = 50 mL/100 g/min; ischemic blood flow = 15 mL/100 g/min

Intracranial Pressure (ICP)

- ICP = cranial (closed space) pressure on brain, CSF, & blood components
- Brain components: Brain mass/cells (80%); blood (10%); CSF (10%)
- Normal range: 0–10 mmHg; CSF: 150 mL normal volume; 450 mL/d
- Increased ICP can lead to herniation & severe neurologic sequelae
  - Acute ↑—shunting of CSF to spinal canal; ventricular compression
  - Further ↑—compress brain tissue, mass effect, neuro deterioration
  - Severe ↑—**Cushing triad** (↑↑ BP + ↓↓ HR + irreg. resp.)
    Herniation—pupil asymmetry, ocular paresis, obtundation, nausea, decerebrate posturing, hemiplegia

Management of Increased ICP

- **Hyperventilation**
  - Vasoconstriction of cerebral vasculature ↓ inflow
  - ↓ Intracerebral H^+ conc promotes flow out of brain tissue
  - Equilibration over a period of hours will negate long-term benefits
  - ↓ O_2 delivery > ↓ brain volume at $PaCO_2$ <26 mmHg
  - May be especially deleterious in traumatic brain injury
  - Rapid normalization of $PaCO_2$ → brain edema & ↑ ICP
- **Head position**
  - Head-up position (15–30°) for drainage from jugular venous system
  - *Often one of most effective interventions to ↓ brain volume*
  - Avoid extremes of neck rotation/venous engorgement or outflow obstruction
- **Direct drainage:** Ventriculostomy, lumbar drain
- **Blood pressure control:** Avoid hypertension (& extreme hypotension)
- **Pharmacologic agents**
  - Avoid potent agents when ICP is a concern
  - Propofol, thiopental—↓ cerebral blood flow and CMR
  - Diuretics—IV furosemide (0.1–1.0 mg/kg)
  - *Potentiate effects of osmolar agents (block ion reuptake + diuresis)*
- **Osmotic therapy**
  - Relies on intact blood–brain barrier
  - Mannitol (0.5–2 g/kg total dose) or hypertonic saline (HTS)
    - Comparative efficacy remains controversial
    - Hypertonic saline may be better in trauma resuscitation with hypovolemia/shock
    - Caution: Impaired cardiac fx (transient ↑ in ECV) or unstable aneurysm
    - Maintain osmolar gap (mannitol) <20 or serum osmolarity <320 mOsm/kg
    - Mannitol—ability to scavenge radicals or HTS/mannitol ↓ viscosity ↑ O_2 delivery

Potential Complications of Hyperosmolar Therapy
• Leakage of hyperosmolar soln into brain tissue with resulting ↑ in brain edema (late)
• Hypernatremia, hypokalemia; rare hyperkalemia with mannitol use
• Rapid overcorrection of a pre-existing hyponatremia → central pontine myelinolysis
• Renal failure (from osmotic load to impaired kidneys)
• Pulmonary edema (due to intravascular fluid overload with impaired cardiac fx)
• Hypovolemia (from mannitol/furosemide diuresis + concomitant blood loss)

CRANIOTOMY

Anesthetic Management

Evoked Potentials

Types of potentials:
- EEG—depth of anesthesia, burst-suppression, isoelectric EEG, ischemia
  - Aneurysm clipping, AVM resection, CEA
- Somatosensory evoked potentials (SSEPs)—dorsal tracts & somatosensory cortex
  - Generated by peripheral nerve stimulation & central detection
  - Reliable but may not detect loss of motor function
  - Used in range of spine & intracranial procedures
  - Measurement compatible with most anesthetics
    (*Inhaled potent agents suppress more than IV agents*)
- Brainstem auditory evoked potentials (BAEPs)—depth of anesthesia & VIII
  - Posterior fossa craniotomy, acoustic neuroma resection
  - Easy to monitor via sounds directly applied to ear
  - Difficult to suppress
- Visual evoked potentials (VEPs)—monitor visual cortex/optic nerve
  - Most sensitive to suppression, rarely used, LED generators evolving technology
- Transcortical motor–evoked potentials (TcMEPs)—motor function (ventral pathways) from cortex to motor endplate (muscle)
  - Widely used in spine surgery, brainstem lesion resection
  - Craniotomy near motor cortex or descending tracts (e.g., internal capsule)
  - Need to avoid long-acting muscle relaxation
  - Generally avoid inhalational agents; propofol infusion commonly used
  - Etomidate (10–20 mcg/kg/min) or ketamine (0.25 mg/kg/h) infusion may enhance amplitude—may be especially useful when baseline signals poor
  - Low-dose dexmedetomidine (0.2–0.4 mcg/kg/h, no bolus) allows ↓ dose of IV agents and may improve analgesia and ↓ hemodynamic lability especially on emergence
- EMG—motor potentials from spinal cord/nerves
  - Compatible with all agents except muscle relaxants

Sensitivity to anesthetic agents:
Cortical > deep brain > spine
Visual > TcMEP > deep motor > spinal motor > SSEPs > BAEP

Suppressant effects of anesthetic agents:
- Inhalational agents > propofol > etomidate > ketamine > opioids
- N₂O generally tolerated up to 50% when conc **STABLE** during monitoring
- Consider TIVA (propofol/etomidate + narcotic) for easily suppressed potentials
- Benzos in moderate doses → minimal effects on monitored potentials
- Low-dose dexmedetomidine (<0.4 mcg/kg/h) is compatible with all monitoring modes but may suppress TcMEP at higher doses

EEG Frequency Ranges	
Delta rhythm (0–3 Hz)	Deep sleep, deep anesthesia, or pathologic states (e.g., brain tumors, hypoxia, metabolic encephalopathy)
Theta rhythm (4–7 Hz)	Sleep and anesthesia in adults; hyperventilation in awake children and young adults
Alpha rhythm (8–13 Hz)	Resting, awake adult with eyes closed, predominantly seen in occipital leads
Beta rhythm (>13 Hz)	Mental activity, light anesthesia

Source: From Bendo AA, Hartung J, Kass IS, et al. Neurophysiology and neuroanesthesia. In Barash PG, Cullen BF, Stoeling RK, eds. *Clinical Anesthesia.* 2nd ed. Philadelphia, PA: Lippincott; 1992:871–918.

General Features

- Mayfield pins & horseshoe headrest both commonly used
  - Pinning is highly stimulating
  - Anesthesiologist must anticipate (rather than react to) stimulation
  - Best to place invasive arterial monitoring before pinning
  - May inject pin sites with local anesthetic before pinning
  - May need to deepen anesthesia/control BP in anticipation of pinning (*may give IV propofol, nicardipine, or opioid [remifentanil] 30–60 s prior*)
- Airway/head usually rotated away from anesthesiologist
- Soft bite block should be placed immediately between molars before draping
  - Tissue edema from tongue biting can form during surgery
  - Can prevent tube kinking from biting or positioning
- Eye protection
  - Secure taping eyelids; consider ophthalmic ointment or Tegaderm to avoid corneal abrasion (note surgeon removal of eye tape during image guidance registration)
    - Posterior fossa craniotomy: Arm positioning & brain stem reflexes
- Plan early for IV access (arms out or tucked)
  - Decide early on need & site for intraop infusions
  - Infuse via visible IV (if possible) to ↓ unnoticed infiltration
- Main times of stimulation: Intubation/pinning/incision/drilling/dural incision
- Avoid coughing/bucking/movement at any time
- Rapid blood loss is possible during any craniotomy (esp if sinus near incision)
- Immediate postop assessment of neurologic function is crucial
  - Inability to perform neuro exam → immediate postop CT imaging
  - Avoid routine use of adjunct sedatives (*confound postop assessment*)
- Opioids: Used as part of a balanced-anesthesia technique
  - Aggressive use of narcotics may lead to delayed emergence
  - Give opioid dose early (i.e., induction, pinning, incision)
    - Fentanyl = short-acting & titratable (5–10 mcg/kg total dose)
    - Hydromorphone = longer-acting, give for postop analgesia
    - Morphine = sedating, slow emergence; avoid in intracranial proc. (*Morphine metabolites may accumulate in renal failure*)
    - Remifentanil (0.1–0.5 mcg/kg/min) & sufentanil (1–2 mcg/kg bolus + 0.1–0.2 mcg/kg/h) can be used as infusions
  - Consider oral or IV acetaminophen for adjunctive analgesia
    - Consider scalp block as an opioid reduction strategy in selected shorter cases
    - Discuss with surgeons blocks (e.g., supraorbital) can cause ecchymoses
- Tight control of BP via invasive monitoring in most cases
  - Avoid significant drops in BP in setting of hemorrhage/elevated ICP
    - Special cases: MoyaMoya dz, AVM with large venous drainoff BP drops can be especially deleterious
- Fluid resuscitation
  - Physiologic solutions (e.g., LR) advantage over normal saline (↑↑ Cl^- → acidosis)
  - Avoid hypotonic or glucose containing fluids (can inc brain swelling/injury)
  - Colloid used as indicated by clinical context (limit albumin in traumatic brain inj)
- Periop antibiotics usually indicated
- Anticonvulsant therapy
  - Indications for anticonvulsant & steroids vary with each pt
  - May potentiate neuromuscular blockers (acute) or antagonize NMB (chronic)
  - Anticonvulsant often used if contact with cortical tissue anticipated
    - IV phenytoin (Dilantin) loading dose: 18 mg/kg in 250 mL NSS at 25 mg/min
    - *Caution: Rapid bolus dosing of phenytoin may cause significant cardiac arrhythmia, hypotension, & cardiovascular collapse*
    - *Renal failure—low albumin and uremia ↑ free levels*
  - Fosphenytoin (a phenytoin prodrug with ↓ side effects) loading dose: 15–20 phenytoin equivalent mg/kg in 250 mL NSS @ 50–100 PE mg/min
  - IV levetiracetam (Keppra) with a loading dose: 1,000 mg/100 mL NSS; 15–30 min
  - IV dexamethasone (10 mg bolus, repeat 4 mg q6h) for edema when indicated
    - Usually reserved for cases with intracranial lesion, elevated ICP, edema
    - Also used routinely for dual PONV prophylaxis

Induction

- Controlled induction with hemodynamic stability
- Moderate hyperventilation in setting of ↑ ICP
- Combination of propofol 1–2 mg/kg, fentanyl 2–4 mcg/kg, & nondepolarizing muscle relaxant is one approach

- Rapid, short-acting anti-HTN agents (esmolol, nicardipine) should be available
- Succinylcholine-associated muscle fasciculation may result in transient ↑ ICP
- Coughing, bucking, or sympathetic surge during laryngoscopy with ↑ BP may cause sudden & untoward ↑ ICP (can use lidocaine 1 mg/kg, additional propofol, remifentanil, or rapidly acting BP agents to prevent/treat)
- Physiologic manifestations of light anesthesia contraindicated in pts with intracranial aneurysm susceptible to rupture
  - Consider invasive monitoring prior to induction of anesthesia
  - Consider topical lidocaine spray during airway management

Maintenance
- Avoid high-dose inhalational agent ↑ brain volume
- Opioid bolus as needed—generally avoid high doses and load earlier in the procedure
- Consider TIVA if monitoring evoked potentials or if need to ↓ brain volume
- Consider using a processed EEG monitor to guide TIVA dose
- Common strategy
  - Propofol infusion for amnesia & brain relaxation
    Stop infusion once 1° resection complete to expedite emergence (especially age >70, processed EEG not used, or long infusion)
  - Narcotic infusion for analgesia & immobility
    (especially if muscle relaxation contraindicated because of monitoring)
- Provided an appropriate anesthetic depth has been reached, HTN should be liberally treated with labetalol or nicardipine to ↓ emergence hypertension
- Closely monitor urine output & replete (especially with mannitol administration)
- Monitor glucose & treat glucose >160 mg/dL with insulin, consider infusion
- Hyperglycemia may exacerbate neurologic injury
- If not contraindicated by monitoring requirements, maintain muscle relaxation TOF $^1/_4$ with bolus or infusion of nondepolarizing muscle relaxant
- Maintain MAP within 20% of baseline
- N_2O may be used with several caveats:
  - May complicate EEG or potential monitoring if level not constant
  - May ↑ cerebral blood flow & contribute to brain swelling/↑ ICP
  - May contribute to pneumocephalus (particularly in posterior fossa proc) or pneumothorax expansion (esp in trauma)
  - May have deleterious effects on neuronal cells (under investigation)

Emergence
- BP control is critical
  - HTN episodes at emergence & postop may cause ↑ bleeding or edema
  - Treat with labetalol or nicardipine
  - A background dexmedetomidine infusion may reduce emergence phenomenon and reduce total sedative dose
- Dual prophylaxis for nausea/vomiting recommended (ondansetron)
  - Avoid promethazine, droperidol, diphenhydramine (can be sedating)
- Emergence should begin *after* Mayfield pins have been removed
- Time should be allowed (5 min) for head wrapping before extubation
- Extubation: Reaches baseline mental status
- Small boluses of propofol (10–40 mg) or remifentanil (0.2–1 mcg/kg)
- Continuous monitoring of vital signs and neuro exam during transport
- Anesthesia team should participate in postextubation neuro exam

Special Features of Operations Involving the Posterior Fossa
- ↑ ICP commonly a concern (due to obstruction by a posterior fossa mass)
  - Consider aggressive treatment of ICP prior to induction
  - In severe cases, consider ventriculostomy under local anesthesia
  - ↑ ICP may occur if head down during positioning/surgical prep
- Prone, head-up position—concern for air embolus
  - Minimal access to IVs, infusions
  - Evaluate thoroughly after positioning, hand may provide better access
- Potential for postop, compressive pneumocephalus
- Kinking of ETT, or mainstem intubation with neck flexion in pins (**MUST place bite block**)
  - Postextubation macroglossia, tongue ischemia/injury
- Proximity to critical neurologic structures involving regulatory centers
  - Brainstem/medulla/pons regulatory centers
  - Bradycardia, apnea, rapid swings in BP may occur
  - Possibility for new postop CN or brainstem deficits [consider extubation risks]

- Small operative window may lead to inc brain swelling
  - Jugular venous drainage/head position, TIVA

Sitting Craniotomy: Lounge chair, back elevated 60°; hips & knees flexed

Advantages
- Operative exposure with ↓ brain swelling/volume, used for:
  - Posterior fossa lesions/cerebellar tumors
  - Pineal gland tumor resection
- Avoidance of prone position & improved ventilation dynamics

Disadvantages
- Risk of air embolus & paradoxical air embolus (PFO/septal defect)
  - Signs: Drop in $ETCO_2$, hypotension, tachycardia, ↑ ETN_2 (rarely available)
  - Monitoring: Precordial Doppler or continuous TEE
  - Access: Place central venous access (for air extraction)
    - May be placed via antecubital vein
    - Multiorifice catheter preferred (more effective for aspiration of air)
- Quadriplegia from extreme neck flexion & ↓ perfusion
- Hypotension from venous pooling & head elevation may result in brain ischemia (within apparently acceptable BP limits)
  - Transduce arterial BP at level of tragus (middle of ear) not right atrium
  - Maintain BP ± 20% baseline MAP; processed EEG may detect hypoperfusion
  - Consider support stockings to ↓ venous pooling
- Nerve injury due to positioning (legs, arms, neck/brachial plexus)

Awake Craniotomy
- Used for resection of tumors (motor or speech cortex) & epileptic foci
- Team approach with emphasis on communication, patience, & experience
- Critical to set pt & surgeon expectations
- Awake with variable sedation versus "asleep → awake → asleep" with LMA/ETT
  - Preference varies by center & experience
  - Simplest method is to avoid airway instrumentation
  - Only period of intense stimulation is opening/drilling/dural incision
- Pt comfort
  - Positioning with padding/pillows & warming blanker for optimal comfort
  - Vasoactive substances (nitroglycerin) may cause profound headache
  - Placement of Mayo stand over head to lift drapes off of the awake pt
- Preparation
  - IV access, monitors, & arterial line prior to blocks
  - Consider lidocaine coated bilateral nasal trumpets (28–34 Fr) connected to O_2 for airway management (↓ obstruction, facilitate supportive oxygenation/ventilation)
  - *Topical anesthetic, vasoconstrictors to nares, and sedation prior to placement*
- Consider peripheral nerve blocks
  - CNV_1—supraorbital, supratrochlear n
  - CNV_2—auriculotemporal, zygomaticotemporal n
  - Cervical branches—posterior auricular, greater & lesser occipital n
  - Remifentanil infusion for analgesia during blocks; PONV prophylaxis at start
  - Choice of local: Use long-acting ropivacaine 0.375% with 1:200,000 epi
  - Bupivacaine in large volume may have increased risk of cardiac toxicity
  - Allow for additional local to be infiltrated by surgeons
  - Consider metoprolol prior to block to blunt epinephrine induced tachycardia
- Maintenance
  - Deeper sedation only during drilling & opening of bone flap
  - Minimize sedation just before dural incision
  - Monitor CO_2—hypercarbia can contribute to brain swelling
  - Low dose Propofol/remifentanil with spontaneous ventilation
  - Dexmedetomidine infusion is a useful adjunct
    - *Minimal resp depression, can cause hypotension/bradycardia*
    - *Treat with glycopyrrolate (0.2 mg) if bradycardia is clinically significant*
    - *Load 1 mcg/kg over 10 min & infuse 0.3–1 mcg/kg/h*
  - Neuromonitoring
    - Map functional cortex—usually speech area
    - Requires continuous pt feedback, communication, visual observation

INTRACRANIAL VASCULAR SURGERY: ANEURYSM CLIPPING & RESECTION OF ARTERIOVENOUS MALFORMATIONS (AVMs)

Preoperative Evaluation
- Where is the aneurysm? Has pt had subarachnoid hemorrhage (SAH)? GCS?
- Determine surgical approach & location of incision; near sinus? Difficult access?
- Need for CSF drainage (improve access/visualization)?
- Need for intraop angiography?
- Evidence of cerebral salt wasting or SIADH after SAH (electrolytes, urine output)?
- Document baseline ECG: Changes common with SAH
  - *(May be associated with ↓ cardiac fx—esp Q waves)*
- In emergent surgery for hemorrhage: FFP, PCC or platelets for clinical indications (e.g., chronic anticoagulation: Antiplatelet or direct thrombin inhibitor)

Induction & Pinning
- Avoid profound HTN or light anesthesia
- Consider laryngotracheal lidocaine during laryngoscopy
- Lidocaine (without epinephrine) at pinning sites prior to Mayfield application
- Potential for catastrophic bleeding: Ensure large-bore IV access
- Lumbar drain or ventriculostomy may facilitate brain decompression & better surgical access (rate & timing of CSF drainage must be coordinated with surgeon)

Maintenance
- BP management = critical
  - A-line mandatory (often preinduction) maintain ±10% baseline BP during dissection
  - If HTN → inhalational, nicardipine, esmolol, nitroprusside, NTG
  - If hypotensive → phenylephrine, ephedrine (test with small doses)
  - ↓ BP at surgical request during direct aneurysm manipulation
  - ↑ BP to baseline MAP during ischemic periods (e.g., temporary clipping)
  - Avoid extreme hypo- or hypertension at all points
  - Consider brief, deliberate hypotension or cardiac standstill with adenosine (12–24 mg) during massive bleeding to facilitate surgical localization & control
- Many surgeons utilize both EEG & intraoperative cerebral angiography
  Some centers use intravenous indocyanine green (infrared spectroscopy) which is injected by the anesthesiologist at the time of imaging (unless hx of iodine allergy)
  - Preop placement of vascular sheath in femoral artery (±sedation)
  - Sheath must be monitored & transduced at all times (including transport)
  - Preop embolization of feeding vessels to AVM may be performed
    (May limit potential for massive blood loss)
- Debate over transfusion thresholds in aneurysm surgery with vasospasm
  - Vasospasm usually occurs d (3–10) after initial bleed/trauma
  - Hemodilution (↓ blood viscosity) vs. transfusion (↑ O₂ delivery) vs. angiography with intra-arterial vasodilator (papaverine, nimodipine)
- Profound, deep anesthesia may be neuroprotective during periods of ischemia
  - Strategy for periop brain protection controversial
  - Burst suppression may be protective in regional ischemia
    - Can use high-dose propofol titrated to EEG
  - High-dose sedative–hypnotics to achieve burst suppression may result in
    - Hypertriglyceridemia & metabolic acidosis (propofol)
    - Propylene glycol toxicity (etomidate)
    - Delayed emergence (all agents)
    - Hypotension (all agents)
- Data inconclusive regarding deliberate hypothermia
  - Pt populations, cooling, & rewarming strategies highly variable
  - Hypothermia (35–36°C) may be an option if intraoperative brain ischemia is anticipated or witnessed global ischemia prior to OR
  - Rewarm prior to extubation/emergence
  - Avoid hyperthermia (↑ CMR/injury)

VENTRICULOPERITONEAL SHUNT PLACEMENT/OMMAYA RESERVOIR

VP shunt: Catheter in lateral ventricle to relieve ↑ ICP by continuous CSF drainage
- Proximal catheter placed into ventricle via burr hole
- Distal catheter (shunt only) placed into peritoneal cavity
- Requires GA, usually with muscle relaxation
  (Submucosal catheter must be passed from neck to abdomen)
- Minimal narcotic requirements for postop pain control (Cons. remifentanil)
- Goal = prompt recovery of preop mental status with extubation

Ommaya reservoir: Intraventricular catheter for CNS delivery of chemotherapeutic agents
- May be performed under local with sedation or GA
- Removal rarely requires more than local with light sedation

EPIDURAL, SUBDURAL, & INTRACEREBRAL HEMORRHAGE (ICH)

- Wide range of etiologies for intracranial bleed
- Trauma—may present with wide range of hemorrhage
  - Consider other injuries
  - ICP often severely ↑ requiring immediate decompression
  - Blood–brain barrier often disrupted
  - Normal autoregulatory mechanisms may be dysfunctional
- Subdural—often present in older pts from vein shearing after fall
- Epidural almost always surgical emergency
- ICH may represent sentinel bleed from aneurysm, AVM, or other pathology/trauma
  - Categorized by Hunt/Hess grade
  - Grade I = asymptomatic/minimal headache; Grade V = deep coma, decerebrate rigidity
  - May have prognostic value, influences timing of surgery
- Be prepared for ongoing blood loss & need for resuscitation/transfusion
- Consider preop volume loading
- Potential for severe pre- & postop brain swelling
- Intracerebral blood = strong stimulus for vasospasm
- "Triple H" therapy (empiric institution of HTN, hypervolemia, hemodilution)
  (Target: Hgb 9 g/dL) may be indicated for ICH (Benefit controversial)
  - Maintain MAP 30–50% above baseline
  - Maintain CVP at high normal levels
  - Raise transfusion threshold (unless ↑ cardiovascular risk)
  - Exercise caution in setting of unstable aneurysm/AVM

TRAUMATIC BRAIN INJURY

- Unique mechanism of injury (diffuse & focal brain damage)
- Unique pathophysiology of dz
  - BBB disruption, vasoplegia, stress response
  - Associated cardiovascular instability
  - Associated pulm failure (ARDS, lung/cardiac contusion, edema)
- Often present with multiple life-threatening injuries
- ICU management crucial for good outcomes
- Glasgow Coma Scale score characterizes severity & may predict outcome
- Usually present for decompression or clot evacuation

Glasgow Coma Scale (3–15 Points)		
Best Eye Opening	**Best Verbal Response**	**Best Motor Response**
Spontaneous – 4	Oriented – 5	Obeys commands = 6
To speech = 3	Confused = 4	Localizes pain = 5
To pain = 2	Inappropriate = 3	Withdrawals = 4
None = 1	Incomprehensible = 2	Flexion to pain = 3
	None = 1	Extension to pain = 2
		None = 1

Score of ≤8 indicates coma & requires intubation
Age-adjusted normal scores: 0–6 mo = 9; 6–12 mo = 11; 1–2 y = 12; 2–5 y = 13; >5 y = 14

- ↑ ICP usually a pressing concern
  - May present to OR for emergency decompressive hemicraniectomy or clot evacuation (epidural/subdural/parenchymal hematoma)
  - Maintenance of CPP: Aggressive fluid resuscitation & BP management
  - Avoid hyperventilation except in case of emergency/decompensation
  - Intractable ↑ ICP common & requires aggressive intervention
  - Regional brain tissue oximeters (e.g., Licox) of unproven clinical utility
  - No uniformly defined target CPP, individualize to clinical context (common goal >60)
- Central diabetes insipidus a common finding
  - Monitor for high-volume urine output (>300 mL/h), rising serum sodium
  - Measure serum/urine osmolarity, serum sodium
  - May treat empirically with arginine vasopressin

- May consider institution of hypothermia for brain protection
  - Early hypothermia may be protective (developing literature)

ELECTROCONVULSIVE THERAPY (ECT)

Goals
- Amnesia, pt immobility, hemodynamic stability
- Provide conditions for therapeutic seizure duration (>30 s)
- Treat prolonged seizure (2–3 min) with pharmacologic agents
- Rapid recovery for discharge from recovery area

Agents
- Many short-acting hypnotic agents have been used
  - Usually avoid benzos (raise seizure threshold)
  - Propofol (may shorten seizure duration), methohexital, thiopental, etomidate, sevoflurane, remifentanil have all been used
    - First line: Methohexital (0.75–2 mg/kg) or etomidate (0.15–0.3 mg/kg)
  - Short-acting muscle relaxation with succinylcholine (1 mg/kg) unless contraindicated
  - Seizure threshold usually ↑ with number of treatments
  - Propofol or benzodiazepines are reasonable choices to treat prolonged seizure

Management
- If pt has received prior ECT treatment with adequate seizure activity
  - Consider using same anesthetic regimen (must document!)
- Preop eval as with any other general anesthetic
  - Pts with cardiac dz → the sympathetic surge (HTN/tachycardia) after seizure must be controlled
  - Pts with ↑ ICP → may be at risk for acute decompensation (sudden ↑ in cerebral blood flow associated with ECT)
  - Consider hyperventilation prior to stimulus
  - Pts with cerebral aneurysm → need tight BP control
  - Hx of "awareness" with prior procedure should be fully evaluated
    Processed EEG monitors may be useful
- Excessive anesthesia may ↑ seizure threshold or ↓ seizure duration
- Inadequate anesthesia may lead to awareness under anesthesia
- Monitors should include all routine monitors + end-tidal CO_2 sampling
- Emergency drugs & airway equipment must be immediately available
- Preoxygenation/denitrogenation as with any general anesthetic
- Inflate BP cuff on calf of one leg **prior** to admin of succinylcholine
  - Allows monitoring of seizure activity
- **Place bite blocks between molar teeth on both sides prior to stimulation**
- Confirm loss of consciousness prior to administration of muscle relaxant
- Post-ECT confusion/memory loss/agitation is common
- Bradycardia is common during electrical stimulus
  - Hx of bradycardia may be (pre)treated with glycopyrrolate
  - In pregnant pts, ECT may induce a transient fetal bradycardia
    - Fetal heart rate monitoring often used in the 3rd trimester
    - ECT may induce labor & require tocolysis
    - Unless pt is in active labor, late-stage pregnancy, or has other risk factors for aspiration, intubation not typically required
- HTN/tachycardia common after ECT
  - May treat with IV labetalol, esmolol, & nicardipine
  - If pt has known profound hemodynamic response, consider pretreatment
- Some pts display profound salivation after ECT
  - Glycopyrrolate (0.1–0.2 mg) pretreatment may limit this effect
  - Use of atropine may exacerbate postictal confusion/memory loss

---

INTERVENTIONAL RADIOLOGY

- Procedures: Diagnostic, cerebral angiogram, intra-arterial thrombolysis (tPA) & thrombectomy for stroke, embolization/coiling of spinal/cerebral AVM or cerebral aneurysm, carotid stenting for stenosis, intra-arterial vasodilator for vasospasm
- MAC vs. GA can be considered depending on procedure and pt condition; sedation if continuous neurologic testing essential or for most diagnostic angiograms
  Blood pressure control paramount (invasive in most cases with intervention)
  Femoral (MAP only, via sheath) or radial

Deliberate Hypertension
- May be necessary to help radiology catheters flow to desired location
- Usually 20–40% above baseline; phenylephrine infusion may be useful

Deliberate Hypotension
- May be required in carotid endarterectomy/arteriovenous malformation (AVM) procedures; neuromonitoring (EEG/SSEP may be employed)
- Various approaches may be used (↑ anesthesia, labetalol, vasodilators—nitroprusside/ nitroglycerin/hydralazine)

Embolization of Arteriovenous Malformation (AVM)
- Polyvinyl alcohol (PVA) injected into feeding vessels of AVM
- Approach: MAC (can continuously monitor neuro status) or GA
- Systemic heparinization may be required
- Complications: Hemorrhage 2° to anticoagulation (can reverse with protamine), hemorrhage 2° to thrombus (can ↑ BP by 20–40 mmHg); ↑ ICP (treat with hyperventilation, head ↑, mannitol, furosemide)

Cerebral Aneurysms
- Uses balloons, coils, or liquid polymer solution to endovascularly treat the aneurysm
- GA or light sedation (pt cooperation + surgeon end); a-line should be placed
- Important to have OR available in case of rupture & urgent need for surgical repair

Central Intra-arterial Thrombolysis/Thrombectomy
- Treatment of stroke if <8 h from onset of symptoms
- MAC (if neurologic assessment is desirable, ? improved outcome) vs. GA (controversy over MAC vs GA for best outcome as numerous can affect it)
- Generally maintain SBP >140 < 180
- Avoid hyperglycemia (<140 mg/dL) and hypoglycemia
  - http://pubs.societyhq.com/SNACC-StrokeConsensusStatement/

SPECIFIC NEUROLOGIC DISORDERS

Myasthenia Gravis (MG)
Etiology: Autoimmune antibodies against nicotinic cholinergic receptors
Symptoms/Signs: Laryngeal weakness → dysphagia, dysarthria; extraocular muscle weakness → diplopia, ptosis; skeletal muscle weakness → worsens with activity
Treatments: Anticholinesterases, steroids, plasmapheresis, thymectomy

Risk Factors for Postoperative Respiratory Failure	
Coexisting lung dz; vital capacity <2.9 L	Dz duration >6 y
Pyridostigmine dose >750 mg/d	Poorly controlled dz

Preoperative Considerations:
- Assess degree of weakness & duration of symptoms; maintain anticholinesterase therapy
- Anticholinesterase overdose → *cholinergic crisis* → further weakness
  Treatment: Anticholinergic administration (i.e., edrophonium)

Anesthetic Management:
- Minimize sedatives/respiratory depressants; consider regional
- Consider rapid sequence induction (pts at ↑ risk of aspiration)
- Avoid muscle relaxants if possible & delay extubation if needed
- Use caution when using neostigmine (↑ risk of cholinergic crisis)

Multiple Sclerosis
Symptoms: Visual disturbances, limb weakness, paralysis, respiratory failure, bulbar palsy
  ↑ risk of aspiration + ↓ airway reflexes = risk of postop resp failure
Neuraxial blockade (spinal) associated with worsening symptoms; epidurals are *not* contraindicated
- Avoid hyperthermia

Guillain–Barré Syndrome
Symptoms: Ascending paralysis, may require vent. support, ↑ aspiration risk, autonomic dysfx
Consider RSI, avoid succinylcholine, minimize muscle relaxants & opioids

Parkinson Disease
Loss of dopaminergic fibers → unopposed acetylcholine activity
Avoid dopamine antagonists (Haldol, promethazine, prochlorperazine, metoclopramide, droperidol); may observe transient exacerbation of symptoms after general anesthesia

Note: In pts with neurologic dz, determination of baseline TOF response prior to dosing of nondepolarizing neuromuscular blockade will inform interpretation of recovery

OTOLARYNGOLOGY (ENT) AND OPHTHALMOLOGY

JOSHUA H. ATKINS

PROCEDURES IN OTOLARYNGOLOGY

Functional Endoscopic Sinus Surgery (FESS)
- Surgery performed via nasal passages
- Usually short surgical procedure (longer for complex surgical indications)

Indications
- Recurrent sinusitis, abnormal transnasal breathing (deviated septum)
- Epistaxis/AVM (e.g., hereditary hemorrhagic telangiectasia)
- Resection of skull base tumor
- Rhinorrhea for repair of CSF leak
- Anatomic access for resection of pituitary adenoma (with neurosurgery)

Special Considerations
- Real-time CT guidance (e.g., Brain Lab) or possibly intraop CT scanning
- Position: Head always rotated away from anesthesiologist, arms tucked for surgeon access, ensure careful padding of ulnar n, ensure ETT & circuit not under tension
- EBL: Usually minimal, ↑ for skull base tumor resection/epistaxis treatment
- Transient hypertension associated with the use of transnasal vasoactive substances
  - Oxymetazoline pledgets, lidocaine with epi, topical cocaine
  - Use intraop β-blockers with caution in conjunction with nasal vasoconstrictors
- Deliberate hypotension/controlled normotension in appropriate candidates
- Surgical instruments close to cribriform plate, optic nerve, carotid artery
- Pain: Low postop opioid needs; consider adjuncts such as PO acetaminophen or lidocaine infusion
- May need periop corticosteroid supplementation in pituitary surgery

Anesthetic Management
- GA with ETT (standard or midline oral RAE tube), controlled ventilation
  - Provides airway protection from blood & irrigation
  - Inhaled potent agent or total intravenous anesthesia (TIVA) is acceptable
- Flexible LMA or MAC anesthesia may be used in selected candidates
  - Movement during MAC or spontaneous ventilation with LMA can interfere with alignment of real-time CT guidance system; difficulty with clearing blood
- Surgeons need full access to nares (no trumpets, NG tubes, nasal temp probes)
  - Oral temp probe may be inaccurate owing to irrigation
  - Ophthalmic ointment to eyes (often no taping for surgeon access)
- Avoid tape across mandible (secure to L side) or consider midline RAE tube
- Warming blanket & Foley catheter for longer procedures
- Periop antibiotics & dexamethasone may be indicated
- Short closure times
- Nasal packing may impair postop breathing
- Consider surgically placed & sutured nasal airway if obese/OSA
- Monitor for postextubation bleeding into posterior oropharynx/hypopharynx
- Thorough oropharyngeal suctioning +/– passage of OG tube **prior** to extubation to evacuate surgical debris & blood
- Avoid noninvasive/PP mask vent (risk of pneumocephalus) unless nasal airway

---

TIVA or Potent Agent for ENT Procedures

Advantages of total intravenous anesthesia
- May ↓ bleeding in operative field
- May ↓ operative time spent clearing field to achieve adequate visualization
- May ↓ emergence coughing & avoid disruption of homeostasis/dural repair
- May ↓ PONV & facilitate avoidance of muscle relaxants if propofol is used

Disadvantages of total intravenous anesthesia
- Depth monitoring: ↑ Pharmacodynamic & pharmacokinetic variability
- May ↑ risk of awareness if muscle relaxation employed
- Undetected IV infiltration → potential for awareness & soft tissue necrosis
- ↑ Cost of infusion medications

One approach
- Propofol (65–150 mcg/kg/min) + remifentanil (0.1–0.3 mcg/kg/min) infusions
  Lidocaine gtt (IBW, 1–3 mg/kg/h, 1–2 mg/kg bolus) as adjunct for ERAS
- + Low-dose potent agent (e.g., 0.3 MAC desflurane) if higher risk awareness
- Agents to support BP (e.g., phenylephrine infusion) as needed
- ± Muscle relaxant as needed for surgeon/pt needs

CSF Leak Repair
Often performed via FESS approach for spontaneous leak with rhinorrhea
- Usually requires intrathecal injection of fluorescein (aids in localization under FESS)
- Usually place lumbar drain for dye injection + 48–72-h postop CSF drainage
- CSF opening pressure may be of prognostic utility (LP kit during drain placement)
- Frequently obese, consider IR placement of drain under fluoroscopy
- Risk of herniation if over drainage, ideally continuously monitor CSF pressure
- Never pressurize, flush, or inject drain tubing
- Consider meningococcal meningitis prophylaxis (e.g., ceftriaxone)

Microdirect/Suspension Laryngoscopy (MDL) & Transbronchoscope ENT Procedures
- Employs specialized surgical laryngoscopes (e.g., Dedo, Jackson)
- Procedure is highly stimulating for relatively brief periods
- Pts often have difficult airways (e.g., radiation/tumor) & significant comorbidities

Indications
- Tumors of larynx, oral cavity, pharynx, hypopharynx
  - Biopsy, laser ablation, robot-assisted microresection (TORS)
  - TORS: Deep muscle relaxation, wire-reinforced tube, eye goggles
  - May involve tongue base epiglottis; consider delayed extubation (48–72 h)
- Vocal cord surgery (typically same d)
  - Vocal cord polyp; collagen injection for cord paralysis; voice prosthesis
- Tracheal stenosis—dilation/ablation of lesions
- Laser ablation/direct chemotherapy of papilloma

Special Considerations
- Formal preop airway discussion with surgeon, consider surgeon in OR at induction
- Potentially difficult airway
  - Prior surgery with scarring or postradiation changes (immobile larynx)
  - Supraglottic/laryngeal masses or tracheal abnormalities (stenosis/web)
  - Friable tissue → bleeding
  - Consider surgeon NPL exam ± awake look with videolaryngoscope in OR
  - Consider awake tracheostomy for nonreassuring assessment above
- Positive-pressure mask ventilation may be challenging/impossible
- Airway = operative field & bed = rotated away
- Anesthetic gases may leak to environment/surgeon (open system)
- Intermittent apnea may be required for surgical access to larynx
- ETT may distort surgical anatomy, impede surgical access, fire substrate
- Laser ablation may be used (requires ↓ FiO$_2$)
  - Use jet ventilation, apneic technique, high-flow nasal cannula, or laser tube
  - Fill laser tube balloons with methylene blue saline
- Metallic laser tubes rigid & no markings use caution with depth of insertion
  - Use airway fire protocol
- Include high fire risk in time out & COMMUNICATE with surgeon
- Surgeon may desire spontaneous ventilation (assess vocal cord movement)
- Intense but fleeting/intermittent stimulus (deep anesthesia)
- Requires constant communication between surgeon & anesthesiologist

Anesthetic Management
- GA usually indicated (owing to intense procedure stimulus)
- Sedation & spontaneous ventilation in selected cases (with cooperative pts)
  - Requires anxiolysis & meticulous topicalization with local anesthetic
- Usually limited to ablation/biopsy of small lesions, biopsy, dilation, or cord injection
- Anesthesiologist often induces GA & shares airway management with surgeon
  - Surgeon should be present prior to induction of anesthesia
- Airway management includes a variety of options
  - ETT (e.g., 4.0–6.0 mm ID) placed under laryngoscopy
  - Catheter for jet ventilation placed under direct visualization (text box, p. 24-6)
  - Intermittent apnea with mask ventilation

High-flow nasal cannula (HFNC) oxygen can also be considered
Consider transcutaneous CO_2 monitoring with jet ventilation
- Airway device (if used) may be periodically removed for surgical access
- TIVA technique preferable to inhaled agent
  - ↓ OR contamination with inhalation gas
  - More consistent depth of anesthesia; profound suppression of airway reflexes
  - Propofol & titratable, short-acting narcotic (e.g., remifentanil) often used
- Muscle relaxation must be individualized for each case
- Inhalational induction may be considered for difficult airway
- Videolaryngoscopy may be helpful even if surgical DL view is poor

Medialization Thyroplasty (Vocal Cord Medialization)
- Procedure performed to treat vocal cord paralysis/bowing
- Partial resection of thyroid cartilage & prosthesis placement

Special Considerations
- Pt cooperation = important component
- Anesthesia best provided with sedation & local injection
  - Pt able to phonate on command during surgery
  - Vocal cord movement observed under nasopharyngeal laryngoscopy
  - Surgical incision similar to partial thyroidectomy
  - Dexmedetomidine load + infusion is an excellent option for cooperative sedation
  - Fire risk high: Air-oxygen blender & low FiO_2

PROCEDURES ON THE INNER EAR AND MASTOID

Indications
- Mastoidectomy/tympanoplasty for recurrent infection
- Cochlear implant for neurodegenerative hearing loss
- Myringoplasty/myringotomy tubes for infection
- Stapedectomy for conductive hearing loss/otosclerosis

Special Considerations
- Multimodal prophylaxis for high risk of nausea and vomiting (e.g., scopolamine patch, dexamethasone, ondansetron, TIVA, fluid loading, minimized long-acting opioids)
- Nerve monitoring (VII/VIII)
- N_2O off (if used) before tympanic membrane closure
  - Potential for rapid expansion of airspace by N_2O diffusion
- Preop & postop communication challenges with hearing loss
  - Replace hearing aid in nonoperative ear/use hand gestures/preop coaching

Anesthetic Management
- Best performed with GA & ETT (except for stapedectomy)
  - LMA can be used in selected pts; especially if no mastoidectomy (drilling)
- Position: Table usually 180° away from anesthesiologist; airway covered/inaccessible
- Surgical manipulation of head must be expected during procedure
- Surgeon infiltration of local anesthetic (lessens need for opioids)
  Oral acetaminophen, IV NSAID, and lidocaine gtt can be considered for analgesia
- Muscle generally avoided to facilitate nerve monitoring

Stapedectomy
- Often light sedation with local anesthesia (GA for selected pts)
- Sedation allows for intraop testing of hearing acuity (Dex, propofol, remi, benzo)
- Excessive sedation may lead to disinhibition & movement
- Snoring/obstruction impairs operating under microscope due to vibrations

Myringotomy Tube Placement (Placement of Ear Tubes)
- Very short procedure, usually performed in pediatric pts under mask GA
- IV access not necessary; can use IM analgesics (ketorolac & fentanyl)

TONSILLECTOMY/PAROTIDECTOMY/UVULOPALATOPHARYNGOPLASTY

Tonsillectomy and Adenoidectomy
Indications
- Recurrent infection
- Obstructive sleep apnea due to hypertrophic tonsillar/adenoid tissue
- Radical tonsillectomy/pharyngectomy for cancer (may be robotic, see MDL)

- Potential for difficult mask/airway—particularly in adults
- Usually GETA with oral RAE tube, secure in midline
- Procedure usually indicated owing to recurrent infection
- May be semiurgent even in the setting of active infection
- Short procedure necessitates careful titration of muscle relaxants when used
- Surgeon removal of mouth gag may result in extubation—monitor closely
- Multimodal PONV prophylaxis critical
- "Bring back" tonsil for bleeding common
  - Aggressive preinduction volume resuscitation (esp pediatric pts)
  - RSI or plan for potentially difficult airway (blood in airway & edema)
  - Pediatric pts with sleep study evidence of recurrent hypoxemic episodes & adults with OSA may demonstrate increased sensitivity to opiate therapy
  - Exogenous opiate requirements to provide effective postop analgesia may be reduced by up to $1/2$ normal per kg dosing
  - Consider scheduled titration of opioids and extended cardiopulmonary monitoring (including possible overnight admission to monitored unit with continuous oximetry or exhaled CO_2) to ↑ effective surveillance of postop respiratory events (especially OSA)

Parotidectomy
- GA with ETT; consider nasal RAE if deep lobe is to be resected (consult surgeon)
  - Nasal tube precautions (oxymetazoline to nares, gentle dilation, tube sizing)
  - Consider bougie-guided nasal intubation to minimize bleeding/trauma
- Facial nerve monitoring; avoid additional muscle relaxation after induction

Uvulopalatopharyngoplasty (UPPP)
- Performed for treatment of obstructive sleep apnea
- Airway management: Mask ventilation/intubation may be difficult
- Review sleep study results—apnea/hypopnea index for severity
- Denitrogenate with CPAP/Pressure Support
- Consider RAMP/HELP positioning for obese pts
- Consider continuous pulse oximetry/CO_2 while inpatient
- Non-opiate analgesia wherever possible

TRACHEOSTOMY

Indications
- Ventilator-dependent respiratory failure
- Chronic aspiration
- Airway pathology with airway compromise or difficult trach/reintubation

Special Considerations
- If already intubated: Vent settings, O_2 & PEEP required, prior airway mgmt
- If not intubated: Consider awake (difficult airway) vs. asleep tracheostomy
- If in resp failure/ARDS: May require special ventilator settings
  - Conventional OR ventilator limited (consider ICU vent)
  - Pt may not tolerate vent disconnect (loss of PEEP) or dec FiO_2 during electrocautery
- Considerable bleeding is rare but possible (aberrant vasculature) intraop or post op

Anesthetic Management
- Awake tracheostomy (see box below)
- GA: Inhalational or TIVA; muscle relaxation generally optimizes surgical conditions
- Potential for ETT balloon puncture upon tracheal incision
  - Deflate ETT balloon prior to tracheal incision
  - Consider advancing ETT (balloon) prior to tracheal incision
  - Or withdrawal to just above tracheotomy site under direct surgical visualization
- Do not fully extubate until tracheostomy is in place & secured
  - If tracheostomy lost, ETT can be quickly readvanced distal to tracheostomy
- Lower FiO_2 (<30%) if monopolar cautery to be used after tracheotomy
- Consider bronchoscopic confirmation of trach tube placement if difficult or nonstandard tube (pXLT, dXLT)

Management of Existing Tracheostomy
- Does tracheostomy have a balloon/cuff?
- Will positive-pressure vent be required? (*Limited with uncuffed tracheostomy*)
- Will unusual positioning be required?
- Is tracheostomy <7 d old?

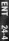

ENT 24-4

Management of Mature Tracheostomy (>7 d)
- Suction existing cannula
- Denitrogenate with 100% O_2 via tracheostomy
- Inhaled induction with potent agent (e.g., sevoflurane) or IV induction
- Consider transtracheal lidocaine (2–4%, 3–5 mL)
- Exchange tracheal tube with a lubricated, wire-reinforced ETT that has the same inner diameter or 1 size smaller than tracheostomy tube
- Advance tube & adjust depth: Check for bilateral breath sounds, confirm CO_2
- Replace tube with clean tracheostomy tube, confirm CO_2 at case completion after resumption of spontaneous ventilation if uncuffed trach

Management of Fresh Tracheostomy
- Fresh tracheostomy (<7 d) requires interdisciplinary management
- Percutaneously placed tracheostomy may be especially challenging
- Should generally not be removed outside OR (no tract)
- Never bag ventilate through a tracheostomy if intratracheal position cannot be confirmed by CO_2, fiberoptic inspection, or passage of suction catheter
- Fresh tracheostomy dislodgement = surgical emergency
  - Call for surgical support, trach tray, & fiberoptic bronchoscope
  - Put sterile gloves on & plug tracheostomy site with finger
  - Do **not** attempt blind replacement of tracheostomy
    - Risk of subcutaneous placement, bleeding, & trauma
  - Attempt mask ventilation from mouth/nose only
  - Place LMA if failed/difficult mask ventilation
- Attempt orotracheal intubation by laryngoscopy
  - Consider fiberoptic intubation if unsuccessful
  - Advance ETT balloon past tracheotomy
- If intubation fails & ventilation is adequate, proceed to OR
  - Tracheostomy replacement via trans-LMA fiberoptic or videolaryngoscopic guidance only in stable clinical circumstances with experienced personnel
- If above efforts fail, surgical re-exploration at bedside
- See also http://www.tracheostomy.org.uk/ safe tracheostomy project

Awake Tracheostomy	
Indications • Acute stridor/upper airway obstruction • Severe airway trauma • Obstructing glottic tumor • Severe tracheomalacia	**Key Points** • Psychological preparation/counseling • Pt must be able to cooperate • Head-up position • Note fire risk if cautery • Supplemental O_2 as needed with expiratory CO_2 monitoring
Blocks (see Chapter 4, Airway Management) • Superficial cervical plexus block • Transtracheal block • Superior laryngeal nerve block • Local field block	• Sedative meds for anxiolysis only • Maintain spontaneous vent • May induce GA after trach in place • Asleep with flexible LMA & spont vent may be an option
Potential Sedatives (use sparingly) Dexmedetomidine, remifentanil, droperidol, ketamine, midazolam	

Laser Surgery and Airway Fires	
Airway Fire Algorithm • Detect fire or smoke in airway *Cease ventilation & extubate* • Mask ventilation with O_2 • Inspect airway for injury • Reintubate • Perform fiberoptic inspection of airway • Consider trach if significant burn injury • Measure carboxyhemoglobin level in blood	*Precautions* • Goggles—including pt • Laser sign on door • Use of laser-resistant tube • ↓ O_2 flows—FiO_2 <30% optimal • N_2O may support combustion • Surgeon communication • Moist pledgets/packing at laser site • Monitor laser power/duration

Lasers (Light Amplification Stimulated Emission of Radiation)

- Light → medium (gas/solid matrix) → amplification → high-energy photon output
- *Types of laser* (↓λ, ↑W): Argon > KTP > Nd-YAG > CO_2 (Mixed CO_2, He/N_2)
- *Laser use*: Laryngeal papilloma, endometrial, endobronchial mass ablations; skin resurfacing, ophthalmologic procedures; coagulation, TURP
- *Risks*: Pt & provider injury from direct, scattered, & reflected laser light & environmental contamination by vaporized tissue (e.g., papilloma surgery)
  - Retinal damage (Argon, Nd-YAG), corneal damage (CO_2)
- Colored goggles (Argon [o], Nd-YAG [g], KTP [r], or glasses [CO_2]) for staff & pt airway fire (moist pledgets in airway & around cuff; laser tube, low FiO_2, avoid N_2O), vaporized infectious/tumor particles (high-efficiency mask)
- *Advantages*: Focused over small area (high power density) with limited collateral tissue damage (depth in mm)

Introduction to Jet Ventilation

- Used frequently in complex airway surgery
- Jet ventilation catheter (e.g., metal, Hunsaker) eliminates need for ETT
- Subglottic & supraglottic approaches (depends on procedure & anatomy)
- Safe jet ventilation requires open airway for entrained air to escape during exhalation
- Jet ventilation can achieve effective oxygenation & ventilation
  - Brief low-volume, high-frequency pulses of O_2 exiting the jet catheter entrain ambient air → deliver larger tidal volume
- Advanced devices (e.g., Monsoon/Mistral) safer than manual (e.g., Sanders)
  - Set FiO_2, humidity, driving pressure (DP), frequency (f), & inspiratory time (IT)
  - Example settings: FiO_2 = 100%; hum = 40%; DP = 22; psi = 120 bpm; IT = 40%
  - Peak airway pressure can be measured & alarms set
  - $ETCO_2$ can be checked intermittently via placement of ETT by surgeon or use of a continuous transcutaneous CO_2 monitor
- High-flow nasal cannula oxygen is emerging as a potential alternative to HFJV

Applications	Potential Complications	Devices
Suspension laryngoscopy	Barotrauma	Mistral
Tracheal resection	Hypercarbia	Monsoon
Limit motion in field (thoracic)	Airway desiccation	Bird
Difficult airway	Hypoxemia	Manual/Sanders
Strategies		
Trans-LMA; supraglottic; sub/transglottic		

PROCEDURES IN OPHTHALMOLOGY

Special Considerations

- Extremes of age (pediatrics—strabismus repair) (geriatrics—cataract surgery)
  - Geriatric pts small doses of sedatives may induced general anesthesia
  - Geriatrics—Increased risk of perioperative delirium/cognitive impairment
  - Caution with multiple sedative combinations in the geriatric pt
- Many ophthalmologists perform regional blocks themselves
- Complications from movement may result in blindness
- Appropriate precautions (see above) for laser surgery
- Access to airway is limited during surgery

Special Medications in Ophthalmologic Population

- Echothiophate for glaucoma
  - Acetylcholinesterase inhibitor → prolongs action of succinylcholine
  - Systemic effects include bronchospasm, bradycardia, hypertension
- Sulfur hexafluoride gas for retinal surgery
  - Pt may have intravitreal gas bubble up to 21-d postop
  - Avoid N_2O due to potential for catastrophic air expansion
- Consider avoidance of succinylcholine in selected circumstances
  - Globe injury → increased intraocular pressure with fasciculation (*succinylcholine is **not absolutely** contraindicated*)
  - Prolonged contracture of ocular musculature after dosing may interfere with forced duction test (FDT) in strabismus surgery
- Pilocarpine & carbachol
  - Drugs that promote efflux of aqueous humor by producing miosis

- Parasympathomimetics (cholinergic agonist)
  - Systemic effects = parasympathetic effects (bradycardia)
- Epinephrine
  - Systemic effects may lead to tachycardia/angina
- Acetazolamide
  - Carbonic anhydrase inhibitor
  - Systemic effects include metabolic acidosis, hypokalemia, ↓ ICP
- Timolol
  - β-blocker
  - Systemic effects include bradycardia, hypotension, bronchospasm
- Oral glycerol side effects: Nausea, vomiting, hyperglycemia
- Mannitol side effects: Volume overload, renal failure

Cataract Surgery: Clear Corneal Phacoemulsification
- Pts often elderly with multiple comorbidities
- Continuous exhaled CO_2 monitoring is standard of care during sedation
- Procedures usually <1 h
- Anesthetic goals
  - Akinesia of the eye & eyelid; adequate analgesia & pt cooperation & avoidance of oculocardiac reflex
- Sedation with regional block or topicalization = preferred method
  - Local infiltration with sedation
  - Regional block with local infiltration & sedation (see Table—Oculocardiac Reflex)
    - Provided by surgeon or anesthesiologist
    - Brief deepening of anesthesia facilitates block placement
    - Options include retrobulbar block; peribulbar block, subtenon's block
    - Block complications: Retrobulbar hemorrhage, globe perforation, optic nerve damage, brainstem anesthesia
  - GA for selected pts (complex procedures/unable to cooperate or stay supine)

Strabismus Surgery
- Indication: Reposition muscles to treat ocular malalignment
- Surgery almost exclusively performed in pediatric pts
- ↑ Incidence of postop nausea & vomiting
- ↑ Risk of intraop oculocardiac reflex (see box below)
- Usually performed under GA with ETT
- Nondepolarizing muscle relaxation may aid diagnostic utility of FDT & surgical operating conditions

Other Procedures
- Repair of ruptured globe
  - Frequently emergent procedure with aspiration risk concerns (full stomach, head, & associated injuries)
  - Commonly requires GA with ETT
  - Consider LMA in select circumstances (pts often have full stomach)
  - Emphasis on control of intraocular pressure (succinylcholine may ↑ IOP)
  - Avoid coughing or bucking during induction & intubation
- Intraocular surgery: Enucleation, vitrectomy, corneal transplantation, glaucoma decompression, repair retinal detachments
  - Control of eye movement & intraocular pressure critical
  - GA preferred
  - Intraocular epinephrine may be used to aid papillary dilatation
    - Monitor for systemic effects
- Detachment repair injects intraocular air or sulfur hexafluoride gas
  - Avoid N_2O or discontinue well before injection
  - Avoid N_2O for subsequent surgery within 3 wk

Oculocardiac Reflex	
Cardiac reflex (bradycardia, sinus arrest, arrhythmia) with multiple triggers: (1) Ocular pressure, (2) ocular muscle stretch, (3) intense stimulation of empty orbit extremely common in pediatric strabismus surgery	
Mechanism:	Afferent-trigeminal
	Efferent-vagus
Treatment/Prevention:	Anticholinergic (pre)treatment (e.g., glyco/atropine). Use of regional block with local anesthetics
	Release ocular pressure/stop stimulation
	↑ Anesthetic depth

Blocks for Ophthalmologic Surgery

- *Contraindications (regional):* Uncooperative pt or pt with severe medical comorbidities that prevent positioning/immobility, trauma to eye, blindness in nonoperative eye, glaucoma, anticoagulation (relative)
- Advantages of local blocks over GA
  - Avoids complications/side effects of GA (e.g., decreased hemodynamic effects)
  - Useful for day surgery/office procedures (fast recovery)
  - Produce good eye akinesia & surgical analgesia
  - Minimal effect on IOP
- Disadvantages of local blocks:
  - Not suitable for all pts (children, language barrier, mentally handicapped)
  - Depends on skills/experience of anesthesiologist/ophthalmologist performing block
  - Not suitable for all types of surgery (open-eye surgery)
  - Complications (see below)
- Choice of technique varies with surgeon
- Most blocks currently performed by ophthalmologists

Block	Agent	Complications
Superficial application	Lidocaine 2%	Toxicity (high levels): Seizure/cardiac effects Epinephrine: Tachycardia
Subtenon's block	Lidocaine 1–2% w/ epinephrine (1:400,000)	Subarachnoid injection: Apnea
Peribulbar block Retrobulbar block (highest risk)	Bupivacaine 0.375–0.75% w/epinephrine (1:400,000)	Intravascular injection: Seizure Globe rupture: Proptosis/agitation Intraneural: Optic nerve damage/blindness Chemosis Oculocardiac reflex Vessel injury—hemorrhage/ecchymosis ↑ intraorbital pressure/proptosis Central retinal artery occlusion Extraocular muscle injury

Peribulbar Block (25G–27G, 25-mm needle)
- Safer (needle inserted outside of extraocular muscle cone), but slower onset
- Primary gaze position → 2 injections above & below globe
- Inject ≈ 5 mL local into superonasal orbit & ≈ 5 mL inferotemporally between lateral & medial of lower orbital margin

Retrobulbar Block (25G–27G, 3-cm needle)
- Faster onset; must anesthetize conjunctiva before needle introduction
- Insert needle halfway between lateral canthus & lateral limbus in lower conjunctiva
- Direct needle straight back until the tip is beyond globe, → then direct needle toward apex of orbit to enter space behind globe between inferior & lateral rectus muscles
- Insert to depth of 25–35 mm; inject 4 mL local

Subtenon's Block (25G needle)
- Injection of local anesthetic directly into posterior aspect of subtenon's space
- Insert needle to contact conjunctiva between eyeball & semilunaris fold (depth <1 mm)
  Advance needle anteroposteriorly with globe directly slightly medially by needle until "click" is felt, at a depth of 15–20 mm (episcleral location)
- Return globe to primary position; aspirate → inject local
- Stop at sign of chemosis (conjunctival edema) & apply ocular compression

RENAL SYSTEM AND UROLOGIC SURGERY

JESSE M. EHRENFELD • RICHARD D. URMAN

EVALUATION OF RENAL FUNCTION

- Urinalysis
  - Specific gravity reflects kidney's ability to concentrate urine
  - Hematuria may occur with intrinsic renal d/o (fever, UTI, kidney stones, urologic tumors, trauma, & coagulopathy)
  - Proteinuria may occur with intrinsic renal d/o, fever, CHF, exercise
- BUN
  - Normal: 10–20 mg/dL
  - Unreliable measure of GFR (↑ in dehydration, high-protein diet, GI bleeding, & increased catabolism)
- Creatinine
  - End product of skeletal muscle metabolism, excreted by kidneys
  - Proportional to skeletal muscle mass
  - Inversely related to GFR
  - Normal: 0.8–1.3 in men, 0.6–1.0 in women (↓ in pregnancy)
  - Less reliable measure of renal function in elderly (GFR ↓ with age but muscle mass also ↓: Can result in a normal Cr despite abnormal renal function)
- Creatinine clearance
  - GFR best indicator of renal fx, difficult to measure; CrCl most reliable estimate of GFR
  - CrCl can be measured using 2- or 24-h urine collection
- Normal: 80–130 mL/min for women; 100–140 mL/min for men

$$\text{Estimated CrCl} = \frac{(140 - \text{age})(\text{body weight in kg})(0.85 \text{ in women})}{(\text{serum Cr})(72)}$$

Acute Kidney Injury

- ↑ Cr by ≥0.3 mg/dL in 48 h, ↑ Cr by 1.5× baseline in 7 d, or urine <0.5 mL/kg/h for 6 h (KDIGO definition)

	Prerenal	Intrinsic	Postrenal
Urine Na$^+$	<10 mEq/L	>20 mEq/L	>20 mEq/L
Urine osmolarity	>500	<350	<350
FE$_{Na}$	<1%	>2%	>2%
BUN/Cr	>20	<10–15	<10–15
Urine Cr/Serum Cr	>40	<20	<20

Prerenal
- Renal hypoperfusion resulting in ↓ GFR
- Causes
  - Hypovolemia, ↓ cardiac output, liver failure, sepsis
  - Renal vasoconstriction (ACE/COX inhibitors)
- Intrinsic (renal)
  - Damage to renal parenchyma
  - Causes
    - Acute tubular necrosis (ATN)—causes include ischemia & toxins (aminoglycosides, myoglobin, IV contrast)
    - Acute interstitial nephritis (AIN)—usually caused by drugs (NSAIDs, β-lactams, sulfonamides, rifampin)
    - Glomerulonephritis
    - DIC
    - TTP
- Postrenal
  - Outflow obstruction (must have bilateral obstruction, unilateral obstruction if only one kidney present, kinked Foley)
  - Causes
    - Nephrolithiasis, BPH, prostate cancer, neurogenic bladder

- Treatment
  - Treat underlying d/o
  - Avoid nephrotoxic drugs
  - Fenoldopam & low-dose dopamine (controversial) may help prevent or treat ARF by dilating renal arteries & ↑ RBF & GFR
- Dialysis if indicated due to:
  - Acidosis
  - Electrolyte disturbances (hyperkalemia)
  - Intoxication (methanol, ethylene glycol)
  - Volume overload
  - Uremia

Chronic Renal Failure
- Either GFR <60 mL/min/1.73 m^2 or evidence of kidney damage (abnormal urinalysis, imaging, or histology) for ≥3 mo
- Causes:
  - Hypertension
  - Diabetes mellitus
  - Glomerulonephritis
  - Polycystic kidney dz
  - Renovascular dz

Stages of CRF		
Stage	Degree of Impairment	GFR
1	Normal	>90
2	Mild	60–89
3	Moderate	30–59
4	Severe	15–29
5	Renal failure	<15

- Treatment
  - ACE inhibitors/ARBs may slow progression of diabetic renal dz
  - Erythropoietin for anemia
  - Dialysis as indicated (hemodialysis/peritoneal dialysis)
  - Phosphate binders for hyperphosphatemia
  - Renal transplantation

Clinical Features of CRF	
System	Manifestations
Neurologic	Peripheral/autonomic neuropathy, encephalopathy
Cardiovascular	Hypervolemia, HTN, CHF, uremic pericarditis, pericardial effusion, accelerated atherosclerosis
Pulmonary	Pulmonary edema
Gastrointestinal	Delayed gastric emptying
Hematologic	Anemia, platelet*/leukocyte dysfunction
Metabolic	Hyperkalemia, hypermagnesemia, hyperphosphatemia, hypocalcemia, hypoalbuminemia, metabolic acidosis
Endocrine	Glucose intolerance, hypertriglyceridemia
Musculoskeletal	Osteoporosis, osteomalacia

*Platelet dysfunction does not improve with platelet transfusion; give DDAVP or cryoprecipitate (vWF activates platelets).

For a list of commonly used diuretics, see Chapter 2H, Clinical Characteristics of Commonly Encountered Diuretics

Diagnostic Guide for Serum and Urine Electrolytes

Condition	Serum Values					Urine Values			
	Na+ (mEq/L)	K+ (mEq/L)	Osmolality (mOsm/L)	Bun (mg/dL)	Creatinine	Na+ (mEq/L)	K+ (mEq/L)	Osmolality (mOsm/L)	Urea (mg/dL)
Primary aldosteronism	140	↓	280	10	N	80	60–80	300–800	Low
Secondary aldosteronism	130	↓	275	15–25	↓	<20	40–60	300–400	
Na+ depletion	120–130	N or ↑	260	>30	N or ↑	10–20	40	600+	800–1,000
Na+ overload	150+	N	290+	N or ↑	N	100+	60	500+	300
H₂O overload	120–130	↓	260	10–15	↓	50–80	60	50–200	300
Dehydration	150	↓	300	30 or N	N or ↑	40	20–40	800+	800–1,000
Inappropriate ADH	<125	↓	<260	<10	↓	90	60–150	U > Posm	300
Acute tubular necrosis									
Oliguric	135	↑	N or ↑	↑↑	↑	40+	20–40	300	300
Polyuric	135	N or ↑	275	↑	↑	20	30	300	100–300

Source: From Link D. Fluids, electrolytes, acid–base disturbances, and diuretics. In: Todres ID, Fugate JH, eds. *Critical Care of Infants and Children*. Boston, MA: Little, Brown; 1996:410–435.

ANESTHESIA FOR PATIENTS WITH RENAL DISEASE

Effects of Anesthesia on Renal Function
- Reversible ↓ in RBF, GFR, urine production during regional & general anesthesia can occur despite maintenance of normal BP/volume status
- RBF & GFR will usually return to normal within several h postop

Indirect Effects of Anesthesia
- Anesthetic agents & sympathetic blockade (during regional techniques)
- → Hypotension & myocardial depression → ↓ RBF & GFR
- Hydration before anesthesia may lessen hypotension and changes in RBF

Direct Effects of Anesthesia
- Fluorinated agents can cause direct renal toxicity (fluoride impairs kidney's ability to concentrate urine & causes tubular necrosis)
  - Fluoride production negligible with halothane, desflurane, & isoflurane
  - Sevoflurane & enflurane release fluoride (no clinical evidence of renal damage)
- Sevoflurane reacts with carbon dioxide absorbents to form compound A (shown to cause renal damage in rat models)
  - Low fresh gas flows should be avoided with sevoflurane (use flows of ≥1 L/min)
  - Consider avoiding sevoflurane in pts with renal insufficiency (theoretical risk of nephrotoxicity)
- Common IV agents do not cause changes in GFR

MEDICATIONS TO AVOID OR USE WITH CAUTION IN RENAL FAILURE

- Lipid-insoluble, ionized drugs, & water-soluble metabolites of hepatically metabolized drugs are renally excreted & may accumulate in renal failure
- Highly protein-bound drugs can accumulate if pt is hypoalbuminemic

Opiates	Morphine	Active metabolites may accumulate & have prolonged effects
	Meperidine	Active metabolites may accumulate & cause both prolonged effects & seizures
Benzodiazepines	Diazepam	Active metabolites may accumulate & cause sedation
Muscle relaxants	Pancuronium	Prolonged effect
	Rocuronium	Prolonged effect (inc duration, reduced clearance)
	Vecuronium	Typically safe with single dose but may accumulate with repeated doses/infusion
	Succinylcholine	May be used if K^+ <5–5.5 mEq/L; same amount of K^+ released in pts with nl renal function (0.5–1 mEq/L)
	Cisatracurium	No significant effect
Reversal agents	Neostigmine Edrophonium Pyridostigmine	May have prolonged effects (however, anticholinergics may also be prolonged)
	Sugammadex	No dosage adjustment in mild/moderate renal impairment; not recommended in severe renal impairment/dialysis pts (FDA)
Cardiovascular agents	Digoxin	Levels may be ↑ due to ↓ clearance; danger for digoxin toxicity
	Nitroprusside	Accumulation of thiocyanate (neurotoxic)
	α-Agonists (phenylephrine)	Constrict renal vasculature
Barbiturates	Thiopental Methohexital	↑ Available drug in hypoalbuminemic pts; may need smaller induction dose
Antibiotics	Aminoglycosides Vancomycin	Need renal dosing to avoid toxic levels

UROLOGIC SURGERY

Cystoscopy/Ureteroscopy/TURBT
General Considerations
- Indications: Need for biopsies, laser lithotripsy, extraction of stones, placement of ureteral stents

- Pts commonly elderly with comorbid medical conditions
- Irrigation fluids often used to improve visualization & for flushing
  - **Sterile water:** Hypotonic, causes hemolysis & hyponatremia when absorbed systemically; safe with electrocautery
  - **Nonelectrolyte solutions (glycine, sorbitol, mannitol):** Slightly hypotonic, can cause hyponatremia if absorbed in large volumes; safe with electrocautery
  - **Electrolyte solutions (NS, LR):** Isotonic, do not cause hemolysis when absorbed systemically; cannot be used with electrocautery

Anesthetic Technique
- Positioning: Lithotomy
- Usually GA, can use local/MAC/regional (T10 level necessary for instrumentation of lower GU tract), consider using LMA
- Muscle relaxation not usually necessary (consider ETT with relaxation if surgeon anticipates working near obturator nerve)
- Minimal to no postop pain; short-acting opioids (fentanyl) usually sufficient

Complications
- Peroneal nerve injury from lithotomy position (causes foot drop)
- Bladder perforation: Extraperitoneal perforation is more common; signs and symptoms include nausea, diaphoresis, & inguinal, retropubic, or lower abdominal pain

Transurethral Resection of the Prostate (TURP)
General Considerations
- Indications: Relief of bladder obstruction from enlarged prostate (typically BPH)
- Typically elderly pts with comorbid medical conditions
- Opening of venous sinuses may lead to absorption of large amounts of irrigation fluid (see cystoscopy above) & can result in TURP syndrome (see below); fluid absorption dependent on duration of procedure, number of sinuses opened (related to prostate size), peripheral venous pressure, & height of irrigation fluid

Anesthetic Technique
- Positioning: Lithotomy
- General or regional (T10 level necessary)
- Base choice on pt's preference, coexisting dz
- Regional anesthesia allows for evaluation of TURP syndrome during procedure
- Muscle relaxation not required, although pt movement should be avoided (prevent further bleeding/perforation of prostate)
- Postop pain usually not significant

Complications
- TURP syndrome
  - Results from absorption of large volumes of irrigant fluid through venous sinuses of prostate
    - $\rightarrow$ Hyponatremia & volume overload
  - Signs/symptoms: Headache, confusion, nausea/vomiting, HTN, angina, seizures, coma, cardiovascular collapse
  - May also result from toxicity from absorption of irrigant solutes
  - Glycine: Can cause transient blindness, seizures
  - Ammonia: Can cause delayed awakening, encephalopathy
  - Hyperglycinemia may result in CNS toxicity & circulatory collapse
  - Treatment: Fluid restriction & diuretics to correct hyponatremia & volume overload; if pt has seizures/is comatose $\rightarrow$ consider hypertonic saline
- Bladder perforation
- Coagulopathy: Dilutional thrombocytopenia from excessive fluid absorption & DIC
- Bacteremia: Since prostate is colonized by bacteria, bacteremia may result after instrumentation
- Prophylactic antibiotics may $\downarrow$ risk of bacteremia/septicemia

Alternatives to TURP
- Medical management with alpha blockers
- Vaporization of prostate tissue with electrocautery/laser/thermocoagulation (avoid danger of TURP syndrome)

Urologic Laser Surgery
General Considerations
- Indications: Condyloma acuminatum; ureteral strictures; BPH; ureteral calculi; & superficial carcinomas of penis, ureter, bladder, or renal pelvis

- Different lasers may be used (CO_2/argon/pulsed dye/Nd-YAG/KTP-532)
- Safety concerns
  - Goggles should be worn by OR personnel & pt to protect eyes from an inadvertent break in laser fiber
  - Lasers should be used intermittently to prevent thermal injuries
  - Special masks should be worn to prevent inhalation of active HPV particles when condyloma are being treated

Anesthetic Technique
- Positioning: Lithotomy
- Local with MAC, general, or regional anesthesia

Open Prostatectomy
General Considerations
- Indications: BPH that can't be resected transurethrally; radical prostatectomy for prostate ca
- Pts often elderly with comorbid medical conditions; blood loss can be significant
- Retroperitoneal lymph node dissection is performed for staging in prostate cancer
- Bilateral orchiectomy may be performed in symptomatic, advanced dz

Monitoring/Access
- Standard monitors; large-bore IV

Anesthetic Technique
Open Prostatectomy
- Positioning: Supine
- Anesthesia: Regional, general, or combined general/epidural
- Epidural may ↓ blood loss, improve postop pain relief, & result in recovery of bowel function more quickly
- Experienced surgeons typically able to perform procedure under general anesthesia with minimal blood loss/small incisions
- Surgeon may ask for methylene blue/indigo carmine to assess integrity of urinary tract
  - Indigo carmine: Can cause hypertension (α-agonism)
  - Methylene blue: Can cause hypotension/interfere with SpO_2 readings

Laparoscopic and Robotic-Assisted Laparoscopic Prostatectomy (RALP)
- Advantages: Less blood loss (vs. open), smaller incisions with less postop pain
- Positioning: Lithotomy; steep Trendelenburg
- Anesthesia: General endotracheal anesthesia
- Complications after RALP include corneal abrasion and ischemic optic neuropathy → Recommend limit time in steep t-burg; restrict intraop IV fluid; use eyelid covers; risk of peripheral nerve injuries from positioning

Cystectomy
General Considerations
- Indications: Simple cystectomy for benign bladder dz (hemorrhagic/radiation cystitis); radical cystectomy for invasive bladder tumors
- Pts often elderly with comorbid conditions; given the association between smoking & bladder cancer, pts may be at risk for CAD & COPD
- After cystectomy, a urinary diversion must be constructed
  - → Piece of ileum can be formed into an ileal conduit (brought out to the abdominal wall as a stoma)
  - → Bladder suspension more involved operation (piece of bowel is formed into a pouch & connected to the urethra)
  - Significant blood & fluid loss may occur

Monitoring/Access
- Standard monitors; consider arterial line, central line given potential for large blood loss & fluid shifts; large-bore IV

Anesthetic Technique
- Positioning: Supine or lithotomy
- General or combined general/epidural anesthesia

Nephrectomy
General Considerations
- Indications: Neoplasm, transplantation, chronic hydronephrosis/infection, trauma
- Pts undergoing nephrectomy for renal cell carcinoma, will undergo preop staging to determine if tumor involves IVC or right atrium
  - Tumor may partially/completely obstruct IVC (reduces venous return & may cause hypotension); IVC may need to be clamped during resection

- Tumor may embolize to pulmonary vasculature (signs: ↓ SpO_2, hypotension, supraventricular arrhythmias)
- Complications: Venous air embolus, diaphragmatic injury (causing pneumothorax)
- May be performed open or laparoscopically

Monitoring/Access
- Standard monitors; consider arterial line
- Large-bore IV (potential for significant blood loss)

Anesthetic Technique
- Positioning: Lateral decubitus position for retroperitoneal approach/supine for transabdominal approach
- General anesthesia or combined general/epidural anesthesia (T7–T9 level)
- Hydration to preserve renal blood flow

ORTHOPEDIC SURGERY

ALEXANDER NGUYEN • ROBERT HSIUNG

GENERAL VS. REGIONAL ANESTHESIA

* Choice based on location, surgical duration, surgeon, & pt preference
* Regional anesthesia may ↑ analgesia & pt satisfaction, ↓ opioid requirement and side effects (ileus, sedation), ↓ length of stay. No clear mortality or DVT benefit over GA.
* GA has greater speed, reliability, and amnesia
* Multimodal pain regimens can be used regardless of technique: COX inhibitors (ketorolac, celecoxib), acetaminophen, anticonvulsants (gabapentin, pregabalin), intra-articular corticosteroid/local anesthetic injection

POSITIONING

* Important to prevent tissue & nerve injury, especially in pts with arthritis & spine dz
* Common peripheral nerve injuries occur with the following frequency: Ulnar > brachial plexus > lumbosacral root > spinal cord
* Supine—most surgeries, including knee, hip, pelvis, arm, hand, foot
* Prone
  * Check pressure points—face/eyes, breasts/genitalia, brachial plexus, abdomen; excess pressure can ↑ venous compression, ↑ airway pressure, & ↓ FRC
  * Endotracheal tube dislodgement & kinking can occur
  * Stretcher should be immediately available for emergent flipping
  * ↑ Risk of perioperative blindness
    * Mechanism: Unknown, may include anterior & posterior ischemic optic neuropathy (AION, PION), central retinal artery occlusion (CRAO), and central retinal vein occlusion (CVAO)
    * Risk factors: Spine surgery, prolonged surgical time (>6 h), blood loss (>40% EBV), prone position, preop anemia, obesity, smoking, DM2
    * Consider using colloids with crystalloids for intravascular volume. Keep head level with or above the heart. Avoid direct pressure on eye orbits to ↓ risk of CRAO & venous congestion
* Lateral
  * Need to protect pressure points & maintain neutral neck alignment
  * Keep pressure off the axilla with an "axillary roll" (placed inferior to axilla, not in it)—this protects the brachial plexus & vasculature in dependent arm
* Sitting/beach chair—shoulder, clavicle surgeries
  * Provides full surgical access to the shoulder, ↑ risk of air embolism (5–25%) Adjust BP goal to ensure adequate perfusion of brain (20 cm H_2O ≈ 15 mmHg)
* **Extremity Surgery** (also see Chapter 6, Regional Anesthesia)
  * Consider regional anesthesia, especially continuous catheter techniques
  * Combined general/regional may maximize speed, amnesia, & analgesia
  * See Table—Anesthetic Options for Extremity Surgery

SPINE SURGERY

Cervical Spine Surgery
* Indications: Instability (trauma, tumor), arthritis/osteophytes, spinal stenosis
* Intubation precautions
  * Consider fiberoptic intubation or techniques that avoid neck hyperextension (intubating LMA, videoscope) although *almost all airway instrumentation does cause some degree of cervical spine movement*. For extremely unstable spine, may even consider "awake" intubation or tracheostomy
  * See Chapter 17: Trauma, Burn, and Critical Care Management for further notes

Thoracic/Lumbar Spine Surgery
* Laminectomy/laminotomy: Excision of vertebral lamina to relieve nerve pressure
* Fusion: Instrumentation with hardware to stabilize spine until bony fusion can occur (6–12 mo postop)
* Indications: Spondylolisthesis, scoliosis, recurrent disc herniation, spinal instability
* Often large operations with large blood loss & periop complications (Consider A-line, good IV access, blood & cell saver)

Anesthetic Options for Extremity Surgery			
Procedure	Anesthetic Options	Positioning	Notes
Upper Extremity			
Shoulder surgery	• General • Interscalene	Beach chair, lateral	Often requires general anesthetic or heavy sedation as pt may be covered in drapes for hours
Elbow surgery	• General • Supraclavicular • Infraclavicular • Axillary	Supine, lateral, or prone	Consider infraclavicular catheters, supplemental intercostobrachial nerve block for proximal medial upper arm innervation
Wrist and hand surgery	• General • Axillary • Supraclavicular • Infraclavicular • Bier block • Digital n. block • Local + MAC	Supine	Typical surgeries include carpal tunnel release, distal radius ORIF, trigger finger release, & ganglion cyst excision
Lower Extremity			
Knee arthroscopy	• General ± saphenous n. block • Spinal • Epidural • Intra-articular local + MAC	Supine	General usually chosen unless Hx of chronic opioid use or pt wants to watch the procedure
Total knee arthroplasty	• General ± femoral (single shot or catheter) ± sciatic (rescue) • Spinal ± femoral catheter • Epidural • Lumbar plexus + sciatic	Supine	Multiple combination nerve blocks possible; Adductor (saphenous) nerve catheters have been replacing femoral nerve catheters for postop pain due to less motor involvement. Tourniquet use common → EBL can be >500 mL after deflation.
Hip fracture	• General ± femoral nerve block (postop analgesia) • Spinal • Epidural	Supine	Femoral nerve blocks have been shown to ↓ delirium in hip fractures by decreasing opioid requirements
Hip arthroplasty	• General ± lumbar plexus (postop analgesia) or ± femoral nerve block • Spinal • Epidural	Lateral	Risk of embolization-induced hypotension/hypoxemia/arrest during cementing: Rx = supportive resuscitation
Ankle	• General • Spinal • Epidural • Popliteal ± saphenous	Supine, lateral, or prone	Epidural may take 30+ min to set in sacral region
Foot, toe, bunion surgery	General Ankle Popliteal ± saphenous (sciatic nerve)	Supine	Medial part of foot is innervated by the saphenous n. (femoral n.). The rest of innervated by sciatic n.

NEUROMONITORING (ALSO SEE CHAPTER 23, NEUROSURGERY AND ECT)

• Indication: Detection of neural pathway compromise during surgery helps guide intraop surgical decision-making
• Definition: Evoked potentials are measurements of nerve conduction in response to stimulation of a neural pathway

- Technique: Waveforms evaluated for amplitude, latency, & morphology; baseline measurements performed after anesthetic stabilized (*avoid boluses/rapid changes in anesthetic depth → infusions can be beneficial*)
- Outcomes: No evidence of improved outcomes in lumbar decompression or lumbar fusion for degenerative spine dz according to the American Association of Neurological Surgeons/Congress of Neurological Surgeons

Types of Monitoring

Somatosensory Evoked Potentials (SSEP)
- Detect injury/ischemia to dorsal columns of spinal cord (sensory tract) supplied by posterior spinal arteries
- Stimulation of common peripheral nerves (posterior tibial, median, ulnar) recorded at scalp (sensory strip)
- Rare false negatives but common false positives
- Does not directly monitor motor tracts
  → Motor injury is possible with normal SSEPs
  → Artery of Adamkiewicz supplies lower 2/3 of spinal cord via anterior spinal artery
- Results may be delayed (20 min)

Corticospinal Motor–Evoked Potentials (MEP)
- Monitors integrity of spinal cord motor tracts (supplied by anterior spinal artery)
- Used for aortic, intramedullary spinal cord tumor, spinal deformity, posterior fossa tumor, & intracranial aneurysms
- Scalp or epidural lead placement to stimulate upper & lower extremities
- *Muscle relaxants should be avoided*
- Immediate results
- Safety issues: Burns, movement-induced injuries, seizures, bite injuries (0.2%), contraindicated with pacemakers

Electromyography (EMG)
- Measures electrical activity of muscles
- Continuous monitoring of spontaneous activity used to monitor for excessive nerve manipulation or blunt trauma to nerve
- Triggered potentials used to identify nerves and identify malpositioned implants (i.e., pedicle screws)
- Used in tethered cord release, tumor excision, acoustic neuroma resection, & facial nerve procedures
- *Muscle relaxants should be avoided*

Factors Affecting Monitoring
- Baseline measurements may be poor, consider prepositioning measurements
- MEPs more sensitive to anesthetics than SSEPs
  - *Muscle relaxants relatively contraindicated in MEPs, but enhance SSEP signals by ↓ EMG artifact*
- ↑ Latency or ↓ amplitude may indicate neurologic dysfunction
  - Bilateral & equal changes likely 2° to temp, hypotension, or anesthetic effects
  - Unilateral changes likely 2° to ischemia/technical factors
- Temperature (SSEP): Hypothermia: ↔ amplitude, ↑ latency
  - Hyperthermia: ↓ Amplitude, ↔ latency
- Hypoxia (SSEP): ↓ Amplitude, ↑ latency
- CO_2 (SSEP): $PaCO_2$ 25–50 with minimal changes
  $PaCO_2$ >100 ↓ amplitude, ↑ latency
- Anemia: ↓ Amplitude
- Hypotension (SSEP): Rapid BP ↓ will ↓ amplitude, ↔ latency
- Positioning: Unstable spine or cervical movement may change signals
- Anesthetic agent (SSEP): IV anesthetic effects < volatile anesthetic effects
- Sensitivity to anesthetics: Visual > TcMEP > deep MEP > spinal MEP > SSEP > BAEP

Effect of Anesthetics on SSEPs		
↓ Amplitude	**Minimal**	**↑ Amplitude**
Barbiturates (↑ latency)	Propofol	Ketamine
Volatile anesthetics (↑ latency)	Opioids	Etomidate
Magnesium	Midazolam	
	Droperidol	
	Clonidine	
	Dexmedetomidine	

- Anesthesia techniques in monitored surgeries (SSEP/MEP)
  - Halogenated anesthetics vs. TIVA
    - Propofol/opioid (i.e., remifentanil) infusions have little or no interference with neuromonitoring (SSEP and MEP) at steady state
    - Infusions can ↓ amount of volatile agent used up to <0.5 MAC
  - Deliberate hypotension
    - Reducing MAP 20–30% below baseline to ↓ blood loss & improve surgical exposure
    - Risks: ↓ Perfusion & O_2 to vital organs (heart, brain, spinal cord)
    - No longer recommended as a safe technique due to risk of stroke
- Postoperative pain management becomes harder as more vertebrae are involved
  - Intraoperative bolus of methadone has been shown to ↓ postoperative opioid consumption and pain scores
  - High-dose ketorolac associated with nonunion of spinal fusions. Further studies required for other NSAIDs
  - Multimodals including gabapentin and acetaminophen are effective
  - Intraoperative and postoperative ketamine, lidocaine, and dexmedetomidine infusions are being studied to reduce opioid use and prevent chronic opioid use
- **Wakeup test**
  - Most reliable assessment of intact spine
  - Involves gentle, slow wakeup with continued analgesia coordinated with surgical team following instrumentation
  - Pt asked to follow commands upon emergence with re-establishment of general anesthesia after neuro-assessment
  - Plan should be outlined with pt prior to surgery (*explain possibility of intraop recall*)
  - Common techniques for rapid awakening include TIVA (propofol, remifentanil, and/ or dexmedetomidine), N_2O-narcotic, short-acting inhalational agent

COMPLICATIONS IN ORTHOPEDIC SURGERY

- Methyl methacrylate bone cement
  - Expands into cancellous bone when applied, can result in ↑ intramedullary pressures → displacement of intramedullary fat → **fat embolism**
  - Cement monomers can cause profound ↓SVR/↓BP with ↓CO, hypoxia (shunting), pulm HTN, and arrhythmia if enters systemic circulation
  - Therapy: High FiO_2, euvolemia, & hemodynamic support
- Fat embolus syndrome (FES)
  - Often occurs with long bone fractures and intramedullary reaming
  - Risk ↑ 24-h postinjury without proper bone fixation
  - Signs: Petechiae, rash, urine fat globules, hypotension, tachycardia, hypoxia/dyspnea, altered mental status, lung infiltrates on CXR. Keep in mind you may not have any physical exam findings at all.
  - Therapy: Supportive to correct hypoxia & hemodynamic instability; intubation with PEEP for refractory hypoxemia; steroids controversial
- Management of blood loss in orthopedic surgery
  - Intraoperative blood salvage/cell saver
  - TXA reduces blood loss and transfusion requirement. Contraindicated in those at high risk of thromboembolic events (coronary stents, Afib, Hx of unprovoked PE)
  - Tourniquet for extremity surgery (see table below)
  - Acute normovolemic hemodilution—pt's blood collected at start of surgery with concomitant replacement with IV fluids; blood is returned to pt at the end of surgery
  - Autologous blood donation collected several weeks prior to elective procedure
  - Preop erythropoietin
- DVT/PE
  - Major cause of perioperative morbidity/mortality in orthopedic surgery (0.3–2% incidence of symptomatic PE)
  - Risk factors: Prolonged surgery, hip/knee replacement, tourniquet use, ↓ mobility postop, age >60
  - Prophylaxis:
    - Encourage early ambulation/physical therapy
    - Use intermittent leg-compression devices throughout perioperative period
    - Consider initiating low-dose anticoagulation (warfarin/LMWH) preoperatively
    - Consider prophylactic IVC filter in high-risk pts

Complications of Intraoperative Tourniquet Use	
Ischemic injury	• Prolonged inflation >2 h can cause neural/tissue ischemia with possible permanent injury • If longer duration, tourniquet should be deflated, perfusion restored, and reinflated after 10–15 min
Tourniquet pain	• Progressive hypertension occurring 30–60 min after cuff inflation, even with adequate regional anesthetic blockade (spinal, epidural, peripheral nerve block) • Mechanism unknown; thought to be mediated through unmyelinated C fibers resistant to local anesthetic blockade • Rx: IV analgesia frequently ineffective; vasodilators can be used to lower BP; tourniquet deflation and reinflation as above
Reperfusion injury following tourniquet deflation	• Acidic metabolites & emboli generated in ischemic limb re-enter systemic circulation, causing hypotension, hypoxia, hypercarbia, pulmonary HTN, embolism, and/or metabolic acidosis • Usually transient → Rx may include fluids & vasopressors; calcium & bicarbonate prn for hyperkalemia & severe acidosis, respectively
Relative contraindications	• Sickle cell, severe peripheral vascular dz, severe crush injury, diabetic neuropathy

ENDOCRINE SURGERY

JESSE M. EHRENFELD • RICHARD D. URMAN

THYROID GLAND

Hyperthyroidism
Anesthesia for Hyperthyroidism
- **Preop**
  - General: Euthyroid status preferred (risk of thyroid storm), check TFTs, continue antithyroid meds & β-blockers to the d of surgery
  - Airway: Check for compression, tracheal deviation, & substernal thyroid mass; consider awake fiberoptic intubation if airway looks challenging
- Benzodiazepines for preop sedation
- **Intraop**
  - General: Avoid/use sympathetic nervous system stimulants cautiously (epinephrine, ketamine, ephedrine, phenylephrine) → severe HTN/tachycardia
  - Ensure pt eye protection (pt often has exophthalmos)
  - Thiopental possesses antithyroid activity in high doses
  - Watch for signs of thyroid storm (hyperthermia, tachycardia, ↑ BP)
  - Autoimmune thyrotoxicosis may be associated with myopathies
- **Postop**
  - Complications: Hormonal disturbances & airway management issues
  - Thyroid storm: Life-threatening condition, can develop 6–24 h after surgery; caused by massive release of T_3 & T_4
    Signs: Tachycardia, fever, confusion, vomiting, dehydration, CHF, agitation (*unlike MH, not associated with ↑ CPK, muscle rigidity, or acidosis*)
  - Parathyroid gland damage/removal → hypocalcemia in 24–72 h postop
  - Recurrent laryngeal n. damage → causes hoarseness if unilateral, stridor if bilateral *diagnosis by fiberoptic laryngoscopy*
  - Neck hematoma → partial/complete upper airway obstruction *Treatment = prompt opening of neck wound & drainage*

Hypothyroidism
Anesthesia for Hypothyroidism
- **Preop**
  - Thyroid supplements should be continued through surgery
  - Delay elective surgeries in case of untreated hypothyroidism (*risk of cardiovascular instability & myxedema coma*)
  - Subclinical hypothyroidism **not** associated with ↑ surgical risk
  - In emergency cases: Consider pretreatment with IV thyroxine & steroids
  - Pts usually obese, may have large tongue, short neck, delayed gastric emptying
- **Intraop**
  - Hypothyroid pts sensitive to narcotics & sedatives
  - Induction: Maintain stable hemodynamics (consider ketamine or etomidate)
  - Hypotension due to abnl baroreceptor fx, ↓ cardiac output, hypovolemia
  - Hypothermia develops very fast & difficult to treat
  - Metabolic disturbances common: ↓ Na & ↓ blood sugar
  - Hypoventilation common (blunted response to hypoxia)
  - Myxedema coma (severe form of decompensated hypothyroidism) can occur (see table below)
- **Postop**
  - Hypothermia, slow drug metabolism, & resp depression may delay extubation
  - Extubation should be done in awake & normothermic pt
  - Regional anesthesia & ketorolac = preferable for pain control (use opioids with caution)

PARATHYROID GLANDS

Hyperparathyroidism
Anesthesia for Hyperparathyroidism
- ECG: Short PR & QT intervals, cardiac conduction d/o (↑ Ca levels)
- Maintain hydration & good urine output
- Consider using lower doses of nondepolarizing muscle relaxants in weak/somnolent pts

Hypoparathyroidism

Anesthesia for Hypoparathyroidism

- **Preop**—serum & ionized Ca should be normalized, especially for pts with cardiac symptoms
- **Intraop**—pre-existing hypocalcemia may augment neuromuscular block
  - Blood products containing citrate (as well as 5% albumin) will ↓ serum Ca level
- **Postop**—hypocalcemia may cause prolonged recovery from neuromuscular blockade

Pheochromocytoma

- May be associated with autosomal dominant multiple endocrine neoplastic synd (MEN types 2a & b)
- Secretes epinephrine, norepinephrine, & occasionally dopamine
  - Secretion may be intermittent or continuous
  - Change in tumor blood flow, direct pressure, & meds can trigger catecholamine release

Anesthesia for Pheochromocytoma

- **Preop:** Goal = control BP & restore of intravascular volume
  - Start α-blockade 10–14 d prior to surgery & **prior** to β-blockade
    - If one accidentally starts β-blockade prior to α-blockade → severe HTN from unopposed α-stimulus
  - Phenoxybenzamine = α-antagonist of choice (another option is prazosin)
    - Starting dose = 10 mg qd or bid, then inc dose by 10–20 mg in divided doses every 2–3 d as needed to control BP (goal final dose = 20–100 mg qd)
  - Propranolol 10 mg qid (should be initiated 3–4 d prior to the surgery)
  - Ca-channel blockers—nicardipine 30 mg bid to supplement α- and β-blockade if BP is poorly controlled
  - Hydrate all pts with pheochromocytoma—carefully in pts with signs of CHF
  - Nitroprusside infusion (also phentolamine IV) for treatment of acute HTN crisis
  - Metyrosine—catecholamine synthesis inhibitor, sometimes used preop
- **Intraop**
  - GA vs. regional—no influence on pt outcome
  - Avoid desflurane, sympathetic stimulants (ketamine, ephedrine), & hypoventilation (cause nonneurogenic release of catecholamines), atracurium, & morphine (histamine release)
  - Prepare nitroprusside & phenylephrine infusions in advance
  - A-line before induction, ± central line (assessment of intravascular volume), ± PA line
  - **Gentle** induction—intubation may cause massive release of catecholamines
  - Tumor manipulation—may cause massive catecholamine release → HTN crisis
  - Suprarenal vein ligation → acute drop in blood catecholamine level → cause hypotension (*treat with fluid administration and direct sympathomimetics*)
  - Catecholamine-resistant vasoplegia: Can also use vasopressin to reverse
  - Refractory tachycardia: Treat with esmolol (25–300 mcg/kg/min)
- **Postop**
  - Maintain normal BP; in about 50% pts BP will remain elevated
  - Bilateral adrenalectomy → steroid support may be necessary

---

DIABETES MANAGEMENT

- **Preoperative**
  - Check type, duration, and severity of diabetes—the more severe, poorly controlled, and long-standing the dz, the higher is the risk of long-term complications
  - Check current therapy for type and dose (diet, oral hypoglycemic drug, or insulin)
  - Morning blood sugar and HbA1c assay help to assess status of diabetic control. Creatinine level and electrolytes may reflect degree of nephropathy
  - Check for the presence of coronary artery dz, HTN, cerebrovascular dz, and peripheral vascular dz; check EKG for presence of rhythm disturbances and prior MIs
  - Consider Na bicitrate and metoclopramide in pts with GERD and gastroparesis
  - Severe peripheral neuropathy may preclude the use of regional anesthesia
  - Long-acting insulins should be stopped and substituted by protamine and lente insulins
  - Long-acting sulfonylurea drugs such as chlorpropamide should be stopped and substituted by short-acting agents. Metformin stopped if concern for intraop metabolic acidosis. Type-2 diabetic pts with marked hyperglycemia on oral treatment should be switched to insulin before operation

- **Emergency surgery**
  - Stabilize metabolic control/volume status as much as possible (delay surgery if possible)
  - Maximize glucose, electrolyte, acid–base status—insulin & glucose infusions
  - Saline infusion if volume is depleted (depending on renal function & cardiac status)
  - K+ infusion if renal function is normal & serum K+ normal or low
  - Bicarbonate infusion **only** in pts with severe acidosis
- **Intraoperative management**
  - Monitoring blood sugar = mandatory for all insulin-dependent pts & poorly controlled pts
  - Pts on neutral protamine Hagedorn (NPH) or protamine zinc insulin (PZI)
    - ↑ Risk for anaphylactic protamine reactions (2° to prior sensitization)
    - Insulin requirements in diabetics vary during surgery; must individualize
- **Postop**
  - Treat N/V in pts with gastroparesis with metoclopramide as pts have increased risk of infection, MI, hyper/hypoglycemia, CV, and renal dysfunction
- **Diabetic emergencies**
  - *Diabetic ketoacidosis:* Usually triggered by trauma or infection in Type I DM
    - Nausea, vomiting, dehydration, polyuria, polydipsia, somnolence → coma
    - Hyperglycemia, wide anion gap metabolic acidosis, ketones in blood & urine, ↓ K+
  - Management: Place A-line, consider intubation for severe CNS depression
    - Start insulin infusion (10 U IV, then 5–10 U/h)
    - Normal saline at 5–10 mL/kg/h (fluid deficit of 3–8 L not uncommon), *add 5% glucose when blood sugar <250 mg/dL*
    - Replenish K (0.3–0.5 mEq/kg/h)
    - Bicarbonate **not** usually required
  - *Hyperosmolar, hyperglycemic, nonketotic coma* (usually type II DM)
    - Severe dehydration & associated with acute hyperglycemia (>600 mg/dL)
    - Treatment: Correct hypovolemia & hyperglycemia
      - Fluid resuscitation with 0.45% saline
      - Give 10 U regular insulin IV stat → insulin drip (see protocol above)
  - *Hypoglycemia*—result of stress, missed meal, exercise, alcohol consumption
    - Hypoglycemia is much more dangerous in unconscious pt than hyperglycemia *(safer to err on the side of hyperglycemia)*
    - Symptoms: Diaphoresis, tachy, impaired cognition, confusion, loc, & seizures
    - Treatment: 50% IV glucose, initial dose 25 mL

Day Before Surgery Insulin Regimens Based on Oral Intake Status								
	Glargine or Detemir		NPH or 70/30 Insulin		Lispro, Aspart, Glulisine, Regular		Non-insulin Injectables	
Day Before Surgery Insulin Regimens	**AM Dose**	**PM Dose**	**AM Dose**	**PM Dose**	**AM Dose**	**PM Dose**	**AM Dose**	**PM Dose**
Normal diet until midnight (includes those permitted clear liquids until 2 h before surgery)	Usual dose	80% of usual dose	80% of usual dose	80% of usual dose	Usual dose	Usual dose	Usual dose	Usual dose
Bowel prep (and/or clear liquids only 12–24 h before surgery)	Usual dose	80% of usual dose	80% of usual dose	80% of usual dose	Usual dose	Usual dose	Hold when starting clear liquid diet/bowel prep	Hold when starting clear liquid diet/bowel prep

NPH, neutral protamine Hagedorn.
From Duggan, DW, Carlson, K, Umpierrez, GE Perioperative hyperglycemia management: An update. Anesthesiology 2017;126:547–60.

Day of Surgery Insulin Regimens

Day of Surgery Insulin Regimens	Glargine or Detemir	NPH or 70/30 Insulin	Lispro, Aspart, Glulisine, and Regular	Non-insulin Injectables
	80% of usual dose if patient uses morning only or twice daily basal therapy	50% of usual dose if BG 120 mg/dL* Hold for BG <120 mg/dL	Hold	Hold

*6.6 mM.

BG, blood glucose; NPH, neutral protamine Hagedorn.

From Duggan, DW, Carlson, K, Umpierrez, GE Perioperative hyperglycemia management: An update. Anesthesiology 2017;126:547–60.

Variable Rate Continuous Insulin Infusion

BG mg/dL (mM)	If BG Increased from Previous Measurement	BG Decreased from Previous Measurement by Less Than 30 mg/dL	BG Decreased from Previous Measurement by Greater Than 30 mg/dL
>241 (13.4)	Increase by 3 U/h	Increase rate by 3 U/h	No change in rate
211–240 (11.7–13.4)	Increase by 2 U/h	Increase rate by 2 U/h	No change in rate
181–210 (10–11.7)	Increase by 1 U/h	Increase rate by 1 U/h	No change in rate
141–180 (7.8–10)	No change in rate	No change in rate	No change in rate
110–140 (6.1–7.8)	No change in rate	Decrease rate by 1/2 U/h	No change in rate
100–109 (5.5–6.1)	1. Hold insulin infusion 2. Recheck BG hourly 3. Restart infusion at 1/2 the previous infusion rate if BG >180 mg/dL (10 mM)		No change in rate Hold insulin infusion
71–99 (3.9–5.5)	1. Hold insulin infusion 2. Check BG every 30 minutes until BG >100 mg/dL (5.5 mM) 3. Resume BG checks every hour 4. Restart infusion at 1/2 the previous infusion rate if BG >180 mg/dL (10 mM)		
70 (3.9) or lower	If BG = 50–70 (2.8–3.9 mM), 1. Give 25 mL D50 2. Repeat BG checks every 30 min until BG >100 mg/dL (5.5 mM) If BG <50 mg/dL (2.8 mM), 1. Give 50 mL D50 2. Repeat BG every 15 min until >70 mg/dL (3.9 mM) 3. When BG >70 mg/dL, check BG every 30 min until >100 mg/dL (5.5 mM). Repeat 50 mL D50 dose if BG <50 mg/dL a second time and start D10 infusion 4. After BG >100 mg/dL (5.5 mM), resume hourly BG check Restart infusion at 1/2 the previous infusion rate if BG >180 mg/dL (10 mM)		

Perioperative target blood glucose (BG) 140–180 mg/dL (7.8–10 mM).

1. If BG >180 mg/dL (10 mM), start insulin infusion.
2. Consider bolus dose (BG = 100/40).
3. Start rate at BG/100 = U/h.
4. Check BG hourly and correct per table.

D10, 10% dextrose solution; D50, 50% dextrose solution.

From Duggan, DW, Carlson, K, Umpierrez, GE Perioperative hyperglycemia management: An update. Anesthesiology 2017;126:547–60.

ADRENAL INSUFFICIENCY

Anesthesia for Adrenal Insufficiency

- **Preop**—administer stress dose of corticosteroid (usually 50–100 mg hydrocortisone IV), especially if on ≥5 mg daily dose of prednisone
- **Intraop**
  - Risk of poor fluid loading tolerance, hypoglycemia, ↑ K^+, dysrhythmias

- Unexplained hypotension (that is unresponsive to fluids & vasopressors) → Treat with glucocorticoid
- Avoid etomidate (suppresses adrenal function)
- **Postop**
  - Provide adequate corticosteroid supplementation

Excess of Corticosteroids (Cushing Syndrome)
- **Causes**
  - 1°—Adrenal adenoma/hyperplasia
  - 2°—ACTH-secreting pituitary microadenoma (Cushing dz), ACTH-secreting tumors, exogenous steroid usage
- **Clinical features:** Moon facies, buffalo hump, central obesity, hirsutism, skin atrophy, osteoporosis, easy bruising, diabetes, proximal myopathy, aseptic hip necrosis, mental status changes, pancreatitis, polyuria/polydipsia

Anesthesia for Cushing Syndrome
- **Preop:** Risk of hypokalemia & glucose intolerance (check both)
  - Cushingoid pts may have HTN, CHF, fragile skin, osteoporosis
  - Use stress dose steroids in case of iatrogenic Cushing syndrome
- **Intraop**
  - Obese (potentially difficult airway/IV access), often HTN
  - Special attention to positioning (skin breaks down easily)
  - High-dose opioids may cause resp depression & difficulty with extubation
- **Postop course**
  - Poor ventilatory performance (↓ FRC), poor mobilization, pressure sores, ↑ infections

Hyperaldosteronism (Conn Syndrome)
- **Causes**
  - 1°—(Conn syndrome) excess secretion of aldosterone by an adrenal adenoma (60%), bilateral adrenal hyperplasia (30%), carcinoma (rare)
  - 2°—high plasma levels of renin & aldosterone (due to CHF/liver cirrhosis)
- **Clinical features**
  - Malignant HTN (centrally mediated or aldosterone-induced)
  - ↓ K^+ often severe & may be exacerbated by diuretics → weakness & tetany
  - HTN pts often hypovolemic (hypovolemia & ↓ K^+ indicate severe total K^+ deficit)
  - Metabolic alkalosis from H^+ loss

Anesthesia for Conn Syndrome
- **Preop:** Correct ↑ BP, metabolic alkalosis, hypokalemia
  - Spironolactone (up to 400 mg qd) may control HTN & moderate hypovolemia/↓ K^+
- **Intraop:** If CHF, uncontrolled HTN, hypovolemia present → place A-line
  - Surgical manipulation of adrenal may release catecholamines → CV instability
  - Give corticosteroid & mineralocorticoids in cases of bilateral adrenalectomy
- **Postop:** Goal = maintain normal BP, electrolyte balance
  - Continue corticosteroid & mineralocorticoids in cases of bilateral adrenalectomy

POSTERIOR PITUITARY GLAND
- Posterior pituitary releases oxytocin & antidiuretic hormone (ADH, vasopressin)
- ADH stimulates kidneys to conserve water
  - Low ADH → diabetes insipidus
  - High ADH → syndrome of inappropriate antidiuretic hormone (SIADH) secretion

Diabetes Insipidus (DI)
- **Causes:** Central DI—insufficient ADH by pituitary (damage from head injuries, genetic d/o, infections, vascular dz, tumors)
- Nephrogenic DI—lack of kidney response to ADH (from drugs, chronic kidney dz)
- **Clinical features:** Thirst, polyuria (up to 20 L/d), low BP, & dehydration
- **Diagnosis:** Urine specific gravity of ≤1.005, urine osmolality <200 mOsm/kg, random plasma osmolality >287 mOsm/kg
- **Treatment:** SQ/nasal/PO vasopressin analogues (desmopressin), chlorpropamide, carbamazepine, thiazide diuretics
- **Anesthetic management**
  - **Preop**—restore intravascular volume, nasal desmopressin 10 mcg bid–tid
  - **Intraop**
    - Total lack of ADH: 100 mU vasopressin before surgery followed by infusion (100–200 mU/h titrated to urine output)

- Partial ADH deficiency: No vasopressin (unless plasma osmolality >290)
- **Postop**—continue desmopressin & monitor electrolyte balance

Syndrome of Inappropriate Antidiuretic Hormone (SIADH) Secretion
- **Clinical features:** ↓ Na superimposed upon symptoms of underlying pathology
  - ↓ Na due to a dilutional effect, **not** Na depletion (may be no clinical symptoms)
  - Symptoms: May include nausea, weakness, anorexia; Na <110 mmol/L → coma
- **Diagnosis:** Must distinguish SIADH from other causes (such as dilutional hyponatremia) (*causes of dilutional ↓ Na: Excess infusion of dextrose/saline drips/use of diuretics*)
  - Diagnosis confirmed by serum Na <130 mmol/L, plasma osmolality <270 mOsm/L, urinary Na >20 mEq/L, & elevated urine osmolality
- **Treatment:** Address underlying problem
  - Release of ADH (from hypophysis or tumor) cannot be suppressed by medical therapy
  - Symptomatic relief: Water intake restriction to 500–1,000 mL per 24 h (plasma & urine osmolality should be measured regularly)
  - Fluid restriction may not be appropriate in SAH—may promote vasospasm
  - Demeclocycline: When fluid restriction is difficult
- **Anesthetic management**
  - Correct hyponatremia, monitor volume status by CVP or PA catheter
  - Monitor electrolytes (urine osmolarity, plasma osmolarity, serum Na) (*including immediately after surgery*)

OBSTETRIC AND GYNECOLOGIC ANESTHESIA

JEANETTE R. BAUCHAT

INTRODUCTION

Morbidity and Mortality in Obstetrics

- Pregnancy-related deaths in the United States are steadily increasing and are currently the highest of the developed nations at 17.2 deaths/100,000 live births
- 3 in 5 pregnancy-related deaths are preventable and implementation of Maternal Safety Bundles through the National Partnership for Maternal safety can reduce maternal morbidity/mortality
- Anesthesia-related deaths are very rare and declining, but mortality from arrest following neuraxial techniques is on the rise due to increasing use of neuraxial techniques to avoid general anesthesia

Source: https://www.cdc.gov/reproductivehealth/maternalinfanthealth/pregnancy-mortality-surveillance-system.htm; https://www.cdc.gov/vitalsigns/maternal-deaths/index.html; https://safehealthcareforeverywoman.org/safety-action-series/overview-of-the-national-partnership-for-maternal-safety/; *Obstet Gynecol* 2011;117:69–74.

	Physiologic Changes of Pregnancy	Implications for Anesthesia
Metabolism and respiration	• Oxygen consumption ↑ • TV ↑↑ and RR ↑ (progesterone) • FRC, RV, and ERV ↓ • ↓ ERV and RV, but TLC same • Pco_2 ↓ to 28–32 mmHg incompletely compensated respiratory alkalosis • ↓ O_2 content (anemia)	• Rapid desaturation with apnea • Increased time to denitrogenation • Increased minute ventilation requirements • Increased pulmonary shunt when supine
Airway Changes	• Upper airway edema • Worsening Mallampati as labor progresses	• ↑ Risk of failed intubation • ↑ Risk of upper airway trauma • Utilize smaller ETT
Circulation	• CO and blood volume ↑ • Uterine perfusion ↑ to 700–900 mL/min (20% CO) • BP ↓, SVR ↓, HR ↑ • Aortocaval compression (supine, gravid uterus compresses the vena cava and aorta) • Hemodynamics postpartum: CO ↑ 75%, return to prelabor values by 48 h, prepregnancy values by 12–24 wk • ↑ Volume of distribution	• Increased CO can worsen underlying cardiac maternal morbidity • Aortocaval compression can ↓ CO, ↓ uterine perfusion
Hematology and coagulation	• Blood volume ↑ 50%, ↑ in plasma volume > ↑ in RBC mass → relative anemia • Plasma cholinesterase conc. ↓ by 25% • Hypercoagulable state in pregnancy: ↑ Platelet turnover, clotting, and fibrinolysis • ↑ 2,3 DPG → right shift of oxyhemoglobin curve → ↑ O_2 delivery	• Anemic pts are at risk during hemorrhage or if surgical intervention is needed • ↑ Risk of DVT and Pulmonary embolism
GI	• Uterine enlargement, labor, and opioids ↓ gastric emptying • ↓ LES tone, ↑ gastric pressure	↑ Risk of aspiration
CNS	• MAC ↓ by 20–40% • ↓ Vasopressor response • ↓ Requirement for epidural & spinal local anesthetics	• Higher vasopressor requirements • Lower local anesthetic dosing for anesthesia and analgesia

Stages of Labor		
Stage of Labor	**Events**	**Innervation**
1st	Onset of regular painful contractions to 10 cm cervical dilation	T10–L1
2nd	Complete dilation to delivery of infant	S2–S4
3rd	Delivery of infant to delivery of placenta	S2–S4

Labor Analgesia and Anesthesia for Cesarean Delivery

- Nonpharmacologic labor analgesia choices: Hypnotherapy, hydrotherapy, and transcutaneous electrical nerve stimulation (TENS)
- Pharmacologic labor analgesia choices: Nitrous oxide, parenteral opioid analgesia (fentanyl, remifentanil), pudendal block, paracervical block, neuraxial analgesia
- Neuraxial analgesia is the most effective form of labor analgesia

Contraindications to Neuraxial Techniques	
Absolute	Pt refusal Severe coagulopathy Sepsis or infection at puncture site Severe hypovolemia Increased intracranial pressure
Relative	Coagulopathy Valvular cardiac lesions (severe AS or MS) Thrombocytopenia Neurologic dz Previous back surgery

Source: *Cochrane Database Syst Rev* 2011;(12):CD000331.

Complications of Neuraxial Techniques	
Minor	Nausea/vomiting Hypotension Itching Shivering
Moderate	Failed/partial blockade Unintentional dural puncture
Major	Needle trauma to nerve Infection (abscess, meningitis) Hematoma Spinal cord ischemia/Cauda equina syndrome Peripheral nerve injury High neuraxial blockade Cardiovascular collapse/death

Adapted from: https://www.nysora.com/techniques/neuraxial-and-perineuraxial-techniques/spinal-anesthesia/

Labor Analgesia

- Labor analgesia should be initiated at maternal request with no consideration to cervical dilation
- Routine platelet count is not necessary in healthy women with regular prenatal care and without prior concerns of coagulation abnormalities *(Anesthesiology 2016;124(2):270–300.)*

Choice of Neuraxial Techniques for Initiation of Labor Analgesia		
Technique	**Advantages**	**Disadvantages**
Combined spinal epidural (CSE)	• Rapid onset compared with epidural, typically used in multiparous women in active labor • Improved overall maternal satisfaction compared with epidural analgesia • Lower probability of failed epidural catheters	• Cannot diagnose a nonfunctional catheter until spinal recedes • Increased pruritus compared with epidural analgesia • High rates of fetal heart rate decelerations

Dural puncture epidural (DPE)	• DPE provided faster onset than epidural • Greater sacral analgesia than epidural • Less asymmetric blocks compared with a standard epidural • Less hypotension and pruritus compared to CSE	• Dural puncture with no medication administered
Epidural	• Ability to slowly titrate level • Ability to diagnose a functional catheter after placement (important for parturients with bad airways, morbid obesity)	• Slower onset than CSE or DPE • High concentrations of local anesthetic may lead to motor blockade
Continuous spinal catheter	• Ability to titrate level • Rapid onset	• These techniques should be reserved in cases of accidental dural puncture • Increased risk of medication error and postdural puncture headache compared to CSE/DPE/epidural

Source: Adapted from F1000Res. 2017;6:1211; Anesthesiology 2001;95:913–920.

Common Medications and Dosing for Neuraxial Labor Analgesia	
Scenario	**Common Regimens**
Common test dose regimens	• Lidocaine 1.5% + epi 1:200,000 (2–3 mL) • Fentanyl 100 mcg • Air (1 mL) while monitoring precordial Doppler • 3% 2-chloroprocaine (2–3 mL)
Initiation of labor analgesia with CSE technique	• 25 mcg fentanyl or 10 mcg sufentanil • 2.5 mg bupivacaine with 15 mcg fentanyl
Initiation of labor analgesia with DPE/epidural technique	Common initial epidural dosing regimens include local anesthetic ± fentanyl 50–100 mcg or sufentanil 1–2 mcg: • Bupivacaine 0.125% (10 mL) • Ropivacaine 0.1–0.2% (10 mL) • Lidocaine 1% (6–10 mL)
Maintenance of labor analgesia with epidural catheter	• Delivery via continuous or programmed intermittent bolus (5–12 mL q1h) +/– pt-controlled epidural bolus (5 mL q10min) • Bupivacaine 0.04–0.125% with fentanyl 1–2 mcg/mL at 8–15 mL/h+/– epinephrine • Bupivacaine 0.125% plain at 8–15 mL/h
Rescue/top-off bolus	• Bupivacaine 0.125–0.25% → 5–10 mL • Consider adding adjuvants for density: Fentanyl 50–100 mcg; Clonidine 50–100 mcg
Maintenance of labor analgesia with intrathecal catheter	• Bupivacaine 0.0625% at 2–3 mL/h, may titrate if breakthrough pain

Labor Neuraxial Analgesia Management	
Typical Sequence of Events	**Remarks**
1. Request for analgesia from pt	No evidence to support delay of epidural placement until an arbitrary cervical dilation
2. Perform preanalgesia evaluation, including physical examination, obtain consent	Per ASA practice guidelines for OB anesthesia: A focused H&P may be associated with ↓ maternal, fetal, & neonatal complications
3. Place BP cuff and pulse oximeter, monitor BP every 2–3 min	Consider administration of a co-load of fluid
4. Perform Neuraxial Technique	Use aseptic technique Perform a timeout prior to all procedures See Table—Choice of Neuraxial Techniques for Initiation of Labor Analgesia and Common Medications and Dosing for Neuraxial Analgesia

5. Start Maintenance infusion for labor analgesia	Maintenance regimens include continuous infusion of programmed intermittent epidural bolus dosing of medications ± PCEA. See Table—Common Medications and Dosing for Neuraxial Analgesia & Anesthesia
6. Monitor BP for 15–20 min after initiation of labor analgesia	Both phenylephrine and ephedrine are acceptable vasopressors for use in L&D
7. Monitor maternal vital signs, motor blockade & level of analgesia every 2–4 h	If inadequate analgesia, check epidural function and administer rescue/top-off bolus. See Table—Common Medications and Dosing for Neuraxial Analgesia & Anesthesia

Source: Adapted from N Eng J Med 2005;352:655–665; Anesthesiology 2016;124(2):270–300.

Anesthetic Considerations in Labor

Anesthesia for Multiple Gestation Deliveries	
↑ Maternal complications	• ↑ Risk of preterm labor, PROM • ↑ Risk of preeclampsia • ↑ Perineal trauma • ↑ Risk of uterine atony, antepartum, & postpartum hemorrhage (PPH)
↑ Fetal complications	• ↑ Risk of preterm birth • Risk to twin B of cord prolapse, unstable lie, breech delivery

Anesthetic management for vaginal delivery	• Epidural analgesia should be used for labor due to the risk of STAT CD or breech extraction for twin B
	• If cord prolapse occurs, anesthesia must be immediately initiated (either neuraxial or GA)
	• Breech extraction of twin B requires:
	  • Sacral anesthesia extending to T10 sensory dermatome to facilitate delivery
	  • Uterine/cervical relaxation to avoid head entrapment of breech twin B; IV nitro or GA with high-dose volatile agents can be used to facilitate uterine relaxation

Anesthetic management for cesarean delivery	• Regional techniques are preferable. See Table—Management of Neuraxial Anesthesia for Cesarean Delivery

Implications for Trial of Labor After Cesarean Delivery (TOLAC)
• 1% risk of uterine rupture—signs include fetal distress, abdominal pain, uterine tenderness, cessation of uterine contractions, palpable fetal parts in abdomen • Continuous FHR monitoring, consider intrauterine pressure monitoring • Consider: Additional IV access and blood sample in the blood bank • Epidural analgesia is *not* contraindicated; breakthrough abdominal or shoulder pain not associated with uterine contractions may be indicative of uterine rupture

Anesthesia for Cervical Cerclage Placement or Postpartum Tubal Ligations	
Cerclage placement	T10 to sacral sensory level needs to be achieved. Common intrathecal regimens include • Bupivacaine 0.5–0.75% 10–15 mg ± fentanyl 15–20 mcg • Lidocaine 5% 50–75 mg + fentanyl 15–20 mcg
Postpartum tubal ligation	Immediate PPTL Advantages: • Ease of access to fallopian tubes (uterus & ovaries are out of pelvis) • Lower risk of bowel laceration, vascular injury • Lower cost (compared to outpatient procedure) Anesthetic Implications: • NPO guidelines should be followed • Pt must be stable with no signs of PPH • Regional preferred (spinal or epidural if in situ) Local anesthetic requirement; returns to prepregnancy value after 12–36 h postpartum Risk of epidural catheter failure ↑ if delivery to surgery interval >8–10 h

Fetal Heart Rate Decelerations

Type of Deceleration	Timing Relative to Contraction	Etiology
Early	Simultaneous with contractions	Vagal reflex to head compression
Late	Onset: 10–30 s after contraction begins. End: 10–30 s after contraction ends with slow recovery to baseline	Uteroplacental insufficiency, hypoxemia, fetal circulatory decompensation
Variable	Variable in depth, shape, duration	Head or cord compression
Response to prolonged FHR deceleration	<ul><li>Activate emergency team response</li><li>Turn off oxytocin/administer fluid bolus</li><li>Change maternal position</li><li>Check BP/administer vasopressor (ephedrine) if indicated</li><li>For uterine tachysystole, administer nitroglycerin (250 mcg IV, 800 mcg sublingual) or terbutaline IM</li></ul>	

Anesthesia for Cesarean Delivery
- Consider implementation of Enhanced Recovery After Cesarean Delivery protocols to improve perioperative outcomes
- Clear communication with the obstetrician to determine the timing of cesarean delivery is critical to favorable maternal and fetal outcomes.
- Pt Safety Checklist should be performed prior to all anesthetic techniques and obstetric surgical procedures.
- Regional anesthesia is the preferred method for nonemergent cesarean delivery

Anesthesia for Cesarean Delivery		
Situation	Choices for Anesthesia	Advantages
Scheduled cesarean delivery	<ul><li>Spinal</li><li>CSE/Epidural (for prolonged surgery)</li><li>GA only if contraindications to neuraxial technique</li></ul>	<ul><li>Parents experience the birth of their child</li><li>Ease of administration of neuraxial opioids for postoperative analgesia</li><li>Avoidance of placental transfer of anesthetic agents to neonate</li><li>Avoidance of potentially difficult airway or aspiration</li></ul>
Urgent cesarean delivery	<ul><li>Spinal</li><li>CSE/Epidural (for prolonged surgery)</li><li>GA for nonfunctional indwelling labor epidural catheters and urgency not allowing time for replacement</li></ul>	<ul><li>If pt has an epidural or spinal catheter for labor *analgesia*, it may be dosed for surgery</li><li>A spinal may be performed as time allows or if there is a contraindication to regional anesthesia, in which case a general anesthetic should be performed</li></ul>
Emergency cesarean delivery	<ul><li>Spinal/CSE may be considered, but a true emergency may not allow time to perform and achieve a T4 surgical block</li><li>Labor epidural may be dosed with a fast-acting local anesthetic and sensory level evaluated upon arrival to OR</li><li>GA is the fastest anesthetic and may be required</li><li>Local anesthetic block by surgeon (in case of inability to perform #1–3)</li></ul>	<ul><li>The decision regarding mode of anesthesia requires communication with the obstetrician regarding maternal & fetal status</li><li>The advantages/disadvantages need to be weighed in the emergency situation of neuraxial anesthesia vs. general anesthesia</li></ul>

Common Medications and Dosing for Neuraxial Anesthesia for Cesarean Delivery	
Scenario	**Common Regimens**
Spinal for cesarean delivery	Local anesthetic: Hyperbaric bupivacaine 10–15 mg or lidocaine 70 mg with fentanyl 15 mcg Prolongation with ± epinephrine 100–200 mcg Consider clonidine 20–50 mcg for women with opioid use d/o
Epidural for cesarean delivery	3% 2-chloroprocaine or 2% lidocaine with bicarbonate & 1:200,000 epinephrine (15–20 mL total)
Neuraxial opioids for postoperative analgesia (most effective analgesia)	Spinal: Preservative-free morphine 100–150 mcg or hydromorphone 50–75 mcg Epidural: Preservative-free morphine 2–3 mg or hydromorphone 0.6 mg
Multimodal analgesia	Scheduled Acetaminophen 1 g PO or IV q6–8h Scheduled NSAIDs: Ketorolac 30 mg IV ×24 h, then scheduled PO NSAIDs If preservative-free morphine fails or is contraindicated: Transversus abdominis plane (TAP) blockade: Ropivacaine 0.5% 3 mg/kg up to 40 mL (20 mL per side)

Source: Best Pract Res Clin Anaesthesiol 2017;31(1):69–79.

Management of Neuraxial Anesthesia for Cesarean Delivery	
Typical Sequence of Events	**Remarks**
1. Perform preanesthetic evaluation, including physical examination, obtain consent; assess need for lab work & blood availability	Per ASA guidelines for OB anesthesia, a focused H&P may be associated with ↓ maternal, fetal, & neonatal complications Consider performing a prebrief with the obstetrician, nursing, OR teams prior to proceeding to the OR
2. Administer antacid prophylaxis	Pts should receive an H2 receptor antagonist, proton pump inhibitor, metoclopramide, and/or a nonparticulate antacid
3. Perform neuraxial technique or	Apply ASA standard monitors Use aseptic technique Perform a timeout prior to all procedures Pt positioning is critical to success See Table—Common Medications and Dosing for Neuraxial Anesthesia for Cesarean Delivery
3a. If the pt has an indwelling epidural catheter, dose the epidural catheter	See Table—Common Medications and Dosing for Neuraxial Anesthesia for Cesarean Delivery
4. Administer fluid co-load and vasopressors	10–15 mL/kg crystalloid should be administered at the time of neuraxial block placement Consider vasopressor infusion with phenylephrine or norepinephrine with rescue boluses of phenylephrine 100–200 mcg or ephedrine 5–10 mg
5. Administer antibiotics	Investigate your individual institutional guidelines
6. Place pt in **left uterine displacement** position (LUD)	Use a wedge or a towel or tilt the OR table
7. Ascertain sensory level & document	T4–6 sensory level should be obtained prior to surgical incision
8. After the umbilical cord is clamped, administer oxytocin	ED_{90} for oxytocin infusions is 0.29 IU/min

Source: Adapted from Anesthesiology 2010;112:530–534; Anesth Analg 2010;110:154–158; Anesthesiology 2016;124(2):270–300.

Management of Anesthesia for Emergency Cesarean Delivery	
Typical Sequence of Events	**Remarks**
1. Discuss urgency of procedure with obstetricians	Based on urgency, decide if there is time for a regional anesthesia. If so, see Table—Management of Neuraxial Anesthesia for Cesarean Delivery
2. Maximize placental perfusion & oxygenation en route to OR	**Ensure LUD** on transport & in OR Administer 100% O_2 on arrival in OR

3. Perform focused Hx and physical examination, including an airway examination	Administer a nonparticulate antacid ASAP
4. If time allows for a regional anesthetic	See Table—Management of Neuraxial Anesthesia for Cesarean Delivery
4a. If a general anesthesia is performed: Rapid sequence induction after confirmation of surgical team readiness	Propofol, etomidate, and ketamine, all suitable for induction. Succinylcholine or high dose of NMBD if there is a contraindication to succinylcholine
5. Maintain anesthesia with 1 MAC halogenated agent prior to delivery; 0.5 MAC halogenated agent after delivery	Administer antibiotics when they become available After delivery, supplement with ≥50% nitrous oxide or propofol infusion Opioids & benzodiazepines may be administered after delivery of the infant
6. Extubate and follow routine postoperative cesarean delivery orders	Multimodal analgesia and TAP block may be indicated for emergency CD

APGAR SCORE

Assessment of the Newborn: Apgar Score			
Score	0	1	2
Color	Pale or white	Pink body, peripheral acrocyanosis	Pink
HR	Absent	<100	>100
Response to stimulation	None	Grimace	Cough, sneeze
Muscle tone	Flaccid	Some movement	Moving
Respiration	None	Weak, irregular	Crying, regular
APGAR SCORE: Needs resuscitation: 0–3; Moderate impairment: 4–6; Normal: 7–10			

POSTDURAL PUNCTURE HEADACHE (PDPH)

Differential dx: Nonspecific tension headache, caffeine withdrawal, migraines, lactation headaches, cortical vein thrombosis, meningitis, subdural hematoma, subarachnoid hemorrhage

H&P and +/− neuroimaging necessary for correct diagnosis

Postdural Puncture Headache		
Symptoms	Onset & Duration	Treatment
Positional headache: frontal, occipital, or generalized Associated symptoms include diplopia, tinnitus, photophobia, nausea, vomiting, neck pain	Onset of headache typically 24–48 h after dural puncture; duration usually 7–14 d	Conservative management includes: • Maintain euvolemia • Caffeine intake • Oral analgesics such as acetaminophen, NSAIDs, opioid Gold standard: Epidural blood patch: Ideally 20 mL blood sterilely injected into epidural space; relief often immediate, can take 24 h

ANTEPARTUM HEMORRHAGE

- Maternal hemorrhage is an obstetric emergency
- Many causes of antepartum/postpartum hemorrhage can lead to profound disseminated intravascular coagulopathy. Fibrinogen ≤250 mg/dL is an indication of DIC in pregnancy and should be repleted with cryoprecipitate or fibrinogen concentrate.
- Choice of anesthetic technique (GA vs. neuraxial technique) will be dictated not only by urgency of CS but coagulation status and potential for massive transfusion

Antepartum Hemorrhage	
Placenta previa (placenta located over internal os)	• Risk factors: Multiparity, age, previous CS, previous previa • Presents as painless vaginal bleeding in 2nd or 3rd trimester • Diagnosis: US or MRI

Abnormal placentation (abnormally adherent placenta)	• Risk factors: Previous CS, placenta previa
	• 3 subtypes of placenta accrete (abnormally adherent placenta)
	  • Placenta accreta: Adherence to myometrium, not invading uterine muscle
	  • Placenta increta: Placenta invades uterine muscle
	  • Placenta percreta: Placenta invades uterine serosa or other pelvic structures
	• Diagnosis: Antepartum dx can be made with US/MRI or intrapartum dx with difficulty in separating placenta or during surgery for CS

Vasa previa (fetal vessels transverse membranes ahead of fetal presenting part)	• Risk factors: Placenta previa, multiple gestation, abnormal placenta, IVF pregnancy • Diagnosis: US or MRI • Obstetric management: Immediate cesarean delivery if active bleeding (fetal bleeding)
Placental abruption	• Risk factors: Hypertension/preeclampsia, abdominal trauma, cocaine use • Diagnosis: Vaginal bleeding, painful, frequent contractions, fetal distress ± US
Uterine rupture	• Risk factors: Previous uterine surgery, uterine trauma • Presentation: Vaginal bleeding, hypotension, fetal distress, ± pain, fetal loss of station • Treatment: Emergent CS

Postpartum Hemorrhage (PPH)

• Labor and Delivery units should have a system for Management PPH including:
  • Risk stratification of all pts on admission, during labor and postpartum
  • Protocol for management of PPH
  • Multidisciplinary Emergency Response Team that can respond to PPH

Source: https://safehealthcareforeverywoman.org/patient-safety-bundles/obstetric-hemorrhage/

Postpartum Hemorrhage	
Cause	**Comments**
Uterine atony (most common cause of PPH)	• Consider uterine massage • Consider uterotonic agents (see Table—Common Obstetric Drugs)
Retained placenta	• Treatment is manual removal of placenta • Surgical sensory level to T10 or GA for those without epidural
Genital trauma (vaginal, vulvar, & cervical lacerations)	• Surgical sensory level sacral-T10 epidural anesthesia or GA for those without epidural
Uterine inversion	• Surgical sensory level to T10 and uterine relaxation may be necessary for replacement of inverted uterus (consider IV nitroglycerin or volatile anesthetics)

DRUGS USED ON THE LABOR AND DELIVERY UNIT

Common Obstetric Drugs			
Drug	**Indication**	**Mechanism**	**Side Effects**
Oxytocin	Stimulate uterine contractions	Activates myometrial oxytocin receptors, ↑ sodium permeability	Hypotension, tachycardia, flushing, antidiuretic effect
Prostaglandins (15-methyl PGF$_{2\alpha}$)	Cervical ripening, uterine atony	Activates uterine smooth muscle contractions	Bronchoconstriction, vasoconstriction, HTN, nausea, vomiting, diarrhea

Ergot alkaloids (methylergonovine)	Uterine atony	Direct activation of uterine smooth muscle	Arterial and venous vasoconstriction, HTN, coronary vasoconstriction, bradycardia
Misoprostol (prostaglandin E1 analog)	Cervical ripening, Stimulate uterine contractions	Binds to myometrial cells causing increased frequency and intensity of contractions	Nausea, diarrhea, fever
Terbutaline	Inhibit uterine contractions (tocolysis)	β2 receptor agonist	HTN, arrhythmia, myocardial ischemia, pulmonary edema

HYPERTENSIVE DISORDERS OF PREGNANCY

Differential Diagnosis for Hypertension in Pregnancy			
Diagnosis	Time of Diagnosis	Resolution After Pregnancy	Comments
Gestational hypertension (gHTN)	>20-wk gestation	Yes	• 25% of women with gHTN may develop preeclampsia
Chronic hypertension	<20-wk gestation	No	• Pts with chronic hypertension may develop superimposed preeclampsia
Preeclampsia	>20-wk gestation	Yes	• Seizures indicate progression to eclampsia • HELLP syndrome (see Table—Severity of Preeclampsia)

Source: Obstet Gynecol 2013;122(5):1122–1131

https://safehealthcareforeverywoman.org/patient-safety-bundles/severe-hypertension-in-pregnancy/

Preeclampsia
- Pathophysiology: Exact mechanism unknown, may involve imbalance between proangiogenic (VEGF, PlGF) and antiangiogenic factors (sFLT-1, sEng) leading to widespread endothelial dysfunction
- Treatment: IV Magnesium to prevent seizures. Only definitive cure for preeclampsia is delivery of the infant
- Low-dose aspirin may be started in women with a Hx of preeclampsia to prevent onset and reduce severity of preeclampsia as well as prevent intrauterine growth restriction
  (Cardiol Clin 2019;37:345–354)

Severity of Preeclampsia		
	Blood Pressure Criteria	Comments
Preeclampsia without severe features	SBP >140 or 30 mmHg above normal DBP >90 or 15 mmHg above normal AND proteinuria ≥300 mg/24 h or protein/creatinine ratio urine dip 0.3	Mild preeclampsia may progress to severe preeclampsia; Pre-eclampsia can be diagnosed in the absence of proteinuria if symptoms of end-organ dysfunction are present
Preeclampsia with severe features	SBP >160 or DBP >110	End-organ symptoms may include HA, visual changes, RUQ pain, pulmonary edema, lab abnormalities (>LFTs, thrombocytopenia) or oliguria
	HELLP (hemolysis, elevated LFTs, low platelets)	Severe form of preeclampsia; Delivery is the only treatment for HELLP. Resolution of hemolysis/thrombocytopenia may require 24–72 h

Source: Obstet Gynecol 2013;122(5):1122–1131; Cardiol Clin 2019;37:345–354.

Anesthetic Considerations in Preeclampsia		
Issue	Complication	Treatment
Hypertension	Stroke risk: Hemodynamic goals include reduction of SBP <160 and DBP <110 within 1 h while still maintaining adequate placental perfusion	**Follow Institutional Algorithms.** Labetalol, hydralazine, nicardipine PO. If hypertensive emergency not resolved by bolus IV or PO meds, consider ICU admission and nicardipine, sodium nitroprusside, or nitroglycerin gtt
Coagulation status	Thrombocytopenia due to platelet aggregation & consumption may occur and disseminated intravascular coagulopathy	Check platelet count, check coagulation status if elevated LFTs or if platelet count ≤100
Pulmonary edema	Respiratory distress	Consider monitoring via continuous pulse oximetry. Consider treatment with furosemide. Intubation if/when indicated
Renal Impairment	Magnesium toxicity, renal failure	Consider reducing Mg infusion. Avoid renal toxic drugs

Antihypertensive Drugs Used in the Peripartum Period			
Drug	Administration and Dose	Onset and Duration	Properties
Labetalol (β- and α-blocker) (β2-agonist	20–80 mg IV	Onset: 1–2 min Duration 2–3 h	• Easy to administer • Rapid onset • Low risk of side effects • Improves placental blood flow • Unreliable response among pts • Use with caution with underlying pulmonary or cardiac dz
Hydralazine (arterial vasodilator)	5–10 mg IV	Onset: 20–30 min Duration: 2 h	• Easy to administer • Maintains CO • Slow, unreliable onset • Rebound tachycardia • Neonatal thrombocytopenia
Nicardipine (Ca channel blocker)	20–40 mg PO (immediate release IR) Infusion: 5–15 mg/h gtt (↑ by 2.5 mg/h q15min)	Onset PO IR: 30–120 min Duration: 8 h Onset IV: 5 min Duration: Possibly 2 h	• Immediate release PO nicardipine should only be used in pts with no IV access or unresponsive/contraindication to labetalol or hydralazine • Nicardipine gtt should be used if pt is unresponsive/contraindication to labetalol or hydralazine and is being delivered
Nitroglycerin NTG (venodilator) or nitroprusside NTP (arterial dilator)	Continuous NTG IV infusion: 5–50 mcg/min Continuous NTP IV infusion; 0.15–10 mcg/kg/min	Immediate onset and continuous infusion required	• If a laboring woman requires these infusions to control her BP she should be delivered expeditiously, have an arterial line in place, and transferred to an ICU

Nonobstetric Surgery in Pregnancy

- Goals for Nonobstetric Surgery in Pregnancy:
  - Maintain placental perfusion: Avoid maternal hypotension, hypocarbia, hypoxemia, aortocaval compression
  - Monitor FHR: Pre- and postop fetal monitoring, but discuss with obstetrician possibility of intraoperative FHR monitoring for viable fetus
  - Consider neuraxial or regional anesthesia as 1st-line anesthetic, when feasible
  - When GA is used, use antacids and rapid sequence induction

Commonly Used Drugs for Nonobstetric Surgery in Pregnancy			
Drug	Drug	Placental Transfer	Properties
Premedications	Benzodiazepine	Yes	• No evidence of one-time exposure of midazolam having adverse fetal effects • Historical data showed association of benzodiazepine with congenital anomalies; discuss risk/benefit with pt
	Antacids	Yes	• H2 blockers and proton pump inhibitors and nonparticulate antacids are safe in pregnancy
Anesthetic agents	IV induction agents	Yes	• No teratogenicity reported, but concern for fetal neurocognitive dysfunction with multiple exposure to anesthetic agents
	Volatile agents	Yes	• Theoretical concern for teratogenicity with nitrous oxide, avoid in pregnancy • Concern for fetal neurocognitive dysfunction with multiple exposure to anesthetic agents
Paralytics	Nondepolarizing agents	No	• Safe to use in pregnancy. Reversal with sugammadex likely safe but minimal data on teratogenicity
	Depolarizing agents (Succinylcholine)	Minimal	• Reduced plasma concentrations of plasma cholinesterase in pregnancy may prolong duration
Analgesics	Local anesthetics	Lidocaine: Yes Bupivacaine, Ropivacaine, mepivacaine, chloroprocaine: No	• Bupivacaine, ropivacaine, and mepivacaine have high plasma protein binding minimizing transfer • Chloroprocaine is rapidly metabolized in maternal plasma minimizing placental transfer
	Opioid	Yes	• Association with birth defects and neonatal opioid withdrawal symptoms with prolonged use, timing of administration, and amount used
	Acetaminophen	Yes	• Although generally considered safe, data is emerging on an association between acetaminophen and children developing asthma
	NSAIDs	Yes	• Avoid in 1st trimester (increased risk miscarriage) and 3rd trimester (premature closure of ductus arteriosus)

Source: www.pdr.net

ANESTHESIA FOR GYNECOLOGIC SURGERY

- Consider using Enhanced Recovery After Gynecological Surgery protocols to improve maternal outcome
- Gynecologic pts are at high risk of postoperative nausea and vomiting. Use PONV risk stratification and appropriate antiemetic prophylaxis regimen

Anesthetic Considerations for Gynecologic Surgery				
Procedure	**Indication**	**Positioning**	**Choice of Anesthesia**	**Anesthetic Considerations**
Hysteroscopy	• Abnormal uterine bleeding • Infertility	Lithotomy	MAC, GA (LMA or ETT), or neuraxial anesthesia	• Short procedure • Potential for fluid overload (uterus is distended with fluid)
Dilation and curettage (D&C)	• Uterine bleeding • Incomplete or missed abortion	Lithotomy	Paracervical block, MAC, spinal, or GA (LMA or ETT)	• Rare risk of uterine perforation or hemorrhage
Dilation and evacuation (D&E)	• 2nd-trimester abortion (for fetal or maternal indications)	Lithotomy	Paracervical block, MAC, spinal, GA (LMA or ETT)	• Rare risk of uterine perforation or hemorrhage
Conization of the cervix (LEEP procedure)	• Diagnosis & treatment of cervical dysplasia	Lithotomy	MAC, GA (LMA or ETT), spinal	• Often short procedures; do not require anesthesia
Hysterectomy: Vaginal, Laparoscopic, Robotic-assisted, or Total abdominal hysterectomy (TAH) ± BSO	• Uterine or cervical cancer • Fibroid dz • Endometriosis	Supine, lithotomy, or both	GA (ETT) ± regional or neuraxial block for postop analgesia	• If Hx of chemo, consider cardiac & pulm implications • Potential for blood loss—consider IV access, invasive monitoring, and T&S or cross-match
Laparoscopic surgery	May be used for many surgeries (e.g., ectopic pregnancy, hysterectomy, postpartum tubal ligation)	Supine, lithotomy or both with Trendelenburg	GA (ETT)	• Laparoscopic GYN surgery may be an independent risk factor for PONV • ↑ Min ventilation required if insufflation with CO_2
Vulvectomy or other oncologic surgeries	Vulvar cancer or other malignancy	Supine or lithotomy	GA (ETT) ± regional or neuraxial block for postop analgesia	• If Hx of chemo, consider cardiac & pulm implications • Potential for blood loss—consider IV access, invasive monitoring, and T&S or cross-match

PEDIATRIC ANESTHESIA

THOMAS M. ROMANELLI • JONATHAN A. NICONCHUK

ANATOMY

Upper Airway
- Infants & small children
  - Larger tongue & shorter mandible relative to oral cavity
  - Larger & narrower epiglottis, angled away from (not parallel to) tracheal axis (*straight blades may improve epiglottic elevation*)
- Infant glottis = cephalad & anterior, creating more acute angle for laryngoscopy
  - Vocal cords have lower anterior attachment
  - ETT can become caught upon anterior commissure of vocal folds
- Nonexpandable cricoid cartilage = narrowest part of infant airway
  - ETT may pass easily through vocal cords but traumatize area beneath (since this area is smaller than the glottic aperture)
  - Uncuffed ETT used traditionally; no longer recommended
  - Recommend 20–25 cm H_2O air leak to ensure appropriate fit & limit swelling
- Cuffed ETT appropriate for all ages and all procedures
  - Allows for positive-pressure ventilation with minimal leak (PPV)
  - Presence of a cuff ↑ external diameter by up to 0.5 mm (can use microcuffed ETT)
  - Stridor more likely when no air leak exists at 30 cm H_2O
- Neonatal trachea only 4 cm long; care must be taken to avoid mainstem intubation
- Tracheal diameter = 4–5 mm
- Airway resistance & laminar flow worsened by any amount of edema
- Infants described as **obligate nasal breathers** (2° to immature coordination between resp drive & oropharyngeal sensorimotor input)
  - Since larynx is positioned higher (more posterior), tongue rests against hard & soft palates during quiet breathing
  - Infants develop better control by 4–5 mo of age

Vascular Access
- Vascular access often preceded by inhalation induction
  - Limits procedural anxiety & withdrawal reflexes & provides vasodilatation
  - Pts at high risk for aspiration (full stomach) should have IV inserted awake (*parents may be helpful to facilitate this task*)
- Access sites include dorsum of hand, antecubital space, prominent scalp veins in infants, saphenous veins adjacent to medial malleoli; intraosseous → consider in the presence of severe dehydration/trauma (e.g., burns)
- Umbilical vein/artery catheterization allows for rapid vascular access in newborn (*placement should be confirmed by x-ray*)
- All IV lines should be carefully examined to make sure there are no air bubbles (*air may cross PFO & result in embolization*)

PHYSIOLOGY

Transition from Fetal to Neonatal Circulation
- Fetus receives oxygenated blood via umbilical vein
- Series of intracardiac (foramen ovale) & extracardiac (ductus arteriosus & ductus venosus) shunts create parallel fetal circulatory system (Fig. 29-1)
  - Allows blood to bypass high resistance of pulmonary vessels
  - Deoxygenated blood is returned to placenta via umbilical arteries
- Transition to neonatal circulation → occurs when umbilical cord is clamped (increased SVR) & spontaneous breathing begins
  - Pulm vascular resistance drops, changing blood flow from parallel to series
    - Left-sided intracardiac pressures ↑ to close foramen ovale
    - Highly oxygenated blood & ↓ levels of placental prostaglandins stimulate contraction & closure of ductus arteriosus
- Shunts not anatomically closed immediately after birth
  - Some conditions (hypoxia, acidosis, sepsis) lead to persistent fetal circulation

Respiratory
- Major conducting airways established by 16th wk of gestation
  - Acinus & all distal structures continue development until term
  - Alveoli mature after birth, continue to ↑ in number until 8 yo

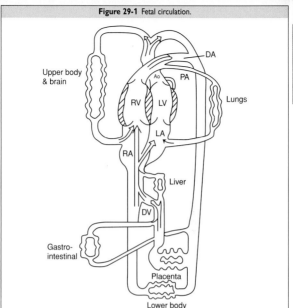

Figure 29-1 Fetal circulation.

Ao, aorta; DA, ductus arteriosus; DV, ductus venosus; LA, left atrium; LV, left ventricle; PA, pulmonary artery; RA, right atrium; RV, right ventricle. (Reproduced with permission from Rudolph AM. Changes in the circulation after birth. In: Rudolph AM, ed. *Congenital Diseases of the Heart*. Chicago, IL: Year Book Medical; 1974.)

- Infant chest wall deforms easily because of cartilaginous structure
  - Accessory muscles provide limited support (poor anatomic rib configuration)
  - Infantile diaphragm contains 20–25% of fatigue-resistant type I muscle fibers → paradoxical chest wall movement when there is ↑ inspiratory effort
  - ↑ Work of breathing → deterioration into resp failure, esp in premature infant
- FRC similar in infants & adults per kg
  - Owing to limited elastic recoil, infant closing capacity may near/exceed FRC: Leads to air trapping when small airways close at end-expiration; cause of age-related changes in PaO_2
- ↑ Tracheal compliance in infants can lead to dynamic tracheal collapse
- Changes in PaO_2, $PaCO_2$, & pH control ventilation by acting on chemoreceptors
  - Degree of response directly related to gestational & postnatal age
  - Hypoxia stimulates newborn resp effort; high conc of O_2 may depress it
  - Nonspecific factors (blood glucose, Hct, temp) also affect infant breathing

Cardiovascular
- Infant/neonatal myocardium contains less contractile tissue than adult heart
  - Neonatal ventricle less compliant during diastole & generates less tension
  - Infant ventricle cannot adequately ↑ stroke volume when metabolic needs ↑
  - Cardiac output proportional to changes in heart rate
    - Bradycardia → ↓ cardiac output; factors contributing to bradycardia (hypoxia, hypercarbia, surgical manipulation) should be corrected
- Consider empiric anticholinergic (atropine) to offset laryngoscopy-induced bradycardia

Renal
- Kidneys very active in utero & produce copious amounts of urine (*contribute to maintenance of amniotic fluid volume*)

- At birth GFR = 15–20% of adult levels; reaches 50% within 2 wk & 100% by 1 y (*low GFR = infants cannot excrete excessive fluid loads/renal cleared drugs*)
- Ability to excrete organic acids poorly developed in neonates (*causes observed "physiologic acidemia" of newborn*)
- Newborns can concentrate urine only to 600–800 mOsm/kg

Hepatic
- Gluconeogenesis & protein synthesis begin at 12 wk gestation (*liver structure near similar to adults; functional development lags*)
- Preterm & small for gestational age infants usually have diminished glycogen stores
  → Prone to hypoglycemic episodes after delivery
  → Treat hypoglycemia promptly (D10 at 4 mL/kg/h)
- Albumin levels in preterm infants are often low and affect drug binding & availability
- **Physiologic jaundice:** Due to RBC breakdown & ↑ enterohepatic circ of bilirubin
  → As opposed to pathologic jaundice (e.g., encephalopathy from kernicterus)

Gastrointestinal
- Low esophageal tone in many newborns; reaches adult level ≈6 wk
  → Projectile vomiting after feeding = classic sign of pyloric stenosis
- Meconium (water, pancreatic secretions + intestinal epithelial cells) usually passed a few hours following delivery
  - Premature infants often have delayed evacuation
    - May also indicate GI dz (meconium ileus/intestinal atresia)

Hematopoietic
- Neonatal estimated blood volume = 85–90 mL/kg at term, gradually ↓ with age
- HbF: Most prevalent after birth, greater O_2 affinity than HbA (adult)
  - "Physiologic anemia of infancy" due to HbF (replaced with HbA by 3 mo)
  - Hg levels rise to 12–13 g/dL by age 2; in adults, they reach 14 for females & 15.5 for males
- Vit K–dependent coag factors ≈40% adult levels (2° to immature liver synthesis)
  - Prolonged PT normally seen in both preterm & full-term infants

Neurologic
- Brain growth phases: Neuronal cell division (15–20 wk gestation) then glial cell division (25 wk–2 y); myelination continues to 3 y
- Malnutrition, disruption of blood–brain barrier, & trauma may affect development
- Developmental milestones represent average rate of neurologic maturation
  - Deviations from norm do **not** necessarily indicate significant problems
  - Premature infant's developmental delay may be considered normal (*depending on degree of prematurity*)

Temperature Regulation
- Infants lose heat rapidly 2° to ↑ surface area:wt ratio, lack of adipose/SQ tissue
  - Infants rely on nonshivering thermogenesis
    - Catecholamine-mediated ↑ in brown fat metabolic activity → pulm & peripheral vasoconstriction, ↑ O use, hypoxia, acidemia
- Effective methods for limiting heat loss include ↑ ambient room temp, cover infant with thermal insulator, use of heat lamp

---

PHARMACOLOGY

Body Fluid Composition
- TBW in newborns ≈85%, ≈60% by 1 y of age; extracellular water (ECW) ↓ faster than intracellular water (ICW)
- Fat, muscle, organ wt are age dependent, affect pharmacodynamics/kinetics
- Infants have greater ECW than adults → volume of distribution for drugs is expanded
  - Drugs with limited tissue uptake may require higher wt-based dosing

Organ System Maturity
- Enzyme systems involved in biotransformation relatively immature
  - Drugs may have prolonged elimination half-lives

Protein Binding
- Often only unbound drug is clinically active (many drugs are protein bound)
  - Albumin is the major binding protein for acidic drugs (e.g., benzos & barbiturates)
  - Neonatal albumin quantitatively & qualitatively deficient → ↓ binding capacity

Receptors
- Age-related variations in response to drugs may be 2° to receptor sensitivities

PREOPERATIVE EVALUATION

Psychological Assessment
- Use clear, simple language to discuss potential risks
- Psychological goals of the preoperative interview:
  - Identify specific causes of anxiety & evaluate potential benefit of preop sedation
  - Address potential risks pertinent to procedure
  - Describe reasonable expectations for postop discomfort, side effects
  - Reassure both parents & pt
- Child-life specialists can facilitate pt education & relieve anxiety; data suggest that beginning expectation training in days prior to surgery is beneficial
  - Comfort objects may accompany pt into OR
  - Parental presence may be useful, but depends on parental anxiety level

Age-based Guidelines for Interacting with Pediatric Pts	
Neonates & infants <9 mo	Typically do not fear strangers & separation is usually uncomplicated; preop sedation usually unnecessary & may prolong emergence
Toddlers	Aware of their environment but limited reasoning ability & reality testing Benefit *most* from preop sedation & parental participation at induction
School-age children	Often do not deal well with loss of control; may admit to fear of waking up during surgery; may be reluctant to ask questions
Adolescents	Often focus on cosmetic side effects & altered body image after surgery Preop anxiolysis may expand to include meditation or music

Suggested Preoperative Sedation Drugs and Dosing			
Drug	Route	Dose (mg/kg)	Onset Time (min)
Midazolam	IV	0.01–0.03	<5
	Oral	0.5–0.75	15–30
	Nasal	0.1–0.2	15–30
	IM	0.05	5–10
	PR	1–3	10
Fentanyl	IV	0.001–0.005	<5
	Oral ("Actiq")	0.010–0.020	15–20
Ketamine	IV	1–2	1–2
	Oral	5	20–45
	IM	2–3	5–10
Methohexital	PR	20–30	5–10
Chloral hydrate	PO, PR	30–100	30–60

Nonopioid Analgesics for Children			
Drug	Dose	Interval	Route
Ibuprofen	4–10 mg/kg	q6–8h	PO
Naproxen	5–7 mg/kg	q6–8h	PO
Ketorolac	First dose: 1 mg/kg Repeat dose: 0.5 mg/kg	q6h	IV or IM
Acetaminophen	10–15 mg/kg 15–20 mg/kg	q4h q4h	PO or IV PR

Source: Adapted from Kahan M. Pain management in the critically ill child. In: Hamill RJ, Rowlingson JC, eds. *Handbook of Critical Care Pain Management*. New York: McGraw-Hill; 1994:507–521.

Neurotoxicity of Anesthetic Agents
- Some concern over potential relationship between anesthetic exposure in young pts and adverse neurodevelopmental outcomes
- To date, no studies have provided definitive evidence to change current clinical practice, especially for single anesthetic exposures under 2 h
- Consensus statement (International Anesthesia Research Society & FDA) recommends "children requiring surgery essential to their health should proceed as directed by their physician"

Preoperative Evaluation of Pediatric Pts with a Systems Focus

History	Important Questions and Pertinent Findings
Prenatal care & delivery	Gestational age; length of hospital stay; duration of intubation & ventilatory support; congenital conditions (BPD, cyanotic heart dz); freq of hospitalizations; review of growth curves; h/o apnea/bradycardia
Airway	Dysmorphic features (e.g., Pierre Robin = assoc with difficult airway); micrognathia; loose teeth; advanced caries
Respiratory	Symptoms of acute/recent URI; asthma; fever; sick contacts; 2nd-hand smoke exposure; presence of wheezing, stridor, nasal flaring, cyanosis; sleep apnea
Cardiac	Murmurs assoc with PFO, PDA, congenital heart dz; freq/duration of cyanotic spells; tachypnea; feeding intolerance; poor growth
Gastrointestinal	Repetitive vomiting; delayed meconium passage; abd distention
Hematologic	Bruising; pallor; family Hx of sickle cell/thalassemia
Neurologic	Patterns of seizure activity; developmental delay; motor weakness; hypotonia; evidence of ↑ ICP

Estimated Pediatric Vital Sign Parameters

Age	RR	HR	SBP	DBP
Preterm	55–60	120–180	45–60	20–45
Neonate	40–55	100–160	55–75	20–60
Infant (<6 mo)	30–50	80–140	85–105	55–65
1 y	30–35	80–120	90–105	55–65
6 y	20–30	75–110	95–105	50–70
10 y	20–30	80–100	95–110	55–70
16 y	15–20	60–80	110–125	65–80

OR EQUIPMENT AND SETUP

- Oral ETT size ≈ (age/4) + 4; depth ≈ (ETT internal diameter × 3)

Suggested ETT Size Selection & Appropriate Insertion Depths

Age/Weight	Internal Diameter (mm)	Depth (oral, cm)	Depth (nasal, cm)
<1.5 kg	2.5	9.0–10.0	12.0–13.0
1.5–3.5 kg	3.0	9.5–11.0	13.0–14.0
Term	3.5	10.0–11.5	13.5–14.5
3–12 mo	4.0	11.0–12.0	14.5–15.0
12–24 mo	4.5	12.0–13.5	14.5–16.0

Recommended Laryngoscopic Blade & LMA Sizes

Age	Blade	Weight (kg)	LMA Size
Premature	Miller 0	<5	1
Neonate	Miller 0	5–10	1.5
1–4 y	Miller 1	10–20	2
4–10 y	Miller 2, Mac 2	20–30	2.5
Adolescent	Miller 2, Mac 3	>30	3
Normal/large adults	Miller 2, Mac 3–4	60–90	3–5
Large adults	Miller 2–3, Mac 3–4	>90	5

Intravenous Fluids
- Fluid replacement: Based on NPO deficit, ongoing maintenance requirement, blood loss, & potential for surgically induced fluid shifts (3rd spacing)
- Lactated Ringer's often appropriate
- Normal saline advised for pts with renal dysfx, mitochondrial myopathy, or neurosurgical procedures
- Dextrose soln for neonates (limited glycogen stores) & diabetic pts who received hypoglycemic meds

- "Buretrol" or other metered device often used for children <6 mo
  - Allows careful control of fluid admin
  - Older children may receive IV fluids through a 60 drop/mL gravity infusion set
  - **Remove all air bubbles** (risk of PFO) from IV tubing & injection ports

Emergency Drugs
- All emergency drugs should have 1.5 in 22G needle for emergency IM injection

Suggested Doses of Common Emergency Drugs		
Drug	IV	IM/(SQ)
Atropine	0.01–0.02 mg/kg	0.02 mg/kg
Succinylcholine	1–2 mg/kg	3–4 mg/kg
Ephedrine	0.1–0.2 mg/kg	
Epinephrine	10 mcg/kg	10 mcg/kg

ANESTHESIA TECHNIQUES

Induction

Comparison of Pediatric Induction Methods and Commonly Used Drugs		
Technique	Advantages	Disadvantages
Mask induction (sevoflurane)	Brief onset (2–3 min) Avoids awake IV Spontaneous respiration Parental participation possible Facilitates IV start via vasodilation	Breath holding/laryngospasm Contraindicated for full stomach/MH Unprotected airway Gases are cold & dry Requires good seal
Intravenous (propofol)	Rapid onset (<30 s) Minimizes duration of unprotected airway	Anxiety about "shots" Pain upon injection Malfunction Extravasation
Intramuscular (ketamine)	Brief (2–4 min) Can inject at multiple sites Does not require cooperation	Pain upon injection Difficulties with obese children Secretions with ketamine Unprotected airway
Rectal (methohexital)	Rapid onset (1–2 min) Quick clearance	Useful only in young children No prepackaged delivery device Unprotected airway

Maintenance
- Volatile agents or TIVA-based techniques can be used
  - Drug selection guided by coexistent dz & surgery duration
- "4–2–1 rule" can guide fluid replacement
  - Neonates & infants require additional care to avoid fluid overload (metered devices) & provide glucose supplementation
  - EBV should always be calculated to guide fluid when surgery has high EBL
  - While children tolerate lower Hct, they also have ↑ metabolic rates & O_2 needs

Pediatric Maintenance Fluid Calculations ("4–2–1")	
Weight (kg)	Rate
<10	4 mL/kg/h
10–20	40 mL/h + 2 mL/kg/h for each kg >10 kg
>20	60 mL/h + 1 mL/kg/h for each kg >20 kg

Estimated HCT and EBV		
Age	HCT (%)	EBV (mL/kg)
Premature	45–60	90–100
Neonate	45–60	80–90
3–6 mo	30–33	70–80
6 mo–1 y	32–35	70–80
1–12 y	35–40	70–75
Adult	38–45	60–70

CLINICAL CONDITIONS

Respiratory

Apnea of Prematurity
- Newborns <34 wk gestational age ↑ risk for perioperative resp complications
  - Immature response to hypoxia & hypercarbia → central apnea
- GA or regional both associated with postop spells; other contributing factors include hypoglycemia, hypothermia, anemia
- Therapies: Positioning (avoid mechanical airway obstruction), resp stimulants (methylxanthine/caffeine 10 mg/kg) in high-risk pts, appropriate monitoring
- Usually premature newborns <60-wk postconception need continuous cardiorespiratory monitoring for 24 h postop (*no outpatient procedures*)

Prematurity—Perioperative Concerns
• ↑ Risk of hypothermia
• Unable to regulate glucose control
• ↑ Risk of postop apnea (esp if <50-wk postconceptual age)
• Retinopathy of prematurity (esp if <44-wk postconceptual age)
• Pulmonary dysfunction

Meconium Aspiration
- Presence of thick, meconium-stained amniotic fluid during delivery ↑ aspiration risk; may result in profound resp distress & hypoxemia
- Suction nares & oral cavity immediately after delivery
  - Transfer newborn to a radiant warmer & assess
  - Routine intubation no longer advocated, though still may be necessary
- PPV should not be used initially → can spread meconium distally into bronchial tree
  - If bradycardia/cyanosis develop → gentle PPV with 100% O_2

Bronchopulmonary Dysplasia (BPD)
- Lung dz of newborn; problematic to accurately define as presentation has varied
- Initially described as lung injury from aggressive mech ventilation and high FiO_2
  - Develop smooth muscle hypertrophy, airway inflammation, pulm HTN
  - Exogenous surfactant, steroids, & gentler vent modes → improved survival (*overall dz incidence has not decreased*)
- Babies <30-wk gestational age → immature lung parenchyma & dysfunctional alveoli
- Pulm dysfx will be persistent to varying degrees (may affect later management)
  - Airway hyperreactivity & resp infections common
  - Supportive care in the OR → gentle ventilation, limit barotrauma, β2-agonists
  - Consider need for postop ICU admission

Congenital Diaphragmatic Hernia (CDH)
- Diaphragmatic defect → presents at birth with cyanosis, resp distress, scaphoid abd
  - Herniation of abd contents into thorax → lung & pulm vessel hypoplasia
  - **Not** simply lung compression & atelectasis
- Surgical correction often postponed to optimize cardiopulmonary status
  - Severe defects require more support (ECMO or nitric oxide)
- Anesthetic management:
  - Intubation (awake, inhalation, or RSI) should minimize gastric distention
  - Maintenance usually volatile + narcotic (avoid N_2O → risk of pneumothorax)
  - A-line + CVP for blood sampling/fluid resuscitation; temp maintenance important
  - Maintain low PVR → avoid hypoxia & hypercarbia
- Sudden CV collapse & ↓ lung compliance → think contralateral pneumothorax
- Postop: Transfer to NICU intubated

Asthma
- Triad of airway inflammation, reversible flow defects, airway hyperreactivity
- Signs & symptoms: Wheezing, dyspnea, chest tightness, coughing
- Preop interview: Freq of episodes, current meds, hospital admissions, steroid use
- Severe bronchospasm can restrict airflow so much that wheezing disappears
- Anesthetic management: Supplemental O_2, bronchodilators, anticholinergics
  - Epinephrine may be required to treat severe episodes
- Avoid ETT use (may precipitate bronchospasm) for noninvasive procedures

Epiglottitis and Croup

	Epiglottitis	Croup
Etiology	H. flu (bacterial)	Viral
Age	1–8 y	6 mo–6 y
Timing	Fast onset	Gradual onset
X-ray findings	"Thumb sign" (swollen epiglottis)	"Steeple" sign (edematous narrowing of subglottic inlet)
Signs & symptoms	High fever, stridor, drooling	Mild fever, "barking" cough, cyanotic
Anesthetic management	Surgery on standby for emergent surgical airway, usually inhalational induction (sitting position) while pt breathing spontaneously; no awake laryngoscopy (risk of laryngospasm)	Cool mist, racemic epi (nebulized), steroids If needed, perform intubation in OR, consider mask induction
Use smaller-than-normal ETT (due to edema)		

Foreign Body Aspiration

- Airway manipulation (even minor) can convert partial into complete obstruction
- Supraglottic foreign body: Careful inhalational induction & gentle upper airway endoscopy to remove foreign body
- Subglottic foreign body: RSI or inhalational induction followed by rigid bronchoscopy or ETT + flex bronch
- Good communication between surgeon & anesthesiologist essential

Tetralogy of Fallot

Definition	Pulmonary stenosis, VSD, overriding aorta, RVH
TET spell management	↑ Ventricular outflow tract obstruction & PVR → inc R-to-L shunt through VSD → cyanosis; hyperventilation to ↓ PVR, phenylephrine to ↑ SVR (>PVR) → causes L–R shunt; also can give fluids, propranolol
Anesthetic management	**Goals:** ↓ R-to-L shunt (avoid ↑ PVR, ↓ heart contractility) **Techniques:** Hydration, continuation of β-blockade, avoidance of crying **Induction:** Ketamine (maintain SVR) vs. inhalational induction (risk of ↑ PVR due to hypoxia & hypercarbia)
SVR/PVR management	↓ SVR: Potent volatile agent, histamine-releasing drugs, α-blockers ↑ PVR: Acidosis, hypercarbia, hypoxia, PPV/PEEP, N₂O

Upper Respiratory Tract Infections (URIs)
- Children have ≈6–8 URIs/y; most caused by rhinovirus
  - Croup, influenza, strep pharyngitis, & allergic rhinitis may mimic URIs
- URIs ↑ airway reactivity for 4–6 wk following onset of symptoms
  - Potential complications from GA → laryngospasm, bronchospasm, & desat
- Risk factors for resp events: H/o prematurity, coexistent reactive airway dz, 2nd-hand smoke exposure, ETT, nasal congestion/secretions, airway surgery
- **Not** practical to cancel all children with recent URI; reschedule elective surgery if:
  - Purulent nasal discharge, productive cough, fever >100°F, change in func status
- LMA acceptable technique to avoid unnecessary airway manipulation; also consider IV induction if feasible, which may ↓ airway events
  - Consider deep extubations (spontaneously breathing under ≥2 MAC of sevo) to minimize airway irritation during emergence

Secondary Smoke Exposure
- 2nd-hand smoke leads to ↑ risk of adverse resp events under GA → laryngo-/bronchospasm, breath holding, airway obstruction, ↑ oral secretions

Cardiac
Patent Foramen Ovale (PFO)
- Intracardiac shunt permits fetal circulation in utero (interatrial communication)
  - Usually closes during delivery, soon after infant's 1st breath
  - Pulm vascular resistance falls & L atrial pressures exceed R → closes flap
- Conditions which ↑ R atrial pressures may reopen conduit → hypoxia, hypercarbia
- Paradoxical air embolism: Can occur in pts with PFO if precautions are not taken

Atrial & Ventricular Septal Defects (ASD/VSD)
- ASD & VSD → L-to-R shunts, do not present with systemic hypoxemia unless defects large & volume overload severe
- Small defects usually asymptomatic & hemodynamically stable
  - Over time, shunt flow may lead to R-heart volume overload & CHF
  - Corrective procedures usually timed according to dz severity
- Anesthetic management
  - Avoid hypoxia & hypercarbia (increased PVR)
  - Conditions which ↑ R-sided heart pressure above L side may provoke shunt reversal & critical hypoxemia

Metabolic
Mitochondrial Disease (MD)
- Diverse group of enzyme complex defects that adversely affect energy metabolism
  - Incidence 1 in 5,000 with variable age of onset & presentation
- Abnl ATP production affects brain, heart, & muscle; can lead to:
  - Seizures, spasticity & developmental delay, hypotonia, cardiomyopathy, arrhythmias, chronic GI dysmotility, delayed growth
- No proven assoc between MD & malignant hyperthermia
  - Pts may be sensitive to propofol, but no clear guidelines regarding its use
  - Be aware of potential for metabolic acidosis
- Normal saline generally recommended for maintenance fluids
  - Lactate admin may cause worsening of symptoms
  - Fluid requirements may be elevated
  - Children may also require glucose supplementation & serial monitoring

Gastrointestinal
Pyloric Stenosis
- Obstruction of pyloric lumen usually age 5 wk → persistent, bile-free projectile vomiting
- Medical (not surgical) emergency (i.e., correct electrolytes before surgery)
  - Infant may be severely dehydrated & have concurrent abnl electrolytes
  - Emesis is H^+ ion rich → hypokalemic, hypochloremic metabolic alkalosis
- ↑ Risk for aspiration
  - Need gastric decompression (NG) immediately before induction
  - Rapid-sequence IV induction with succinylcholine often employed
- Procedure usually brief; long-acting muscle relaxation unnecessary; consider PR acetaminophen and avoidance of opioids

Tracheoesophageal Fistula (TEF)
- Most common presentation (85%) = Type C (proximal esoph atresia w/distal fistula)
- Symptoms: Coughing, excessive drooling, & cyanotic episodes
  - Failure to pass soft-tipped suction catheter into stomach is diagnostic
  - Presence of blind esophageal pouch confirmed by x-ray
- Preop assessment: Focused on resp support, aspiration precautions, & identification of other congenital abnl (echo to rule out endocardial cushion defects)
- Anesthesia management: A-line usually placed
  - Position pt on 30° wedge to avoid passive aspiration of gastric fluid
  - Induction goal to minimize aspiration risk (awake intubation or RSI)
  - Avoid PPV prior to intubation
    - May cause significant gastric distention, diaphragmatic elevation, & hypoxia
    - Can perform gastrostomy to relieve intrathoracic pressure if decompensating
  - Deliberate R-sided mainstem intubation → limit transmission of air across fistula
  - Pass ETT distal to fistula, then withdraw until bilateral breath sounds obtained
  - Lung isolation indirectly achieved by surgical compression of nondependent lung
    - May be poorly tolerated (V/Q mismatch); consider intermittent lung reinflation
    - Hypotension may occur → distortion of mediastinal structures & ↓ venous return
  - Extubate stable pts (with good pain control) to avoid pressure on tracheal suture line
    - If pt remains intubated, only suction with a premeasured catheter that does not extend beyond distal tip of ETT

Gastroschisis & Omphalocele
- Involve defects of anterior abdominal wall with herniation of visceral components

Comparison of Gastroschisis and Omphalocele

	Gastroschisis	Omphalocele
Etiology	Omphalomesenteric artery occlusion	Failed gut migration from yolk sac to abdomen
Incidence	1:15,000	1:6,000
Presentation	Lateral to umbilicus	Midline
Hernial sac	Absent	Present
Bowel function	Abnormal	Normal
Associated anomalies	Prematurity	Beckwith–Wiedemann syndrome; congenital heart dz; bladder exstrophy

- Cover exposed viscera to avoid evaporative heat loss & limit infection
  - Large fluid shifts occur; fluids should be aggressively replaced
  - Serial electrolyte & glucose monitoring important (consider A-line/CVC)
- Anesthetic technique
  - Awake intubation or RSI; avoid N_2O
- Defect closure may → ↑ intra-abdominal pressures which may cause ↑ peak airway pressure, ↓ venous return, hypotension, lower-extremity ischemia
- Postop often require mech vent support

Necrotizing Enterocolitis
- Etiology multifactorial: Pts usually present with bowel distention & bloody feces
  - Preterm infants <2-wk gestational age at highest risk
- Intestinal hypoperfusion & ischemia → weakened intestinal wall
- Anesthesia management: Place A-line & CVC
  - Resuscitation should include crystalloid & blood products
  - Monitor urine output, avoid N_2O
  - DIC, thrombocytopenia may occur
- Pts often return to OR for re-exploration

Pediatric Congenital Syndromes

Syndromes and Their Anesthetic Implications

Name	Description	Anesthetic Implications
Adrenogenital syndrome	Inability to synthesize hydrocortisone. Virilization of female	Need hydrocortisone even if not salt-losing. Check electrolytes
Apert syndrome	Craniofacial abnormalities, syndactyly and potential developmental delay	Possible hydrocephalus and elevated intracranial pressures. Potential difficult airway
Ataxia–telangiectasia	Cerebellar ataxia. Skin and conjunctival telangiectasia. Decreased serum IgA and reticuloendothelial malignancy	Defective immunity; recurrent chest and sinus infections. Bronchiectasis
Beckwith–Wiedemann syndrome	Birth weight >4 kg Macroglossia and omphalocele	Persistent severe neonatal hypoglycemia. Airway problems
Cherubism	Tumorous lesion of mandibles and maxillae with intraoral masses. May cause respiratory distress	Intubation may be extremely difficult. May require tracheostomy
Congenital iodine deficiency syndrome (cretinism)	Absent thyroid tissue or defective synthesis of thyroxine and goiter	Airway problems; large tongue, goiter. Respiratory center very sensitive to depression. CO_2 retention common. Hypoglycemia, hyponatremia, hypotension. Low cardiac output. Transfusion poorly tolerated
Cri-du-chat syndrome	Chromosome 5P abnormal. Abnormal cry, microcephaly. Micrognathia. Congenital heart dz	Airway problems; stridor, laryngomalacia. Possibly difficult intubation

Down syndrome (trisomy 21)	60% have congenital heart dz. Duodenal atresia in some. Cervical spine abnormalities	Difficulty airway; large tongue, small mouth. Risk of laryngospasm, especially on extubation. Bradycardia. Sequelae of cardiac anomalies
Duchenne muscular dystrophy	Muscular dystrophy with frequent cardiac muscle involvement. Usually die in the 2nd decade. Amount of skeletal muscle involvement and cardiac involvement unrelated	Same as congenital myotonia plus cardiac involvement. Reduce drug doses. Avoid respiratory depressants, muscle relaxants. Postoperative ventilatory support may be required
Edward syndrome (trisomy 18)	Congenital heart dz in 96%. Micrognathia in 80%. Renal malformations 50–80%. Usually die in infancy	Possible difficult intubation. Care with renally excreted drugs
Ehlers–Danlos syndrome	Collagen abnormality with hyperelasticity and fragile tissues. Dissecting aortic aneurysm. Fragility of other blood vessels. Possible bleeding diathesis	CVC—spontaneous rupture of vessels. Angiogram 1% mortality. ECG conduction abnormalities. IV difficult to maintain; hematoma. Poor tissues and clotting defects lead to hemorrhage, especially GI tract. Spontaneous pneumothorax
Familial periodic paralysis	Muscle dz. Hypokalemia, attacks of quadriplegia	Monitor serum K^+. Limit use of dextrose. Monitor ECG. Avoid relaxants
Fanconi syndrome (renal tubular acidosis)	Usually $2°$ to other dz. Proximal tubular defect. Acidosis, K^+ loss. Dehydration	Impaired renal function. Treat electrolyte and acid–base abnormalities. Look for $1°$ dz (galactosemia, cystinosis, etc.)
Homocystinuria	Inborn error of metabolism. Thromboembolic phenomena due to intimal thickening. Ectopia lentis. Osteoporosis. Kyphoscoliosis	Dextran often used to reduce viscosity and platelet adhesiveness; ↑ peripheral perfusion. Angiography may precipitate thrombosis, especially cerebral
Primary ciliary dyskinesia (Kartagener syndrome)	Dextrocardia, sinusitis, and bronchiectasis. Abnormal immunity	Chronic respiratory infections, structural heart dz
Klippel–Feil syndrome	Congenital fusion of two or more cervical vertebrae, leading to neck rigidity	Difficulty airway and intubation
Frontonasal dysplasia	Varying degrees of cleft face. Frontal lipomas. Dermoids	Cleft nose, lip, and palate may cause intubation difficulties
Marfan syndrome (arachnodactyly)	Connective tissue d/o. Dilated aortic root leads to AI. Aortic, thoracic, or abdominal aneurysm. Pulmonary artery, mitral valve involved. Kyphoscoliosis, pectus excavatum, lung cysts. Joint instability and dislocation	Care with myocardial depressant drugs. Beware possible dissection of aorta. Lung function poor. Possible pneumothorax. Care in positioning; easily dislocated joints
Myasthenia congenita	Similar to adult myasthenia gravis	Avoid respiratory depressants, muscle relaxants. May require postop ventilation. Problems with anticholinesterase therapy pre- and postop if necessary. Pulmonary complications due to poor cough
McArdle dz	Glycogen storage dz V	Muscles affected including cardiac muscle; care with cardiac depressant drugs

Pierre Robin syndrome	Cleft palate, micrognathia, glossoptosis. Associated congenital heart dz may occur	Anticipate difficult airway. Micrognathia & glossoptosis may lead to resp distress, requiring trach or tongue suture to relieve postoropharyngeal obstruction
Porphyria	Intermittent porphyria most common autosomal dominant form. Often latent before puberty. Abd pain, neurologic dysfx, electrolyte imbalances & psychiatric disturbances characterize acute episodes	Avoid barbiturates (thiopental, methohexital). Ketamine, etomidate, & propofol appear safe. Maintenance of anesthesia with narcotics, volatile agents, & nondepolarizing muscle relaxants is recommended. Avoid regional anesthesia in the presence of existing neurologic deficit
Prader–Willi syndrome	Neonate—hypotonia, poor feeding, absent reflexes. 2nd phase—hyperactive, uncontrollable polyphagia, developmental delay	Obesity of extreme proportions leading to cardiopulmonary failure
Scleroderma	Diffuse cutaneous stiffening. Plastic surgery required for contractures and constrictions	Facial and oral scarring; difficult airway and intubation. Chest restriction; poor compliance. Diffuse pulmonary fibrosis, hypoxia. Veins often invisible and impalpable. Cardiac fibrosis or cor pulmonale. Hx of steroid therapy
Stevens–Johnson syndrome	Erythema multiforme; urticarial lesions; and erosions of mouth, eyes, and genitalia. Possible hypersensitivity to exogenous agents/drugs	Oral lesions; avoid intubation and esophageal stethoscope. Monitoring difficult because of skin lesions but essential. ECG—fibrillation, myocarditis, pericarditis occur. Temperature control—febrile episodes. Intravenous access—essential but avoid cut-down because of infection. Consider ketamine. Pleural blebs and pneumothorax may occur
Tay–Sachs dz	Gangliosidosis. Blindness and progressive dementia and degeneration of central nervous system	No described anesthetic hazard. Progressive neurologic loss leads to respiratory complications. Supportive measures are only treatment
Treacher Collins syndrome (mandibulofacial dysostosis)	Micrognathia and aplastic zygomatic arches. Microstomia, choanal atresia. Congenital heart dz may occur	Possible airway and intubation difficulties. Less severe than Pierre Robin deformity, but airway worsens over time
Von Hippel–Lindau syndrome	Retinal or CNS hemangioblastoma (posterior fossa or spinal cord) Associated with pheochromocytoma & renal, pancreatic, or hepatic cysts	Problems due to associated pheochromocytoma, renal and hepatic pathology
Neurofibromatosis type 1 (Von Recklinghausen dz)	Café-au-lait spots. Tumors in all parts of CNS. Peripheral tumors associated with nerve trunks. Increased incidence pheochromocytoma. Honeycomb cystic lung changes. Renal artery dysplasia and hypertension	Screen for pheochromocytoma (urinary VMA) and lung function. Tumors may occur in the larynx and right ventricular outflow tract. Care with renally excreted drugs if kidneys involved

Wilson dz (hepatolenticular degeneration)	Decreased ceruloplasmin causes abnormal copper deposits, especially in liver and CNS motor nuclei. Renal tubular acidosis	Hepatic failure 2° to fibrosis. IV induction (propofol, ketamine, etomidate) acceptable. Apnea uncommon with succinylcholine administration, despite pseudocholinesterase deficiency. Consider reduced dosing of renally excreted drugs
Wolff–Parkinson–White syndrome	ECG abnormality—short PR, prolonged QRS with phasic variation in 40%. Associated with many cardiac defects. Anomalous conduction path between atria and ventricles. Delta wave may be present on ECG	Scopolamine preferred to atropine as antisialagogue. Tachycardia due to atropine or apprehension may change ECG and suggest infarction, with ST-segment depression. Paroxysmal SVT on induction of anesthesia or during cardiac surgery has been reported. Should be treated with digitalis, propranolol, pacemaker if necessary. Neostigmine may accentuate WPW pattern

Source: Adapted from Pajewski TN. Anesthesiology Pocket Guide. Philadelphia, PA: Lippincott-Raven; 1997.

NEONATAL & PEDIATRIC RESUSCITATION

Neonatal Resuscitation Algorithm
Note: The following summary is not to be a substitute for completion of the Neonatal Resuscitation course as administered by a certified instructor.
- ~10% of newborns require direct assistance to achieve cardiopulmonary stability during transition to extrauterine life. <1% require extensive efforts
- Term neonates with adequate breathing/crying and tone should be dried and kept warm. All others require rapid assessment and the following sequential interventions
- Dry and keep warm, position, airway check, stimulate to breathe
- Ambu-bag ventilation, oximetry monitoring, possible intubation
- Chest compressions
- Medications and volume expansion

New recommendations since 2010:
- Initial evaluation now followed by simultaneous assessment of HR and respirations. Oximetry monitoring should be used early
- For full-term babies, resuscitation should begin with air rather than 100% FiO_2
- Supplemental oxygen should be blended with air with delivered concentration guided by oximetry
- Current evidence neither supports nor contradicts the routine endotracheal suctioning of infants born in the presence of meconium-stained amniotic fluid
- Neonatal chest compression–ventilation ratio should remain 3:1, higher ratio to be applied if neonatal arrest due to cardiac etiology
- Therapeutic hypothermia may be considered for term/near-term infants with evolving hypoxic–ischemic encephalopathy
- It is appropriate to consider cessation of resuscitation efforts if no detectable heart rate for 10 min
- Delay cord clamping for at least 1 min in babies NOT requiring resuscitation

Pediatric Advanced Cardiac Life Support (Also see Chapter 37, Emergency Algorithms)
Note: The following summary is not to be a substitute for completion of the PALS course as administered by a certified instructor.
- Current PALS algorithms (Fig. 29-2) are based upon the identification and appropriate treatment of the precipitating conditions that ultimately lead to pediatric cardiac arrest. The conditions include respiratory distress, respiratory failure, various shock states, and arrhythmias
- The conduct of any algorithm is based upon the "assess, categorize, decide, act" model of healthcare provider team behaviors. The process is iterative
- Assessments progress from general evaluations of pt distress to focused examinations and identification of pathophysiology

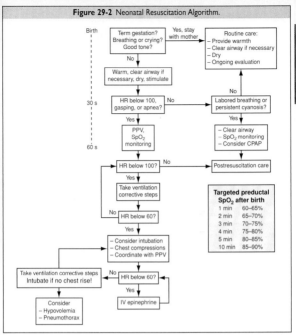

Figure 29-2 Neonatal Resuscitation Algorithm.

- General: Appearance, work of breathing, circulation → determine presence of life-threatening condition
- Primary: Airway, breathing, circulation, disability, exposure → hands-on evaluation including vital signs' measurement and oximetry. Initial treatment may include measures to maintain airway patency, support/provide respirations, and establish IV access and commence fluid resuscitation
- Secondary: SAMPLE format (signs & symptoms, allergies, medications, past medical Hx, last meal, and events) provides mechanism for focused H&P complemented by lab studies (HCT, ABG, CXR, capnography) to guide continuing management efforts
- All PALS treatment efforts should be supported by high-quality CPR when indicated

Important changes to PALS since 2010:
- Defibrillation—initial dose of 2–4 J/kg acceptable. For refractory VF, may ↑ to 4 J/kg. Subsequent energy levels should be at least 4 J/kg, not to exceed 10 J/kg
- Wide-complex tachycardia now identified by QRS width of >0.09 s. This simplifies previous age-assignment of normal QRS measurements. Affect concerns computer interpretations
- Routine administration of calcium is NOT recommended UNLESS there is evidence of hypocalcemia, calcium-channel blocker overdose, hypermagnesemia, or hyperkalemia
- Etomidate is NOT recommended for routine use in pediatric pts with septic shock
- Specific guidelines now address resuscitation management strategies in pts with congenital heart dz and pulmonary hypertension. (Consider early use of ECMO if available.)
- After restoration of effective cardiac output, continuously monitor oxygen saturation. Consider titration of oxygen therapy to maintain SpO_2 ≥94% (reduce risk of oxidative injury from ischemia–reperfusion effect)
- Perform CO_2 detection (capnography or colorimetry) to confirm ETT placement in all settings and during transport
- Therapeutic hypothermia (32–34° for 12–24 h) may be considered for pediatric pts that remain comatose after resuscitation from cardiac arrest. Possible benefit to neurologic recovery.

RICHARD D. URMAN • JESSE M. EHRENFELD

- Incidence: 20–30% of general surgical pts, 70–80% of high-risk pts
- Impact: Accounts for 0.1–0.2% of unanticipated hospital admissions
  - ↑ PACU length of stay & costs, ↓ pt satisfaction

Major Risk Factors for PONV (also see Fig 30-1)		
Patient Factors	**Anesthetic Factors**	**Surgical Factors**
Female	Volatile anesthetics	Surgical procedure
Hx of PONV or motion sickness	Duration of anesthesia	(cholecystectomy, gynecologic, laparoscopy)
Nonsmokers	Postop opioids	Surgical duration
Younger age (<50 y)	Nitrous oxide	
	General vs. regional anesthesia	

Source: Gan TJ, Diemunsch P, Habib A, et al. Society for ambulatory anesthesia. Consensus guidelines for the management of postoperative nausea and vomiting. *Anesth Analg* 2014;118(1):85–113; also 2020 updated guidelines (in press).

Strategies to Reduce Baseline Risk for PONV (also see Fig 30-1)
Avoidance of general anesthesia by the use of regional anesthesia
Use of propofol for induction and maintenance of anesthesia
Avoidance of nitrous oxide
Avoidance of volatile anesthetics
Minimization of intraoperative and postoperative opioids
Adequate hydration
Using sugammadex instead of neostigmine for the reversal of neuromuscular blockade

Source: Gan TJ, Diemunsch P, Habib A, et al. Society for ambulatory anesthesia. Consensus guidelines for the management of postoperative nausea and vomiting. *Anesth Analg* 2014;118(1):85–113; also 2020 updated guidelines (in press).

Simplified Risk Score for PONV			Prediction and Prophylaxis of PONV		
Risk Factors	**Points**		**No. of Points**	**% Risk of PONV**	***Prophylaxis**
Female	1		0	10% (low risk)	2 agents
Hx of PONV/ motion sickness	1		1	21% (low risk)	
Nonsmoker	1		2	39% (mod risk)	2 agents
Postop opioids	1		3	61% (high risk)	Multimodal therapy/ 3-4 agents
			4	79% (high risk)	

Source: Adapted from Apfel CC, Läärä E, Koivuranta M, et al. A simplified risk score for predicting PONV: conclusions from cross-validations between two centers. *Anesthesiology* 1999;91:693–700; *according to 2020 updated PONV guidelines (in press).

- Pharmacologic combination therapy for PONV prophylaxis
  - Aprepitant + dexamethasone
  - 5-HT3 receptor antagonist + dexamethasone
  - 5-HT3 receptor antagonist + haloperidol
  - 5-HT3 receptor antagonist + dexamethasone + haloperidol
  - 5-HT3 receptor antagonist + aprepitant
  - Scopolamine patch and anti-histamines can also be used in combination with above drugs
- PONV rescue strategy
  - If initial agent is ineffective → give drug from a different class
  - Repeat haloperidol and 5-HT3 antagonists q6h (futile to repeat antiemetic given for prophylaxis or treatment any sooner than 6h)
  - Repeat administration of dexamethasone, transdermal scopolamine, aprepitant, and palonosetron is not recommended
- Discharge criteria
  - Often based on formal scoring systems (see Chapter 14, PACU Management and Discharge) or RN/MD assessment
  - Oral intake: Not required prior to discharge
  - Voiding: Only required if pt received neuraxial anesthesia or had gynecologic, hernia, anorectal, or genital surgery
  - Spinal/epidural anesthesia: Pt must have return of sensation & no motor block
  - Nerve blocks: Discharge can occur before full return of motor/sensory function, instruct pt to protect numb limb from injury

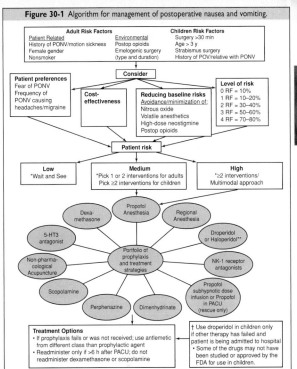

Figure 30-1 Algorithm for management of postoperative nausea and vomiting.

(From Gan TJ, Diemunsch P, Habib A, et al. Society for ambulatory anesthesia. Consensus guidelines for the management of postoperative nausea and vomiting. *Anesth Analg* 2014;118(1):85–113.); *However, the updated 2020 updated PONV guidelines (in press) now recommend 2 interventions in low and medium risk groups and 3-4 interventions in high risk groups; **Amisulpride is now also available.

Antiemetic Drugs				
Class	**Drug**	**Dose**	**Timing**	**Side Effects**
5HT₃ Antagonists	Ondansetron Granisetron Dolasetron[a] Tropisetron[a] Ramosetron[a] Palonosetron	4 mg IV 0.35–3 mg IV 12.5 mg IV 2 mg IV 0.3 mg IV 0.075 mg IV	End of surgery At induction	Headaches Elevated LFT Constipation QT prolongation
NK-1 receptor antagonists	Aprepitant Casopitant[a] Rolapitant[a]	40 mg PO 150 mg PO 70–200 mg PO	At induction	Cytochrome p450 inhibitor, constipation, hypotension, headache
Steroid	Dexamethasone Methyl-prednisolone	4–5 mg IV 40 mg IV	At induction	Hyperglycemia Risk of postop infection

Butyrophenones	Droperidol	0.625–1.25 mg IV	End of surgery	QT prolongation, drowsiness, extrapyramidal effects; amisulpride: **no** QT prolongation
	Haloperidol	0.5–<2 mg IV/IM/PO		
	Amisulpride	5 or 10 mg IV		
Phenothiazines	Promethazine	6.25–12.5 mg IV	End of surgery	
	Prochlorperazine	5–10 mg IV		
	Metoclopramide	>20 mg IV		
Antihistamine	Dimenhydrinate	1 mg/kg IV		Drowsiness, agitation, extrapyramidal effects
	Meclizine	50 mg PO		
Other	Propofol	20 mg IV	In PACU	Resp depression
	Scopolamine	Transpatch	Prior evening or 2 h before surgery	Sedation, confusion, dizziness, dry mouth sedation
	Ephedrine	0.5 mg/kg IM	End of surgery	
	Midazolam	2 mg IV	30 min before end of surgery	
	Gabapentin	600–800 mg PO	1–2 h prior to induction	
	Perphenazine	5 mg IV/IM	At induction	
	Mirtazapine	30 mg PO		
Nonpharma-cologic	PC6 acupoint stimulation; Neuromuscular stimulation over median nerve; hydration; aromatherapy		Pre- or postinduction	

[a]Not available in the United States.

Source: Gan TJ, Diemunsch P, Habib A, et al. Society for ambulatory anesthesia. Consensus guidelines for the management of postoperative nausea and vomiting. *Anesth Analg* 2014;118(1):85–113.

MELISSA L. BELLOMY

GENERAL CONSIDERATIONS AND SAFETY

- Thorough preop evaluation of every pt is essential
- All pts *must* have standard ASA monitors while receiving anesthesia care
- Transport equipment should be available (bag–valve–mask with O_2 tank)
- Emergency drugs should be available & IV access confirmed
- Postop care & standards are the same as for OR-based anesthesia
- Pay attention to possible allergies to contrast dye

ASA Guidelines for Non-OR Anesthetizing Locations
• Reliable O_2 source, including backup supply
• Adequate & reliable suction
• Adequate & reliable gas scavenging system (if anesthetic gases are to be used)
• Self-inflating resuscitator bag capable of delivering 0.9 FiO_2 + PPV
• Adequate drugs, supplies, & equipment for the planned activity
• Adequate monitoring equipment to adhere to ASA monitoring standards
• Sufficient electrical outlets, connected to an emergency power supply
• Sufficient space for equipment and personnel
• Immediate availability of emergency cart with defibrillator & emergency drugs
• Reliable 2-way comm + availability of skilled anesthesia support personnel
• Observation of all applicable building & safety codes and facility standards

Source: Adapted from *ASA Standards for Basic Intraoperative Monitoring.*

CT AND MRI

CT: General Considerations
- Pt should wear lead with thyroid shield at all times while in CT scanner

CT: Monitors
- Standard ASA monitors required if any anesthesia given
- No metallic precautions; however, placement away from field minimizes artifact

CT: Anesthetic Considerations
- Anesthetic options range from mild sedation to general anesthesia
- Pt factors to consider: Pt cooperation, claustrophobia, comorbidities, age, mental status, length of scan, airway exam (limited access to airway in the CT scanner), potential for airway compromise (head/neck trauma)
- Ensure adequate length of IV lines, anesthesia circuit, monitoring wires

Special Procedures in the CT Suite
Stereotactic Brain Biopsy
- Metal frame placed to perform procedure (usually with local + opioid/benzo)
- Technique: MAC, titrate sedation carefully to avoid airway compromise. If GA necessary, awake fiberoptic intubation may be the safest technique

Percutaneous Vertebroplasty
- Indication: Reverse vertebral collapse in osteoporotic pts
- Technique: Usually MAC (or GA if pt in excessive pain)
- Pt is in prone position → consider pelvic/chest support to avoid abdominal compression and impaired ventilation

MRI: General Considerations
- Indications for anesthesia care: Children, mental delay, claustrophobia, respiratory difficulty, hemodynamic instability
- Distinct features of anesthesia in MRI:
  - Powerful magnet
    - Remove ferromagnetic equipment: Stethoscopes, credit cards, USB drives, pens, keys, IDs, beepers, cell phones, wrist watches, infusion pumps
    - Check pt for pacemaker, aneurysm clips, intravascular wires, metal implants
    - Metals safe: Beryllium, nickel, stainless steel, tantalum, & titanium
- Difficulty accessing airway
  - Carefully titrate sedatives & have monitors facing clinician at all times

- Nonferrous monitoring equipment needed, nonmagnetic laryngoscopes
- In emergency, remove pt from MRI scanner immediately and initiate treatment
- Ensure adequate length of IV lines, anesthesia circuit, monitoring wires
- Keep EKG wires uncoiled—can cause T and ST wave artifacts, pt burns

INTERVENTIONAL NEURORADIOLOGY

General Considerations
- Standard ASA monitors; if arterial line necessary, radial or through femoral sheath
  - Femoral sheath a-lines → only MAP is useful, may lose waveform if instrumented
- Technique: GA if motionless state required; local or sedation if rapid neurologic testing necessary or for most diagnostic scans

Embolization of Arteriovenous Malformation (AVM)
- Liquid or particulate embolic agents injected into feeding vessels of AVM
- Approach: MAC (can continuously monitor neuro status) or GA (if extensive)
- Systemic heparinization may be required
- Complications: Hemorrhage (transfuse, reverse anticoagulation, deliberate hypotension); ↑ ICP (hyperventilate, head ↑, mannitol, furosemide, 3% NaCl)

Cerebral Aneurysms
- Uses endovascular stents, coils, or liquid polymer solution to treat aneurysm
- Usually performed under general anesthesia, arterial line should be placed
- Important to have OR available in case of rupture & urgent need for surgical repair

Central Intra-arterial Thrombolysis
- Treatment of stroke if <6 h from onset of symptoms or penumbra visualized on diffusion weighted imaging
- Usually performed under MAC (neurologic assessment is desirable)

ENDOSCOPY AND ERCP

General Considerations
- Most upper and lower endoscopies are performed without an anesthesiologist
- Lateral position for lower endoscopy; lateral/supine for upper endoscopy
- Important to have access to airway at all times

Technique
- Anesthetic options range from mild sedation to general anesthesia
  - Midazolam/fentanyl/propofol combination often used; consider ↓ dose ketamine
- Pt factors to consider: Pt cooperation, comorbidities, age, mental status, length of procedure
- **Upper endoscopy:** Consider pharyngeal topical anesthesia (lidocaine, benzocaine) prior to endoscope insertion
  - Postop pain: Relatively low, usually from air used for inflation
- **Endoscopic Retrograde Cholangiopancreatography (ERCP):** May be performed in supine, lateral, or prone position; pt can have significant pain during bile duct dilatation

Complications
- Airway obstruction, laryngospasm, bronchospasm, inadvertent extubation, aspiration, GI perforation

DAVID A. EDWARDS • JENNA WALTERS

INTRODUCTION

Also see Urman RD, Vadivelu N. *Pocket Pain Medicine.* 1st ed. Philadelphia, PA: Lippincott Williams & Wilkins; 2011.

Pain Durations		
Acute pain	0–6 wk	New onset or exacerbation, normal healing period
Subacute pain	1–3 mo	Prolonged, transitional (acute to chronic)
Chronic pain	>3 mo	Persistent, pathologic, or continuous stimulus induced

Types of Pain		
Nociceptive	An adaptive (protective) pain; pain sensed by pain receptors (nociceptors) that sense thermal, mechanical, or chemical stimuli • *Somatic pain*—musculoskeletal pain (broken bones, unhealed wounds, surgical) • *Visceral pain*—pain from organs (bladder, bowel, ovaries)	Superficial somatic: Sharp, easily localized (burns) Deep somatic: Throbbing, aching, worse with movement, poorly localized (broken bones) Visceral: Pressure, deep, dull, diffuse, poorly localized, referred
Inflammatory	An adaptive (protective) pain; results from local inflammation (arthritis, infection, tissue injury)	Throbbing Ache
Pathologic	A maladaptive pain; damage/dysfunction of nervous system (diabetes, surgical transection, nerve injury) • *Neuropathic pain*—diabetic neuropathy • *Dysfunctional pain*—central sensitization, fibromyalgia, irritable bowel, tension type headache	Electric, burning, fire, stabbing, cutting, pins and needles, tingling, shooting

Definition of Pain Terms	
Pain	"An unpleasant sensory or emotional experience associated with actual or potential tissue damage, or described in terms of such damage" (IASP)
Dysesthesia	Unpleasant abnormal sensation (spontaneous or evoked)
Paresthesia	Abnormal sensation (spontaneous or evoked)
Hyperesthesia	↑ Sensitivity to any stimulus
Hyperpathia	Painful syndrome of ↑ pain in response to a stimulus (especially repetitive stimulus)
Hyperalgesia	Painful stimulus is more painful than expected (pinprick hurts even more) • *Primary hyperalgesia*—painful zone innervated by nerves in region of the lesion • *Secondary hyperalgesia*—expanded area that becomes painful as a result of becoming sensitized • *Opioid-induced hyperalgesia*—acute opioid exposure paradoxically ↑ pain, acute opioid withdrawal ↑ pain sensitivity, or chronic opioid exposure ↑ pain sensitivity
Allodynia	Painful response to nonpainful stimulus (e.g., light touch skin causes pain)
Hypoesthesia	↓ Sensitivity to nonpainful stimulus
Hypoalgesia	↓ Pain in response to normally painful stimulus
Anesthesia	Absence of sensation to painful or nonpainful stimulus
Analgesia	Absence of pain to painful stimulus
Anesthesia dolorosa	Painful sensation in anesthetic area
Meralgia paresthetica	Numbness/pain from lateral femoral cutaneous n. compression

Multimodal analgesia	Principle of combining analgesic modalities (meds, procedures, techniques) at lower individual doses to improve pain tx while decreasing risks/side effects (as opposed to polypharmacy, combining meds at higher doses resulting in increased risks/side effects)
Opioid tolerant	An increased dose of opioid is required for the same effect (NIH definition of opioid tolerant pt = taking 60 mg morphine PO in 24 h ×7 d)
Dependence	A state of normal function in the presence of drug, but a withdrawal syndrome when the drug is removed
Addiction	Compulsive substance use despite negative life interference
Pain	"An unpleasant sensory or emotional experience associated with actual or potential tissue damage, or described in terms of such damage" (IASP)

Chronic Pain in the United States
- Primary reason people see a doctor
- Primary reason people are out of work
- Affects 210 million adults
- Costs $300 billion in direct costs and $330 billion in lost productivity
- More than cancer, diabetes, and heart dz combined (J Pain 2012;13(8):715–724)

Epidemic of Opioid Misuse and Diversion in the US (Source: CDC)
- Risk/benefit assessment of opioid prescription should take into account that the United States is in the midst of an epidemic of misuse and diversion of prescription opioids, and that no robust data currently support improved population outcomes for opioid prescription >6 mo in pts with chronic pain
- Women are more likely to have chronic pain, be prescribed prescription painkillers, be given higher doses, and use them for longer time periods than men
  - Cases of neonatal abstinence syndrome have increased 300% in last decade
- 1 in 20 people >12 y old in the United States use opioids for nonmedical purposes
  - 50% of these people obtain the medication from a friend or family member for free, but 81% of these "free" medications have come from a health-care provider
- Each d, 46 people die from prescription opioid overdose in the United States
  - Epidemiologic risk factors for death include male gender, white/Native American race, rural and Southern location, and middle age (35–55)
  - Combination with benzodiazepines results in higher rates of mortality
- Diversion for financial gain also common; opioids sell for $1/mg on the street
- Red flags for opioid misuse or diversion
  - Refusal to consider other nonopioid options
  - Requesting a specific opioid medication by name
  - Multiple early refills/ER visits
  - Anger, disability, litigation, catastrophizing
- Opioid prescribing guidelines for chronic nonmalignant pain are available to aid prescribers in recognition and risk mitigation; these may vary by state. Common recommendations for screening (and documentation) prior to prescribing controlled substances include:
  - A substance use and psychological Hx
  - A standardized opioid risk assessment tool (e.g., ORT score)
  - Query of the state prescription drug monitoring program (PDMP) database
  - Urine drug screening (UDS)
  - Informed consent agreement about risks of opioid use, including counseling about neonatal abstinence syndrome in women of reproductive age
  - Frequent longitudinal re-evaluation of opioid needs based on level of risk and functional status of pt
- As prescriptions of opioids ↓, the rates of heroin and illicit fentanyl overdose deaths have >quadrupled since 2010
- In this setting, nonopioid pharmacologic and nonpharmacologic options must be considered prior to or concurrent with opioids for any nonmalignant chronic pain

Low Back Pain (LBP)
- Annual US incidence: 80–85% lifetime prevalence; 23% chronic prevalence; 11–12% of the population disabled by low back pain (Lancet 2012;379:9814,482–91)
- Low back pain is the leading cause of disability worldwide, with the majority of cases having no clear etiology (Ann Rheum Dis 2014;73(6):968–974)
- Prognosis: 90% spontaneously recover within 4–6 wk; after 6 mo <50% return to work; after 1 y only 10% return to work

- Risk factors: Smoking, obesity, older age, female gender, sedentary lifestyle, low education, low socioeconomic status, worker's compensation claims, psychological factors (e.g., anxiety, depression, somatization d/o)
- Mechanical factors like lifting and bending are not a clear risk factor for chronicity
- 64% of asymptomatic subjects have MRI abnormalities of the lumbar spine like disc bulges, protrusions, and degeneration (N Engl J Med 1994;331(2):69–73)
- See Figure 32-1 for H&P and Figure 32-2 for Initial Evaluation Algorithm

Differential Diagnosis of Low Back Pain

Mechanical (80–90%)
Intervertebral discs (e.g., degenerative disc dz, herniation)
Intervertebral joints (e.g., facet joint arthropathy), sacroiliac joint (SIJ)
Spinal canal narrowing, neuroforaminal narrowing (stenosis)
Ligamental, muscular sprain (myofascial)
Vertebral fractures
Alignment d/o (scoliosis, kyphosis, spondylolisthesis)

Nonmechanical (1–2%)
Neoplasm, infection, hematoma

Causes of referred pain (1–2%)
Cardiovascular (e.g., aortic dissection/aneurysm)
Hematologic (e.g., sickle cell crisis)
Gastrointestinal (e.g., pancreatitis, cholecystitis)
Renal (e.g., nephrolithiasis, pyelonephritis)
Pelvic dz (e.g., prostatitis, endometriosis, retroperitoneal mass)

Neuropathic (2–4%)
Peripheral or central sensitization syndrome which may include multiple sites, and mood d/o (anxiety, depression, catastrophizing)

Figure 32-1 Low Back Pain History & Physical Exam.

Rule out emergencies (e.g., infection, hematoma, acute neurologic deterioration, tumor progression)

History
1. *Origination*—onset, inciting factors
2. *Location*—where are the sites of the most pain (e.g., left/right/midline, lumbar)
3. *Duration*—how long has it been, frequency, trajectory (e.g., days, weeks, years, daily, occasional, at night, stable, improving, worsening)
4. *Quantification*—how bad is it (e.g., 8/10 on NRS)
5. *Qualification*—what does it feel like (e.g., sharp, dull, ache, pinch, electric)
6. *Radiation*—does the pain radiate (e.g., lateral, down the leg, to the back of the head)
7. *Exacerbation/alleviation*—what makes it worse/better (e.g., rest, leaning forward, meds, mindfulness, yoga, acupuncture, non/interventional treatments)
8. *Modifications*—co-morbid or psych situations that make pain worse (e.g., anxiety, depression, PTSD, non/restful sleep, substance use d/o)
9. *Associations*—rule out emergencies (e.g., infection, hematoma, acute neurologic deterioration, weight loss, etc. denoting cancer progression, bowel/bladder incontinence & perineal numbers denoting critical stenosis)
10. *Considerations*—social situations (e.g., legal proceedings, disability, early retirement)

Physical Exam
1. *Inspection*—scoliosis, deformity, local skin changes (e.g., infection, vascular dz, or complex regional pain syndrome)
2. *Palpation*—identify points of tenderness over spinous processes, paraspinal muscles, muscle insertion points, joint locations (e.g., facet, sacroiliac, dermatomal)
3. *Mobilization*—assess range of motion in extension/flexion/lateral rotation of spine (e.g., pain with flexion may reflect disc dz, pain with extension may reflect facet arthropathy or spinal stenosis, pain with lateral motion may reflect disc dz/herniation or spondylosis, worsening pain with standing/walking may reflect stenosis, assess gait)
   —straight leg raise and lower-extremity exam for signs of radiculopathy
4. *Sensation*—assess temperature, touch, pain (pinprick), balance to evaluate loss of sensation due to nerve compromise
5. *Provocation*—tests (e.g., straight leg raise, Faber's and Gaenslen's), reflexes (e.g., clonus, hyperreflexia, Babinski/Hoffman's denoting myelopathy)

Psychosocial Evaluation (e.g., SOAP, COMM, DAST, ACEs, ORT scores)
Diagnostic Studies—imaging (e.g., x-ray, CT, MRI, SPECT, bone scan, myelography)
   —electrodiagnostic (e.g., EMG/NCS)
   —labs (e.g., usually not needed unless suspect infection, cancer, rheum dz)

Strength Testing

Strength Testing		
Test	Muscles	Innervation
Hip flexion	Iliopsoas muscle	L1–3, lumbar plexus
Hip abduction (abd)/adduction (add)	Abd: Gluteus medius/minimus muscle Add: Adductor longus muscle/brevis/magnus muscle, gracilis muscle	Abd: L4–S1, gluteal nerve Add: L2–4, obturator nerve
Knee flexion (flex)/extension (ext)	Flex: Biceps femoris muscle Ext: Quadriceps muscle	Flex: L5–S2, sciatic nerve Ext: L2–4, femoral nerve
Foot plantar flexion/dorsiflexion	Dorsiflex: Tibialis anterior muscle Plantarflex: Gastrocnemius muscle, soleus muscle	Dorsiflex: L4–5, deep peroneal nerve Plantarflex: S1–2, tibial nerve

0/5, no contraction; 1/5, minimal contraction, no movement; 2/5, movement in horizontal plane, full range of motion if gravity eliminated; 3/5, movement against gravity; 4/5, movement against minimal resistance; 5/5, unrestricted strength, movement against full resistance.

Source: Urman RD, Vadivelu N. *Pocket Pain Medicine*. 1st ed. Philadelphia, PA: Lippincott Williams & Wilkins; 2011:28–32.

Sensory Testing

Sensory Testing	
Nerve	Sensory dermatome (see Chapter 6 for dermatomal map)
L1	Inguinal crease
L2	Upper anterior thigh
L3	Anterior to medial knee
L4	Anterolateral thigh to anterior knee and great toe
L5	Lateral thigh to lateral knee, anterior shin, plantar and dorsal foot
S1	Posterolateral thigh to heel, lateral foot, little toe
S2	Posteromedial thigh to heel
S3–5	Genital/anal area

Source: Urman RD, Vadivelu N. *Pocket Pain Medicine*. 1st ed. Philadelphia, PA: Lippincott Williams & Wilkins; 2011:28–33.

Cervical and Lumbar Disk Herniation Patterns					
Disc	Root	Pain paresthesias	Sensory loss	Motor loss	Reflex loss
C4–C5	C5	Neck, shoulder, upper arm	Shoulder	Deltoid, biceps, infraspinatus	Biceps
C5–C6	C6	Neck, shoulder, lat. arm, radial forearm, thumb, & index finger	Lat. arm, radial forearm, thumb, & index finger	Biceps, brachioradialis	Biceps, brachioradialis, supinator
C6–C7	C7	Neck, lat arm, ring & index fingers	Radial forearm, index & middle fingers	Triceps, extensor carpi ulnaris	Triceps, supinator
C7–T1	C8	Ulnar forearm and hand	Ulnar half of ring finger, little finger	Intrinsic hand muscles, wrist extensors, flexor dig profundus	Finger flexion
L3–L4	L4	Anterior thigh, inner shin	Anteromedial thigh and shin, inner foot	Quadriceps	Patella
L4–L5	L5	Lat. thigh and calf, dorsum of foot, great toe	Lat calf and great toe	Extensor hallucis longus, ± foot dorsiflexion, invers, & evers	None
L5–S1	S1	Back of thigh, lateral posterior calf, lat. foot	Posterolat. calf, lat and sole of foot, smaller toes	Gastrocnemius ± foot eversion	Achilles

Figure 32-2 Algorithm for Initial Evaluation of Low Back Pain

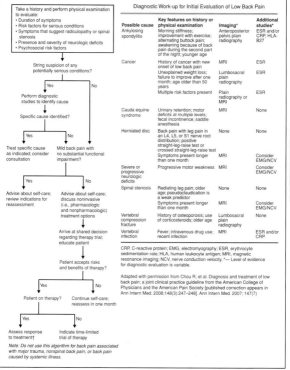

Take a history and perform physical examination to evaluate:
- Duration of symptoms
- Risk factors for serious conditions
- Symptoms that suggest radiculopathy or spinal stenosis
- Presence and severity of neurologic deficits
- Psychosocial risk factors

↓

String suspicion of any potentially serious conditions?

Yes → Perform diagnostic studies to identify cause → Specific cause identified?
- Yes → Treat specific cause as indicated; consider consultation
- No → Mild back pain with no substantial functional impairment?

No → Mild back pain with no substantial functional impairment?
- Yes → Advise about self-care; review indications for reassessment
- No → Advise about self-care; discuss noninvasive (i.e. pharmacologic and nonpharmacologic) treatment options

↓ Arrive at shared decision regarding therapy trial; educate patient

↓ Patient accepts risks and benefits of therapy?

Yes → Patient on therapy?
- Yes → Assess response to treatment†
- No → Indicate time-limited trial of therapy

No → Continue self-care; reassess in one month

Note: Do not use this algorithm for back pain associated with major trauma, nonspinal back pain, or back pain caused by systemic illness.

Diagnostic Work-up for Initial Evaluation of Low Back Pain

Possible cause	Key features on history or physical examination	Imaging*	Additional studies*
Ankylosing spondylitis	Morning stiffness; improvement with exercise; alternating buttock pain; awakening because of back pain during the second part of the night; younger age	Anteroposterior pelvis plain radiography	ESR and/or CRP, HLA-B27
Cancer	History of cancer with new onset of low back pain	MRI	ESR
	Unexplained weight loss; failure to improve after one month; age older than 50 years	Lumbosacral plain radiography	ESR
	Multiple risk factors present	Plain radiography or MRI	ESR
Cauda equine syndrome	Urinary retention; motor deficits at multiple levels; fecal incontinence; saddle anesthesia	MRI	None
Herniated disc	Back pain with leg pain in an L4, L5, or S1 nerve root distribution; positive straight-leg-raise test or crossed straight-leg-raise test	None	None
	Symptoms present longer than one month	MRI	Consider EMG/NCV
Severe or progressive neurologic deficits	Progressive motor weakness	MRI	Consider EMG/NCV
Spinal stenosis	Radiating leg pain; older age; pseudoclaudication is a weak predictor	None	None
	Symptoms present longer than one month	MRI	Consider EMG/NCV
Vertebral compression fracture	History of osteoporosis; use of corticosteroids; older age	Lumbosacral plain radiography	None
Vertebral infection	Fever; intravenous drug use; recent infection	MRI	ESR and/or CRP

CRP, C-reactive protein; EMG, electromyography; ESR, erythrocyte sedimentation rate; HLA, human leukocyte antigen; MRI, magnetic resonance imaging; NCV, nerve conduction velocity. *— Level of evidence for diagnostic evaluation is variable.

Adapted with permission from Chou R, et al. Diagnosis and treatment of low back pain: a joint clinical practice guideline from the American College of Physicians and the American Pain Society [published correction appears in Ann Intern Med. 2008;148(3):247–248]. Ann Intern Med. 2007; 147(7)

(Adapted from Crews JC. Multimodal pain management strategies for office-based & ambulatory procedures. *JAMA* 2002;288:629–32.)

Figure 32-3 Low Back Pain Treatment.

Nonpharmacologic Therapy

Mechanical
- Immobilization, bracing, splinting (in rare cases of instability)
- Cryotherapy (ice)
- Heat
- Physical therapy (musculoskeletal stretching/strengthening)
- Occupational therapy
- Aquatherapy (therapeutic movements in a pool)
- Movement therapies—yoga, tai chi, qi gong
- Lymphedema therapy
- Therapeutic massage
- Transcutaneous electrical nerve stimulation (TENS), iontophoresis
- Therapeutic ultrasound
- Manual therapies (massage, chiropractic treatment)
- Desensitization therapy

Psychology
- Cognitive behavioral therapy (CBT)
- Biofeedback
- Mindfulness, relaxation, distraction techniques

- Distraction techniques
- Co-morbidity management (depression, anxiety, catastrophizing, dependence)
- Lifestyle modification (smoking cessation), avoidance of triggers

Interventional
- Acupuncture, dry needling, trigger point injections
- Epidural/caudal steroid injection (ESI/CSI)
- Paravertebral blocks
- Selective nerve root block (SNRB)
- Facet joint injection (FJI), medial branch block (MBB), radiofrequency lesioning (RFL) of medial branch nerves
- Spinal cord stimulator (SCS)
- Vertebroplasty/kyphoplasty
- Intrathecal drug delivery system (IT pain pump)

Pharmacologic therapy*
Nonopioid
Inflammatory pain
- NSAIDs (ibuprofen, naproxen, ketorolac, diclofenac, etodolac, meloxicam, methyl salicylate/menthol)
- Steroids (oral, intra-articular, perineural, epidural, IM, IV)

Neuropathic & Central pain
- Anticonvulsants (gabapentin, pregabalin)
- SNRIs (duloxetine, milnacipran)
- TCAs (amitriptyline, nortriptyline, desipramine)
- Na^+ channel blockers (lidocaine topical cream/patch/IM/ IV), mexiletine, topiramate)
- NMDA receptor antagonists (ketamine, memantine, dextromethorphan, Mg^{2+})

Nociceptive pain
- Antispasmodics (muscle spasm related pain, e.g., cyclobenzaprine, tizanidine, baclofen, diazepam/lorazepam)
- Acetaminophen and NSAIDs also effective, especially if inflammatory pain is also present

Nonspecific pain
- Acetaminophen
- Alpha agonists (clonidine, dexmedetomidine, guanfacine)

Opioids

*While many of these medications are used commonly for pain treatment by those familiar with their use, evidence for efficacy for pain treatment is mixed and limited for many. This list is not exhaustive.

Interventional Pain Treatment
Blocks
- Can provide significant pain relief but are often temporary and require repeat procedures
- Some procedures can be performed as diagnostic tests (facet injections, MBBs, selective nerve root blocks)

Neuromodulation (Spinal Cord Stimulation [SCS])
- Most effective in radicular pain, rather than axial pain
- Mechanism not clearly understood; initially believed to be "gate control theory" (activation of dorsally located inhibitory neurons and interneurons to counteract excitatory input at the dorsal horn of the spinal cord [the "gate"]); current data suggest alterations in neurochemistry and reduction in hyperexcitability of wide-dynamic range neurons in spinal cord
- Placement of electrodes in the epidural space; a trial using externalized electrode extensions done prior to permanent implantation
- Outcomes vary depending on pt selection

Surgical Procedures
- Discectomy, laminectomy, spinal fusion (open or minimally invasive [MIS]); indicated for acute evacuation of hematoma, acute cauda equina syndrome, progressive/severe neuromotor deficit with definable etiology after 6–8 wk of treatment, infection, trauma/fracture, tumor, severe anatomic deformities

> Nonsurgical interventional procedures should be avoided if the pt is on anticoagulants, has a coagulopathy or infection at the site of the injection. Risks include inadvertent intraneural, epidural, intrathecal, subdural, and intravascular injection, as well as local anesthetic toxicity. ASRA guidelines for interventional procedures in pts on anticoagulation can be found here:

http://journals.lww.com/rapm/Fulltext/2015/05000/Interventional_Spine_and_Pain_Procedures_in.2.aspx (*Reg Anesth Pain Med* 2015;40(3):182–212)

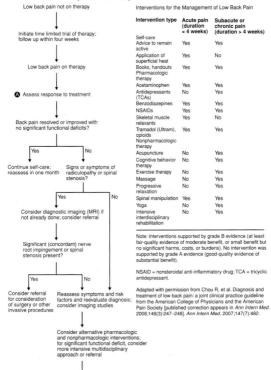

Algorithm for the Management of Low Back Pain in Adults

Low back pain not on therapy

↓

Initiate time limited trial of therapy; follow up within four weeks

↓

Low back pain on therapy

↓

Ⓐ Assess response to treatment

↓

Back pain resolved or improved with no significant functional deficits?

Yes → Continue self-care; reassess in one month

No → Signs or symptoms of radiculopathy or spinal stenosis?

Yes → Consider diagnostic imaging (MRI) if not already done; consider referral

↓

Significant (concordant) nerve root impingement or spinal stenosis present?

Yes → Consider referral for consideration of surgery or other invasive procedures

No → Reassess symptoms and risk factors and reevaluate diagnosis; consider imaging studies

↓

Consider alternative pharmacologic and nonpharmacologic interventions; for significant functional deficit, consider more intensive multidisciplinary approach or referral

↓

Return to assessment of treatment response → Go to **Ⓐ**

MRI = magnetic resonance imaging.

Interventions for the Management of Low Back Pain

Intervention type	Acute pain (duration < 4 weeks)	Subacute or chronic pain (duration > 4 weeks)
Self-care		
Advice to remain active	Yes	Yes
Application of superficial heat	Yes	No
Books, handouts	Yes	Yes
Pharmacologic therapy		
Acetaminophen	Yes	Yes
Antidepressants (TCAs)	No	Yes
Benzodiazepines	Yes	Yes
NSAIDs	Yes	Yes
Skeletal muscle relaxants	Yes	No
Tramadol (Ultram), opioids	Yes	Yes
Nonpharmacologic therapy		
Acupuncture	No	Yes
Cognitive behavior therapy	No	Yes
Exercise therapy	No	Yes
Massage	No	Yes
Progressive relaxation	No	Yes
Spinal manipulation	Yes	Yes
Yoga	No	Yes
Intensive interdisciplinary rehabilitation	No	Yes

Note: Interventions supported by grade B evidence (at least fair-quality evidence of moderate benefit, or small benefit but no significant harms, costs, or burdens). No intervention was supported by grade A evidence (good-quality evidence of substantial benefit).

NSAID = nonsteroidal anti-inflammatory drug; TCA = tricyclic antidepressant.

Adapted with permission from Chou R, et al. Diagnosis and treatment of low back pain: a joint clinical practice guideline from the American College of Physicians and the American Pain Society [published correction appears in Ann Intern Med. 2008;148(3):247–248]. Ann Intern Med. 2007;147(7):482.

Red Flags That May Require Emergent/Urgent Dx and Treatment
New fracture
Major trauma
Minor trauma/heavy lifting in older osteoporotic pts
Age <20 or >50 (in the absence of trauma)
Hx of cancer or constitutional symptoms (e.g., fever, weight loss, fatigue)
Infection risk factors (e.g., immunosuppressed, IV drug abuse, recent invasive proc.)
Severe, unrelenting nighttime pain
Cauda equina syndrome: Saddle anesthesia, bowel/bladder dysfx, rapidly progressing neurologic deficits

Acute low back pain treatment:
- 4–6 wk since onset
- 90% of all pts with back pain have resolution within 6 wk
- Usually myofascial in origin

- Must rule out more serious conditions (see "Red Flags")
- Diagnostic imaging (consider plain film radiography, CT, MRI, depending on severity and urgency of symptoms) is not recommended unless red flags present
- Goal is to return to normal lifestyle quickly
- Usually responds to noninvasive treatment:
- Set expectations, pt education, self-care
- Modification of current activity level, gentle physical therapy
- Develop home exercise program
- Heat or ice
- Pharmacologic therapy (NSAIDs, acetaminophen, muscle relaxants, usually does not require opioid therapy)

Subacute low back pain treatment:
- 4–6 wk to 6 mo since onset
- Goal is to slow and/or stop progression to chronic back pain with return to normal lifestyle
- Diagnostic imaging (plain film radiography, CT, MRI depending on severity and urgency of symptoms)
- Physical therapy, and also develop home exercise program
- Consider referral to spine/pain specialist, psychosocial evaluation
- Nonemergent radiculopathy: Consider surgical evaluation and minimally invasive interventional procedures (e.g., epidural steroid injections)
- NSAIDs, acetaminophen, muscle relaxants, antidepressants, +/– opioids

Chronic low back pain treatment:
- >6 mo since onset
- Detailed Hx and physical examination
- Goal is to limit symptoms with functional improvement
- Diagnostic imaging (plain film radiography, CT, MRI repeat imaging if necessary, e.g., new onset or change in symptoms)
- Rehabilitative therapy, including physical and occupational therapy
- Referral to spine/pain specialist (for interventional procedures)
- Psychosocial evaluation, query for pain in other somatic sites, substance use Hx especially if pt receiving protracted prescriptions for opioids
- Consideration of adjuncts like yoga, acupuncture, cognitive behavioral therapy
- Long-term treatment: Noninvasive and invasive therapy (see Treatment section above)

LUMBAR SPINAL CANAL STENOSIS

Pathophysiology
- Degeneration of discs, joints, and/or vertebrae lead to instability causing osteophyte formation, hypertrophy, and calcification of the posterior longitudinal ligament, leading to narrowing of the spinal canal (central +/– or lateral recess)
- May result either in central canal and/or foraminal stenosis
- Stenosis may stabilize or progress

Evaluation
- Hx and physical examination
- Examination can be relatively normal; result of imaging studies important for diagnosis
- Constant or intermittent low back pain, radiates to one/both lower extremities
- Often pts walk leaning forward ("shopping cart posture")
- Loss of lumbar lordosis
- Pain mainly perceived with walking, especially downhill and/or standing
- Neurogenic claudication (bilateral posterior leg pain worsening with ambulation, relieved with sitting and leaning forward); important to consider vascular claudication in the differential diagnosis
- Central stenosis: Axial and radicular pain, radicular pain usually nondermatomal (e.g., lower extremities ache with walking); otherwise normal lower-extremity neurologic examination
- Foraminal stenosis (can cause radicular pain): May present with sensory, motor, or reflex changes along dermatomal distribution; exacerbating factors: Walking (especially downstairs), standing, extension (buckling of ligamentum flavum and disc protrusion), relieving factors: Rest, sitting/lying down, flexion
- Diagnostic imaging: Very important for diagnosis
- CT: Visualization of bony and ligamentous changes
- MRI: Visualization of spinal cord and nerve root involvement

Treatment
- Noninterventional therapy: Refer to treatment section in introduction
- Interventional therapy:
  - Central canal stenosis: Interlaminar/transforaminal epidural (if single-level stenosis)/caudal steroid injection (if multilevel stenosis)
  - Foraminal stenosis: Epidural steroid injection, SNRB. Nonparticulate steroid and live fluoroscopy should be used with the transforaminal approach to minimize risk of spinal cord injury from vascular damage/embolism
  - Interspinous devices (e.g., X-stop to ↓ extension, disc compression with milder stenosis)
  - MILD procedure (percutaneous lumbar decompression)
  - Spinal cord stimulation (if radicular component)
  - Intrathecal drug delivery system (especially if fractures or stenosis related to malignancy)
  - Surgical procedures

FAILED BACK SURGERY SYNDROME (FBSS)

Pathophysiology
- Diagnosis of failed back surgery syndrome is not a specific diagnosis, *per se*, and is discouraged from use *in lieu* of a more specific diagnosis or combination of diagnoses
- Causes: Scar tissue in the spinal canal, development of adhesions, nerve injury during surgery, recurrent disc herniation, facet joint arthropathy above/below the area of fusion, instrumentation irritation of nerves/bone, CRPS
- Persistence or recurrence of original pain or development of new pain

Evaluation
- Hx and physical examination as above
- Hx of lumbar surgery (obtain preop and postop symptoms, operative findings, and levels of instrumentation are important to evaluate new findings)
- Diagnostic imaging:
  - Plain film radiography: Evaluate bony/instrument changes
  - CT: Evaluate bone and canal space in setting of MRI incompatible hardware
  - MRI: Evaluate soft tissue in setting of MRI-compatible hardware or after surgeries without placement of hardware

Treatment
- Difficult to treat
- Treatment often palliative in nature
- Co-existing mood and sleep d/o common, central sensitization may develop
- Noninterventional therapy: Refer to Treatment section in Introduction
- Interventional therapy:
  - Repeat surgery typically ineffective for chronic symptoms
  - Epidural steroids not durably effective for chronic symptoms
  - Spinal cord stimulator may be useful especially for radicular pain
- Functional rehabilitation programs incorporating intensive outpatient cognitive behavioral therapy and rehabilitative activity may improve function and coping skills long term

OSTEOARTHRITIS VS. RHEUMATOID ARTHRITIS

Osteoarthritis vs. Rheumatoid Arthritis		
	Osteoarthritis	**Rheumatoid arthritis**
Age of onset	Usually >40 y of age	Any age
Speed of onset	Slow (y)	Rapid (wk–mo)
Affected joints	Often limited to one set of joints (monoarticular): Often asymmetrical; DIP and large weight-bearing joints (knee, hip)	Often small (hands, feet cervical spine) and occasionally larger joints (elbow, knee); polyarticular; often symmetrical involvements
Morning stiffness	<1 h: May recur during d	>1 h
Joint pathology	Noninflammatory, "wear and tear"	Inflammatory synovitis
Joint symptoms	Joints painful often without swelling; crepitus; gradual onset, often unilateral	Joints painful, swollen, warm, stiff, more rapid onset; often symmetrical

Associated symptoms	None	Generalized malaise, constitutional symptoms, and involvement of other organ systems
Systemic symptoms	None	Fatigue, generalized malaise

Source: Urman RD, Vadivelu N. *Pocket Pain Medicine*. 1st ed. Philadelphia, PA: Lippincott Williams & Wilkins; 2011:31–36.

PERIPHERAL NEUROPATHIC PAIN

- Causes include diabetes, cancer, herpes zoster, infections, trauma, autoimmune dz, surgery, compression (carpel tunnel, piriformis syndrome, thoracic outlet syndrome)

ALGORITHM FOR MANAGEMENT OF NEUROPATHIC PAIN

	Algorithm for the Management of Neuropathic Pain	
Step 1	Pain assessment, Hx and physical examination, obtain release of information to review previous diagnostic studies, and treatment records	
Step 2	Consider nonpharmacologic modalities (physiotherapies; psychological interventions, such as cognitive behavioral therapy; or early referral for targeted interventional therapy to facilitate diagnosis and effect treatment)	
Step 3	Initiate 1st-line monotherapy (gabapentin or pregabalin or TCA or SNRI)	
Response	*Ineffective or not tolerated*	*Partial treatment response*
Step 4	Switch to alternative 1st-line drug monotherapy (TCA or SNRI or gabapentin or pregabalin)	Consider adding 1st-line drug (TCA or SNRI or gabapentin or pregabalin)
Response	*Ineffective or not tolerated*	*Partial treatment response*
Step 5	Initiate monotherapy with tramadol or opioid analgesic; consider use of opioid risk screening tool, medication management agreement, and informed consent	Consider adding tramadol or opioid analgesic; consider use of opioid risk screening tool, medication management agreement, and informed consent
Response	*Ineffective or not tolerated*	
Step 6	Refer pt to pain specialty clinic for consideration of 3rd-line drugs, interventional treatments, neuromodulation, and pain rehabilitation programs	

Source: Urman RD, Vadivelu N. *Pocket Pain Medicine*. 1st ed. Philadelphia, PA: Lippincott Williams & Wilkins; 2011:26–29.

Peripheral Neuropathy

Pathophysiology
- Most commonly from diabetes and subsequent microvascular injury involving small blood vessels that supply nerves; toxic, metabolic, and infectious (HIV) causes as well
- Associated with sensory, motor, & autonomic symptoms
- >80% of peripheral neuropathy is idiopathic

Symptoms
- *Sensory:* Burning, pricking, pins-and-needle, shooting, electric sensation
- *Motor:* Distal impaired fine coordination & proximal weakness (difficulty climbing stairs)
- *Autonomic:* Vasomotor and sudomotor changes

Evaluation
- Assessment of the appearance of the feet, presence of ulceration, and ankle reflexes
- Normal results on vibration testing (128 Hz tuning fork) or monofilament make large fiber peripheral neuropathy from diabetes less likely
- Nerve conduction tests may show ↓ peripheral nerve fx, but not appropriate routine test

Treatment
- Mostly preventive & symptomatic measures
- Optimize glycemic control if diabetic
- Pharmacologic treatment: Topical (lidoderm patches, capsaicin), tricyclic antidepressants (amitriptyline, nortriptyline, desipramine), selective norepinephrine reuptake inhibitors (duloxetine, venlafaxine), anticonvulsants (pregabalin)

- Physical therapy, including gait training
- *Transcutaneous electrical nerve stimulation* (TENS) and *interferential current* (IFC)
- Other (α-lipoic acid, methylcobalamin, c-peptide, photo energy therapy)

POSTHERPETIC NEURALGIA (PHN)

- Incidence 131/100,000 per y; more likely in elderly or immunocompromised pts; 20% with pain at 3 mo and 15% with pain at 2 y; incidence ↑ with each decade over the age of 50
- Antivirals and steroids in the acute phase lessen symptoms but do not reduce the incidence of PHN
- Live attenuated varicella zoster vaccine reduces incidence of PHN and is recommended for all those over age of 50 and in immunocompromised
- Reactivation of varicella virus in ganglion → ganglionitis & segmental peripheral neuritis

Symptoms
- Most (50%) AHN and PHN occurs in the thoracic dermatomes (especially T4–6)
- Most common sites on head/neck: V1 (10–20%) and cervical dermatomes (10–20%)

Evaluation
- Hx of zoster; although rare, *zoster sine herpete* or PHN without rash, can occur
- Physical examination will reveal allodynia, hyper- or hypoesthesia in dermatomal distribution

Treatment
- Topical lidocaine or capsaicin
- Adjuvant analgesics: Gabapentin, pregabalin, tricyclic antidepressants
- Tramadol and morphine/other opioids
- Alternative therapy for symptom relief (e.g., biofeedback, acupuncture)
- Interventional therapy
  - Stellate ganglion blockade: May provide symptomatic improvement (often combination of local anesthetic and corticosteroid) and prevent PHN
  - Intercostal nerve blockade or neurolysis
  - Spinal cord or peripheral nerve stimulation
  - General reference for above: *N Engl J Med* 2014;371:1526–1533

TRIGEMINAL NEURALGIA

Incidence
- Annual occurrence is 4/100,000
- Onset rare before age 35, usually occurs >50 y of age
- Female-to-male ratio is 1.7:1
- Right side involvement is more common
- Tic douloureux refers to the grimace that occurs with pain attacks

Etiology
- Most commonly idiopathic
- Microneuromas of CNV or vascular compression/pulsation (usually by superior cerebellar artery)
- Other causes include aneurysm, multiple sclerosis (MS), tumor (schwannomas of CN V, extraneural compression by tumor of surrounding tissue), trauma, chronic basal meningitis, diabetes mellitus (DM), congenital anomalies (Note: Aneurysm, MS, tumor, trauma, DM, congenital anomalies should be accompanied by other physical signs and symptoms)

Symptoms
- Severe episodic lancinating, sharp, stabbing, unilateral pain in the distribution of one or more of the trigeminal nerve branches, most often V2
- Unilateral, intermittent
- Although episodes typically last only a few s and come in consecutive chains, each total attack may last up to 15–20 min, occurring daily or several times per wk/mo; attacks triggered by often innocuous contact with trigger zone
- Pts usually asymptomatic between attacks
- With severe attacks, pts can become easily dehydrated from avoiding beverages and food, and suicidality may develop. Important to monitor.

Evaluation
- Hx
- Physical examination is often normal. If there is a sensory deficit, a more peripheral trigeminal neuropathic pain (like from an nerve injury during a dental procedure) should be considered

- Facial pain in the trigeminal distribution that is not typical of classic TGN is atypical facial pain and may be part of a central sensitization syndrome

> Loss of corneal reflexes, sensory changes, pain that crosses the midline and bilateral pain at the same time → rule out other causes

- Diagnostic imaging: Head CT or MRI/MRA

Treatment
- Pharmacologic therapy
  - 80% of pts respond to treatment with carbamazepine (rigid lab monitoring for bone marrow suppression required); improvement sometimes occurs within hours; up to 20% of pts, especially elderly pts, have side effects like ataxia, drowsiness, and confusion; bone marrow depression has also been reported); oxcarbazepine has similar efficacy with less significant side effects
  - Clonazepam, gabapentin, baclofen, tricyclic antidepressants
  - If immediate relief is required, use IV lidocaine or phenytoin until pt is able to tolerate oral medication
  - 2nd line: Consider opioids
  - Alternative therapy (e.g., biofeedback, relaxation therapy, acupuncture)
- Interventional therapy
  - Trigeminal nerve or Gasserian ganglion block (mostly combination of preservative-free local anesthetic and corticosteroid)
  - Neurolysis, percutaneous rhizotomy, gamma knife radiosurgery
  - Percutaneous stereotactic radiofrequency thermal rhizotomy
  - Stereotactic thalamic or motor cortex stimulation
  - Microvascular decompression surgery (e.g., Jannetta procedure)
- Surgical treatment of atypical facial pain in the trigeminal distribution that does not meet criteria for classic TGN and does not have a known compressive lesion typically results in poor outcomes; these cases should be treated like neuropathic pain from other causes

---

COMPLEX REGIONAL PAIN SYNDROME (CRPS)

- **Type I (90%):** No identifiable nerve injury
- **Type II (10%)** (Identifiable inciting nerve injury, also known as causalgia)
- Although initially believed secondary to sympathetic dysregulation, increasing evidence CRPS may be a central nervous system inflammatory process with widespread sensory abnormalities, and abnormal cortical restructuring

Signs and Symptoms of CRPS
- Diagnosis
  - Diagnosis is clinical, using the Budapest Criteria
  - Budapest clinical diagnostic criteria for CRPS
    1. Continuing pain, which is disproportionate to any inciting event
    2. Must report at least 1 symptom in *3 of the 4* following categories:
       - *Sensory:* Reports of hyperesthesia and/or allodynia
       - *Vasomotor:* Reports of temperature asymmetry and/or skin color changes and/or skin color asymmetry
       - *Sudomotor/Edema:* Reports of edema and/or sweating changes and/or sweating asymmetry
       - *Motor/Trophic:* Reports of decreased range of motion and/or motor dysfunction (weakness, tremor, dystonia) and/or trophic changes (hair, nail, skin)
    3. Must display at least one sign at time of evaluation in *2 or more* of the following categories:
       - *Sensory:* Evidence of hyperalgesia (to pinprick) and/or allodynia (to light touch and/or temperature sensation and/or deep somatic pressure and/or joint movement)
       - *Vasomotor:* Evidence of temperature asymmetry (>1°C) and/or skin color changes and/or asymmetry
       - *Sudomotor/Edema:* Evidence of edema and/or sweating changes and/or sweating asymmetry
       - *Motor/Trophic:* Evidence of decreased range of motion and/or motor dysfunction (weakness, tremor, dystonia) and/or trophic changes (hair, nail, skin)
    4. There is no other diagnosis that better explains the signs and symptoms
       Appendix II *(Pain 2010;150(2):266–274)*

- Laboratory or radiographic findings are rarely useful in making the diagnosis or effecting treatment outcomes

Treatment
- Physical therapy to prevent functional loss is the primary treatment goal, and the treatment with the most robust efficacy
- Pharmacologic therapy
  - Evidence is empirical, and efficacy of pharmacologic agents is variable
  - Strongest evidence for IV bisphosphonates, IV lidocaine, and ketamine with variable results
  - Antineuropathic agents (gabapentin, tricyclic antidepressants, mexiletine) can be trialed as for other cases of neuropathic pain
  - Opioid trials reasonable, but little data to support chronic use
- Cognitive behavioral therapy/coping skills/psychological support
- Evidence of efficacy with transcranial magnetic stimulation and graded motor imagery (mirror box therapy)
- Interventional therapy
  - Stellate ganglion or lumbar sympathetic blockade may give symptomatic improvement, strong evidence for durable efficacy is lacking
    - Stellate ganglion located at C7
    - Volumetric local anesthetic blocks may result in Horner syndrome, but this is from incidental blockade of the superior cervical ganglion; sign of successful blockade is increased temperature in the ipsilateral hand
    - Recurrent laryngeal nerve blockade will occur and results in hoarseness; temporary phrenic nerve paralysis also occurs but usually asymptomatic; caution in those with limited pulmonary reserve or contralateral phrenic nerve paralysis
    - Serious complications include pneumothorax, vascular injury/hematoma, or epidural/intrathecal spread resulting in cardiorespiratory collapse
  - Lumbar sympathetic ganglion located between L2 and L4
    - Successful block with local anesthetic will result in temperature ↑ in ipsilateral foot
    - Risks include retroperitoneal hematoma, inadvertent lumbar plexus block with ipsilateral leg weakness, epidural spread with bilateral leg weakness
  - Spinal cord stimulation is effective in carefully selected pts

OCCIPITAL NEURALGIA

Etiology
- Pain can be neuropathic, myofascial, or referred, as well as secondary to osteoarthritic changes of the cervical spine

Symptoms
- Pain in distribution of greater and lesser occipital nerve
- Unilateral constant, dull, achy, with paroxysmal sharp stabbing sensations
- Pain associated with occipital nerve tenderness, myofascial pain, and trigger points in the cervical musculature

Evaluation
- Hx and physical examination
  - Tenderness to palpation/Tinel sign over base of occipital nerve

Treatment
- Pharmacologic therapy
  - 1st line: NSAIDs, anticonvulsants, TCAs
  - 2nd line: Opioids
- Alternative therapy: Biofeedback, relaxation therapy, yoga, acupuncture, TENS
- Interventional therapy
  - Occipital nerve block with preservative-free local anesthetic +/− corticosteroids
  - Upper cervical medial branch block with preservative-free local anesthetic/corticosteroids
  - Upper cervical facet joint injection with preservative-free local anesthetic +/− corticosteroids
  - RFA of C2–4 medial branch or occipital nerve after diagnostic block
  - Botulinum toxin injection in cervical musculature especially for myofascial pain component
  - Occipital nerve neurolysis via alcohol, phenol injection
  - Occipital nerve stimulator
  - Occipital nerve decompression, occipital neurectomy, or C2 ganglionectomy

Primary Chronic Headache Syndromes
- Tension: Most common form; mostly described as constant pressure, often bilateral; can radiate from neck, back, eyes, or other muscle groups
- Migraine: See below
- Medication overuse headache

Clinical Evaluation
- Hx: Quality, severity, location, duration, time of onset, exacerbating/alleviating factors; rule out any secondary headache d/o or underlying pathology ("worst HA ever," awakens from sleep, vomiting, focal neurologic signs, constitutional sx)
- Medication use Hx, substance abuse Hx
- Chronic HA of any type often a part of central sensitization syndromes with associated mood and sleep disturbance; evaluate as per fibromyalgia

Chronic Migraine

Epidemiology
- Migraine in 12% of general population; 2–5% of the general population has chronic migraine diagnosis; F > M; peak incidence ages 20–40
- Risk factors include obesity, mood d/o, and caffeine and medication overuse (>10 d/mo)

Diagnosis
- Chronic migraine defined as >15 headache d per mo for >3 mo, in which >8 d meet diagnostic criteria for migraine with or without aura
- Unilateral (chronic most likely bilateral), retro-orbital, throbbing or pulsatile headache; lasts 4–72 h
- Often accompanied by nausea, vomiting, photophobia, or aura
- "POUNDing": Pulsatile; duration 4–72 h; Unilateral; Nausea & vomiting; Disabling Likelihood ratio (LR) 3.5 if 3 criteria are met, LR 24 if ≥4 criteria are met

Treatment
- Eliminate triggers, modify risk factors
- Prophylaxis: TCA, β-blockers, CCB, valproic acid best for episodic migraine; topiramate and botulinum toxin A best evidence for prophylaxis of chronic migraine
- Cognitive behavioral therapies, exercise, and other nonpharmacologic interventions as per treatment of central sensitization syndromes

(Source: Lipton RB. *Headache* 2011;51(suppl 2):77–83; Diener HC, Solbach K, Holle K, et al. *Clin Med* 2015;15(4): 344–350)

PHANTOM LIMB PAIN

Incidence
- 60–80% experience phantom pain after amputation; severe in 10–15%
- This is different than stump pain, which is pain at the site of amputation, usually related to peripheral neuroma or mechanical issues with prosthetics
- Pre-existing pain (i.e., in vascular amputees) a risk factor for chronicity of phantom pain; psychological factors, especially if amputation traumatic, also play a role in intensity and chronicity of pain

Etiology
- Peripheral, spinal, and supraspinal mechanisms involved
- Peripheral factors like stump neuroma or autonomic hyperexcitability in the stump may exacerbate phantom limb pain
- Hyperexcitability of spinal cord neurons occurs
- Cortical reorganization occurs after amputation, and the amount of reorganization directly correlates with intensity and chronicity of pain

Treatment
- Pharmacologic
  - Treat as per neuropathic pain; results are mixed
- Interventional
  - Prophylactic treatment with epidural analgesia, regional anesthesia, and perioperative antineuropathic agents like gabapentin may reduce immediate postop stump pain, but results on prevention of phantom pain are inconsistent to date
  - Once phantom pain has developed, peripheral nerve blocks, lumbar sympathetic blocks, or spinal cord stimulation may reduce excitatory input from the periphery

into the hyperexcitable spinal cord and abnormally reorganized cerebral cortex, but robust data showing durable significant improvements are lacking
- Nonpharmacologic/noninterventional options
  - Psychological support/CBT
  - Physical therapy/early prosthetic use
  - Graded motor imagery/mirror box therapy to prevent and modulate cortical reorganization

---

VISCERAL PAIN

Incidence
- Primarily chronic pelvic and abdominal pain
- Each affect ~10 million US adults, more common in women
- Visceral afferents become more sensitized in response to injury, inflammation, and stress
  - Incidence of preadolescent physical or sexual abuse/other psychological trauma significantly associated with the development of functional abdominal pain in children and multiple somatic complaints including irritable bowel syndrome, chronic pelvic pain, and fibromyalgia as adults

Symptoms
- Poorly localized secondary to complex innervation and viscerosomatic convergence of somatic and autonomic nervous systems
- Dull, aching, crampy
- Distention and contraction of hollow organs worsen pain
- Visceral autonomic dysfunction (problems with autonomically mediated sexual, urinary, and gastrointestinal function) commonly coexists with pain
- Exacerbated by stress

Evaluation
- Exclude modifiable pathology
  - Hx
    - Hx of past psychological trauma and current psychological distress
    - Presence of bowel, bladder, or sexual dysfunction, including symptoms of interstitial cystitis and irritable bowel syndrome
    - Consider modifiable contribution of opioid-induced bowel dysfunction (pain with distention of intestines secondary to constipation; sphincter dysfunction)
- Examination
  - Evaluate for abdominal wall or pelvic floor (somatic) contributions to pain
    - Rectus sheath, abdominal oblique, pelvic floor spasm, or trigger points
    - Look for sensory deficit or hyperesthesia/allodynia consistent with scar neuroma or intercostal/ilioinguinal/genitofemoral neuralgia from prior surgical intervention
  - Abdominal distention, poorly localized pain, lack of abdominal wall findings more consistent with visceral pain
- Treatment
  - Somatic/neuropathic components from abdominal wall/pelvic floor:
    - If somatic component, use NSAIDs, muscle relaxants, physical therapy, TENS unit, topical lidocaine, trigger point injections
    - Neuropathic source from the abdominal wall/pelvic floor may be treated with antineuropathic medications, peripheral nerve blocks, i.e., ilioinguinal, genitofemoral, pudendal, transversus abdominis plane (TAP) blocks
  - Visceral component
    - Minimize opioids to reduce opioid-induced bowel dysfunction
    - Gabapentin/pregabalin, TCA/SNRIs, other antineuropathics for visceral hypersensitivity
    - Psychological interventions including cognitive behavioral therapy, stress reduction critical
    - Celiac plexus block (pancreatitis, renal dz, upper abdominal surgery, or hypersensitivity)
      - Celiac plexus innervates from GE junction to splenic flexure of colon with sympathetic contributions from T5–12 splanchnic nerves
      - Inferior to crus of diaphragm, anterior to celiac artery at T12 level
      - Local anesthetic blockade results in hypotension and diarrhea from unopposed parasympathetic action
      - Complications include pneumothorax, retroperitoneal bleed, damage to kidneys/bowel, epidural spread

- • Superior hypogastric plexus block (endometriosis, interstitial cystitis, pelvic surgery, or hypersensitivity)
  - • Innervates pelvic viscera, including bladder and reproductive organs
  - • Located anterior to the L5/S1 disc
  - • Complications include L5 paresthesia/injury, retroperitoneal hematoma, bowel/bladder injury
- • Ganglion impar block
  - • Single unpaired terminal sympathetic ganglion located anterior to sacrococcygeal junction
  - • Used for distal rectal, vaginal, urethral, anal pain
- • Neurolytic visceral plexus blocks and neuromodulatory spinal cord stimulation have been used for chronic nonmalignant pain with variable success

FIBROMYALGIA

(JAMA 2014;311(15):1547–1555)

Incidence
- • 2–8% of the general population
- • The 2nd most common d/o seen by rheumatologist (after OA)
- • Female-to-male ratio is **2:1**; family members of affected 8× as likely to have fibromyalgia as well

Etiology
- • Musculoskeletal pain of unknown etiology (genetic, infectious, environmental, hormonal predisposing factors all described); sleep and mood abnormalities the norm
- • Commonly predated by multiple somatic complaints, like functional abdominal pain and headache, in childhood. Abuse, trauma, and/or psychological stress in childhood also ↑ risk of developing fibromyalgia 2-fold
- • Mechanism: Central sensitization resulting in heightened pain sensitivity (blockade of N-methyl-D-aspartate [NMDA] receptors may diminish pain)
- • Other associated findings: Abnormal nonrapid eye movement (REM) sleep, diminished hypothalamic–pituitary axis, growth hormone deficiency, central hypodopaminergia, abnormal serotonin metabolism, muscle disuse, or deconditioning
- • Polymorphisms of genes in serotoninergic, dopaminergic, and catecholaminergic systems; abnormalities in pain processing shown on functional MRI

Symptoms
- • Dz complex entails pain plus three key domains: Mood, sleep, and stress
- • Classic symptoms are widespread/diffuse chronic pain patterns and include allodynia or dysesthesia, frequently symmetric distribution, fatigue, weakness, chronic sleep disturbances, functional bowel disturbances, pelvic pain, headache, TMD, anxiety, depression, PTSD
- • Fibromyalgia is considered a central sensitization syndrome, or centralized pain d/o, reflecting the underlying abnormality in sensory processing by the CNS

Evaluation
- • **ACR Preliminary Diagnostic Criteria** (Arthritis Care & Res 2010;62(5):600–610)
- • Tender points no longer felt to be relevant to diagnosis
- • Laboratory or other diagnostic studies useful only to rule out other rheumatologic/ infectious causes of widespread pain
- • Pt satisfies diagnostic criteria for fibromyalgia if 3 clinical conditions are met:
  - • Widespread pain index (WPI) ≥7 and symptom severity (SS) scale score ≥5 or WPI 3–6 and SS scale score ≥9
  - • Symptoms have been present at a similar level for at least 3 mo
  - • The pt does not have a d/o that would otherwise explain the pain
    - • WPI calculates number of areas in which pt had pain over the last wk (total score between 0 and 19)
    - • The SS scale score is the sum of the severity of the 3 symptoms (fatigue, waking unrefreshed, cognitive symptoms) plus the extent (severity) of somatic symptoms in general. The final score between 0 and 12.
- A sample diagnostic survey incorporating these criteria: Figure 32-4

Treatment
- • Alternative therapy
  - • Education (fibromyalgia knowledge, nutrition, physical and mental health), aerobic exercise, and cognitive–behavioral therapy all have strong evidence for efficacy for durable efficacy and functional improvement

Figure 32-4 Example of patient self-report for the assessment of fibromyalgia based in Criteria in the 2011 Modification of the ACR Preliminary Diagnostic Criteria for Fibromyalgia.

Widespread Pain Index
(1 point per check box; score range: 0–19 points)

(1) Please indicate if you have had pain or tenderness **during the past 7 days** in the areas shown below.
Check the boxes in the diagram for each area in which you have had pain or tenderness.

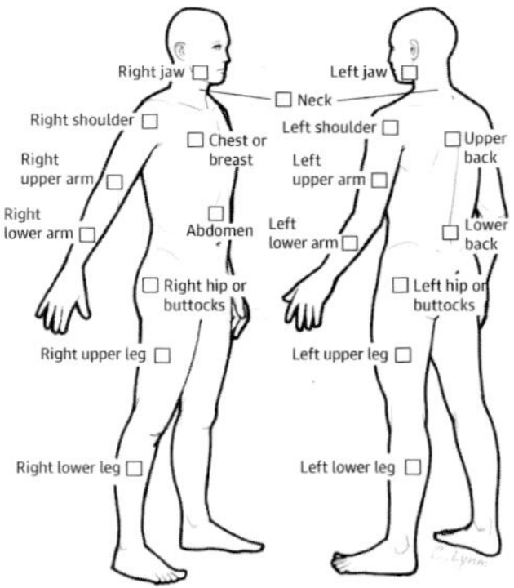

Symptom Severity
(score range: 0–12 points)

(2) For each symptom listed below, use the following scale to indicate the severity of the symptom **during the past 7 days**.

- **No problem**
- **Slight or mild problem**: generally mild or intermittent
- **Moderate problem**: considerable problems; often present and/or at a moderate level
- **Severe problem**: continuous, life-disturbing problems

	No problem	Slight or mild problem	Moderate problem	Severe problem
Points	0	1	2	3
A. Fatigue	☐	☐	☐	☐
B. Trouble thinking or remembering	☐	☐	☐	☐
C. Waking up tired (unrefreshed)	☐	☐	☐	☐

(3) During the **past 6 mo** have you had any of the following symptoms?

Points	0	1
A. Pain or cramps in lower abdomen	☐ No	☐ Yes
B. Depression	☐ No	☐ Yes
C. Headache	☐ No	☐ Yes

Additional criteria (no score)

(4) Have the symptoms in questions 2 and 3 and widespread pain been present at a similar level for at **least 3 mo**?

☐ No ☐ Yes

(5) Do you have a disorder that would otherwise explain the pain?

☐ No ☐ Yes

ACR indicates American College of Rheumatology. Scoring information is shown in Berry Red. The pble score ranges from 0–31 points; a score ≥13 points is consistent with a diagnosis of fibromyalgia. (Adapted from Clauw D. *JAMA* 2014;311(15):1547–1555.)

- Trigger points, yoga, acupuncture, myofascial release, and tai chi all have some evidence of efficacy, although clinical trials limited
- Pharmacologic therapy
  - 1st-line (strong evidence) anticonvulsants (e.g., gabapentin, pregabalin), tricyclic antidepressants (e.g., amitriptyline), SNRIs (e.g., milnacipran, duloxetine, venlafaxine)
  - Secondary to overactive endogenous opioid system in pts, exogenous opioids ineffective, and may lead to hyperalgesia; tramadol may have some efficacy related to its serotonin and norepinephrine uptake
  - NSAIDs and steroids also ineffective for generalized pain of fibromyalgia

---

CANCER PAIN

- Somatic, neuropathic, cancer-related bone pain & visceral pain, or combination
- Multiple etiologies: E.g., plexopathies, metastasis, procedure-related pain (postmastectomy/post-thoracotomy pain syndrome, phantom pain, radiation-induced neuritis, polyneuropathy from chemotherapy)

Treatment
- Treatment should be symptomatic & combined with oncologic treatments like targeted radiation therapy
- **Pharmacologic**
  - Follow the 3-step (plus step 4, interventional procedures) WHO analgesic ladder (Fig. 32-1)
- **Interventional**
  - **Intrathecal drug delivery systems:** Deliver agents into intrathecal space (e.g., commonly used, mostly in combination are opioids [morphine], local anesthetics, clonidine, baclofen, ziconotide)
  - **Tunneled catheters** (e.g., provides neuraxial analgesia) (intrathecal/epidural) frequently used for the treatment of cancer pain with life expectancy <1 mo
  - **Neurolytic procedures** may target any peripheral nerve or plexus of nerves invaded by tumor with injection of alcohol/phenol or RF lesioning; visceral targets include celiac plexus (pancreatic and upper abdominal) superior hypogastric plexus (pelvic) and ganglion impar (rectal)
- **Alternative treatment**
  - Psychological support, critical
  - Acupuncture, yoga/other gentle movement therapy may provide significant symptomatic relief

CHRISTINA JELLY • ROBERT E. FREUNDLICH

NONLIVING DONORS

Cadaveric Organ Grafts
- Donors usually brain dead, without evidence of untreatable infection or extracranial malignancy
- Brain death criteria (also see Chapter 36, Ethical Issues & Event Disclosure)
  - Criteria may vary by hospital
  - Irreversible cessation of brain function
  - Flat electroencephalogram/no flow on transcranial Doppler
  - Comatose without spontaneous movement or response to painful stimuli
    - Rule out causes of reversible cerebral dysfunction
  - Lack of brainstem activity
    - Assess brainstem for lack of brainstem reflexes *Pupillary response to light, corneal reflex, oculocephalic reflex (doll's eye), oculovestibular reflex (cold caloric testing), gag & cough reflex, facial motor response*
    - Apnea test (1) Preoxygenated pt with 100% O_2 for 10 min & confirm normal $PaCO_2$; (2) Turn off ventilator & administer O_2 via T-piece; (3) After 7–10 min, $PaCO_2$ >60 mmHg (or ↑ in $PaCO_2$ of 20 mmHg from baseline value) & no resp effort confirms lack of brainstem control (positive apnea test)
    - Other brainstem activity tests: Cerebral angiography (gold standard), Transcranial Doppler, EEG, AEPs

Non–Heart Beating Organ Donors (NHBD) = Donation after Cardiac Death (DCD)
- Organs removed only after cardiac arrest ensues (longer warm ischemia time)
- Legal & ethical issues complicate widespread acceptance
- Less favorable outcomes in liver transplantation (more graft dysfunction, early graft loss, decreased survival)

Organ Preservation Techniques
- Recommended maximum time limits for cold storage before reperfusion
  Kidney: 1–2 d; heart: 6 h; lungs: 8 h; liver: 18 h
- Ex vivo perfusion may permit extended storage windows

Intraoperative Management of Procurement
- Pathophysiologic changes in brain death
  - Hypotension, ↑ cardiac output, myocardial dysfx, & ↓ SVR (do not give vasoactive drugs to ↑ blood pressure during this period). The autonomic storm phase follows.
  - ↓ Oxygenation from neurogenic pulm edema, diabetes insipidus
  - Electrolyte disturbances: ↑ Na^+, ↓ K^+
  - Hyperglycemia, coagulopathy, hypothermia
  - Hormonal swings requiring therapy (triiodothyronine, methylprednisolone, desmopressin, insulin)
- General anesthetic goals
  - Maintain euvolemia
  - SBP >100 (MAP 70–110 mmHg)
  - Po_2 >100 mmHg
  - $PaCO_2$ 30–35 mmHg
  - Urine output 1–1.5 mL/kg/h
  - Hemoglobin >10.0 g/dL
  - CVP 6–12 mmHg
  - FiO_2 <40% (as tolerated) for lung procurement
  - Maintain sodium <155 mmol/L
- Anesthesia
  - Preop antibiotics
  - General with positive-pressure lung ventilation
  - Long-acting nondepolarizing muscle relaxants
  - Volatile anesthetics & narcotics to control hemodynamics
    - Surgical stimulation may cause hemodynamic responses (i.e., ↑ BP) via spinal cord pathways
    - Brain death criteria pts have no pain perception (analgesia is *not* required)
  - Pressors of choice = dopamine, vasopressin (helps with potential DI)
  - Draw 50–200 mL of blood required for pretransplant testing

- Specific requirements depend on which organs are harvested
  - Pancreas harvest: May need to irrigate oro/nasogastric tube with betadine solution to maintain sterility
  - Lung & heart harvest: Pull back CVP & PA catheter if cross-clamping needed, surgeon may perform bronchoscopy and possibly prostaglandin E_1
  - Liver harvest: Phentolamine or alprostadil usually given just before or during cross-clamping ($\downarrow$ SVR & allows for even distribution of preservation solution)
  - Heparin bolus (350–400 mg/kg) upon request by surgeon

LIVING KIDNEY DONOR

Donor Criteria and Evaluation
- Donor kidney function must be normal without Hx of renal stones or proteinuria
- Must be without significant cardiopulmonary, psychiatric, neurologic dz. Also without diabetes, or uncontrolled hypertension. BMI must be <35.

Anesthetic Considerations
- Preoperative antibiotics
- GA with ETT, 1–2 large-bore IVs
- Can be managed with epidural and combined epidural and spinal techniques
- Positioning: R or L lateral (with table flexed & kidney rest elevated)
- Generous fluid requirements (must place Foley); goal urine output 10–20 mL/kg/h *Mannitol or furosemide* may be used to maintain urine output
- Heparin often given before renal vessels are clamped (3,000–5,000 U IV)
- Protamine may be given after kidney is dissected free & blood supply tied off

Surgical Procedure
- Laparoscopic, rather than open donor nephrectomy, is increasingly preferred
- Potential complications: Pneumothorax, subcutaneous emphysema, & positional complications (pt often lateral and flexed)

LIVING LIVER DONOR

Donor Criteria
- Imaging (CT/MRI) & lab eval (LFTs/coags) to assess liver fx & anatomy
- No consensus on who can donate: Factors associated with poor performance → ↑ donor age, graft steatosis, ↑ graft ischemia times, ↑ ICU d, ↑ inotrope requirement

Pediatric Recipients
- Usually need only L lateral (sometimes performed laparoscopically) or L hepatic lobe

Adult Living Donors
- May need only L lateral, L hepatic, or R hepatic lobe (leaves donor with 1/3 the original liver mass)

Morbidity & Mortality
- Complication rates vary from 0–67%, crude morbidity rate = 37%
- As of 2011, there were 7 US deaths from living liver donation

Surgical Procedure
- R-sided subcostal incision vs. chevron incision
  → Liver mobilized & vascular structures dissected free
  → Liver transected
  → Bile duct & vascular structures oversewn, hemostasis achieved, incision closed

Anesthetic Considerations
- Preop antibiotics
- GA with ETT; 2 large-bore IVs or one 9 Fr catheter; A-line; ± CVP
- PRBCs should be available (although blood loss usually <1 L)
- Low CVP may be preferred to minimize risk of blood loss
- Consider preop thoracic epidural (some do not place—fear auto-anticoagulation after right lobectomy)
- Oro/nasogastric tube for gastric decompression (improves exposure)
- Liver manipulation may cause hypotension from ↓ venous return

LIVING LUNG DONOR

- Recipient usually receives 1-lung lobe from 2 different living donors (1 LLL & 1 RLL)

Morbidity & Mortality

- Morbidity is reported to be low, but with poor follow-up *Complications: Re-exploration, pleural effusion, hemorrhage, phrenic n. injury, pericarditis, pneumonia, ileus*

Anesthetic Considerations

- Preop antibiotics
- GA with ETT; large-bore IV access; A-line
- Positioning: Lateral decubitus
- ± Thoracic epidural catheter
- Heparin given just before lobar artery ligation

Surgical Procedure

- Thoracotomy incision
- Usually take left lower lobe (LLL) or right lower lobe (RLL)

Contraindications to Solid Organ Transplantation	
Absolute Contraindications	**Relative Contraindications**
• Active uncontrolled infection • Severe cardiopulmonary/medical condition (pt unfit for surgery) • Inability to tolerate immunosuppression (AIDS) • Continued drug/tobacco/alcohol abuse • Brain death • Extrahepatic malignancy • Inability to comply with medical regimen • Lack of psychosocial support	• Noncompliance • Hx of drug abuse • Advanced age • Psychological instability • HIV infection

ANESTHESIA FOR KIDNEY TRANSPLANTATION

Indications

- Polycystic kidney dz
- Diabetes mellitus–related kidney failure
- Hypertensive kidney dz
- Glomerular dz
- Tubulointerstitial dz
- Other familial or congenital dz

Preoperative Evaluation

- Check electrolytes the morning of surgery (consider IHD if ↑ K, volume overloaded)
- Should have dialysis within 24 h of surgery
- Typical comorbidities
  - CAD = major cause of death in ESRD pts before & after transplant
  - Electrolyte abnl, HTN, DM, delayed gastric emptying, acidosis, anemia
  - CHF (from vol overload & compensatory concentric cardiomyopathy)
  - Coagulopathies (qualitative platelet defect in uremic pts), pericarditis

Intraoperative Management

- Immunosuppression: Mycophenolate mofetil (PO or IV), solumedrol (500 mg IV × 1 postinduction), and either basiliximab (20 mg IV over 30 min × 1 after induction), or thymoglobulin 1.5 mg/kg IV over 2–3 h (premedicate with acetaminophen and diphenhydramine)
- Cyclosporine, tacrolimus, azathioprine, alemtuzumab, and antithymocyte globulin are options as well depending on institutional protocol
- Preop antibiotics
- Consider antifibrinolytics (epsilon-aminocaproic acid, tranexamic acid)
- Consider ddAVP for uremic platelet dysfunction
- Standard monitors (avoid placing BP cuff, IVs/art line on fistula arm)
- Consider A-line (if indicated by comorbidities)
- Consider central line—CVP monitoring, ability to give thymoglobulin
  May be challenging to place (prior dialysis lines)

Induction & Maintenance

- Usually GA (RSI if gastroparesis suspected—i.e., long-standing diabetes)
- Spinal & epidural not typically implemented (platelet dysfx in uremic pts)
- Paralytics
  - Consider avoiding succinylcholine if K >5.5 mEq/L (may elev K⁺ 0.5 mEq upon induction)
  - Vecuronium & pancuronium may have prolonged effects

- Atracurium & cisatracurium not affected by ESRD (Hoffman degradation and nonenzymatic ester hydrolysis)
- Narcotics
  - Morphine, meperidine, oxycodone metabolites can accumulate & prolong duration
  - Fentanyl, sufentanil, alfentanil, and remifentanil may be safer alternatives

Surgical Procedure
- 10–15 cm arced incision from pubic symphysis to anterior superior iliac spine
- Kidney transplanted into pelvis
- Graft anastamoses usually made to external iliac vein & artery *External iliac artery & vein clamped for anastamoses*
- Graft warm ischemia time is usually about 15–30 min
- Bladder filled via Foley catheter (to facilitate ureteral anastomosis to bladder)
- Native kidney rarely removed (e.g., pt has intractable HTN or chronic infection)

Specific Intraoperative Considerations
- Hypotension may ensue with unclamping of iliac vessels & graft reperfusion Avoid α-adrenergic agents that cause graft vessel vasoconstriction (phenylephrine) Low-dose dopamine (3–5 mcg/kg/min) may be a better option
- Goal SBP coming off clamp >120, maintain throughout reperfusion. Permissive HTN up to 160 may be requested
- Give calcium immediately/empirically for hemodynamic instability, high likelihood of hyperkalemia
- Heparin may be requested before clamping of iliac vessels
- ↑ Preload (CVP of 12–15 & MAP >60) before unclamping/reperfusion by administering 0.9 NS (3–5 L may be needed) or colloid
- Mannitol may act as free radical scavenger & help diurese kidney after reperfusion (furosemide also used); goal urine output >0.5 mL/kg/h
- Target glucose <180 mg/dL.
- Ca-blocker admin before vessel anastomosis may prevent reperfusion injury
- Consider bicarbonate infusion for significant metabolic acidosis (pH <7.2)

Postoperative Management
- Pt usually extubated
- Continue hydration for goal urine output >0.5 mL/kg/h

ANESTHESIA FOR PANCREAS TRANSPLANTATION

Indications
- Mostly type I diabetics with diabetic retinopathy, nephropathy, neuropathy, and vasculopathy. Most (~75%) combined with kidney transplantation.

Preoperative Evaluation
- Baseline lipase and amylase
- Preop cardiac evaluation, EKG, echocardiogram, stress test

Intraoperative Management
- Immunosuppression: Mycophenolate 1 g IV × 1, solumedrol 100 mg every 12 h (Note: Mycophenolate 1 mg PO × 1 may be given preoperatively in lieu of intraop dose and postop management includes thymoglobulin 1.5 mg/kg IV [acetaminophen and diphenhydramine pretreatment] and tacrolimus)
- Antibiotic prophylaxis
- Standard monitors; A-line preinduction; CVP; consider PA catheter & TEE
- Venous access
  - Large-bore peripheral access (RICC line or 8.5 Fr peripheral IV)
  - 8.5 or 9 Fr central venous catheter, consider SLIC

Induction & Maintenance
- Maintain renal blood flow, keep glucose <180
- Usually GA (RSI if gastroparesis suspected—i.e., long-standing diabetes)
- Spinal & epidural not typically implemented (platelet dysfx in uremic pts)

Specific Intraoperative Considerations
- Avoid dextrose-containing IV fluids
- Glucose management: Discontinue insulin, monitor glucose every 30 min with goal >150
- Hydrate and have RBCs available
- Dopamine 3–5 mcg/kg/min for hemodynamics but vasoactives associated with worse outcomes

- Goal during output >30 mg/h
- Heparin before clamping vessels
- Consider bicarb for pH management

Postoperative Management
- Pt usually extubated
- ICU care for fluid management
- Bedrest to avoid twisting of grafts
- No dextrose-containing fluids
- Strict glycemic control
- Octreotide for pancreatitis

(Note: Combined pancreas-kidney transplantation is performed in pts with type 1 diabetes and ESRD. The kidney is performed first. See above for kidney considerations.)

ANESTHESIA FOR LIVER TRANSPLANTATION (ALSO SEE CHAPTER 20, GENERAL SURGERY)

General
- 1-y survival following transplant 80–90%; 5-y survival: 60–80%
- Organ allocation: Based on MELD (model of end-stage liver dz) or PELD (pediatric) score
- Increasing use of Non-heart Beating Donation (NHBD), although still a small minority; also more use of extended donor criteria organs (age >70, DM, HTN, atherosclerotic heart dz) requiring more rapid reperfusion

Preoperative Evaluation
- Underlying diagnoses of recipients
  Hepatitis C (28%), EtOH (18%), cryptogenic cirrhosis (11%), primary biliary cirrhosis (9%), primary sclerosing cholangitis (8%), fulminant (6%), autoimmune (6%), hep B (4%), EtOH + hep C (4%), HCC (2%), metabolic (4%), other (4%)
- Extrahepatic manifestations of liver dz: Correctible problems include coagulopathy (platelet & FFP admin), pleural effusions (thoracentesis), ascites (paracentesis)
- Elevated pulmonary arterial pressure on echo is a contraindication to transplant

	Extrahepatic Manifestations of Liver Dz
Pulm	Portopulmonary HTN, hepatopulmonary syndrome, pleural effusions
CV	Hyperdynamic circulation (↑ cardiac output & ↓ SVR),cirrhotic cardiomyopathy
GI	Portal HTN, esophageal varices, ascites
CNS	Encephalopathy, ↑ ICP (with fulminant hepatic failure)
Heme	Thrombocytopenia (↓ thrombopoietin & hypersplenism), ↓ clotting factors (↓ synthetic fx, DIC, fibrinolysis)
Renal	Oliguria, renal insufficiency, hepatorenal syndrome

Intraoperative Management
- Immunosuppression: Methylprednisolone 500 mg–1 g IV during anhepatic phase
- Standard monitors; A-line preinduction; CVP; consider PA catheter & TEE
- Venous access
  - Large-bore peripheral access (RICC line or 8.5 Fr peripheral IV)
  - 8.5 or 9 Fr central venous catheter
- May need additional access if PA catheter is in lumen of 8.5 or 9 Fr central catheter
  Equipment
  - Stat lab must be close by & available
  - Rapid infuser systems (Level I, Belmont, etc.) set up & available
  - Blood products available (usually 10 U FFP, 10 U PRBCs, & platelets, activated Factor VII)
  - Venovenous bypass machine (with perfusionist) available
  - Cell saver

Induction and Maintenance
- Usually RSI (for "full stomach" precautions) or awake intubation
- Pts often coagulopathic (use care when placing lines, ETT, NG tube)
- Moderate coagulopathy is permissible, provided there is no clinical bleeding
  - Aggressive use of blood products may worsen outcome
  - Conservative fluid management in selected pts
- Maintain normothermia

Postoperative Management
- Peripheral nerve injuries commonly due to positioning
- Following skin closure, pt brought to ICU (usually intubated)

Phases of a Liver Transplant Operation

The Preanhepatic (Dissection) Phase
- Primary purpose: Dissection of porta hepatis & mobilization of native liver
- Hypotension: Surgical bleeding, ascites/effusion drainage, clamping/pressure on abd veins
- Bleeding risks: Portal HTN, coagulopathy, & prior abdominal surgery
- Metabolic alterations: ↑ K^+, metabolic acidosis, ↓ Ca^{2+} (from citrate toxicity)
- Coagulopathy: Underlying factor deficiencies, thrombocytopenia, & dilutional coagulopathies
- Hypothermia (must be prevented or corrected, or will worsen coagulopathy)
- Ensure adequate urine output & euvolemia

The Anhepatic Phase
- Begin = clamping hepatic artery & portal vein; end = reperfusion of donor liver
- Venous return falls by 50%, anticipate hypotension
- Vessels perfusing liver are clamped & old liver removed
- Warm ischemic time: Begins when donor liver removed from ice, ends when reperfused; should limit warm ischemia time to between 30 & 60 min
- Portal vein, inferior vena cava (IVC), & hepatic artery usu clamped during this phase
- Venovenous bypass occasionally required for pts who do not tolerate cross-clamping
  - Blood diverted from portal vein & IVC into SVC, usu via axillary vein
  - Advantages: Avoids renal/splanchnic engorgement, maintains preload, ↑ renal perfusion; may ↓ blood loss, ↓ transfusion requirements
  - Disadvantages: ↑ Risk of air embolus/DVT, seroma, nerve injury, wound lymphocele
- Piggyback technique may obviate need for IVC clamping
  - Native hepatic veins fashioned into a cuff (serves as a receptacle for suprahepatic IVC of the donor liver); cava to cuff anastomosis performed & native IVC need not be clamped
- Preparation for reperfusion: ↑ K^+ & acidosis prevalent in the absence of functioning liver
- Aggressively treat with furosemide, albuterol, ↑ ventilation, insulin/D50 and/or bicarb

Reperfusion
- Begins with allograft reperfusion; ends with completion of biliary anastomosis
- Allograft flushed of air, debris & residual preservative solution
- Unclamping of donor liver → embolic debris, ↑ K^+, metabolic acidosis, ↓ Ca^{2+}, hypovolemia, hypotension, hypovolemia, release of cytokines & other destabilizing agents. Caval reperfusion is usually well tolerated, but portal vein reperfusion often results in hypotension.
- *Postreperfusion syndrome (PRS)* → ↓ MAP of 30% from baseline, lasts ≥1 min, within 5 min of reperfusion
  - Can see arrhythmias, ↓ SVR, ↓ cardiac output, vasodilation, ↑ L ventricular filling pressure, R ventricular dysfx
  - Contributing factors: ↑ K^+, ↓ Ca^{2+}, acidosis, & blood loss
  - Air embolus & thromboembolus may be seen via echo or inferred via PA-line
  - Treatment: Minimize ↑ K^+, ↓ Ca^{2+}, acidosis; usually resolves within 30 min
- *Postreperfusion coagulopathy* → may also follow graft reperfusion
  - Due to (1) release of heparin or (2) tissue plasminogen activator (tPA) → 1° fibrinolysis
  - Heparin effect reversible with heparinase on thromboelastography (TEG)
  - Cryoprecipitate, FFP, & antifibrinolytics (epsilon aminocaproic acid, tranexamic acid) may treat 1° fibrinolysis
  - Protamine will treat heparin effect
  - Refractory coagulopathy may indicate graft failure
- Indicators of good graft function: Resolution of coagulopathy & metabolic acidosis, return of normoglycemia & bile production

---

ANESTHESIA FOR LUNG TRANSPLANTATION

Indications
- COPD, idiopathic pulmonary fibrosis, cystic fibrosis (CF), α_1-antitrypsin deficiency, PPH (primary pulmonary HTN)
- Terminally ill pts with end-stage lung dz
- Less frequently: Sarcoidosis, retransplantation, Eisenmenger syndrome

Indications for Heart–Lung Transplantation (HLT)
- Pts with lung transplant indication & significant left ventricular dz
- Most commonly PPH, CF, & Eisenmenger syndrome

Bilateral Sequential Lung Transplantation (BSLT)
- Infection in both lungs requiring both to be removed. Usually in cystic fibrosis and bronchiectasis to prevent spread of infection from the native to the transplanted lung.
- BSLT = 1 lung transplanted (start with native lung with worse function) followed by a repeat procedure on contralateral side

Living Donor Lung Transplantation (LDLT)
- Recipients have progressive deterioration and cannot wait for a cadaveric donor
- Cystic fibrosis

Preoperative Evaluation
- Lab values: ABO compatibility of donor & recipient, CBC, chemistry, coags
- CXR, echocardiography (RV failure), EKG
- Functional data (including PFTs) & left heart cath (exclude CAD and intracardiac shunt)
- Pts may have difficulty lying flat (poor pulm function)

Intraoperative Considerations
- Immunosuppression: IL-2R antagonist (basiliximab) or antithymocyte globulin pre-op. Methylprednisolone prior to reperfusion of new lung.
- Targeted pre-op antibiotics, especially in Pseudomonas colonized pts (CF)
- Standard monitors, 2 large-bore IVs, A-line, central line, PA catheter; consider TEE (assess RV fx)
- Consider Intraop or postop thoracic epidural placement for pain control
- Lung isolation techniques (fiberoptic scope necessary)
- Be ready for emergent initiation of cardiopulmonary bypass/ECMO

Induction and Maintenance
- Lung isolation: Double-lumen tube, univent tube, or ETT + bronchial blocker
- Avoid N_2O (presence of bullous emphysematous dz, pulm HTN, intraop hypoxemia)
- Fluid management usually conservative (helps with postop management)
- Permissive hypercapnia
- Be vigilant for cardiac instability or pneumothorax on nonoperative side

Surgical Procedure for Single-Lung Transplantation
- Posterolateral thoracotomy position (need for rapid access to cannulation sites for emergent cardiopulmonary bypass may affect positioning)
- Incision usually anterior thoracotomy with partial sternotomy
- Sequence of surgical events:
  1. Structures for lung to be resected are dissected free
  2. Pneumonectomy completed
  3. Bronchial anastomosis first, PA anastomosis, atrial/pulm vein anastomosis last
  4. Pulmonary circulation flushed & ventilation begun
  5. Process repeated for other side during bilateral sequential lung transplantation

Specific Intraoperative Considerations
- Lung recipients susceptible to pulm HTN & R ventricular dysfx during 1-lung ventilation
  - Fluid restriction, use of small tidal volumes (6 mL/kg), PEEP, and lowest acceptable FiO_2
- Hypoxemia common in 1-lung ventilation; consider using:
  - FiO_2 of 100%
  - PEEP of 10 as tolerated to dependent lung
  - CPAP to nondependent lung
- **Nitric oxide (NO)**
  - Advantages:
    - ↓ Pulm vascular resistance & improves oxygenation
    - NO preferentially reaches ventilated areas, causing ↑ blood flow, improvements in mismatch & improved oxygenation
    - ↓ Inflammatory response to surgery or trauma
    - Impedes microbial growth
    - Activates guanylate cyclase in platelets to attenuate platelet aggregation & adhesion
  - Disadvantages:
    - Methemoglobinemia, NO metabolite–related lung injury
    - Rapid discontinuation of NO in pulm vasculature prevents systemic vasoconstriction & results in systemic hypotension
  - May see hypotension with restoration of graft blood flow after anastomosis
  - At end of procedure, eval of pt for tube exchange to single lumen is performed, although high PEEP requirements & oropharyngeal edema may preclude it

- Cardiopulmonary bypass (CPB) indications
  - Adequate oxygenation cannot be maintained despite ventilatory/pharmacologic interventions & PA clamping by surgeons
  - Inability to ventilate
  - Development of severe RV dysfx
  - CI <2 L/min/m^2, SvO$_2$ <60%, MAP <50–60 mmHg, SaO$_2$ <85–90%, pH <7
  - ECMO may be an alternative to CPB
- May see hypotension with restoration of graft blood flow after anastomosis
- At end of procedure, eval of pt for tube exchange to single lumen is performed, although high PEEP requirements & oropharyngeal edema may preclude it

Postoperative Management
- Maintain optimal ventilation, hemodynamics, and pain control
- Use lowest possible FiO$_2$, utilize PEEP
- Minimize peak airway pressures
- Impeccable infection control practices (stopcock care, antibiotics, and central line cleanliness)

ANESTHESIA FOR HEART TRANSPLANTATION

General Information
- 1-y survival = 87%, 2-y survival 80% from 1982–2015
- Poor survival due to paucity of donor organs; devices (e.g., left ventricular-assist devices—LVAD) used to provide a bridge to transplant

Most Common Indications
- New York Heart Association class III/IV heart failure (despite optimal therapy)
- Heart failure survival scores high risk
- Peak VO$_2$ <10 mL/kg/min after anaerobic threshold
- Severely symptomatic ventricular arrhythmias refractory to medical, ICD, surgical Tx
- Severely limiting ischemia unresponsive to interventional or surg revascularization

Possible Contraindications to Heart Transplantation	
Irreversible pulmonary hypertension (>6 Wood units) (orthotopic procedure)	Age >65 y
Continued illicit drug/tobacco use, noncompliance	Uncontrolled malignancy
Significant irreversible renal, hepatic, vascular, or pulm dysfunction	Obesity
Coexisting systemic illness with a poor prognosis	Previous malignancy
Diabetes mellitus with end-organ damage	Signif coagulopathies
Active infective process (hepatitis B & C)	Active peptic ulcer dz
Amyloidosis (cardiac dz may recur)	Pulm infarction lasts 6–8 wk

Source: Adapted from Miller RD. *Miller's Anesthesia.* 6th ed. Philadelphia, PA: Elsevier; 2004.

Preoperative Assessment
- Donor heart function worsens with ischemic time >6 h
- Pt usually not NPO (owing to short notice of graft availability)
- Pt may receive extensive levels of cardiovascular support
  - Meds—warfarin, vasopressor support, ACE inhibitor, dobutamine, milrinone
  - Devices—LVAD, CIED (pacemaker/ICD), IABP

Intraoperative Management
- Immunosuppression: Mycophenolate mofetil (1.5 g IV) preop, may administer basiliximab, 1 g methylprednisolone (IV on bypass)
- Preop antibiotics
- Ensure blood products available
- Consider antifibrinolytics (epsilon-aminocaproic acid, tranexamic acid)
- Large-bore IV access, std monitors, preinduction A-line, CVP & PA catheter, TEE
- Induction and maintenance
  - Commonly etomidate (0.2 mg/kg), fentanyl (1 mcg/kg), succinylcholine
  - Neuromuscular blockade with nondepolarizing agent
  - May need inotropic support upon induction
  - Standard heparin dosing for pre-CPB anticoagulation
  - See Chapter 18, Cardiac Surgery, for detailed notes on CPB
- Separation from CPB
  - Transplanted heart denervated (will not mount tachy-/bradycardic responses)

- Only direct-acting sympathomimetics work for inotropic/chronotropic effects
  - Isoproterenol, epinephrine, milrinone, dobutamine
- LV function is generally adequate; however, RV dysfunction often seen
- Strategies to lower PVR
  - Maintain adequate oxygenation; avoid hypercapnia/hypothermia
  - Optimize airway pressures & tidal volumes
  - Use nitrates, PGE1, prostacyclin, & inhaled NO as indicated
  - Use CVP/TEE to guide fluid management
  - Consider extracorporeal membrane oxygenation (ECMO), intra-aortic balloon pump, or impella

Surgical Procedure
- Incision median sternotomy
- Aortic cannulation high, near the arch
- Recipient heart excised (except for L atrial tissue with pulmonary veins)
- Biatrial approach—excises both atria (mandating bicaval anastomosis)
- Classic approach—atria transected at grooves

Specific Intraoperative Considerations
- Anticipate previous cardiac surgery (redo-sternotomy)
  - Structures may be adhered to sternum & ruptured upon entry
  - Presence of LVAD/RVAD (longer surgery, more bleeding)
- Many have CIED in situ which needs to be reprogrammed preop (antitachycardia functions turned off)
- Pts with hemodynamic instability may need ECMO prior to induction
- No specific anesthetic strategies for post-transplant anesthesia delivery
  - May see a delayed response to catecholamines
  - Anticipate a denervated heart with absence of vagal tone
- Immunosuppressants:
  - Given to prevent graft rejection and loss of allograft
  - Typical triple therapy for solid organ transplantation is usually a calcineurin inhibitor (cyclosporine), a steroid (prednisone) and an antimetabolite (mycophenolate)
  - The dosing chart below provides typical therapy. Dosing may need to be adjusted based upon clearance issues and combination drug management strategies. Check with your institutional pharmacy before administering.

Category	Name	Dose and Delivery	Comment
Calcineurin	Cyclosporine	Postop: 3–6 mg/kg PO daily (IV available)	Renal, liver, heart transplant
Inhibitors	Tacrolimus (FK506)	Postop: 0.05–0.1 mg/kg PO every 12 h (IV available)	Renal, liver, heart transplant
Antimetabolics	Azathioprine	2.5 mg/kg PO daily (IV available)	Renal transplant
	Mycophenolate	Preop: 1 g PO (or can be given intraop) Intraop: 1–1.5 g IV Postop: 1–1.5 g PO or IV every 12 h	Heart, renal transplant
Rapamycin Inhibitors	Sirolimus	Postop: Loading dose of 6 mg PO followed by 2 mg PO daily	Renal transplant (not recommended in liver or lung transplant pts)
Corticosteroids	Methyl-prednisolone	Intraop: 500 mg–1 g IV Postop: 4–48 mg PO daily (IV available)	Liver, renal, lung, heart transplant
	Prednisone	Postop: 5 mg PO daily (dose varies)	Liver, renal, lung, heart transplant
T lymphocyte antagonist	Thymoglobulin	Intraop: 1.5 mg/kg IV over 3–6 h (with acetaminophen and diphenhydramine pretreatment) Postop: 1.5 mg/kg IV daily over 4 h	Renal transplant
	Basiliximab	Preop: 20 mg IV 2 h prior to surgery Postop: 20 mg IV 4 d after transplantation	Renal transplant

MICHAEL C. LUBRANO

GENERAL CONCERNS & CONSIDERATIONS

- Aging means ↑ comorbidities, which ↑ perioperative mortality & morbidity
  - Major adverse cardiovascular events (arrhythmias, MI, stroke)
  - Airway and pulmonary problems (hypoxemia, aspiration, pneumonia, atelectasis)
  - CNS dysfunction (delirium, postop cognitive dysfunction [POCD], CVA)
  - Health care acquired infections

EFFECTS OF AGING ON PHYSIOLOGY

Cardiovascular System
- CVD: In 75% of pts 75+ yo; will ↑ incidence of arrhythmias, CHF, aortic stenosis, diabetes mellitus (small vessel CAD with silent ischemia)
- LVH and/or CAD → ↑ coronary perfusion pressure and time to avoid ischemia
  - Maintain elevated diastolic pressures and heart rate ≤70 bpm
- ↓ Arterial elasticity → ↑ afterload, ↑ systolic HTN → LVH
  - ↑ Sympathetic tone, parasympathetic activity
  - ↓ Baroreflex function + stiffening → orthostatic hypotension, labile BP
- ↑ Diastolic dysfunction (rapid LV filling phase ↓ from >90—<20%)
  - Passive filling ↑ up to 50%—preserve diastolic time (HR ≤70)
  - Atrial systole ↑ up to 50%—maintain sinus rhythm

Pulmonary System
- Hypoxemia with minimal residual weakness or sedation
  - ↑ A-a Gradient: ↓ PaO_2, ↓ SpO_2, ↓ $DLCO_2$ → more likely to require ↑ FiO_2
  - ↓ Carotid body function, ↓ ventilatory response to hypoxia and hypercarbia
- ↑ Central airways, anatomic physiologic dead space
  - ↑ RV, ↑FRC, no changes in TLC; ↓ FVC, ↓ FEV_1
  - ↓ Compliance, ↑ residual volume, ↑ chest wall rigidity
- ↑ Aspiration risk → ↓ airway reflexes, ↓ muscle strength, ↓ coughing
  - ↑ COPD and bronchospastic dz, "silent" pneumonia, atelectasis

Renal System
- ↓ GFR, ↓ muscle mass → normal creatinine but prolonged drug elimination half-lives
  - GFR: 126 mL/min young adult → 60 mL/min by 80 yo
- ↑ Studies requiring contrast media → dye-induced renal insufficiency
- ↑ Incidence of perioperative acute renal failure

Nervous System
- ↑ Carotid dz → need to maintain cerebral perfusion pressure and time
- ↓ Neuronal density → downregulation of opioid, GABA receptors
  - ↓ MAC, ↓ MAC-awake → prolonged emergence

Assessing Frailty and Low Physiologic Reserve
- Frailty is age related and multidimensional→ predicts adverse surgical outcomes
- The Frailty Questionnaire is an assessment tool where ≥3 points is positive for frailty

FRAIL Questionnaire	
• Fatigue • Resistance • Aerobic • Illnesses • Loss of weight	• Are you fatigued (yes = 1 pt) • Can you walk up 1 flight of stairs? (no = 1 pt) • Can you walk 1+ block? (no = 1 pt) • Do you have more than 5 illnesses (yes = 1 pt) • Lost 5%+ of weight in 6 mo (yes = 1 pt)

PHARMACOLOGY IN THE ELDERLY

Factors Complicating Drug Administration
- Macrovascular: ↓ Arterial elasticity so ↓ BP during induction, ↑ BP during emergence
- Medications: ↑ Number of chronic meds; polypharmacy (>10) → ↑ mortality
- Receptors: Poor β-receptor sensitivity; reliant on vascular tone and preload
  - Receptor downregulation of opioids, benzodiazepines

- Pharmacokinetics: ↓ TBWater means ↓ volume of distribution, ↑ blood concentrations
  - ↑ TBFat as reservoir and ↓ GFR → prolonged drug elimination half-lives
  - Induction agents and opioids—dose based on lean body weight (LBW)
  - Neuromuscular blocking agents—dose based on LBW + $1/3$ (TBW – LBW)
- Pharmacodynamics: ↓ MAC and ↓ MAC-awake
  - Loss of consciousness at higher BIS index if ≥65 y of 70 (58–90)

Anesthetic Agent Selection and Administration

Agents to Avoid or Give Cautiously	Agents Requiring Reduced Doses
• Anticholinergics (scopolamine → delirium) • Antihistamines (promethazine, → delirium) • β-Blockers (bronchospasm, bradycardia) • Digitalis (dysrhythmias) • Diuretics (hypokalemia, hypovolemia) • Ketorolac (acute renal failure) • Metoclopramide, droperidol (extra pyramidal side effects) • Morphine (reduced Vd, may accumulate) • Oral hypoglycemics (hypoglycemia) • Pancuronium (prolonged fxn, renal excreted)	• Benzodiazepines—50% or avoid • Etomidate—50% due to disinhibition • Gabapentin—avoid large doses, renal excretion • *Meperidine—10–20 mg IV for shivering ONLY • Opioids—reduce 10% for every decade over 40 yo • Propofol—0.8–1.2 mg/kg for induction

*Meperidine: Effects = toxic metabolite (seizures), anticholinergic (agitation, tachycardia), serotonin syndrome with MAOIs.

- Drug administration: Start with low doses, titrate slowly (most have slower onset)
- MAC: Administer reduced concentrations of inhaled agents with increasing age
  - Over 40 yo, MAC ↓ 6% per decade; MAC for 70–85 yo = 60–85%

Neuromuscular blocking agents
- Prolonged duration with: ↑ Age (if steroid based, hypothermia, inhaled agents)
- Use short- or intermediate-acting agents, consider cisatracurium if ↑ creatinine
- Do not follow rocuronium with cisatracurium (significant potentiation)
- Always fully reverse with neostigmine or sugammadex to avoid respiratory failure

---

ADDITIONAL PERIOPERATIVE CONSIDERATIONS

Neuraxial/Regional Blocks
- ↑ Pain control, ↓ venous thrombosis, ↓ EBL (especially in ortho cases)
  - Higher level of block w epidural and spinals, reduce agent doses & volumes
- Hypotension pronounced, treat with ephedrine/phenylephrine; colloid less effective

Elderly Cognitive Assessment
- 65 yo+ without dementia about 25–33% have probable preop cognitive impairment
- Preop "Mini-Cog" score ≤2 → postop delirium, longer hospital stay, and discharge to location other than home

Mini-Cog Assessment	Mini-Cog Scoring
• Repeat 3 Words • Clock Drawing • Recall 3 Words	• 1 pt for each word spontaneously recalled • 2 pt normal clock, 0 pt for inability or refusal to draw clock • Total points = 5

Postop Delirium (POD) and Periop Neurocognitive Disorder (PND)
- Unclear if propofol-based TIVA or inhalational agents affect incidences of POD, mortality, or LOS because of very low quality of evidence (Miller D. Cochrane Review 2018, Issue 8. Art. No.: CD012317)
- Moderate-quality evidence that EEG monitoring could reduce the risk of POD in patients aged ≥60
- Regional with light sedation (BIS >80) may be preferred to deep sedation
- POD: 15% of elderly, 30–70% for emergent or major surgery; can occur hrs to days/ weeks postop
  - Treat what's reversible: electrolytes, anemia, uremia, sepsis, pain, ETOH withdrawal, cognitive reorientation, early mobility, nutrition, hydration, correction of vision/ hearing impairment
  - If no improvement, standard therapy is low-dose haloperidol
- Delayed Neurocog Recovery: Timeframe of <1 wk and up to 36 months postop
- PND: 10–40% of pts >60 yo
  - Requires: (1) Cog concern by pt, informant, or clinician; (2) Objective evidence of decline (including testing); and (3) ADL impairment of daily function

- Baseline risks: age >60 yo, baseline cognitive impairment, lack of sleep, ETOH/drug withdrawal, diabetes, frailty/functional limitations, major surgery, visual/hearing impairment, neurodegenerative disease
- Associated with ↑ mortality, LOS, non-home discharge, readmission
- Perioperative factors: duration of anesthesia, depth of anesthesia, type of surgery, reoperation, postoperative infection, respiratory complications/hypoxia, dysglycemia, pain, use of vasoactive drugs, use of benzodiazepines

ELECTROCARDIOGRAM (ECG) INTERPRETATION

JESSE M. EHRENFELD • RICHARD D. URMAN

ECG LEAD PLACEMENT & UTILITY

- 12 leads
  - Limb leads: I, II, III, aVR, aVL, aVF
    - II, III, aVF—inferior
    - I, aVL—lateral
  - Precordial chest leads: V1, V2, V3, V4, V5, V6
    - V1, V2—septal
    - V3, V4—anterior
    - V5, V6—lateral
- Coronary arteries
  - LAD: V1, V2, V3, V4, anterior, & septal
  - Circumflex: I, aVL, V5, V6, lateral, & posterior (inferolateral)
  - RCA: II, III, aVF, inferior, & posterior (inferolateral)
- Intraoperative monitoring
  - II = best for detecting arrhythmias
  - V = best for detecting ischemia

STEPS FOR ECG INTERPRETATION

- Rhythm
  - Check for P before every QRS
  - Check PR intervals to assess for AV block
  - Check QRS intervals to assess for bundle branch blocks
- Rate
  Count large boxes between R waves on ECG *(each large box = 0.2 s)*
  - 1 large box = 300 bpm
  - 2 boxes = 150 bpm
  - 3 boxes = 100 bpm
  - 4 boxes = 75 bpm
  - 5 boxes = 60 bpm
  - 6 boxes = 50 bpm
- Examine axis; ST segments; T, Q, and U waves; QRS width & progression, hypertrophy **Axis** = direction of vector which represents heart's overall wave of depolarization

Interpretation of Axis in Vertical Plane		
Lead I	**Lead AVF**	**Axis**
Positive	Positive	Normal
Positive	Negative	Left axis deviation
Negative	Positive	Right axis deviation
Negative	Negative	Extreme right axis deviation

ATRIOVENTRICULAR CONDUCTION SYSTEM

- **1st-degree AV block**—PR interval increased >0.2 s
- **2nd-degree AV block**
  - **Mobitz type I** (Wenckebach)—AV delay (PR interval) ↑ with each beat, until QRS is dropped after P wave
    - Treatment—only if symptomatic: Atropine, isoproterenol, permanent pace
  - **Mobitz type II**—sudden *unpredictable* dropped QRS not associated with progressive PR interval prolongation
    - Caution: May progress to 3rd-degree heart block
    - Treatment—permanent pacemaker
- **3rd-degree AV block** (complete heart block)
  - No relationship between P wave & QRS—"AV dissociation"
  - Treatment—permanent pacemaker

- **Bundle branch block**
  - **Right bundle branch block** (RBBB)
    - Examine QRS in V1 & V2
    - Right ventricular depolarization delayed
    - LBBB makes it difficult to determine infarction on ECG
  - **Left bundle branch block** (LBBB)
    - Examine QRS in V5 or V6
    - Left ventricular depolarization delayed
    - Difficult to determine infarction on ECG
- **Atrial flutter**
  - Regular atrial activity; 180–350 bpm; ventricular rate 150 bpm *(2:1 AV block)*
  - ECG: "F waves," "sawtooth" pattern, flutter waves
  - Treatment
    - Unstable → immediate electrical cardioversion
    - Burst pacing (temporary or permanent pacemaker)
    - Medical therapy (β-blockers, Ca^{2+}-channel blockers)
    - Radio frequency catheter ablation (RFA)
- **Atrial fibrillation**
  - Irregular atrial activity at 350–600 bpm, ventricular rate 160
  - ECG: Wavy baseline, absent P waves
  - Treatment
    - Unstable → immediate electrical cardioversion
    - Chemical cardioversion (Class IA, IV, III antiarrythmics)
    - Antiarrhythmic drugs
    - Anticoagulation
    - Rate control: β- or Ca^{2+}-channel blockers, digoxin
    - Maze procedure
- **Paroxysmal SVT**
  - Ventricular rate 140–250 bpm
  - ECG: Narrow complex, P waves hidden in QRS complexes *(QRS may be slightly widened, not more than 0.14 s)*
  - Treatment: Vagal maneuvers, β- or Ca^{2+}-channel blockers, radio frequency ablation
- **Wolff–Parkinson–White**
  - PR interval shortened, delta wave, wide QRS
  - Treatment: β- or Ca^{2+}-channel blockers, radiofrequency ablation

VENTRICULAR ARRHYTHMIAS

- **Premature ventricular beats**
  - Widened QRS
  - *Couplet*—two in a row; *Bigeminy*—every other beat is PVC
- **Ventricular tachycardia**—3 or more PVCs in a row, 100–200 bpm
  - Nonsustained VT (NSVT)—persists for <30 s
  - Sustained VT—persists for ≥30 s
  - Treatment
    - Symptomatic: Electrical cardioversion followed by antiarrhythmic drugs; follow ACLS protocol
    - Asymptomatic NONSUSTAINED VT: β-blockers, implantable cardioverter-defibrillator (ICD) in pts at high risk
    - Unstable: Defibrillation as if ventricular fibrillation
- **Torsades de pointes**
  - Polymorphic VT with varying amplitudes of QRS twisting about the baseline
  - Treatment: Magnesium 1–2 g IV followed by infusion
- **Ventricular fibrillation**
  - Chaotic irregular appearance without discrete QRS waveforms
  - Treatment: See ACLS protocol; ICD if arrhythmia not associated with acute MI

Bundle Branch Blocks		
Normal	V1 ⌇ V6 ⌇	Initial depol is left-to-right across septum (R in V_1 & Q in V_6; absent in LBBB) followed by LV & RV free wall, with LV dominating (nb—WHAT IS THIS, RV depol later and visible in RBBB)

RBBB	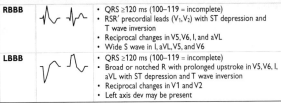	• QRS ≥120 ms (100–119 = incomplete) • RSR′ precordial leads (V$_1$,V$_2$) with ST depression and T wave inversion • Reciprocal changes in V5,V6, I, and aVL • Wide S wave in I, aVL,V5, and V6
LBBB		• QRS ≥120 ms (100–119 = incomplete) • Broad or notched R with prolonged upstroke in V5,V6, I, aVL with ST depression and T wave inversion • Reciprocal changes in V1 and V2 • Left axis dev may be present

Bifascicular block: RBBB + LAHB/LPHB; trifascicular: 1° AVB + RBBB + LAHB/LPHB

Other ECG Abnormalities

Hypertrophy
• **Right atrial hypertrophy**
  • Large, biphasic P wave with tall initial component
• **Left atrial hypertrophy**
  • Large, biphasic P wave with wide terminal component
• **Ventricular hypertrophy**
  • Right ventricular hypertrophy
    • R wave >S in V1 (R wave becomes progressively smaller from V1–V6)
    • S wave persists in V5 & V6
    • Right axis deviation with slightly widened QRS
    • Rightward rotation in horizontal plane
  • Left ventricular hypertrophy
    • S wave in V1 + R wave in V5 >35 mm
    • Left axis deviation with slightly widened QRS
    • Leftward rotation in horizontal plane
    • Inverted T wave that slants downward gradually but upward quickly

Electrolyte Imbalances
• Hypokalemia: Flattened T wave, U waves
• Hyperkalemia: Peaked T waves, wide or flat P wave, wide QRS
• Hypercalcemia: Shortened QT
• Hypocalcemia: Prolonged QT

Drug Effects
• Digitalis toxicity: Inverted or flattened T waves, shortened QT interval

Pulmonary Embolism
• Right axis deviation
• Acute RBBB
• Inverted T waves in V1 to V4 from right ventricular overload
• Wide S in I large Q; and inverted T in III

Pericarditis
• Diffuse ST-segment elevation (looks similar to acute MI, usually more universal in nature)
• May see subsequent inverted T waves (similar to acute MI)

Hypothermia
• J wave or Osborne wave—⏌ point elevation with T wave inversion, especially in the setting of slowed conduction

Biventricular Pacemaker
• Cardiac resynchronization therapy—used to synchronize contraction of right and left ventricles to ↑ cardiac output in pts with heart failure

Cardiac Transplantation
• 2 sets of P waves
• Increased SA node refractory period
• Prolonged atrial conduction
• 1st-degree AV block common

ETHICAL ISSUES & EVENT DISCLOSURE

JESSE M. EHRENFELD • RICHARD D. URMAN

Obtaining Informed Consent
• Informed consent is a process—not simply signing a document
• Consent forms should be read & signed by pt before administering sedatives   → Should contain description of procedure, *specific* potential risks and benefits
• Principle of pt autonomy (pt may accept/refuse treatment)
• Incapacitated pts (under influence, altered consciousness, incompetent, disabled)   → next of kin/health-care proxy/court-appointed guardian should provide consent
• Telephone consent acceptable, preferably cosigned by a witness
• Consent may be waived in an emergency situation
• Resuscitation efforts generally do not require informed consent because they are   considered emergency interventions and consent is implied
• For non-English speakers, use official interpreter (not family) whenever possible

- **Shared decision making** → collaborative process enables pts and providers to make decisions together, while considering medical evidence available + pt values
- **Advance directive** → instructions given by an individual specifying what should be done for his or her health should he or she no longer be able to make decisions
- **Living will** → addresses specific directives regarding treatment course to be taken by caregivers (may forbid certain interventions—e.g., intubation, CPR) if pt unable to give informed consent
- **Health-care power of attorney** → appoints an individual (a proxy) to make health-care decisions should pt become incapacitated
- **Mental competency** → legal term; pt's ability to make rational informed decisions
  - Adults are presumed to be competent
  - **Only a court** can declare a person incompetent
  - **Physician opinion** of incompetency = **opinion only**
- **Brain death**
  - Definition = permanent absence of brain & brainstem function
  - Must rule out confounding factors (*drug/toxins, hypothermia <32°, metabolic derangements, Guillain–Barré syndrome, locked-in syndrome*)

Brain Death Criteria—Adults & Children	
Coma	Absence of gag reflex
Absence of motor responses	Absence of coughing in response to tracheal suctioning
Absence of pupillary responses to light	Absence of sucking and rooting reflexes
Absence of corneal reflexes	Absence of respiratory effort at PaCO$_2$ of 60 mmHg or 20 mmHg > pts nl value
Absence of caloric (vestibulo-ocular) reflexes	

END-OF-LIFE ISSUES

- *DNR/DNI is **not** automatically suspended during surgery*
- In case of DNR/DNI, must clearly document that status & communicate with medical & nursing staff to avoid providing unwanted treatment
- Specific measures not to be performed should be clearly documented by a physician (e.g., intubation, chest compressions, defibrillation, invasive line placement, vasopressors)
- In cases of medical futility: Physician has duty to counsel medical decision maker (next of kin, legal guardian) & explain possibility of DNR/DNI status & potential for withdrawal of life-sustaining measures
- Medical decision maker should receive info about pt's prognosis before making end-of-life decisions for the pt

PEDIATRIC/MINOR (<18 Y) PATIENTS

- Physicians must obtain informed consent from a parent or surrogate before a child can undergo any medical intervention
- Consent for pregnancy termination procedure dependent on state laws
- Pediatric pts' wishes should be included in decision-making process as appropriate

JEHOVAH'S WITNESSES (JW)

- JW pts usually will not accept blood or blood products (even under life-saving circumstances)
- Obtain informed consent, discuss options, & document preoperative discussion with pt regarding products pt will/will not accept
- Special legal considerations may apply to minors, incompetent individuals, emergency procedures
- Physicians may opt out of providing care for a JW pt
- JW may agree to some blood conservation (special cell-saver) techniques
- Generally prohibited
  - Allogenic transfusion of whole blood, red cells, white cells, platelets, plasma
  - Autologous (preoperative donated) blood/blood products
- May be acceptable (discuss with JW)
  - Cell-saver scavenging, cardiopulmonary bypass, dialysis, plasmapheresis
    - If blood does not come out of a continuous circuit with pt
  - Epidural blood patch
  - Blood plasma fractions
    - Albumin, globulins, clotting factors—factors VIII & IX
    - Erythropoietin
    - PolyHeme (blood substitute solution—chemically modified human Hgb)
    - Hemopure (blood substitute solution—chemically stabilized bovine Hgb)

DISCLOSURE AND APOLOGY—COMMUNICATING ABOUT UNANTICIPATED EVENTS

Triggers for Disclosure
• Interception of a potential error (e.g., wrong site identified during time out) • Error with no harm (e.g., drug dosing error) • Adverse/unanticipated event (e.g., failed intubation)

- *National Patient Safety Foundation* guiding principle:
  "When a health care injury occurs, the patient ... is entitled to a prompt explanation of how the injury occurred and its short- and long-term effects. When an error contributed to the injury, the patient ... should receive a truthful and compassionate explanation about the error and the remedies available to the patient. They should be informed that the factors ... will be investigated so that steps can be taken to reduce the likelihood of similar injury to other[s]." (11/14/00)
- *The Joint Commission* accreditation standards: Require the disclosure of sentinel events and other unanticipated outcomes of care

Quick Guide to Breaking Bad News
• Use a quiet, private area free from distractions • Provide a brief review of the event/unanticipated outcome; don't speculate, stick to facts • Be frank, but kind in your delivery of news • Pause after your disclosure; silence is OK; give the pt time to react • Gauge readiness for more information • Invite questions • Assure that physician follow-up is available

- Apologies:
  - *Avoid these ineffective phrases:* "I'm sorry, but..." or "I'm sorry you feel..." → does not show apology for the error, shows sorrow/indifference toward the feelings of the pt/family
  - *Avoid* placing blame
  - Be an active listener and signal general agreement when appropriate "yes, good point," or "I hear what you are saying"
  - *Practice the 3R's:* **R**estate, **R**espect, **R**espond "Let me repeat, your point is..."

Note: If an adverse event occurs, but was NOT the result of an error or omission, there is no need to apologize; review facts, explain findings, and let the pt know it is OK to disagree

CHAD R. GREENE

ADVANCED CARDIAC LIFE SUPPORT (ACLS)

C-A-B (Chest compressions, Airway, Breathing)

- **Compressions:** Begin CPR with 30 chest compressions. If 2 rescuers for infant or child, provide 15 compressions
- Open **Airway:** After chest compressions, open airway (head tilt–chin lift or jaw thrust)
- **Breathing:** If a victim is breathing or resumes effective breathing, place in recovery position. If a victim is *not* breathing, give 2 breaths that make chest rise. Allow for exhalation between breaths. After 2 breaths, immediately resume compressions

Specific Details (Also see Fig. 37-1)

Recommended Pulse Site	
Adult	Carotid
Child	Carotid/femoral
Infant	Brachial

Rescue Breathing	Breaths/min
Adult	10–12
Child	12–20
Infant	12–20

- **Compressions** and circulation
  - Check for a pulse
    - If a pulse is present, continue rescue breathing
    - Reassess pulse every 2 min
    - If a pulse is not present within 10 s or pt shows signs of poor perfusion, begin chest compressions
  - Chest compressions (*should now be before airway/breathing*)
    - Initiate immediately
    - Minimize interruptions between compressions
  - Adult, child, and infant
    - Continuous ventilation @ 8–10 breaths/min
    - Continuous compressions @ 100–120/min
    - Resume CPR immediately after defibrillation
    - Complete chest recoil between compressions
    - If 2 rescuers present, switch roles every 2 min to prevent fatigue
    - Continue cycles of CPR until a defibrillator or additional help arrives
  - Rhythm checks should not be longer than 10 s
    - Should be done after 5 cycles of CPR have been completed (2 min)
  - Pulse checks should be done only if an organized rhythm is restored
  - Drug administration and definitive airway placement should minimally interrupt compressions

Compression Techniques for Adults & Children			
Chest Compressions	Adult (>8 y old)	Child (1 y old– puberty)	Infant (<1 y old)
Location	Center of sternum	Lower $1/2$ of sternum	Lower $1/2$ of sternum
Depth	2 in.	$1/3$–$1/2$ depth of chest	$1/3$ depth of chest
Technique	Heels of both hands	Heels of both hands	2 fingers if alone; thumbs encircling hands if 2 rescuers
Rate (per min)	100–120	100–120	100–120
Compression/ ventilation ratio	1 or 2 rescuers 30:2	1 rescuer 30:2 2 rescuers 15:2	1 rescuer 30:2 2 rescuers 15:2

- **Airway/breathing**
  - Maintain patent airway, give supplemental oxygen
  - Place advanced airway
    - Minimize interruptions of chest compressions during placement
    - Continuous waveform capnography should be used for confirmation & maintenance of ETT placement (if not available, use CO_2 calorimetric detector)

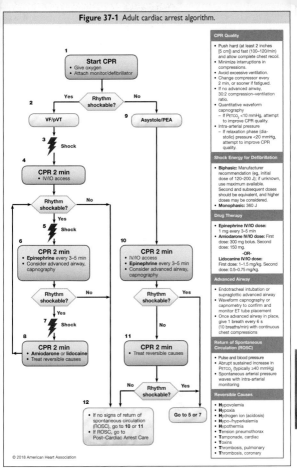

Figure 37-1 Adult cardiac arrest algorithm.

(Reprinted with permission from, *Circulation* 2018;138:e740–9/ © 2018 American Heart Association, Inc.)

- After airway placed, 2 providers should administer continuous CPR (not in cycles)
- **Intravascular access should be obtained**
  - Intravenous—*peripheral* or *central* (faster med onset, but may interfere with CPR)
  - Intraosseous (IO) access—may be safely used if difficult IV access
  - Endotracheal route—not desirable, last resort if IV or IO cannot be obtained
    - Dose: 2–2.5 × standard IV dose diluted in 5–10 mL NS
    - Drugs OK via ETT → lidocaine, atropine, epinephrine, vasopressin, Narcan
- **Defibrillation**
  - Prompt defibrillation is critical when a pt displays a shockable rhythm
    - Initial dose for biphasic is 120–200 J; monophasic is 360 J; 2 J/kg in peds (1–8 y)
- **Differential diagnosis**—diagnose and treat throughout resuscitation

Adult Drug Dosages			
Drug	**Indication**	**IV Dose**	**ETT Dose**
Adenosine	SVT	6 mg, repeat dose with 12 mg	
Amiodarone	SVT, VT/VF, AF/flutter	150 mg over 10 min, then 1 mg/min	
	Pulseless VF/VT	300 mg, repeat with 150 mg	
Atropine	Bradycardia	0.5 q3–5min, max 3 mg	Note: <0.5 mg can lead to paradoxical bradycardia
Calcium	Hypocalcemia, hyperkalemia, hypermagnesemia	Chloride: 5–10 mg/kg Gluconate: 12–30 mg/kg	
Diltiazem	AF with RVR, re-entrant tachycardia	0.25 mg/kg bolus, may repeat bolus 0.35 mg/kg; 5–15 mg/h infusion	
Dobutamine	Systolic heart failure	2–20 mcg/kg/min	
Dopamine	Oliguria	1–5 mcg/kg/min	
	Hypotension, CHF, bradycardia	2–10 mcg/kg/min	2–2.5 mg
Epinephrine	Pulseless VT/VF, asystole	1 mg q3–5min	
	Hypotension, bradycardia	0.1–1 mcg/kg/min	
	Bronchospasm, anaphylaxis	0.1–0.25 mg	
Glucose/dextrose	Hypoglycemia	25–50 g	
Lidocaine	Refractory VT, PVCs	1–1.5 mg/kg IV, repeat 0.5–0.75 mg/kg q5–10min, max 3 mg/kg; 15–50 mcg/kg/min infusion	2–2.5 × IV dose
Magnesium	Hypomagnesemia, Torsades de pointes	1–2 g	
Naloxone	Opioid overdose	0.4–2 mg, titrated q2–3min in 0.2 mg increments	Least desirable route; supported only by anecdotal evidence
Procainamide	Atrial and ventricular arrhythmias	Load: 20 mg/min until toxicity or up to 17 mg/kg; maintenance: 1–4 mg/min	
Sodium bicarbonate	Cardiac arrest	1 mEq/kg (after established ventilation), as per ABG	
	Metabolic acidosis	Base deficit × wt (kg) × 0.2	
Vasopressin	Pulseless VT/VF	40 U × 1 dose	2–2.5 × IV dose
Verapamil	SVT, AF/flutter, WPW	2.5–5 mg over 2 min, repeat 5–10 mg; max total 20 mg	
Isoproterenol	Bradycardia	2–10 mcg/min	

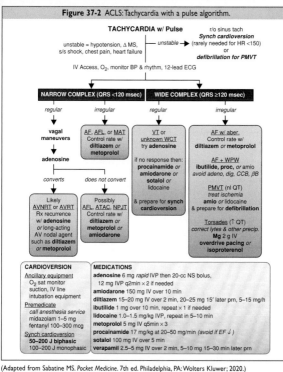

Figure 37-2 ACLS: Tachycardia with a pulse algorithm.

TACHYCARDIA w/ Pulse

unstable = hypotension, Δ MS, s/s shock, chest pain, heart failure — *unstable* → r/o sinus tach *Synch cardioversion* (rarely needed for HR <150) or *defibrillation for PMVT*

IV Access, O₂, monitor BP & rhythm, 12-lead ECG

NARROW COMPLEX (QRS <120 msec)

regular
vagal maneuvers
↓
adenosine
↓
converts / *does not convert*

converts: Likely AVNRT or AVRT Rx recurrence w/ adenosine or long-acting AV nodal agent such as diltiazem or metoprolol

does not convert: Possibly AFL, ATAC, NPJT Control rate w/ diltiazem or metoprolol or amiodarone

irregular
AF, AFL, or MAT Control rate w/ diltiazem or metoprolol

WIDE COMPLEX (QRS ≥120 msec)

regular
VT or unknown WCT try adenosine
if no response then: procainamide or amiodarone or sotalol or lidocaine & prepare for synch cardioversion

irregular
AF w/ aber. Control rate w/ diltiazem or metoprolol

AF + WPW ibutilide, proc, or amio avoid adeno, dig, CCB, βB

PMVT (nl QT) treat ischemia amio or lidocaine & prepare for defibrillation

Torsades (↑ QT) correct lytes & other precip. Mg 2g IV overdrive pacing or isoproterenol

CARDIOVERSION

Ancillary equipment
O₂ sat monitor
suction, IV line
intubation equipment

Premedicate
call anesthesia service
midazolam 1–5 mg
fentanyl 100–300 mcg

Synch cardioversion
50–200 J biphasic
100–200 J monophasic

MEDICATIONS

adenosine 6 mg *rapid IVP* then 20-cc NS bolus, 12 mg IVP q2min × 2 if needed
amiodarone 150 mg IV over 10 min
diltiazem 15–20 mg IV over 2 min, 20–25 mg 15' later prn, 5–15 mg/h
ibutilide 1 mg over 10 min, repeat × 1 if needed
lidocaine 1.0–1.5 mg/kg IVP, repeat in 5–10 min
metoprolol 5 mg IV q5min × 3
procainamide 17 mg/kg at 20–50 mg/min *(avoid if EF ↓)*
sotalol 100 mg IV over 5 min
verapamil 2.5–5 mg IV over 2 min, 5–10 mg 15–30 min later prn

(Adapted from Sabatine MS. *Pocket Medicine*. 7th ed. Philadelphia, PA: Wolters Kluwer; 2020.)

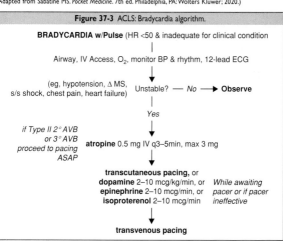

Figure 37-3 ACLS: Bradycardia algorithm.

BRADYCARDIA w/Pulse (HR <50 & inadequate for clinical condition

Airway, IV Access, O₂, monitor BP & rhythm, 12-lead ECG
↓
(eg, hypotension, Δ MS, s/s shock, chest pain, heart failure) — Unstable? — *No* → **Observe**
↓
Yes
↓

if Type II 2° AVB or 3° AVB proceed to pacing ASAP

atropine 0.5 mg IV q3–5min, max 3 mg
↓
transcutaneous pacing, or
dopamine 2–10 mcg/kg/min, or
epinephrine 2–10 mcg/min, or
isoproterenol 2–10 mcg/min

While awaiting pacer or if pacer ineffective

↓
transvenous pacing

(Adapted from Sabatine MS. *Pocket Medicine*. 7th ed. Philadelphia, PA: Wolters Kluwer; 2020.)

PEDIATRIC ADVANCED LIFE SUPPORT (PALS) (ALSO SEE CHAPTER 29, PEDIATRIC ANESTHESIA)

Pediatric resuscitation is recommended for children from age 1 y to start of puberty

RECOGNIZE THE NEED OF CPR

- Sudden cardiac arrest
  - Uncommon in the pediatric population
- Majority of the events are asphyxia, usually not a primary cardiac cause; therefore, ABCs remain
  - Usually present as asystole or bradycardia
  - VF and PEA are less common
    - Likely to be the rhythm in a sudden witnessed collapse
- With an unwitnessed arrest, perform BLS immediately and then obtain an AED (CPR first)
- With a witnessed arrest, defibrillate as soon as possible, then CPR (defibrillate first)
- Regarding the infant (<1 y old) population, there are no data to support or refute the use of defibrillation

Ventricular Fibrillation/Ventricular Tachycardia (Pulseless)
- **Pediatric pulseless arrest algorithm**
  - Designed to minimize interruptions of compressions
  - Rhythm checks are performed after 5 cycles (or 2 min) after shock
    - After a definitive airway is placed, CPR is continuous
  - Diagnose and treat underlying causes throughout resuscitation
- **Pediatric pulseless arrest algorithm sequence**
  - Perform BLS while obtaining a defibrillator
  - If a shockable rhythm is seen, defibrillate
    - 2 J/kg on the first attempt, 4 J/kg on subsequent attempts
    - Paddle size: Adult size for children >10 kg (~1 y old)
      Infant size for children <10 kg
    - Largest paddles that can fit on the chest with a 3 cm distance between the paddles are recommended
  - After 1 shock, immediately resume compressions
    - CPR before subsequent shocks is associated with a higher rate of success of defibrillating the rhythm
  - After 5 cycles of CPR (2 min), check the rhythm
  - If a shockable rhythm is present, defibrillate (4 J/kg) and resume compressions
  - Check the rhythm after 5 cycles and give epinephrine during compressions while charging the defibrillator
    - Drug timing is less important than continuous compressions
    - Standard-dose epinephrine (0.01 mg/kg) should be given every 3–5 min
  - After defibrillation, resume CPR for 5 cycles
  - Check the rhythm and defibrillate if shockable (4 J/kg), then resume CPR and administer amiodarone or lidocaine
    - Amiodarone 5 mg/kg IV
    - Lidocaine 1 mg/kg IV
  - Treat Torsades de pointes with magnesium
    - Magnesium 25–50 mg/kg IV
  - If the pt develops an organized rhythm, check for a pulse
    - If a pulse is present, supportive care should begin
    - When no pulse is palpable, continue CPR
  - If an organized rhythm is achieved but shockable rhythm recurs, give amiodarone during chest compressions before defibrillation

Asystole and PEA
- Similar in causes and treatment
- Grouped together in pediatric pulseless arrest algorithm
- **Pediatric cardiac arrest algorithm**
  - After rhythm is determined, begin CPR
  - Administer epinephrine every 3–5 min, minimizing interruptions of compressions
  - Diagnose and treat underlying factors

Bradycardia with Cardiorespiratory Compromise
- Give supportive care including supplemental oxygen and adequate ventilation
- Evaluate heart rate and perfusion

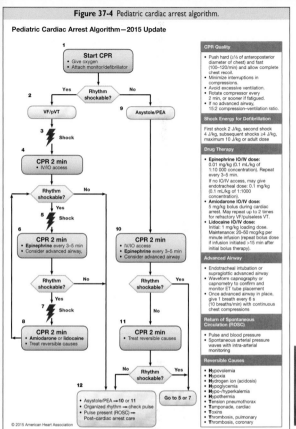

Figure 37-4 Pediatric cardiac arrest algorithm.

Pediatric Cardiac Arrest Algorithm—2015 Update

1
Start CPR
• Give oxygen
• Attach monitor/defibrillator

Rhythm shockable?

2 Yes → **VF/pVT**

No → **9** **Asystole/PEA**

3 Shock

4
CPR 2 min
• IV/IO access

Rhythm shockable? No →

Yes →

5 Shock

6
CPR 2 min
• Epinephrine every 3–5 min
• Consider advanced airway.

Rhythm shockable? No →

Yes →

7 Shock

8
CPR 2 min
• Amiodarone or lidocaine
• Treat reversible causes

10
CPR 2 min
• IV/IO access
• Epinephrine every 3–5 min
• Consider advanced airway

Rhythm shockable? Yes →

No →

11
CPR 2 min
• Treat reversible causes

Rhythm shockable? Yes → **Go to 5 or 7**

No →

12
• Asystole/PEA →**10** or **11**
• Organized rhythm → check pulse
• Pulse present (ROSC) →
• Post–cardiac arrest care

CPR Quality
• Push hard (≥⅓ of anteroposterior diameter of chest) and fast (100–120/min) and allow complete chest recoil.
• Minimize interruptions in compressions.
• Avoid excessive ventilation.
• Rotate compressor every 2 min, or sooner if fatigued.
• If no advanced airway, 15:2 compression-ventilation ratio.

Shock Energy for Defibrillation
First shock 2 J/kg, second shock 4 J/kg, subsequent shocks ≥4 J/kg, maximum 10 J/kg or adult dose

Drug Therapy
• **Epinephrine IO/IV dose:** 0.01 mg/kg (0.1 mL/kg of 1:10 000 concentration). Repeat every 3–5 min.
If no IO/IV access, may give endotracheal dose: 0.1 mg/kg (0.1 mL/kg of 1:1000 concentration).
• **Amiodarone IO/IV dose:** 5 mg/kg bolus during cardiac arrest. May repeat up to 2 times for refractory VF/pulseless VT.
• **Lidocaine IO/IV dose:** Initial: 1 mg/kg loading dose. Maintenance: 20–50 mcg/kg per minute infusion (repeat bolus dose if infusion initiated >15 min after initial bolus therapy).

Advanced Airway
• Endotracheal intubation or supraglottic advanced airway
• Waveform capnography or capnometry to confirm and monitor ET tube placement
• Once advanced airway in place, give 1 breath every 6 s (10 breaths/min) with continuous chest compressions

Return of Spontaneous Circulation (ROSC)
• Pulse and blood pressure
• Spontaneous arterial pressure waves with intra-arterial monitoring

Reversible Causes
• Hypovolemia
• Hypoxia
• Hydrogen ion (acidosis)
• Hypoglycemia
• Hypo-/hyperkalemia
• Hypothermia
• Tension pneumothorax
• Tamponade, cardiac
• Toxins
• Thrombosis, pulmonary
• Thrombosis, coronary

© 2015 American Heart Association

ALGORITHMS 37-6

(Adapted from Caen AR, Berg MD, Chameides L. Part 12: Pediatric Advanced Life Support 2015. American Heart Association Guidelines Update for Cardiopulmonary Resuscitation and Emergency Cardiovascular Care. *Circulation.* 2015;132[suppl 2]:S526–S542.)

• If heart rate is below 60 bpm and poor perfusion is still evident after ventilation is supported, start CPR
• If still persistent after 2 min, consider drug therapy (epinephrine atropine) or transthoracic or transvenous pacing
• If stabilized, give supportive care and observe
• If pulse is absent, follow recommendations for pulseless arrest

Tachycardia with Cardiorespiratory Compromise
• Give supportive care including supplemental O_2
• Evaluate rhythm and QRS complex
  • **Narrow complex tachycardia (≤0.09 s)**
    • Sinus
      • Diagnose and treat cause
    • Supraventricular tachycardia (SVT)
      • Vagal stimulation

- Adenosine
- Synchronized cardioversion (0.5–1 J/kg, repeat 2 J/kg)
- Amiodarone or procainamide (if unresponsive to above treatments)
- Consider cardiology consultation
- **Wide complex tachycardia (>0.09 s)**
  - Ventricular tachycardia (VT)
  - Adenosine (to differentiate narrow vs. wide complex)—use only for a regular rhythm and monomorphic QRS in a stable pt
  - Synchronized cardioversion (same dose as above)
  - Amiodarone or procainamide
  - Consider cardiology consultation

Acute coronary syndromes: see Figure 37-5

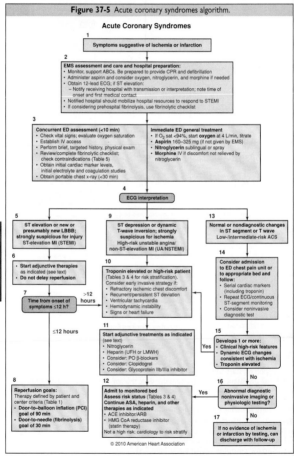

Figure 37-5 Acute coronary syndromes algorithm.

© 2010 American Heart Association

(Adapted from Neumar RW, Otto CW, Link MS, et al. 2010. American Heart Association guidelines for cardiopulmonary resuscitation and emergency cardiovascular science. Part 8. Adult advanced cardiovascular life support. *Circulation* 2010;122:S729–67.)

VASCULAR ACCESS/DRUG ADMINISTRATION

- Intravenous
  - Preferred route
- Intraosseous
  - Safe and effective if intravenous cannot be achieved
  - Onset of action is similar to IV route
  - Recommended in cardiac arrest when IV access is not yet established
- Endotracheal
  - Can be used if other routes are not accessible
  - Drugs that can be administered through ETT
    - Lidocaine
    - Atropine
    - Epinephrine
    - Narcan supported only by anecdotal evidence
  - Recommended dose = 2.5 × standard dose in 5 mL normal saline followed by 5 ventilations
    - Optimal doses unknown
      - ETT size for children ages 1–8 y = (age in y + 4)/4

Pediatric Drug Dosages			
Drug	Indications	IV dose	ETT dose
Adenosine	SVT	0.1 mg/kg, 2nd dose: 0.2 mg/kg (maximum 12 mg)	
Amiodarone	Pulseless VT/VF	5 mg/kg; up to 15 mg/kg or 300 mg	
Atropine	Bradycardia	0.02 mg/kg q5min, max total 1 mg child, 2 mg adolescent *Note:* <0.1 mg can lead to paradoxical bradycardia	0.04–0.06 mg/kg ETT
Calcium chloride	Hypocalcemia, hyperkalemia, hypermagnesemia	20 mg/kg Maximum single dose: 2 g	
Dobutamine	Systolic heart failure	2.5–15 mcg/kg/min	
Dopamine	Hypotension	1–20 mcg/kg/min	
Epinephrine	Cardiac arrest	0.01 mg/kg (0.1 mL/kg 1:10,000) q3–5min, max 1 mg	0.1 mg/kg (0.1 mL/kg 1:1,000) in 1–2 mL diluent, max 10 mg
	Hypotension	0.1–1 mcg/kg/min	
	Anaphylaxis	0.01 mg/kg q20min	
Glucose/ dextrose	Hypoglycemia	0.5–1 g/kg	
Lidocaine	Refractory VT	1 mg/kg, max 100 mg	2–3 mg/kg
	PVCs	20–50 mcg/kg/min	
Magnesium	Hypomagnesemia, Torsades de pointes	25–50 mg/kg over 10–20 min, max 2 g	
Naloxone	Narcotic overdose	Full reversal: ≤20 kg: 0.1 mg/kg ≥5 y or >20 kg: 2 mg	Least desirable route; supported only by anecdotal evidence
Procainamide	Atrial and ventricular arrhythmias	15 mg/kg	
Sodium bicarbonate	Cardiac arrest	1 mEq/kg (after established ventilation)	
	Metabolic acidosis	Base deficit × wt (kg) × 0.3	
Verapamil	SVT	<1 y old: 0.1–0.2 mg/kg over 2 min q30min 1–15 y old: 0.1–0.3 mg/kg, max 5 mg, repeat 15 min, max 10 mg	

COMMON MEDICAL PHRASES IN SPANISH

MANUEL CAVAZOS • JESSE M. EHRENFELD

INTRODUCTION

Initial Evaluation/Preop	
What is your name?	¿Cuál es su nombre?
What surgery are you having today?	¿Qué cirugía va a tener hoy?
Where does it hurt?	¿Dónde le duele?
How old are you?	¿Cuántos años tiene?
How much do you weigh in pounds?	¿Cuánto pesa en libras?
Are you pregnant?	¿Está embarazada?
Are you allergic to anything?	¿Tiene alguna alergia?
Do you take any medications regularly?	¿Toma medicamentos regularmente?
Have you ever been hospitalized?	¿Ha estado alguna vez hospitalizado?
Have you had surgery in the past?	¿Ha tenido alguna cirugía en el pasado?
Do you have any heart problems?	¿Padece de problemas cardíacos?
Do you get chest pains?	¿Padece de dolor de pecho?
Have you ever had a heart attack?	¿Alguna vez tuvo un ataque cardíaco?
Can you walk two flights of stairs?	¿Puede subir dos pisos por las escaleras?
Do you have problems with your lungs?	¿Padece de problemas en los pulmones?
Do you have asthma?	¿Padece de asma?
Do you feel short of breath when walking?	¿Al caminar siente que le falta el aire?
Do you have acid reflux?	¿Padece de reflujo?
Do you feel nauseous?	¿Siente náuseas?
Have you vomited? When was the last time?	¿Ha vomitado? ¿Cuándo fue la ultima vez que vomitó?
Do you have diabetes?	¿Padece de diabetes?
Do you have any problems with your kidneys?	¿Tiene algún problema en sus riñones?
Has anyone told you it was difficult to place a breathing tube?	¿Alguna vez le han dicho que fue difícil intubarlo para poder respirar?
Have you ever had any problems with anesthesia?	¿Ha tenido problemas con la anestesia en el pasado?
Has anyone in your family ever had problems with anesthesia?	¿Algún miembro de su familia ha tenido problemas con la anestesia?
When did you last eat or drink?	¿Cuándo fue la última vez que comió o bebió algo?
What questions do you have about the anesthesia plan today?	¿Qué preguntas tiene acerca del plan de anestesia de hoy?

Physical Examination	
Open your mouth, please.	Abra la boca, por favor.
Do you have full range of motion of your neck?	¿Puede mover el cuello para todos lados?
Move your toes, please.	Por favor, mueva los dedos de sus pies.
Squeeze my hands, please.	Por favor, apriete mis manos.
Breathe deeply through your mouth.	Respire profundo por la boca.

Induction	
If possible, can you move over to the OR table?	Si le es posible, ¿Puede pasarse a la mesa de operaciones?
We can assist you if needed.	Si es necesario lo podemos ayudar.
Don't worry.	No se preocupe.
Take a deep breath.	Respire profundo.
Please breathe normally through this mask. It's just oxygen.	Por favor respire normal a través de esta mascarilla. Solo es oxígeno.

You might feel some burning in your IV. This is normal.	*Tal vez sentirá un poco de ardor en la línea intravenosa. Esto es normal.*
You will start to feel sleepy now.	*Ahora va a empezar a sentirse con sueño.*
You're going to feel some pressure on your neck.	*Va a sentir un poco de presión en el cuello.*
Everything is OK.	*Todo está bien.*
We will take good care of you.	*Lo vamos a cuidar muy bien.*

Emergence	
Open your eyes.	*Abra sus ojos.*
Take a deep breath.	*Respire profundo.*
Squeeze my left hand/right hand.	*Apriete mi mano izquierda/derecha.*
Do you have any pain? Where?	*¿Tiene algún dolor? ¿Dónde?*
Your surgery is over.	*Ya termino su cirugía.*
You are still in the operating room.	*Todavía está en la sala de operaciones.*
We are going to the recovery room now.	*Ahora vamos a la sala de recuperación.*

APPENDIX A: FORMULAE AND QUICK REFERENCE

CARDIOLOGY

Fick Cardiac Output

Oxygen consumption (L/min) = CO (L/min) × arteriovenous (AV) oxygen difference

CO = oxygen consumption/AV oxygen difference

Oxygen consumption must be measured (can estimate w/125 mL/min/m² but inaccurate)

AV oxygen difference = Hb (g/dL) × 10 (dL/L) × 1.36 (mL O_2/g of Hb) × (SaO_2 – SvO_2)

SaO_2 is measured in any arterial sample (usually 93–98%)

SvO_2 (mixed venous O_2) is measured in RA, RV, or PA (assuming no shunt) (normal ~75%)

$$\therefore \textbf{ Cardiac output (L/min)} = \frac{\text{Oxygen consumption}}{\text{Hb (g/dL)} \times 3.6 \times (SaO_2 \times SvO_2)}$$

Shunts

$$Q_P = \frac{\text{Oxygen consumption}}{\text{Pulm vein } O_2 \text{ sat – Pulm artery } O_2 \text{ sat}} \text{ (if no R} \rightarrow \text{L shunt, PV } O_2 \text{ sat} \approx SaO_2)$$

$$Q_S = \frac{\text{Oxygen consumption}}{SaO_2 \text{ – Mixed venous } O_2 \text{ sat}} \text{ (MVO}_2 \text{ drawn proximal to potential L} \approx \text{R shunt)}$$

$$\frac{Q_P}{Q_S} = \frac{SaO_2 - MV\ O_2 \text{ sat}}{PV\ O_2 \text{ sat} - PA\ O_2 \text{ sat}} \approx \frac{SaO_2 - MV\ O_2 \text{ sat}}{SaO_2 - PA\ O_2 \text{ sat}} \text{ (if only L} \rightarrow \text{R and no R} \rightarrow \text{L shunt)}$$

Valve Area

$$\text{Gorlin equation:} \quad \frac{\text{CO/(DEP or SEP)} \times \text{HR}}{44.3 \times \text{constant} \times \sqrt{\Delta P}} \text{ (constant = 1 for AS, 0.85 for MS)}$$
Valve area

$$\text{Hakki equation: Valve area} = \frac{\text{CO}}{\sqrt{\Delta P}}$$

Coronary Artery Anatomy (see Fig. A-1)

Figure A-1 Coronary arteries.

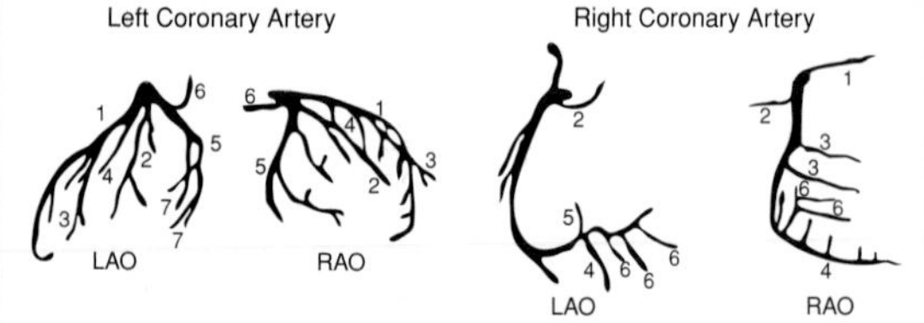

Left Coronary Artery · Right Coronary Artery

LAO · RAO · LAO · RAO

1. **Left anterior descending artery (LAD)**
2. Ramus medianus artery
3. Diagonal branches
4. Septal branches
5. **Left circumflex artery (LCx)**
6. Left atrial circumflex artery
7. Obtuse marginal branches

1. Conus artery
2. SA node artery
3. Acute marginal branches
4. Posterior descending artery (PDA)
5. AV node artery
6. Posterior left ventricular artery (PLV)

(From Grossman WG. *Cardiac Catheterization and Angiography*. 4th ed. Philadelphia, PA: Lea & Febiger, 1991, with permission.)

PULMONARY

Dead space = Lung units that are ventilated but not perfused
Intrapulmonary shunt = Lung units that are perfused but not ventilated
Alveolar gas equation:

$$P_AO_2 = [F_IO_2 \times (760 - 47)] - \frac{P_aCO_2}{R} \text{ (where R} \approx 0.8)$$

$$P_AO_2 = 150 \frac{P_aCO_2}{0.8} \text{ (on room air)}$$

A-a gradient = $P_AO_2 - P_aO_2$ [normal A-a gradient ≈ 4 + (age/4)]
Minute ventilation (V.E) = Tidal volume (V_T) × Respiratory rate (RR) (normal 4–6 L/min)
Tidal volume (V_T) = Alveolar space (V_A) + Dead space (V_D)
Fraction of tidal volume that is dead space

$$\left(\frac{V_D}{V_T}\right) = \frac{P_aCO_2 - P_{expired}CO_2}{P_aCO_2}$$

$$P_aCO_2 = k \times \frac{CO_2 \text{ production}}{\text{Alvelor ventilation}} = k \times \frac{\dot{V}_{CO_2}}{RR \times V_T \times \left(1 - \frac{V_D}{V_T}\right)}$$

NEPHROLOGY

Anion gap (AG) = Na − (Cl + HCO_3) (normal = [alb] × 2.5; typically 12 ± 2 mEq)
Delta-delta (ΔΔ) = [ΔAG (i.e., calc. AG − expected)/Δ HCO_3 (i.e., 24 − measured HCO_3)]
Urine anion gap (UAG) = (U_{Na} + U_K) − U_{Cl}

$$\textbf{Calculated osmoles} = (2 \times Na) + \left(\frac{glc}{18}\right) + \left(\frac{BUN}{2.8}\right) + \left(\frac{EtOH}{4.6}\right)$$

Osmolal gap (OG) = Measured osmoles − Calculated osmoles (normal <10)

$$\textbf{Estimated creatinine clearance} = \frac{[140 - age(y)] \times wt \text{ (kg)}}{\text{serum Cr (mg/dL)} \times 72} (\times 0.85 \text{ in women})$$

$$\textbf{Fractional excretion of Na} (FE_{Na}, \%) = \left[\frac{\dfrac{U_{Na}(mEq/L)}{P_{Na}(Eq/L)} \times 100\%}{\dfrac{U_{Cr}(mg/mL)}{P_{Cr}(mg/dL)} \times 100\% \text{ (mL/dL)}}\right] = \dfrac{\dfrac{U_{NA}}{P_{NA}}}{\dfrac{U_{Cr}}{P_{Cr}}}$$

Corrected Na in hyperglycemia
Estimate in all pts: Corrected Na = Measured Na +

$$\left[2.4 \times \frac{\text{(measured glc} - 100)}{100}\right]$$

However, Δ in Na depends on glc *(Am J Med 1999;106:399)*
Δ is 1.6 mEq per each 100 mg/dL ↑ in glc ranging from 100–440
Δ is 4 mEq per each 100 mg/dL ↑ in glc beyond 440
Total body water (TBW) = 0.60 × IBW (× 0.85 if female and × 0.85 if elderly)

$$\textbf{Free } H_2O \textbf{ deficit} = TBW \times \left(\frac{[Na]_{serum} - 140}{140}\right) \approx \left(\frac{[Na]_{serum} - 140}{3}\right) \text{(in 70 kg Pt)}$$

$$\textbf{Transtubular potassium gradient (TTKG)} = \dfrac{\dfrac{U_K}{P_K}}{\dfrac{U_{Osm}}{P_{Osm}}}$$

Heparin for Thromboembolism	
80 U/kg bolus	
18 U/kg/h	
PTT	**Adjustment**
<40	Bolus 5,000 U, ↑ rate 300 U/h
40–49	Bolus 3,000 U, ↑ rate 200 U/h
50–59	↑ Rate 100 U/h
60–85	No Δ
86–95	↓ Rate 100 U/h
96–120	Hold 30 min, ↓ rate 150 U/h
>120	Hold 60 min, ↓ rate 200 U/h

(*Circulation* 2001;103:2994.)

Heparin for ACS[A7]	
STEMI w/fibrinolysis	
60 U/kg bolus (max 4,000 U)	
12 U/kg/h (max 1,000 U/h)	
UA/NSTEMI	
60–75 U/kg bolus (max 5,000 U)	
12–15 U/kg/h (max 1,000 U/h)	
PTT	**Adjustment**
<40	Bolus 3,000 U, ↑ rate 100 U/h
40–49	↑ Rate 50 U/h
50–70	No Δ
71–85	↓ Rate 50 U/h
86–100	Hold 30 min, ↓ rate 100 U/h
101–150	Hold 60 min, ↓ rate 150 U/h
>150	Hold 60 min, ↓ rate 300 U/h

- PTT q6h after every change (half-life of heparin is ~90 min)
- PTT qd or bid once PTT is therapeutic
- CBC qd (to ensure that Hct and plt counts are stable)

OTHER

Ideal body weight (IBW) = [50 kg (men) or 45.5 kg (women)] + 2.3 kg/in. over 5 ft

$$\text{Body surface area (BSA, m}^2) = \sqrt{\frac{\text{height (cm)} \times \text{weight (kg)}}{3,600}}$$

SENSITIVITY AND SPECIFICITY CALCULATIONS

		Disease	
		Present	**Absent**
Test	⊕	a (true ⊕)	b (false ⊕)
	⊖	c (false ⊖)	d (true ⊖)

$$\text{Prevalence} = \frac{\text{All diseased}}{\text{All patients}} = \frac{a + b}{a + b + c + d}$$

$$\text{Sensitivity} = \frac{\text{True positives}}{\text{All diseased}} = \frac{a}{a + c} \quad \text{Specificity} = \frac{\text{True negatives}}{\text{All healthy}} = \frac{d}{b + d}$$

$$\oplus \text{ Predictive value} = \frac{\text{True positives}}{\text{All positives}} = \frac{a}{a + b}$$

$\ominus$ **Predictive value** $= \dfrac{\text{True negatives}}{\text{All negatives}} = \dfrac{d}{c + d}$

Accuracy $= \dfrac{\text{True positives} + \text{True negatives}}{\text{All patients}} = \dfrac{a + d}{a + b + c + d}$

$\oplus$ **Likelihood ratio** $= \dfrac{\text{True positives rate}}{\text{False positive rate}} = \dfrac{Se}{1 - Sp}$

$\ominus$ **Likelihood ratio** $= \dfrac{\text{False negative rate}}{\text{True negative rate}} = \dfrac{1 - Se}{Sp}$

Posttest odds $= \text{Pretest odds} \times \text{LR}$

APPENDIX B: ANESTHESIA MACHINE CHECKOUT & SETTING UP THE OR

ANESTHESIA MACHINE CHECKOUT

Checkout only valid for an anesthesia system that conforms to current standards and includes an ascending bellow ventilator and the following monitors: Capnograph, pulse ox, oxygen analyzer, spirometer, and breathing pressure monitor w/high- & low-pressure alarms

- Verify backup ventilation equipment is available and functioning*
- High-pressure system
  - Check oxygen cylinder supply*
  - Check central pipeline supplies*
- Low-pressure system
  - Check initial status of low-pressure system*
  - Perform leak check of machine low-pressure system*
  - Turn on machine master switch and all other necessary electrical equipment*
  - Test flowmeters*
- Adjust and check scavenging system*
- Breathing system
  - Calibrate O_2 monitor*
  - Check initial status of breathing system
  - Perform leak check of breathing system
- Test manual and automatic ventilation systems and unidirectional valves
- Check, calibrate, and/or set alarm limits of all monitors
- Check final status of the machine
  - Vaporizers off*
  - APL valve open
  - Selector switch to "Bag"
  - All flowmeters to zero
  - Pt suction level adequate
  - Breathing system ready to use

*Note: If an anesthesia provider uses the same machine in successive cases, the steps denoted by an asterisk need not be repeated or may be abbreviated after the initial checkout

SETTING UP THE OR FOR A CASE: "SOAP M"

S: Suction
Make sure suction is on, plugged in tightly to the canister, on at full blast

O: Oxygen
Check that pipeline supply is between 50 and 55 psi and connected to the wall
Check that the cylinder in the back of the machine has adequate oxygen (>1,000 psi)
Calibrate O_2 sensor
Make sure a self-inflating bag–valve–mask is available

A: Airway
Check all laryngoscopes and handles
Choose appropriate ETT and check cuff for leaks. Have an ETT stylet available
Make sure an LMA is available
Oral airway, bite block, and tape
Stethoscope

P: Pharmacy
Draw up drugs needed for the case (including a sedative, induction agent, paralytics)
Make sure emergency drugs (epinephrine, atropine, extra succinylcholine) are available
Make sure vaporizers are adequately filled
Make sure appropriate antibiotics are available
Set up appropriate drips and have a functioning drug infusion pump

M: Machine/Monitors
Check the machine (see Anesthesia Machine Checkout above)
Check the monitors: BP cuff present and of appropriate size; pulse oximeter functioning; EKG cables & electrodes available; nerve stimulator present & functioning
Fluid & pt warmers available; A-line, CVP, PA, and EEG monitors as indicated

APPENDIX C: MANAGEMENT OF MALIGNANT HYPERTHERMIA (ALSO SEE CHAPTER 11)

MH Hotline 1-800-644-9737 or 1-315-464-7079; website: WWW.MHAUS.ORG

DIAGNOSIS VS. ASSOCIATED PROBLEMS

Signs of MH
- Increasing EtCO$_2$
- Rigidity—trunk or total body rigidity; masseter spasm or trismus
- Tachycardia/tachypnea
- Mixed respiratory and metabolic acidosis
- Increased temperature (may be a late sign)
- Myoglobinuria

Sudden/Unexpected Cardiac Arrest in Young Patients
- Presume hyperkalemia and initiate treatment (see #6 below)
- Measure CK, myoglobin, ABGs, until normalized
- Consider dantrolene
- Usually secondary to occult myopathy (e.g., muscular dystrophy)
- Resuscitation may be difficult and prolonged

Trismus or Masseter Spasm with Succinylcholine
- Early sign of MH in many pts
- If limb muscle rigid, begin treatment with dantrolene
- If surgery is emergent, continue with nontriggering agents, evaluate & monitor pt
- Check CK immediately and at 6 h intervals until returning to normal. Observe for dark or cola-colored urine. If present, liberalize fluid intake and test for myoglobin

ACUTE PHASE TREATMENT

1. GET HELP. GET DANTROLENE—Notify Surgeon
- Discontinue volatile agents and succinylcholine
- Hyperventilate with 100% oxygen at flows of 10 L/min or more
- Stop surgery as soon as possible; if emergent, continue with nontriggering agents
- Do not waste time changing the circle system and CO$_2$ absorbent

2. Dantrolene
- *New formulation*: **Ryanodex** (dantrolene sodium)
  - Mix each 250 mg ampule with 5 cc of sterile water (not saline)
  - IV push, 2.5 mg/kg
  - Additional bolus (if needed) up to max cumulative dose 10 mg/kg
- *Original formulation*: **Dantrium/Revonto** (dantrolene sodium)
  - Mix each 20 mg ampule with 60 cc sterile water (not saline)
  - IV push, 2.5 mg/kg IV every 5 min until symptoms subside
  - Continue administering up to 10 mg/kg

3. Bicarbonate for metabolic acidosis
- 1–2 mEq/kg if blood-gas values are not yet available

4. Cool the pt if core temp >39°C. Lavage body cavities, stomach, bladder, rectum. Apply ice to surface. Infuse cold saline IV. Stop cooling if <38°C & falling to prevent drift <36°C

5. Dysrhythmias usually respond to treatment of acidosis and hyperkalemia
- Use standard drug therapy except calcium channel blockers, which may cause hyperkalemia or cardiac arrest in the presence of dantrolene

6. Hyperkalemia—treat with hyperventilation, bicarbonate, glucose/insulin, calcium
- Bicarbonate: 1–2 mEq/kg IV
- Insulin: For **pediatric**, 0.1 units insulin/kg and 1 mL/kg 50% glucose or for **adults**, 10 units regular insulin IV and 50 mL 50% glucose
- CaCl 10 mg/kg or Ca gluconate 10–50 mg/kg for life-threatening hyperkalemia
- Check glucose levels hourly

7. Follow EtCO$_2$, electrolytes, blood gases, CK, core temperature, urine output and color, coagulation studies. If CK and/or K+ rise more than transiently or urine output falls to <0.5 mL/kg/h, induce diuresis to >1 mL/kg/h and give bicarbonate to alkalinize urine to prevent myoglobinuria-induced renal failure (see D below)
- Venous blood gas (e.g., femoral vein) values may document hypermetabolism better than arterial values
- Central venous or PA monitoring as needed and record minute ventilation
- Place Foley catheter and monitor urine output

POSTACUTE PHASE

A. Observe the pt in ICU for at least 24 h, due to risk of recrudescence

B. Dantrolene 1 mg/kg q4–6h or 0.25 mg/kg/h for at least 24 h

C. Follow vitals and labs as above (see #7 above)
- Frequent ABG as per clinical signs
- CK every 8–12 h; less often as the values trend downward

D. Follow urine myoglobin and institute therapy to prevent myoglobin precipitation in renal tubules and the subsequent development of renal failure. CK levels above 10,000 IU/L is a presumptive sign of rhabdomyolysis and myoglobinuria. Follow standard ICU therapy for acute rhabdomyolysis and myoglobinuria (urine output >2 mL/kg/h by hydration and diuretics along with alkalinization of urine with Na-bicarbonate infusion with careful attention to both urine and serum pH values)

E. Counsel the pt and family regarding MH and further precautions; referral to MHAUS

JULIE K. FREED

INTRODUCTION

- Global pandemic in 2020 caused by SARS-CoV-2 (coronavirus), results in COVID-19
- Predominantly lower respiratory illness (COVID-19)
- Origin of outbreak was in Wuhan, China (December 2019)
- Transmission via droplets/fomites and possibly aerosols in patients +/– symptoms
- <24-hr survival of viral particles on paper surfaces, <72-hr survival on plastic or steel
- Incubation period: Median 4 days (common range 2–7 days), up to 14 days
- Ro for COVID-19 is 2.0–2.5 (compared to influenza 1.2–1.6)

Clinical Signs and Symptoms (% of pts reporting)	
Systemic	Fever (44–98%)
Pulmonary	Dry cough (46–82%)
	Shortness of breath (20–64%) Upper respiratory symptoms (congestion) (5–25%)
GI	Nausea, diarrhea (unknown)
ENT	Anosmia (unknown)

POOR PROGNOSTIC INDICATORS

- **Demographics:** Age >65 yrs old, males
- **Comorbidities:** Cardiovascular disease (including HTN), diabetes, pulmonary disease, cancer, immunosuppression
- **Lab Findings:** Severe lymphopenia, elevated troponins, creatinine, LDH, CRP, and d-dimer

Disease Course	% of COVID-19 Patients
Mild–moderate symptoms not requiring ICU admission	~80%
Respiratory bacterial superinfection	~10–20%
Respiratory viral coinfection	~2–25%
Acute respiratory distress syndrome (ARDS)	~20%
Acute renal injury requiring dialysis	~5%
Cardiomyopathy or cardiogenic shock	Anecdotal reports

PERIOPERATIVE CONSIDERATIONS

- Necessary precautions are required during an outbreak to prevent transmission
- Aerosolization of sputum in the perioperative setting is a source of exposure
- **Highest risk** of exposure for anesthesiologist is during **intubation and extubation**
- To mitigate risk of transmission the healthcare worker should:
  - Practice frequent hand washing (most important hygiene measure)
- Use personal protective equipment (PPE) for all known or suspected cases
- N95 mask to be worn for all known or suspected cases and asymptomatic open airway cases (e.g., bronchoscopy)
- Limit the number of providers in OR during intubation and extubation to anesthesia providers only wearing appropriate PPE
- An antiviral HME filter should be placed between the ETT and reservoir bag

AIRWAY RECOMMENDATIONS (OR AND OUT-OF-OR)

- Designate the most experienced anesthesia professional to perform the intubation
- Avoid awake fiberoptic intubations and consider using video laryngoscope

---

[†]This information was collected through April 3, 2020 during the global pandemic caused by SARS-CoV-2 (COVID-19). The author would like to note that protocols and/or recommendations offered here may have changed since publication.

- Preoxygenate for minimum 5 min 100% FiO$_2$, Perform RSI
- Avoid mask ventilation, LMA for difficult airway, then consider surgical airway
- Resheath the laryngoscope immediately post intubation (double gloving technique)
- Doff all PPE in the room with exception of N95 mask, wash hands immediately

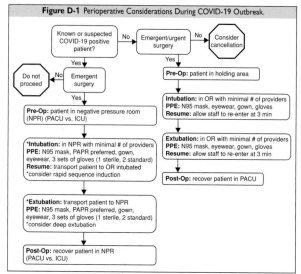

Figure D-1 Perioperative Considerations During COVID-19 Outbreak.

(Adapted from guidelines provided by the Anesthesia Patient Safety Foundation (APSF) on Perioperative Considerations for the 2019 Novel Coronavirus (COVID-19)).

INDEX

Note: Page number followed by f indicates figure and A indicates appendix respectively.